SLEEP DEPRIVATION

LUNG BIOLOGY IN HEALTH AND DISEASE

Executive Editor

Claude Lenfant
Former Director, National Heart, Lung, and Blood Institute
National Institutes of Health
Bethesda, Maryland

1. Immunologic and Infectious Reactions in the Lung, *edited by C. H. Kirkpatrick and H. Y. Reynolds*
2. The Biochemical Basis of Pulmonary Function, *edited by R. G. Crystal*
3. Bioengineering Aspects of the Lung, *edited by J. B. West*
4. Metabolic Functions of the Lung, *edited by Y. S. Bakhle and J. R. Vane*
5. Respiratory Defense Mechanisms (in two parts), *edited by J. D. Brain, D. F. Proctor, and L. M. Reid*
6. Development of the Lung, *edited by W. A. Hodson*
7. Lung Water and Solute Exchange, *edited by N. C. Staub*
8. Extrapulmonary Manifestations of Respiratory Disease, *edited by E. D. Robin*
9. Chronic Obstructive Pulmonary Disease, *edited by T. L. Petty*
10. Pathogenesis and Therapy of Lung Cancer, *edited by C. C. Harris*
11. Genetic Determinants of Pulmonary Disease, *edited by S. D. Litwin*
12. The Lung in the Transition Between Health and Disease, *edited by P. T. Macklem and S. Permutt*
13. Evolution of Respiratory Processes: A Comparative Approach, *edited by S. C. Wood and C. Lenfant*
14. Pulmonary Vascular Diseases, *edited by K. M. Moser*
15. Physiology and Pharmacology of the Airways, *edited by J. A. Nadel*
16. Diagnostic Techniques in Pulmonary Disease (in two parts), *edited by M. A. Sackner*
17. Regulation of Breathing (in two parts), *edited by T. F. Hornbein*
18. Occupational Lung Diseases: Research Approaches and Methods, *edited by H. Weill and M. Turner-Warwick*
19. Immunopharmacology of the Lung, *edited by H. H. Newball*
20. Sarcoidosis and Other Granulomatous Diseases of the Lung, *edited by B. L. Fanburg*

21. Sleep and Breathing, *edited by N. A. Saunders and C. E. Sullivan*
22. *Pneumocystis carinii* Pneumonia: Pathogenesis, Diagnosis, and Treatment, *edited by L. S. Young*
23. Pulmonary Nuclear Medicine: Techniques in Diagnosis of Lung Disease, *edited by H. L. Atkins*
24. Acute Respiratory Failure, *edited by W. M. Zapol and K. J. Falke*
25. Gas Mixing and Distribution in the Lung, *edited by L. A. Engel and M. Paiva*
26. High-Frequency Ventilation in Intensive Care and During Surgery, *edited by G. Carlon and W. S. Howland*
27. Pulmonary Development: Transition from Intrauterine to Extrauterine Life, *edited by G. H. Nelson*
28. Chronic Obstructive Pulmonary Disease: Second Edition, *edited by T. L. Petty*
29. The Thorax (in two parts), *edited by C. Roussos and P. T. Macklem*
30. The Pleura in Health and Disease, *edited by J. Chrétien, J. Bignon, and A. Hirsch*
31. Drug Therapy for Asthma: Research and Clinical Practice, *edited by J. W. Jenne and S. Murphy*
32. Pulmonary Endothelium in Health and Disease, *edited by U. S. Ryan*
33. The Airways: Neural Control in Health and Disease, *edited by M. A. Kaliner and P. J. Barnes*
34. Pathophysiology and Treatment of Inhalation Injuries, *edited by J. Loke*
35. Respiratory Function of the Upper Airway, *edited by O. P. Mathew and G. Sant'Ambrogio*
36. Chronic Obstructive Pulmonary Disease: A Behavioral Perspective, *edited by A. J. McSweeny and I. Grant*
37. Biology of Lung Cancer: Diagnosis and Treatment, *edited by S. T. Rosen, J. L. Mulshine, F. Cuttitta, and P. G. Abrams*
38. Pulmonary Vascular Physiology and Pathophysiology, *edited by E. K. Weir and J. T. Reeves*
39. Comparative Pulmonary Physiology: Current Concepts, *edited by S. C. Wood*
40. Respiratory Physiology: An Analytical Approach, *edited by H. K. Chang and M. Paiva*
41. Lung Cell Biology, *edited by D. Massaro*
42. Heart–Lung Interactions in Health and Disease, *edited by S. M. Scharf and S. S. Cassidy*
43. Clinical Epidemiology of Chronic Obstructive Pulmonary Disease, *edited by M. J. Hensley and N. A. Saunders*

44. Surgical Pathology of Lung Neoplasms, *edited by A. M. Marchevsky*

45. The Lung in Rheumatic Diseases, *edited by G. W. Cannon and G. A. Zimmerman*

46. Diagnostic Imaging of the Lung, *edited by C. E. Putman*

47. Models of Lung Disease: Microscopy and Structural Methods, *edited by J. Gil*

48. Electron Microscopy of the Lung, *edited by D. E. Schraufnagel*

49. Asthma: Its Pathology and Treatment, *edited by M. A. Kaliner, P. J. Barnes, and C. G. A. Persson*

50. Acute Respiratory Failure: Second Edition, *edited by W. M. Zapol and F. Lemaire*

51. Lung Disease in the Tropics, *edited by O. P. Sharma*

52. Exercise: Pulmonary Physiology and Pathophysiology, *edited by B. J. Whipp and K. Wasserman*

53. Developmental Neurobiology of Breathing, *edited by G. G. Haddad and J. P. Farber*

54. Mediators of Pulmonary Inflammation, *edited by M. A. Bray and W. H. Anderson*

55. The Airway Epithelium, *edited by S. G. Farmer and D. Hay*

56. Physiological Adaptations in Vertebrates: Respiration, Circulation, and Metabolism, *edited by S. C. Wood, R. E. Weber, A. R. Hargens, and R. W. Millard*

57. The Bronchial Circulation, *edited by J. Butler*

58. Lung Cancer Differentiation: Implications for Diagnosis and Treatment, *edited by S. D. Bernal and P. J. Hesketh*

59. Pulmonary Complications of Systemic Disease, *edited by J. F. Murray*

60. Lung Vascular Injury: Molecular and Cellular Response, *edited by A. Johnson and T. J. Ferro*

61. Cytokines of the Lung, *edited by J. Kelley*

62. The Mast Cell in Health and Disease, *edited by M. A. Kaliner and D. D. Metcalfe*

63. Pulmonary Disease in the Elderly Patient, *edited by D. A. Mahler*

64. Cystic Fibrosis, *edited by P. B. Davis*

65. Signal Transduction in Lung Cells, *edited by J. S. Brody, D. M. Center, and V. A. Tkachuk*

66. Tuberculosis: A Comprehensive International Approach, *edited by L. B. Reichman and E. S. Hershfield*

67. Pharmacology of the Respiratory Tract: Experimental and Clinical Research, *edited by K. F. Chung and P. J. Barnes*

68. Prevention of Respiratory Diseases, *edited by A. Hirsch, M. Goldberg, J.-P. Martin, and R. Masse*

69. *Pneumocystis carinii* Pneumonia: Second Edition, *edited by P. D. Walzer*

70. Fluid and Solute Transport in the Airspaces of the Lungs, *edited by R. M. Effros and H. K. Chang*

71. Sleep and Breathing: Second Edition, *edited by N. A. Saunders and C. E. Sullivan*

72. Airway Secretion: Physiological Bases for the Control of Mucous Hypersecretion, *edited by T. Takishima and S. Shimura*

73. Sarcoidosis and Other Granulomatous Disorders, *edited by D. G. James*

74. Epidemiology of Lung Cancer, *edited by J. M. Samet*

75. Pulmonary Embolism, *edited by M. Morpurgo*

76. Sports and Exercise Medicine, *edited by S. C. Wood and R. C. Roach*

77. Endotoxin and the Lungs, *edited by K. L. Brigham*

78. The Mesothelial Cell and Mesothelioma, *edited by M.-C. Jaurand and J. Bignon*

79. Regulation of Breathing: Second Edition, *edited by J. A. Dempsey and A. I. Pack*

80. Pulmonary Fibrosis, *edited by S. Hin. Phan and R. S. Thrall*

81. Long-Term Oxygen Therapy: Scientific Basis and Clinical Application, *edited by W. J. O'Donohue, Jr.*

82. Ventral Brainstem Mechanisms and Control of Respiration and Blood Pressure, *edited by C. O. Trouth, R. M. Millis, H. F. Kiwull-Schöne, and M. E. Schläfke*

83. A History of Breathing Physiology, *edited by D. F. Proctor*

84. Surfactant Therapy for Lung Disease, *edited by B. Robertson and H. W. Taeusch*

85. The Thorax: Second Edition, Revised and Expanded (in three parts), *edited by C. Roussos*

86. Severe Asthma: Pathogenesis and Clinical Management, *edited by S. J. Szefler and D. Y. M. Leung*

87. *Mycobacterium avium*–Complex Infection: Progress in Research and Treatment, *edited by J. A. Korvick and C. A. Benson*

88. Alpha 1–Antitrypsin Deficiency: Biology • Pathogenesis • Clinical Manifestations • Therapy, *edited by R. G. Crystal*

89. Adhesion Molecules and the Lung, *edited by P. A. Ward and J. C. Fantone*

90. Respiratory Sensation, *edited by L. Adams and A. Guz*

91. Pulmonary Rehabilitation, *edited by A. P. Fishman*

92. Acute Respiratory Failure in Chronic Obstructive Pulmonary Disease, *edited by J.-P. Derenne, W. A. Whitelaw, and T. Similowski*

93. Environmental Impact on the Airways: From Injury to Repair, *edited by J. Chrétien and D. Dusser*

94. Inhalation Aerosols: Physical and Biological Basis for Therapy, *edited by A. J. Hickey*

95. Tissue Oxygen Deprivation: From Molecular to Integrated Function, *edited by G. G. Haddad and G. Lister*

96. The Genetics of Asthma, *edited by S. B. Liggett and D. A. Meyers*

97. Inhaled Glucocorticoids in Asthma: Mechanisms and Clinical Actions, *edited by R. P. Schleimer, W. W. Busse, and P. M. O'Byrne*

98. Nitric Oxide and the Lung, *edited by W. M. Zapol and K. D. Bloch*

99. Primary Pulmonary Hypertension, *edited by L. J. Rubin and S. Rich*

100. Lung Growth and Development, *edited by J. A. McDonald*

101. Parasitic Lung Diseases, *edited by A. A. F. Mahmoud*

102. Lung Macrophages and Dendritic Cells in Health and Disease, *edited by M. F. Lipscomb and S. W. Russell*

103. Pulmonary and Cardiac Imaging, *edited by C. Chiles and C. E. Putman*

104. Gene Therapy for Diseases of the Lung, *edited by K. L. Brigham*

105. Oxygen, Gene Expression, and Cellular Function, *edited by L. Biadasz Clerch and D. J. Massaro*

106. Beta$_2$-Agonists in Asthma Treatment, *edited by R. Pauwels and P. M. O'Byrne*

107. Inhalation Delivery of Therapeutic Peptides and Proteins, *edited by A. L. Adjei and P. K. Gupta*

108. Asthma in the Elderly, *edited by R. A. Barbee and J. W. Bloom*

109. Treatment of the Hospitalized Cystic Fibrosis Patient, *edited by D. M. Orenstein and R. C. Stern*

110. Asthma and Immunological Diseases in Pregnancy and Early Infancy, *edited by M. Schatz, R. S. Zeiger, and H. N. Claman*

111. Dyspnea, *edited by D. A. Mahler*

112. Proinflammatory and Antiinflammatory Peptides, *edited by S. I. Said*

113. Self-Management of Asthma, *edited by H. Kotses and A. Harver*

114. Eicosanoids, Aspirin, and Asthma, *edited by A. Szczeklik, R. J. Gryglewski, and J. R. Vane*

115. Fatal Asthma, *edited by A. L. Sheffer*

116. Pulmonary Edema, *edited by M. A. Matthay and D. H. Ingbar*

117. Inflammatory Mechanisms in Asthma, *edited by S. T. Holgate and W. W. Busse*

118. Physiological Basis of Ventilatory Support, *edited by J. J. Marini and A. S. Slutsky*

119. Human Immunodeficiency Virus and the Lung, *edited by M. J. Rosen and J. M. Beck*

120. Five-Lipoxygenase Products in Asthma, *edited by J. M. Drazen, S.-E. Dahlén, and T. H. Lee*

121. Complexity in Structure and Function of the Lung, *edited by M. P. Hlastala and H. T. Robertson*

122. Biology of Lung Cancer, *edited by M. A. Kane and P. A. Bunn, Jr.*

123. Rhinitis: Mechanisms and Management, *edited by R. M. Naclerio, S. R. Durham, and N. Mygind*

124. Lung Tumors: Fundamental Biology and Clinical Management, *edited by C. Brambilla and E. Brambilla*

125. Interleukin-5: From Molecule to Drug Target for Asthma, *edited by C. J. Sanderson*

126. Pediatric Asthma, *edited by S. Murphy and H. W. Kelly*

127. Viral Infections of the Respiratory Tract, *edited by R. Dolin and P. F. Wright*

128. Air Pollutants and the Respiratory Tract, *edited by D. L. Swift and W. M. Foster*

129. Gastroesophageal Reflux Disease and Airway Disease, *edited by M. R. Stein*

130. Exercise-Induced Asthma, *edited by E. R. McFadden, Jr.*

131. LAM and Other Diseases Characterized by Smooth Muscle Proliferation, *edited by J. Moss*

132. The Lung at Depth, *edited by C. E. G. Lundgren and J. N. Miller*

133. Regulation of Sleep and Circadian Rhythms, *edited by F. W. Turek and P. C. Zee*

134. Anticholinergic Agents in the Upper and Lower Airways, *edited by S. L. Spector*

135. Control of Breathing in Health and Disease, *edited by M. D. Altose and Y. Kawakami*

136. Immunotherapy in Asthma, *edited by J. Bousquet and H. Yssel*

137. Chronic Lung Disease in Early Infancy, *edited by R. D. Bland and J. J. Coalson*

138. Asthma's Impact on Society: The Social and Economic Burden, *edited by K. B. Weiss, A. S. Buist, and S. D. Sullivan*

139. New and Exploratory Therapeutic Agents for Asthma, *edited by M. Yeadon and Z. Diamant*

140. Multimodality Treatment of Lung Cancer, *edited by A. T. Skarin*

141. Cytokines in Pulmonary Disease: Infection and Inflammation, *edited by S. Nelson and T. R. Martin*
142. Diagnostic Pulmonary Pathology, *edited by P. T. Cagle*
143. Particle–Lung Interactions, *edited by P. Gehr and J. Heyder*
144. Tuberculosis: A Comprehensive International Approach, Second Edition, Revised and Expanded, *edited by L. B. Reichman and E. S. Hershfield*
145. Combination Therapy for Asthma and Chronic Obstructive Pulmonary Disease, *edited by R. J. Martin and M. Kraft*
146. Sleep Apnea: Implications in Cardiovascular and Cerebrovascular Disease, *edited by T. D. Bradley and J. S. Floras*
147. Sleep and Breathing in Children: A Developmental Approach, *edited by G. M. Loughlin, J. L. Carroll, and C. L. Marcus*
148. Pulmonary and Peripheral Gas Exchange in Health and Disease, *edited by J. Roca, R. Rodriguez-Roisen, and P. D. Wagner*
149. Lung Surfactants: Basic Science and Clinical Applications, *R. H. Notter*
150. Nosocomial Pneumonia, *edited by W. R. Jarvis*
151. Fetal Origins of Cardiovascular and Lung Disease, *edited by David J. P. Barker*
152. Long-Term Mechanical Ventilation, *edited by N. S. Hill*
153. Environmental Asthma, *edited by R. K. Bush*
154. Asthma and Respiratory Infections, *edited by D. P. Skoner*
155. Airway Remodeling, *edited by P. H. Howarth, J. W. Wilson, J. Bousquet, S. Rak, and R. A. Pauwels*
156. Genetic Models in Cardiorespiratory Biology, *edited by G. G. Haddad and T. Xu*
157. Respiratory-Circulatory Interactions in Health and Disease, *edited by S. M. Scharf, M. R. Pinsky, and S. Magder*
158. Ventilator Management Strategies for Critical Care, *edited by N. S. Hill and M. M. Levy*
159. Severe Asthma: Pathogenesis and Clinical Management, Second Edition, Revised and Expanded, *edited by S. J. Szefler and D. Y. M. Leung*
160. Gravity and the Lung: Lessons from Microgravity, *edited by G. K. Prisk, M. Paiva, and J. B. West*
161. High Altitude: An Exploration of Human Adaptation, *edited by T. F. Hornbein and R. B. Schoene*
162. Drug Delivery to the Lung, *edited by H. Bisgaard, C. O'Callaghan, and G. C. Smaldone*
163. Inhaled Steroids in Asthma: Optimizing Effects in the Airways, *edited by R. P. Schleimer, P. M. O'Byrne, S. J. Szefler, and R. Brattsand*

164. IgE and Anti-IgE Therapy in Asthma and Allergic Disease, *edited by R. B. Fick, Jr., and P. M. Jardieu*

165. Clinical Management of Chronic Obstructive Pulmonary Disease, *edited by T. Similowski, W. A. Whitelaw, and J.-P. Derenne*

166. Sleep Apnea: Pathogenesis, Diagnosis, and Treatment, *edited by A. I. Pack*

167. Biotherapeutic Approaches to Asthma, *edited by J. Agosti and A. L. Sheffer*

168. Proteoglycans in Lung Disease, *edited by H. G. Garg, P. J. Roughley, and C. A. Hales*

169. Gene Therapy in Lung Disease, *edited by S. M. Albelda*

170. Disease Markers in Exhaled Breath, *edited by N. Marczin, S. A. Kharitonov, M. H. Yacoub, and P. J. Barnes*

171. Sleep-Related Breathing Disorders: Experimental Models and Therapeutic Potential, *edited by D. W. Carley and M. Radulovacki*

172. Chemokines in the Lung, *edited by R. M. Strieter, S. L. Kunkel, and T. J. Standiford*

173. Respiratory Control and Disorders in the Newborn, *edited by O. P. Mathew*

174. The Immunological Basis of Asthma, *edited by B. N. Lambrecht, H. C. Hoogsteden, and Z. Diamant*

175. Oxygen Sensing: Responses and Adaptation to Hypoxia, *edited by S. Lahiri, G. L. Semenza, and N. R. Prabhakar*

176. Non-Neoplastic Advanced Lung Disease, *edited by J. R. Maurer*

177. Therapeutic Targets in Airway Inflammation, *edited by N. T. Eissa and D. P. Huston*

178. Respiratory Infections in Allergy and Asthma, *edited by S. L. Johnston and N. G. Papadopoulos*

179. Acute Respiratory Distress Syndrome, *edited by M. A. Matthay*

180. Venous Thromboembolism, *edited by J. E. Dalen*

181. Upper and Lower Respiratory Disease, *edited by J. Corren, A. Togias, and J. Bousquet*

182. Pharmacotherapy in Chronic Obstructive Pulmonary Disease, *edited by B. R. Celli*

183. Acute Exacerbations of Chronic Obstructive Pulmonary Disease, *edited by N. M. Siafakas, N. R. Anthonisen, and D. Georgopoulos*

184. Lung Volume Reduction Surgery for Emphysema, *edited by H. E. Fessler, J. J. Reilly, Jr., and D. J. Sugarbaker*

185. Idiopathic Pulmonary Fibrosis, *edited by J. P. Lynch III*

186. Pleural Disease, *edited by D. Bouros*

187. Oxygen/Nitrogen Radicals: Lung Injury and Disease, *edited by V. Vallyathan, V. Castranova, and X. Shi*
188. Therapy for Mucus-Clearance Disorders, *edited by B. K. Rubin and C. P. van der Schans*
189. Interventional Pulmonary Medicine, *edited by J. F. Beamis, Jr., P. N. Mathur, and A. C. Mehta*
190. Lung Development and Regeneration, *edited by D. J. Massaro, G. Massaro, and P. Chambon*

ADDITIONAL VOLUMES IN PREPARATION

Long-Term Intervention in Chronic Obstructive Pulmonary Disease, *edited by R. Pauwels, D. S. Postma, and S. T. Weiss*

Sleep Deprivation: Clinical Issues, Pharmacology, and Sleep Loss Effects*, edited by C. A. Kushida*

Pneumocystis Pneumonia: Third Edition, Revised and Expanded, *edited by P. D. Walzer and M. Cushion*

Ion Channels in the Pulmonary Vasculature, *edited by J. X.-J. Yuan*

Asthma Prevention, *edited by W. W. Busse and R. F. Lemanske, Jr.*

The opinions expressed in these volumes do not necessarily represent the views of the National Institutes of Health.

SLEEP DEPRIVATION

Basic Science, Physiology, and Behavior

Clete A. Kushida
Stanford University
Stanford, California

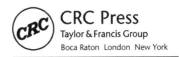

CRC Press is an imprint of the
Taylor & Francis Group, an **informa** business

CRC Press
Taylor & Francis Group
6000 Broken Sound Parkway NW, Suite 300
Boca Raton, FL 33487-2742

First issued in paperback 2019

© 2010 by Taylor & Francis Group, LLC
CRC Press is an imprint of Taylor & Francis Group, an Informa business

No claim to original U.S. Government works

ISBN-13: 978-0-8247-5949-0 (hbk)
ISBN-13: 978-0-367-39352-6 (pbk)

Visit the Informa Web site at
www.informa.com

and the Informa Healthcare Web site at
www.informahealthcare.com

Introduction

The second half of the past century was a time of remarkable scientific expansion and knowledge explosion. Biology and health fields were the beneficiaries of many genuine observations and discoveries and, as a result, the health of individuals and the public as a whole improved markedly. The area of sleep and sleep disorders illustrates the advances in knowledge that occurred.

Sleep is a topic that has long been addressed by writers—but much more frequently by poets than by researchers. As an example, in the beginning of the nineteenth century, Samuel Taylor Coleridge gave us this verse:

> Oh, Sleep! It is a gentle thing,
>> Beloved from pole to pole

Unquestionably, during the last few decades the study of sleep and its biology in health and disease has moved to the forefront of research, and it has revealed a wealth of observations. At the same time, it has attracted the interest of many investigators with expertise in diverse basic disciplines and clinical areas.

The association of sleep disorders with other clinical fields such as cardiology, neurology, mood and attention disorders, and pneumology is well recognized. Sleep deprivation is a medical issue, but also a social one. As a consequence, we have seen a number of societal and regulatory changes to ensure that appropriate sleep time is available.

This series of monographs, *Lung Biology in Health and Disease*, includes a number of volumes on sleep, the first one having been published in 1984. Seven of these volumes have been exclusively about one or another aspect of sleep, and others, on different subjects, included components related to sleep. However, *lack* of sleep did not achieve stardom in this series until Dr. Clete Kushida from the world-famous Stanford Sleep Disorders Clinic and Research Center accepted the invitation to edit this volume on *Sleep Deprivation: Basic Science, Physiology, and Behavior.*

This volume and its companion on *Sleep Deprivation: Clinical Issues, Pharmacology, and Sleep Loss Effects* are true landmarks in the area of sleep biology and medicine. Dr. Kushida enrolled contributors who have pioneered exploration of the field, and I am grateful to them all for the opportunity to introduce this volume to the readership.

Claude Lenfant, M.D.
Bethesda, Maryland

Preface

"That we are not much sicker and much madder than we are
is due exclusively to that most blessed and blessing
of all natural graces, sleep."

—Aldous Huxley

"Be alert. The world needs more lerts."

I remember this prominent sticker posted on the office door of Dr. Mary Carskadon, when she was at Stanford University. Since her office was next to the entrance of the Sleep Research Laboratory where I conducted undergraduate sleep research, this was the first item I saw when I entered and exited the lab. Needless to say, these words became forever stamped on my mind and, in a modern society in which increased work and family commitments threaten sleep, these are undoubtedly words to live by.

The field of sleep research is experiencing an enviable period of growth since the discovery of REM sleep in 1953. Yet there are still fundamental questions in our field that remain unanswered; many of these questions are within the realm of sleep loss and sleep deprivation. Fortunately, there are many talented investigators who have assumed the responsibility of answering some of these questions, and we look forward to their important breakthroughs.

This work is a direct outcome of the vision and efforts of Dr. Claude Lenfant at the National Heart, Lung and Blood Institute. This monograph could not exist without the outstanding contributions of the talented group of international authors; their diligent work is greatly appreciated. I am deeply indebted to the renowned and true pioneers of our field, Drs. William C. Dement and Allan Reschtschaffen, who provided both direct and indirect supportive expertise for this project. In all of my endeavors, I can always count on my parents, Samiko and Hiroshi Kushida, to assist me; this monograph was no exception.

Lastly, the major theme of this work is that sleep deprivation has profound repercussions on the well-being of the individual and society. It is my sincere hope that the reader becomes proactive and participates in our field's crusade to eliminate sleep loss. The following goals may serve to guide the reader in this crusade:

- To strive to eliminate personal sleep debt, and to encourage others to do the same.
- To prevent those who are sleep deprived from operating motor vehicles or hazardous machinery, or otherwise placing themselves or others in unsafe situations.
- To advise those who are persistently sleepy to seek medical opinion.
- To educate the public on the importance of sleep, and to advocate social change in educational and professional situations where sleep deprivation is currently the norm.

Clete A. Kushida
Stanford, California

Contributors

Joel H. Benington
St. Bonaventure University, St. Bonaventure, New York, U.S.A.

Carlo Blanco-Centurion
West Roxbury Veterans Administration Medical Center,
and Harvard Medical School, West Roxbury, Massachusetts, U.S.A.

Michael H. Bonnet
Dayton Department of Veterans Affairs Medical Center, Wright State
University, Kettering Medical Center, and the Wallace Kettering Neuroscience
Institute, Dayton, Ohio, U.S.A.

Monte Buchsbaum
Mount Sinai School of Medicine, New York, New York, U.S.A.

William Bunney
University of California–Irvine, Irvine, California, U.S.A.

Julie Carrier
Hôpital Sacré-Cœur and University of Montreal, Montréal, Québec, Canada

Judy Chang
Stanford University, Stanford, California, U.S.A.

Wynne Chen
Stanford University, Stanford, California, U.S.A.

Chiara Cirelli
University of Wisconsin–Madison, Madison, Wisconsin, U.S.A.

Camellia P. Clark
University of California–San Diego, San Diego, California, U.S.A.

William C. Dement
Stanford University, Stanford, California, U.S.A.

Frank Desarnaud
West Roxbury Veterans Administration Medical Center,
and Harvard Medical School, West Roxbury, Massachusetts, U.S.A.

Mohammad Faisal
School of Life Sciences, Jawaharlal Nehru University, New Delhi, India

Luca A. Finelli
The Salk Institute, La Jolla, California, U.S.A.

Jonathan A.E. Fleming
University of British Columbia, Vancouver, British Columbia, Canada

Geneviève Forest
University of Ottawa, Ottawa, Ontario, Canada

Hélène Gaudreau
McGill University and Hôpital Sacré-Coeur, Montréal, Québec, Canada

Dmitry Gerashchenko
West Roxbury Veterans Administration Medical Center,
and Harvard Medical School, West Roxbury, Massachusetts, U.S.A.

J. Christian Gillin
Veterans Admistration Medical Center and University of
California–San Diego, San Diego, California, U.S.A.

Roger Godbout
University of Montréal and Hôpital Rivière-des-Prairies, Montréal,
Québec, Canada

Joan C. Hendricks
Ryan Veterinary Hospital of the University of Pennsylvania,
Philadelphia, Pennsylvania, U.S.A.

Michael Irwin
University of California–Los Angeles, Los Angeles, California, U.S.A.

Tracy F. Kuo
Stanford University, Stanford, California, U.S.A.

Clete A. Kushida
Stanford University, Stanford, California, U.S.A.

Carol A. Landis
University of Washington, Seattle, Washington, U.S.A.

Rachel Leproult
University of Chicago, Chicago, Illinois, U.S.A.

Vibha Madan
School of Life Sciences, Jawaharlal Nehru University, New Delhi, India

Birendra N. Mallick
School of Life Sciences, Jawaharlal Nehru University, New Delhi, India

Robert W. McCarley
Harvard Medical School, Boston VA Healthcare System, Brockton, Massachusetts, U.S.A.

Sarosh J. Motivala
University of California–Los Angeles, Los Angeles, California, U.S.A.

Eric Murillo-Rodriguez
West Roxbury Veterans Administration Medical Center, and Harvard Medical School, West Roxbury, Massachusetts, U.S.A.

Barbara L. Parry
University of California–San Diego, San Diego, California, U.S.A.

June J. Pilcher
Clemson University, Clemson, South Carolina, U.S.A.

Paul J. Shaw
The Neurosciences Institute, San Diego, California, U.S.A.

Priyattam J. Shiromani
West Roxbury Veterans Administration Medical Center, and Harvard Medical School, West Roxbury, Massachusetts, U.S.A.

Karine Spiegel
Université Libre de Bruxelles, Campus Hôpital Erasme, Brussels, Belgium

Bwanga-Mukishi Tchiteya
Hôpital Sacré-Coeur and University of Montreal, Montréal, Québec, Canada

Mahesh M. Thakkar
Harvard Medical School, Boston VA Healthcare System, Brockton, Massachusetts, U.S.A.

Giulio Tononi
University of Wisconsin–Madison, Madison, Wisconsin, U.S.A.

Eve Van Cauter
University of Chicago, Chicago, Illinois, U.S.A.

Kenneth P. Wright, Jr.
University of Colorado, Boulder, Colorado, U.S.A.

Joseph C. Wu
University of California–Irvine, Irvine, California, U.S.A.

Contents

Introduction   Claude Lenfant . . . . *iii*
Preface . . . . *v*
Contributors . . . . *vii*

1. Perspectives *1*
   Wynne Chen and Clete A. Kushida
   I. Introduction *1*
   II. Methods and Limitations of Sleep Deprivation *3*
   III. Lessons Learned from the Regulation of Sleep *8*
   IV. Early Theories on the Function of Sleep *11*
   V. More Current Theories on the Function of Sleep *17*
   VI. A Look to the Future *22*
      References *23*

2. History of Sleep Deprivation *31*
   William C. Dement, Clete A. Kushida, and Judy Chang
   I. Introduction *31*
   II. Early Studies of Sleep Deprivation *32*
   III. Psychiatric Consequences of Selective REM Sleep Deprivation *37*

IV. Sleep Loss and Daytime Sleepiness *39*
V. The Function(s) of Sleep *39*
VI. Confounds of Experimental Methodology *43*
VII. Conclusions *43*
    References *44*

3. **Animal Models of Sleep Deprivation** **47**
Joan C. Hendricks
  I. Introduction *47*
 II. Historical Overview: What Models Have Been Used to Study Sleep
    Deprivation? *48*
III. Influences on the Use of Higher Vertebrates for Sleep Research *49*
IV. Cost-Benefit Analysis: Choosing a Model *50*
 V. Use of Mammalian Models *52*
VI. Newer "Simple" Models *54*
VII. Even Simpler Models? *56*
VIII. Interpretive and Methodological Issues Raised in Comparative
    Studies of Sleep Deprivation *56*
 IX. Concluding Thoughts *58*
    References *58*

SLEEP DEPRIVATION/FRAGMENTATION PARADIGMS

4. **Total Sleep Deprivation** **63**
Chiara Cirelli and Giulio Tononi
  I. Introduction *63*
 II. TSD Methods: Advantages and Disadvantages *63*
III. Effects of Total Sleep Deprivation *69*
IV. Yoked Control *70*
 V. Sleep Deprivation and Stress *71*
VI. Sleep Deprivation and the Noradrenergic System *73*
VII. NREM vs. REM Rebound After Sleep Deprivation *74*
VIII. Conclusions *75*
    References *76*

5. **Partial and Sleep-State Selective Deprivation** **81**
Carol A. Landis
  I. Introduction *81*
 II. Definitions of Partial Sleep and Sleep-State Selective
    Deprivation *81*
III. Experimental Studies in Humans *82*
IV. Experimental Studies in Animals *85*

  V. Perspectives and Limitations for Interpretation of Findings *92*
 VI. Conclusions *95*
     References *96*

 6. Sleep Fragmentation ***103***
     Michael H. Bonnet
   I. Introduction *103*
  II. Relationship Between Various Schedules of Sleep
      Fragmentation and Daytime Alertness *105*
 III. Experimental Control for Sleep Fragmentation Parameters *107*
  IV. Sleep Fragmentation and Other Physiological and
      Behavioral Measures *109*
   V. Sleep Fragmentation Compared with Sleep Deprivation *111*
  VI. Different Types of Arousal *112*
 VII. Clinical Effects of Sleep Fragmentation: Sleep Apnea and Periodic
      Limb Movements *115*
VIII. Future Research *116*
      References *117*

     **EXTRINSIC FACTORS AFFECTING SLEEP
     LOSS/DEPRIVATION**

 7. Environmental Influences on Sleep and Sleep Deprivation ***121***
     Kenneth P. Wright, Jr.
   I. Introduction *121*
  II. Assessment of Human Sleep and Performance *122*
 III. Sensory Neurophysiology and Behavioral Responsiveness
      During Sleep *122*
  IV. Environmental Factors that Influence Sleep *127*
   V. Sleep in Altered Environments *133*
  VI. Effects of Environmental Factors on Performance During Sleep
      Deprivation *141*
 VII. Conclusions and Future Directions *142*
      References *145*

 8. Shift Work ***157***
     June J. Pilcher
   I. Introduction *157*
  II. Normal Day Shifts *159*
 III. Permanent Shifts *159*
  IV. Rotating Shifts *161*
   V. Shift Length *163*

  VI. Conclusions *164*
      References *164*

9. Medications, Drugs of Abuse, and Alcohol *167*
    Jonathan A.E. Fleming and Clete A. Kushida
    I. Introduction *167*
   II. Medications and Other Substances with a Primary
      Central Effect *168*
  III. Medications and Other Substances with a Secondary
      Central Effect *178*
  IV. Conclusions *181*
      References *181*

10. Factors Affecting Test Performance *191*
    Tracy F. Kuo and Clete A. Kushida
    I. Introduction *191*
   II. Subject Factors *191*
  III. Testing Environment *194*
  IV. Summary and Conclusions *197*
      References *198*

INTRINSIC FACTORS AFFECTING SLEEP LOSS/DEPRIVATION: COGNITIVE, PHYSIOLOGIC, AND MOLECULAR ASSOCIATIONS

11. Attention and Memory Changes *199*
    Geneviève Forest and Roger Godbout
    I. Introduction *199*
   II. Brief Review of Sleep Organization *200*
  III. Brief Review of Physiological Functions of Sleep *201*
  IV. Cognitive Functions *202*
   V. Conclusions *213*
      References *214*

12. Cortical and Electroencephalographic Changes *223*
    Luca A. Finelli
    I. Introduction *223*
   II. Basic Electrophysiology of the Waking State *224*
  III. Changes in Alertness and Performance with the Progression of
      Time Awake *228*
  IV. Electrophysiological Changes with the Progression of
      Time Awake *232*

V. Electroencephalographic Markers of Sleep Propensity for Wakefulness and Sleep *239*

VI. Neural Correlates of Alertness and Cognitive Performance During Prolonged Wakefulness: PET Studies *246*

VII. Neural Correlates of Alertness and Cognitive Performance During Prolonged Wakefulness: fMRI Studies *248*

VIII. Concluding Remarks and Perspectives *251*
References *255*

13. **Physiological and Neurophysiological Changes** **265**
Mahesh M. Thakkar and Robert W. McCarley

I. Introduction *265*

II. Physiological Effects of Sleep Deprivation *266*

III. Neurophysiological or Psychological Effects of Sleep Deprivation *269*

IV. Total Sleep Deprivation *270*

V. REM Sleep Deprivation *278*

VI. Selective NREM Sleep Deprivation *281*

VII. Conclusions *282*
References *282*

14. **Metabolic and Endocrine Changes** **293**
Karine Spiegel, Rachel Leproult, and Eve Van Cauter

I. Introduction *293*

II. Influences of Sleep-Wake Cycle and Circadian Rhythmicity on Endocrine and Metabolic Functions *294*

III. Sleep Following Acute Sleep Deprivation and During Chronic Partial Sleep Restriction *298*

IV. Impact of Acute and Chronic Partial Sleep Deprivation on Hypothalamo-Pituitary Hormones *301*

V. Impact of Sleep Deprivation on Leptin and Ghrelin Levels and Appetite Regulation *306*

VI. Impact of Sleep Deprivation on Glucose Metabolism *308*

VII. Possible Mechanisms Mediating Adverse Effects of Sleep Deprivation on Endocrine and Metabolic Functions *310*
References *312*

15. **Thermoregulatory Changes** **319**
Paul J. Shaw

I. Introduction *319*

II. Body Temperature Regulation *320*

III. Sleep Deprivation *325*

IV. Conclusions *333*
References *334*

16. Biochemical Changes *339*
    Birendra N. Mallick, Vibha Madan, and Mohammad Faisal
    I. Introduction *339*
    II. Sleep Deprivation and Biochemical Changes *340*
    III. Sleep Deprivation–Induced Changes in Biomolecules and
         Physiological Functions *347*
    IV. Could There Be a Biomolecular Marker to Identify
         Sleep Loss? *349*
    V. Summary and Conclusions *350*
    References *350*

17. Immunologic Changes *359*
    Sarosh J. Motivala and Michael Irwin
    I. Introduction *359*
    II. Sleep and Immunity *362*
    III. Sleep Deprivation and Immunity *369*
    IV. Sleep Loss and Immunity: Clinical Samples *378*
    V. Conclusions *381*
    References *381*

18. Changes in Gene Expression *387*
    Chiara Cirelli
    I. Introduction *387*
    II. Global Brain Changes of RNA and Protein Content Related to
         Sleep and Sleep Deprivation *387*
    III. Gene Expression in Sleep and Wakefulness *388*
    IV. Gene Expression and Neuromodulatory Systems *392*
    V. Genes Induced by Long Periods of Sleep Deprivation *393*
    VI. Long-Term Sleep Deprivation, Brain Cell Death, and
         Oxidative Stress *393*
    VII. Conclusions *394*
    References *395*

19. Criteria for Classifying Genes as Sleep or Wake Genes *399*
    Priyattam J. Shiromani, Dmitry Gerashchenko, Carlo Blanco-Centurion,
    Eric Murillo-Rodriguez, and Frank Desarnaud
    I. Introduction *399*
    II. Using Gene Expression to Delineate Sleep-Wake Circuitry *401*
    III. Sleep and Genetics in *Drosophila* *406*
    IV. Criteria for Classifying Genes as "Sleep Genes" *407*

V. Conclusions *409*
References *410*

INTRINSIC FACTORS AFFECTING SLEEP
LOSS/DEPRIVATION: PSYCHIATRIC ASSOCIATIONS

20. Mood Changes **415**
  Camellia P. Clark
  I. Continuous Sleep Deprivation *415*
 II. Effects of Sleep Disruption and Deficiency *416*
III. Personality Factors Affecting Response to Sleep Deprivation *417*
IV. Sleep Deprivation in Children and Adolescents *417*
 V. Interaction Between Emotional Response to Sleep
    Deprivation and Performance *417*
VI. Mechanisms of Mood Response to Sleep Deprivation: Potential
    Clues from Animal and Pharmacology Studies *418*
VII. Areas for Future Study *419*
    References *419*

21. Antidepressant Effects **421**
  Joseph C. Wu, Monte Buchsbaum, William Bunney, and J. Christian Gillin
  I. Introduction *421*
 II. Metabolic Activity in Specific Brain Regions in Depressed Sleep
     Deprivation Responders *422*
III. Role of Neurotransmitter Systems in the Antidepressant Effects of
     Sleep Deprivation *423*
IV. Conclusions *427*
    References *428*

22. Personality/Psychopathologic Changes **431**
  Camellia P. Clark, J. Christian Gillin, and Barbara L. Parry
  I. Personality *431*
 II. Psychopathologic Changes *432*
    References *437*

OTHER INTRINSIC FACTORS AFFECTING SLEEP
LOSS/DEPRIVATION

23. Age and Individual Determinants of Sleep Loss Effects **441**
  Hélène Gaudreau, Julie Carrier, and Bwanga-Mukishi Tchiteya
  I. Introduction *441*
 II. Ontogeny of Sleep Modifications *442*

  III. Age-Dependent Changes in Sleep Regulatory Mechanisms *444*
  IV. Individual Differences in Sleep and Wakefulness *450*
   V. Conclusions *466*
      References *467*

24. Homeostatic and Circadian Influences *481*
    Joel H. Benington
   I. Introduction *481*
  II. Evidence for Sleep Homeostasis *482*
  III. Modeling Sleep Homeostasis *484*
  IV. Implications of Sleep Homeostatic Models *489*
   V. Effects of Sleep Deprivation on Sleep Structure *492*
  VI. Circadian Rhythms and Sleep Deprivation *495*
 VII. Conclusions *500*
      References *501*

Index *507*

1

Perspectives

WYNNE CHEN AND CLETE A. KUSHIDA

Stanford University, Stanford, California, U.S.A.

"The term 'function' in the biological literature is a slippery idea. Whether we think in terms of genes, cells or organisms, these entities are not functionally discrete. Despite their differences, each operates seamlessly within a system to achieve survival in the face of environmental challenges, while also carrying the constraints of the evolutionary past and the capacity of future change."

Kenneth S. Kosik—*Beyond phrenology, at last* (1)

I. Introduction

What is sleep? Sleep scientists might define sleep as a period of behavioral quiescence and non-responsiveness to the environment that is electroencephalographically, physiologically, and behaviorally distinct from the waking state. Sleep is divided into two states, rapid-eye-movement (REM, or "paradoxical" sleep in animals) and non-REM (NREM) sleep that are also electroencephalographically, physiologically, and behaviorally distinct from one another. NREM sleep is further subdivided into four stages 1–4 (or I-IV), corresponding to the depth of sleep, and the presence of specific electrophysiologic markers.

What is sleep deprivation? The deprivation of sleep is the partial or near-complete removal of sleep in an organism. There can never be a complete absence of sleep, due to the fact a "perfect" sleep deprivation procedure has not been developed that is technologically capable of eliminating all sleep. With sleep deprivation, especially over a long period, there is a progressively-accumulating sleep debt that results in greater and greater efforts, bordering on the heroic, to maintain wakefulness in the subject. Microsleeps, which are often too brief to detect and prevent, are an inevitable consequence of sleep deprivation, and the accumulation of these very brief sleep periods may add up to significant amounts of sleep as the deprivation period progresses. There are several types of sleep deprivation. Besides "total" sleep deprivation, there is partial sleep deprivation, which typically can refer to two different paradigms. The first is where sleep is restricted to a level less than baseline sleep amounts, irrespective of sleep state or stage. For example, partial sleep deprivation may involve restricting a human subject to 4 hours of sleep per night, in contrast to his or her baseline sleep amounts of 8.5 hours of sleep per night. The second paradigm for partial sleep deprivation refers to the following. Sleep deprivation may be sleep state specific, where the subject may be specifically deprived of NREM or REM sleep, or sleep stage specific, where the subject may be specifically deprived of any of the stages of NREM sleep. It is impossible to deprive a subject of a state or stage of sleep without affecting the other state or stages of sleep. For example, deprivation of REM sleep will inevitably result in a decrease in NREM sleep amounts, and vice versa. Subjects may also be acutely or chronically sleep deprived, with increased effort required, as discussed earlier, for the longer periods of deprivation. Sleep fragmentation, a different method of sleep deprivation, involves awakening the subject during their sleep, and can either be sleep state/stage specific (e.g., awaking a subject only during REM sleep) or not. A subject can also be naturally deprived of sleep by the presence of sleep disorders or medical conditions that disrupt or fragment sleep.

What it is the function of sleep? In the field of behavioral neurosciences, this question is rather unique in being so familiar, yet so difficult to define scientifically (2). It is clear that sleep has an important physiologic function, given its widespread presence in the animal kingdom, and its persistence among species despite the attendant risks taken during such recurrent periods of reduced awareness, which is characteristic of the sleep state (3). Molecular and behavioral conservation indicate that sleep likely conferred a selective advantage in ancestral mammals, and sleep deprivation experiments in animals have clearly shown that sleep is required for survival (4). However, the specific function or functions of sleep have not been so easily defined, as evidenced by the several reviews and conferences on the subject (2,5,6). While several putative functions for sleep have been proposed, as Rechtschaffen has opined (5), such theories have suffered from a lack of parsimony; it has been difficult to explain diverse data gathered by different methods among different populations. Indeed, the evidence on sleep function may be inconsistent and incongruous because sleep makes several partial contributions to several different functions. No single contribution may be so essential or ubiquitous across species and age groups, that a succinct statement about its function can be made (5). Furthermore, such functions may not be well reflected at the organ or system level. Specifically, the observable system characteristics of sleep might be relevant only in that it permits more essential molecular processes to occur (4). For example, it has been proposed that the muscular hypotonia of sleep may allow for the endogenous reinforcement of motor circuits by synaptic activation (7).

Yet, the past decade has proven an especially exciting time in the field of sleep research, characterized by intense investigation into the biochemical and genetic mechanisms of sleep (8). Innovations in technology have allowed researchers to examine the sleeping brain using quantitative electrophysiology, functional neuroimaging, and genetic techniques. Furthermore, the ability to monitor and record the awake and sleeping brain with electroencephalography (EEG) outside of the laboratory setting, has led to knowledge, which would have been impossible to acquire previously (9). It has been possible to map upwards from the level of neuromodulatory systems to the functional geography of the human brain and, finally to cognition (10–12). We now know that the control mechanisms of sleep are manifested at every level of biological organization, from genes and intracellular processes, to neuronal cell networks, and involve systems that control movement, behavior, cognition, and autonomic functions (13). Studies utilizing sleep deprivation protocols have been instrumental in much of this progress, and what follows will be an overview of the role of sleep deprivation in this ongoing search for the function(s) of sleep. In the end, while no one prevailing theory about the function of sleep emerges the victor, how and why the various theories emerged and evolved should become evident, as should how the aforementioned technological advances have made basic sleep deprivation techniques more powerful than the earliest researchers in the field of sleep medicine, could have ever imagined.

II. Methods and Limitations of Sleep Deprivation

The very first sleep deprivation studies (see also Chap. 2) were conducted in puppies (14), but were soon followed by human studies. In 1896, three young subjects (15) were crudely studied while being kept awake for 88 to 90 hours. Physiological and psychological assessments revealed increases in weight; impairments in reaction time and voluntary motor ability; and memory deficits. One participant also experienced visual hallucinations and a gradual decrease in body temperature, although circadian rhythmicity was preserved. Recovery sleep lasted 10.5 to 12 hours, and all subjects seemed to be normal after their recovery night of sleep. However, more than fifty years would pass until more sophisticated methods of physiologic monitoring allowed the discovery of REM sleep (16). Soon after, Dement (17) performed the first human selective REM sleep deprivation experiment in which more frequent attempts at entering REM sleep and an increased percentage of REM sleep rebounds during recovery sleep were observed, as well as psychological disturbances, which included anxiety, irritability, and difficulty in verbal communication.

This led to more refined techniques in selective REM sleep deprivation in animal models, which have included the cat, mouse and rat; the rat being the most extensively studied to date. The rat is perhaps the most ideal animal model for physiologists (18); three major procedures have been used to enforce sleep deprivation in the rat (19). Requiring relatively modest labor and instrumentation, the most commonly employed method has been that involving continuously enforced locomotion. However, there has been controversy over whether this method of stimulation—locomotion—contributes to rebounds from short-term total sleep deprivation (20–24). Yet, subsequent studies using "gentler" methods of sleep deprivation, such as "hand-deprivation" (21,25), proved equally if not more problematic. It seemed impractical if not impossible to enforce chronic total sleep deprivation with such a method, as it required several experimenters, and rats could adapt quickly even to the most novel of methods of gentle stimulation. For example, one study maintained deprivation by "non-putative" procedures, but ultimately, immersion in water was frequently required to help maintain wakefulness (26); even then, there was some evidence of decreased attentiveness on the part of the experimenters themselves.

Therefore, in an attempt to reduce both the motor activity and sensory stimulation necessary to induce sleep deprivation, Rechtschaffen and colleagues (27,28) at the University of Chicago, devised the "disk-over-water" (DOW) method (Figures 1 and 2; see also chapters 4,5). In this method, both experimen-

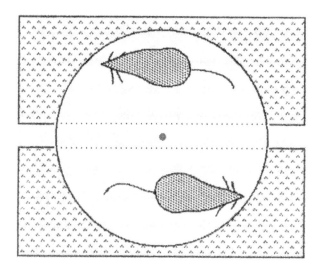

Figure 1   Schematic diagram of the "disk-over-water" apparatus used by Rechtschaffen's group at the University of Chicago. This diagram shows an experimental (sleep deprived) rat and yoked control rat on opposite sides of the same disk. The disk is placed over shallow pans of water.

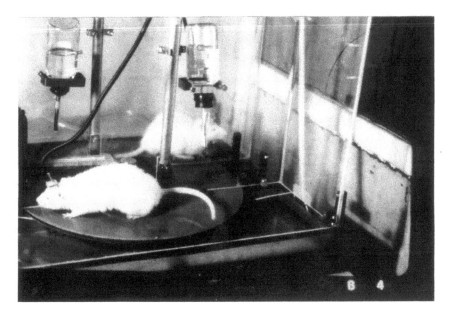

Figure 2 Photograph of the "disk-over-water" apparatus showing an experimental (sleep deprived) rat and yoked control rat. Each rat has a headplug that anchors a recording cable to the skull; the cable allows the transfer of electrical signals derived from implanted electrodes to the polysomnographic equipment. The rats are shown atop the disk over shallow pans of water and surrounded by Plexiglas® cages. Water bottles and stainless steel food tubes are shown attached to the cage walls.

tal and control rats were subjected to similar sensory stimulation and a similar light locomotor load (i.e., the disk usually rotated at only about 20–30% of the day for a total of about 1.0 kilometers per day, which was comparatively less than the daily 3.0 kilometers per day that the rats would normally run) (24). Therefore, an advantage of the DOW method was that the effects of the deprivation method were controlled for by the use of a yoked-control rat, which received almost the exact type of physical stimulation as the sleep-deprived rat. Whatever stress was induced by the deprivation method per se would theoretically be experienced by both the sleep-deprived and control rats, and would equally affect their sleep patterns during recovery sleep (19). Indeed, sleep-deprived rats studied in this manner showed either minimal or none of the traditional "stress" indicators. These include the development of stomach ulcers, adrenal hypertrophy, increases in ACTH and corticosterone, decreased food intake, expression of stress-response genes, an initial decrease in metabolic rate, or initial hypothermia and later fever (totally sleep-deprived rats showed the opposite). However, these profoundly sleep-deprived rats did exhibit a unique syndrome consisting of a progressive increase in energy expenditure, a debilitated appearance (Figs. 3 and 4), the development of distinctive skin lesions (Figs. 5 and 6), and thermoregulatory

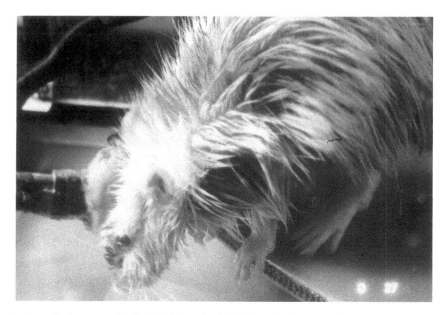

Figure 3   Photograph of a REM (paradoxical)-sleep-deprived rat after 27 days of deprivation. This photograph was taken a few hours before the rat died. Note the debilitated ungroomed appearance, discolored fur, and the swollen paws.

changes, and eventual death—which had never been documented in any conventionally stressed rats in an experimental setting (4).

Such animal models of sleep deprivation have been important in the field of sleep medicine research, as it has been impossible to chronically and profoundly sleep deprive humans to a similar extent, for obvious reasons. In fact, most human total sleep deprivation studies have been carried out for only 5 days or less, with the most notable exception being one study in which sleep deprivation was extended to 11 days (29). Partial sleep deprivation studies have similarly been limited to 16 consecutive nights, and have also revealed no damaging physiological symptoms. Yet, as will be discussed in some detail later, one interesting model of chronic partial sleep deprivation has been that of pharmacologically-induced REM sleep deprivation among individuals taking antidepressants [such as monoamine oxidase inhibitors (MAOIs) or tricyclic antidepressants (TCAs)]. On review of the available literature on human sleep deprivation (29,30), it appears that the major point of correspondence with rat total sleep deprivation experiments is that of increased hunger in human subjects (31). A study using a 72-hr total sleep deprivation protocol in humans revealed markedly increased urea excretion, which parallels the increase in plasma urea nitrogen in the Chicago totally and partially sleep-deprived rats. Apart from this however, there has been no substantial evidence suggesting that total sleep deprivation in humans results in the same physiological changes seen in the Chicago experiments, either

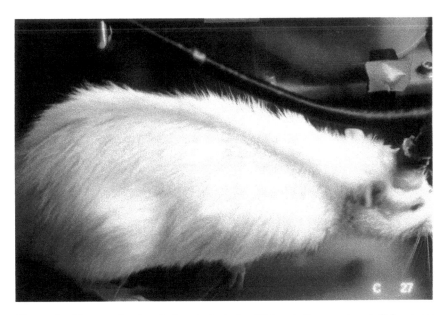

Figure 4 Photograph of a yoked control rat after 27 days in the experiment. This rat was paired with the REM-sleep-deprived rat depicted in Figure 3. This yoked control rat and the REM-sleep-deprived rat were placed on opposite sides of the same disk; however, the REM-sleep-deprived rat was not allowed to enter REM sleep since the disk would rotate each time the deprived rat tried to enter into this forbidden sleep state. The yoked control rat in this figure was allowed to sleep whenever the disk was stationary; this amounted to over 90 percent of time in which this rat could obtain sleep *ad libitum*. Note that this rat appears healthy compared to the deprived rat depicted in Figure 3.

in weight, body metabolism, or other biochemical measures. With regards to REM sleep deprivation, while increased appetite has also been observed (17,32), human studies have generally tended to emphasize the psychological, behavioral, and central, rather than systemic effects of deprivation. Thus, it is difficult to compare the findings of studies performed in animals with those of humans.

Despite these limited data, it has been postulated that deprivation-induced changes probably occur at different rates among different species (33), and if one assumes that daily sleep amounts (13.6 hr in rats; 8.0 hr in humans) reflect sleep need and associated vulnerability to sleep loss, then it would be expected that rats would develop total sleep deprivation symptoms about 1.7 times faster than humans. By parallel extrapolation, rats should also develop REM sleep deprivation symptoms 1.3 times faster than humans. If, as the Chicago experiments indicated, the lethal effects of sleep loss are related to increments in energy expenditure (EE), and if the increments were proportional to basal oxygen consumption (0.86 cm^3/g/hr in rats, and 0.22 in humans), humans would be expected to survive sleep loss about 3.9 times longer than rats. As will be discussed, one of the earlier theories regarding the func-

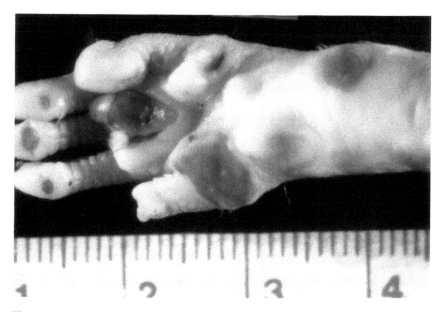

Figure 5   Skin lesions on the hind paw of a REM-sleep-deprived rat at the end of the experiment. Note the deep ulcer in the center of the rat's paw, the lesions on the pressure areas, and the lesions on the tips of the digits.

tion of sleep involved the hypothesis that some of the major effects of sleep loss were mediated by excessive heat loss. Since rats have a larger ratio of surface area to body mass than humans (940 versus 155 cm^2/kg), they might be six times more vulnerable than humans to such heat loss effects of sleep deprivation (33).

Yet, it must be emphasized from the start that despite the popularity of these sleep deprivation techniques, they are in the end, only correlational (4,5). Stimuli are administered which lead to a reduction of sleep time, and accompanying physiologic and/or behavioral changes. These changes cannot be confidently interpreted to be the direct results of sleep loss or deprivation, until other putative mediators of change that are produced (like stress) can be discounted by the experimental situation (4). While the issue of stress has been for the most part resolved, issues of completeness of sleep deprivation (particularly total sleep deprivation) remain controversial, as illustrated in the studies examining the regulation of sleep.

III.   Lessons Learned from the Regulation of Sleep

Intuitively, it is a common belief that sleep has a restorative function. An integral concept to this theory has been that of sleep regulation, about which much has been learned in recent years (34). Sleep deprivation protocols have played an important role in this research, and a closer examination of pertinent studies in

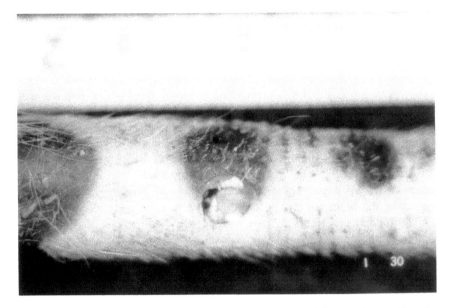

Figure 6 The tail of a REM-sleep-deprived rat at the end of the experiment. Note the large lesions scattered along the surface of the rat's tail. A circular punch biopsy sample was removed from the margin of the center lesion.

basic sleep homeostasis would be prudent before any further discussion regarding the possible functions of sleep.

Indeed the very fabric of sleep medicine (34), the concept of sleep homeostasis was initially articulated in the basic principle of sleep-cycle control proposed by Borbély in his "Two-Process Model" of sleep regulation (35,36). In recent years, much has been learned about the circadian processes regulating sleep (see also Chap. 24), but intricacies regarding the molecular mechanisms behind the homeostatic drive (Process S) and the ultradian NREM-REM oscillator, remain incomplete (13). Yet, the homeostatic regulation of NREM sleep has been well-studied, consisting of changes in both its duration and intensity (34); slow oscillations in the delta frequency range (0.75 to 4 Hz band) are characteristic of the EEG during slow-wave sleep (SWS), which reflect the burst-pause firing patterns of hyperpolarized thalamocortical and corticothalamic neurons (37–40). The EEG slow-wave activity (SWA or "delta power") as assessed by spectral analysis, has been traditionally considered to be the electrophysiological correlate of homeostatic sleep drive, or Process S (34). It is believed that SWA reflects qualitative sleep "intensity", as delta power is negatively correlated with the response to arousing stimuli (41) and SWS fragmentation (25). However, delta power is also quantitatively related to prior sleep and wakefulness in mammals, including humans (37); it displays a monotonic decay over the first three NREM-REM sleep cycles (42), increases during wakefulness (37,43,44), and is reduced after excess sleep (45).

Daytime naps reverse the buildup of delta power, leading to its reduction in later nocturnal sleep (46). Conversely, partial or total sleep deprivation results in an increase in SWA during recovery sleep, the extent of which is a function of the prior waking duration (42,47,48). Furthermore, correlation of the temporal progression of sleep pressure to its regional distribution in the surface EEG along the antero-posterior axis (9,49) has revealed a fronto-occipital power gradient, with the more frontal areas being specifically involved in sleep homeostasis (50,51). Greater SWA has also been observed in frontal rather than parietal and occipital regions during the first NREM period of the night in human sleep (52).

This anterior predominance has been found to be even greater in the recovery sleep that follows total sleep deprivation (49,52,53), and thus it has been posited that SWA might indicate an especially high need for recovery sleep in the region of the brain responsible for executive function and working memory (9,52). Furthermore, frontal deficits are especially characteristic of sleep disruption resulting from experimental deprivation from other disorders such as obstructive sleep apnea (OSA) (9,54,55). Finally, positron emission tomography (PET) scanning has revealed that frontal areas lag behind more posterior ones in reactivation after awakening (56), and thus, the frontal areas might be the first part of the cortex to fall asleep (9,57). These topographical differences in sleep homeostatic processes confirm that at least some aspects of the processes regulating human NREM sleep are local in nature (49).

Once asleep, NREM and REM sleep compete for expression at the expense of each other (34). Suppression of SWS during the first 3 to 5 hours of sleep through auditory stimulation, leads to significant enhancement of SWS and delta power in the subsequent hours of undisturbed sleep (58,59). However, studies have also shown that NREM sleep deprivation leads to increases in REM sleep pressure (47,60–63). The process underlying this essentially regular NREM-REM sleep alternation is thought to be a sleep-dependent oscillator (61,64–73), which acts more like an hourglass, rather than a clock. Furthermore, while the homeostatic sleep drive and this ultradian oscillator interact to regulate the timing and intensity of NREM sleep, they operate independently, as shown in suprachiasmatic nuclei (SCN)-lesioned rats (74–76) and in humans subjected to forced desynchrony protocols (77).

However, what regulates the amount of NREM versus REM sleep within this ultradian oscillator remains controversial, and it is here that the issue of "completeness" of sleep deprivation arises. Franken (34) has proposed that like NREM sleep, the deficits in REM sleep are mainly compensated for by increases in REM sleep time as observed in selective REM and total sleep deprivation studies in mammals—at least in the short term. Specifically, studies in cats, mice and rats suggest that REM sleep increases during recovery from REM sleep deprivation, varying in length from 1 to 24 hours, and is proportional to the loss incurred by that deprivation (21,22,25,78–83). However, in the long term, Franken has proposed that REM sleep propensity increases in the absence of REM sleep—in both waking and NREM sleep. Specifically, REM sleep recovery is more "complete" the longer the total sleep deprivation. Short episodes of total sleep deprivation are followed by either no REM rebounds or rebounds which represent only a fraction of the REM sleep lost, while longer periods of total sleep deprivation produce REM rebounds that recover a greater fraction of the REM sleep that is lost. Thus the apparent need for REM sleep, and subsequent compensatory response during recovery sleep, is greater after a 24-hour period of sleep deprivation, when compared to only 12 hours.

However, more than a few hours of total sleep deprivation is inevitably less than "total" for two reasons. First, there may be a delay in stage identification by experimenters or an overwhelming and unrelenting drive to sleep in experimental subjects, such that short, identifiable sleep episodes occur; these have been referred to as either "NREM (or) REM error sleep" periods. As well, NREM sleep-like processes may increase during waking, at times detectable as low-amplitude SWA scattered in the awake EEG. This phenomenon has been referred to as "NREM sub-sleep"; similarly, the inferred but unobserved REM sleep processes during the awake state or NREM sleep, have been termed "REM sub-sleep" (84). Accordingly, Benington (85) has alternatively hypothesized that the finding of more complete REM sleep recovery with longer total sleep deprivation is better explained by this accumulation of NREM sub-sleep, rather then REM sleep itself. Analogous to SWA and homeostatic sleep drive, it is postulated that pre-REM events (PREs), or NREM-to-REM sleep transitions (NRTs) represent a measure of REM sleep pressure, which increases exclusively during NREM (34,65). These discrete EEG events in NREM precede transitions to REM sleep, and increase in number as NREM sleep progresses; thus, REM sleep may be controlled solely by NREM sleep, and it has been posited that REM sleep somehow subserves NREM sleep function (34,65). Furthermore, it has been argued that this theory is more intuitively satisfying and more physiologically sensible, given the fact that waking and REM sleep are neurophysiologically very similar, as compared to NREM and REM sleep. Therefore, this NREM-dependent accumulation of REM sleep propensity during the deprivation period would not occur if total sleep deprivation was truly "total" or complete (86).

This must therefore be kept in mind when examining studies regarding the theories about the possible functions of sleep. These theories have historically fallen into two classes—those that support the premise that sleep serves bodily functions, and others which suggest that sleep functions more centrally, in maintaining, repairing, and consolidating brain synapses. While the former represented some of earliest theories regarding the function of sleep, such hypotheses failed to explain why loss of vigilance would be necessary in the sleep state, which in itself is a maladaptive behavior (87).

IV. Early Theories on the Function of Sleep

Theories based on the Chicago experiments (88), focused on the examination of proximal causes of death. While imperfect, it was felt at the time that such examination could potentially identify functional targets for sleep. While no severe, uniformly occurring histological abnormalities were found in the systemic organs or in the brains of severely sleep-deprived rats, two important theories regarding the possible function of sleep did emerge from these sentinel experiments.

A. Thermoregulation

A candidate function of sleep was thermoregulation (see also Chap. 15), as hypothermia was suspected as a proximal cause of death in the sleep-deprived rats, who all exhibited an eventual decline in intraperitoneal temperature (T_{ip}). In fact, a decline of more than $1°C$ below baseline proved a reliable indicator of impending death within a day or two. However, totally sleep-deprived rats kept warm by exogenous heat still died, whereas cold-stressed control rats survived much lower body temperatures than the totally sleep-deprived rats (89). Furthermore, attenuation of the T_{ip} decline in hyperthyroid totally sleep-deprived rats did not lengthen their survival and acceleration of the decline in hypothyroid totally sleep-deprived rats or totally sleep-deprived rats with lesions of the pre-optic anterior hypothalamus (PoAH), did not shorten their survival. Thus, the T_{ip} decline was not necessarily the cause of death in otherwise untreated sleep-deprived rats (4). Regarding energy expenditure (EE), T_{ip} fell despite a doubling of EE, and near the end of sleep deprivation, rats chose initial ambient temperatures of more than $50°C$ (hot to the touch) in a thermal gradient and operantly maintained a mean cage temperature of $37°C$ (compared to a baseline mean of $26°C$). Subsequent experiments using pharmacological agents (acetylsalicylic acid and naltrexone) to manipulate either T_{set} or EE, were unhelpful in further explaining these observations. Lesions to the PoAH were similarly unrevealing, and suggested that PoAH impairment alone could not have accounted for the thermoregulatory changes seen in the sleep-deprived rats. Other studies failed to identify any peripheral mechanisms for the initial excessive heat loss, and thus it is possible that routing of food energy to non-thermal forms might have made it difficult for experimental rats to efficiently maintain body temperature in spite of huge increases in food intake. However, it is still unknown as to what these alternative non-thermal forms could have been. Food energy did not go into storage (weight) and was not dissipated into locomotion (above control levels). Furthermore, it was not excessively dissipated into wastes, and loss of heat to the water under the disk was ruled out as a sufficient explanation of energy loss by water-exposed control rats (4).

In humans, few studies have provided data concerning the issue of thermoregulation, due mainly to ignorance as to its possible importance (90). However, a few interesting observations have been made, including the fact that while the circadian body temperature rhythm remains intact during human total sleep deprivation (91), the average daily temperature has been reported to shift downward (29). Subjects also feel cold more during these protocols (90,92), but unfortunately as they were allowed to put on more clothing, this confounded the assessment of any true change in core temperature. To date, no studies have controlled for these behavioral counter measures. Regarding energy metabolism, there have been interesting reports of subjects experiencing increased hunger during the first 1 or 2 days of total sleep deprivation, particularly during the early morning (31). Food intake well exceeds that predicted by the increased energy requirement through being awake rather than asleep, and the desire for food seems truly "physiological" rather just a manifestation of boredom. It has been reported (93) that 72 hours of total sleep deprivation produces significant changes in blood electrolyte levels and increased urea production, with the claim that these changes reflect metabolic disturbances. But the findings were confounded by *ad libitum* feeding, and by only a "limit" to smoking and caffeine intake by subjects. Other studies have suggested impairment of activation of various enzymes involved in the metabolic pathways within muscle after 120-hour total sleep deprivation (94), as well as small fluctuations of protein oxidation (urea formation) (95). No total sleep deprivation study has carefully monitored body weight, although several have claimed little or no change (29). Alternatively, the efficiency of energy metabolism can roughly be assessed through the physiologic capacity to perform at a fixed physical workload. Studies (96–98) have assessed O_2 uptake and CO_2 production, and energy substrate utilization (respiratory quotient- RQ) at various workloads over 33–72 hours of total sleep deprivation. None have reported any adverse effects, and although exercise endurance can fall, this seems to be due to psychological rather than physiological factors (96,99). In the setting of frank exercise, thermoregulatory impairment has been reported in subjects during 33 hours of total sleep deprivation (100), with evaporative and dry heat loss dropping significantly. Total sweat rate declined by 27 percent, further increasing the normal rise of esophageal temperature. A drop in resting core temperature during total sleep deprivation was also noted.

Therefore, on balance, the available evidence does point to some apparently minor problems with thermoregulation and energy metabolism in animals and humans, but probably of a CNS rather than a more systemic nature. For a relatively large mammal like man, a decrement in the ability to conserve heat would seem much less important to survival than it would be to a rat, which has a small thermal capacity and a relatively large surface area (90).

B.   Immune Function and Cytokines

Another major candidate for a proximal cause of death in the Chicago experiments was organ failure secondary to systemic infection (4). In fact, it is a commonly held belief, anecdotally, that sleep loss increases one's susceptibility to disease and that conversely, sleep is important in recovery from illness. One proposed hypothesis is that sleep is essential for the proper functioning of host defense systems, and that the loss of sleep leads to impairment of the immune system (see also Chap. 17). Conversely, it has also been suggested that sleep may augment immune functions upon activation by pathogens (101).

There may be some basis to both of these hypotheses, as the brain and host defense systems are capable of bidirectional communication; specifically, nervous system changes can influence the immune system through direct innervation and control of cellular recirculation patterns. Conversely, neurons and glial cells have specific receptors for regulatory substances derived from host defense systems (101).

As has been reviewed (101), host immune systems in higher organisms are complex and multilayered, and involve relatively fixed, anatomical barriers (such as skin, mucosal surfaces, secretions, and cilia) as well as active components; the latter include nonspecific and specific defenses, which are further subdivided into cellular and humoral components. Given this complexity, studies examining the connection between immunity and sleep have been limited for several reasons. First, host defenses to pathogens usually involve interactions among multiple cellular and humoral components acting locally and systemically. While local coordination is achieved through direct cell-to-cell interactions and through soluble factors and cytokines, systemic coordination involves the neuroendocrine and autonomic nervous system as well as a complex cytokine network. Therefore, to study the effects of sleep on host defenses, it would be ideal to assess multiple components simultaneously, but in practice, this has proven impossible; thus, most studies focus on sampling one or at most a few isolated host defense measures or surrogates (101). Furthermore, most studies rely on the assessment of cells from peripheral blood samples, which bias interpretation given the fact that conventional immune responses originate from the secondary lymphoid organs (lymph nodes, spleen, etc.) and not from cells in the circulation (101). Finally, studies have not distinguished between the recirculating pool of lymphocytes that mount immune responses in lymph nodes and spleen and cells derived from the mucosa-associated lymphoid tissue (MALT). The latter cells are particularly important, given their size (20–50 percent of the body's total lymphocytes), extensive autonomic innervation of mucosal sites, and local availability of neuropeptides (101).

It is perhaps because of these limitations that studies thus far have been mixed regarding the role of sleep in immunity. As would be expected, animals have been the most extensively studied, as their host defenses can be examined systematically (101). One often cited study in support of the detrimental effects of sleep deprivation on immunity is that by Brown and colleagues (102), who assessed the effects of sleep deprivation on mice challenged with the influenza virus. However, as discussed by Benca (101), while this study suggested that sleep-deprived rats showed an impaired ability to clear a viral challenge, it was impossible to conclude from the provided data whether this was due to an impairment of the immune system per se or whether it was related to secondary effects on viral clearance. However, this study did suggest impairment of some aspect of the host defense system (101). In terminally sleep-deprived rats using the DOW method, Everson and colleagues (103) reported an increased rate of bacteremia in blood cultures from 5 of 6 experimental rats near death. Although the data were highly suggestive of a breakdown of host defenses, it was impossible to assess whether this impairment was an early, primary effect of sleep deprivation, or a late-developing complication in a debilitated animal with multiorgan system failure. Therefore, to examine the temporal relationship between sleep loss and host defense breakdown, Bergmann (104) sleep-deprived rats for 4 days and subsequently examined them for bacterial infection, postmortem. In comparison to yoked controls, cultures showed bacteremia in 3 of 11 sleep-deprived rats and only 1 of 10 control rats, whereas cultures of organs responsible for filtration (kidney, liver and mesenteric lymph nodes) were either free of bacterial growth or had only low numbers of colonies present. Overall, no significant differences in bacterial growth were seen between the experimental and control groups. More importantly, other symptoms of sleep deprivation (increased energy expenditure, increased temperature, and weight loss), were unrelated to the presence of bacteria, suggesting that the physiological syndrome that accompanies sleep deprivation is not necessarily related to infection. Taken together, these studies suggest that bacteremia related to sleep deprivation might be due to the breakdown in barriers and/or alterations in nonspecific defenses rather than to primary effects on the immune system (101). Sleep probably affects the supporting events that regulate the quality and quantity of immune responses; it is well known that primary and secondary lymphoid organs are connected to the sympathetic and parasympathetic systems, and thus the autonomic system and HPA axis do affect immune responses. Key components in this interaction are cytokines, and cellular participants, such as the mast cell. Cytokines as a group likely play an important role in linking the immune and nervous systems; these include pro-inflammatory IL-1 and TNF-α, the neuropoietic cytokines [IL-6, leukemia inhibitory factors [LIF], ciliary neurotrophic factor (CNTF)] and the neurotrophins such as nerve growth factor (NGF) (101). Possible regulatory interactions are suggested by the observation that NGF acts as an autocrine B-cell factor which is required for the development of secondary antibody responses, and that IL-6, which acts on B cells, has properties similar to those of NGF in the CNS (101). Mast cells may participate in these interactions, as they are ideally located around capillary beds through the connective tissue and in all mucosal surfaces, as well as being innervated by afferent autonomic neurons. They can degranulate when stimulated, and contain preformed cytokines including TNF-α. Thus these cells may serve as cellular transducers of autonomic signals, which modulate immune responses. Changes in sleep and wakefulness, which are associated with changes in sympathetic activation, could therefore influence mast cell function and related mucosal defense reactions. For example, the necrotic skin lesions observed in the Chicago experimental rats may have been related to intradermal mast cell activity, and the bacteremia related to sleep-deprivation induced mucosal breakdown (101). However, this must be balanced against isolated reports that sleep deprivation may actually enhance certain aspects of host defenses, as observed in studies involving tumor growth (101,105).

Far fewer human studies have been performed regarding immunity and sleep deprivation, but these have been reviewed (101,106). No consistent effects of sleep deprivation on cytokine activity, mitogen responses, or natural killer (NK) activity have been observed. However, this may have been due to variabilities in measured parameters in the peripheral blood, as well as differences in the circadian time of testing or duration of sleep deprivation protocols. However, it should be kept in mind that the parameters tested based on peripheral blood samples may ultimately prove to be poor surrogates of host immune function; for example, NK activity in the blood may not be functionally important, as NK cells probably are most effective in tissues rather than in the circulation, and a decrease in such peripheral cell activity may actually represent an enhancement of host defenses in the tissues (101).

C. Exogenous and Endogenous Somnogens

It is an interesting observation that sleep often accompanies illness, and this has historically been cited as evidence in support of a connection between sleep and host defenses (101). Humans with common viral infections such as influenza, rhinovirus, and Epstein-Barr virus (EBV) tend to sleep more (107), while other infections tend to be associated with alterations in the distribution rather than the total duration of sleep within a 24-hour period, such as in the case of trypanosomiasis (108). Implicit in this theory is that sleep is somehow helpful or necessary to combat infection. However, this is not necessarily the case, as increased sleep could simply be a side effect of cytokine release without clinically important regulatory effects on host defenses (101). Consistent with this has been the finding that bacterial and viral components have hypnotic effects when injected into a variety of mammalian species (101). Examples include muramic peptides (MPs), which are components of bacterial peptidoglycans and associated with increases in NREM and SWS when injected into the peritoneum and cerebral ventricles of animals, including rats, particularly during their normal period of wakefulness (101). Similarly, other bacterial membrane components such as lipopolysaccharide (LPS, or endotoxin) and virus-derived substances such as double-stranded ribonucleic acid (RNA) have also been found to be somnogenic in several species (101).

However, if components of infectious organisms can induce sleep, what about endogenous substances? One theory regarding the function of sleep has been that wakefulness may lead to the accumulation of potentially toxic substances, which must be cleared during subsequent sleep. This so called "hypnotoxin" theory was perhaps one of the first theories proposed. Ishimori (109) in 1909 and Legendre and Piéron (110) in 1913, independently extracted a hypnogenic substance and hypnotoxin, respectively, from the brain tissues, cerebrospinal fluid (CSF) and blood of sleep-deprived dogs. These extracts were able to induce sleep or sleep-like behavior in their otherwise healthy, awake counterparts. Ishimori felt at that time that "the fact that the cerebral matter of sleep-deprived animals contains a potent hypnogenic substance which can not be detected in the brain of normally sleeping animals, leads to clarify the cause of induction of our normal sleep…" (109). By the 1960s, advanced techniques enables researchers to identify a possible sleep substance in cats and rabbits. In 1977, a novel nonapeptide, delta-sleep inducing peptide (DSIP), was identified (111). Other researchers (112) also attempted to extract substances, such as sleep-promoting substance (SPS) directly from the brain tissues of sleep-deprived rats; in 1983, the active component of SPS, uridine (a pyrimidine nucleoside), was discovered. Later, another active component (the oxidized form of glutathione or GSSG), was also identified: discovery of these blood-, brain- and CSF-derived substances have stimulated further research regarding sleep-modulating activities of several substances, but none has emerged as ideal. Rather, many possible sleep substances representing a variety of body constituents have been proposed (112,113).

V.   More Current Theories on the Function of Sleep

A.   Brain Maturation and Developmental Plasticity

As such, modern theories regarding the function of sleep have been more sophisticated, given technological advances in the field of neurobiology. One of these theories has been that sleep—particularly REM sleep—is required for brain maturation and developmental plasticity (5). Sleep deprivation studies have supported the important role of REM in brain development (3), as evidenced by the reports of greater effects of monocular patching on the lateral geniculate cells (i.e., the cells connected to the patched eye become smaller, those associated with the other eye become larger) of kittens deprived of REM sleep (114).

B. Memory Reinforcement

Much attention has also been placed on REM sleep and its possible role in memory reinforcement and consolidation (see also Chap. 11). Indeed, the physiologic correlates of REM sleep have been found in nearly all mammals (115), and the interest in sleep and memory was intensified by a publication (116) hypothesizing that REM functioned to eliminate unneeded memories. This focus on sleep and learning largely displaced earlier theories associating REM with psychological well-being and mental illness (115). The possible role of NREM sleep has also been examined in the context of learning, focusing on the possible role of synchronized discharges in the reinforcement of synaptic connections in the hippocampus and neocortex (117,118). While relatively fewer studies have been performed examining NREM sleep, most animal studies of REM sleep deprivation have used some form of NREM sleep deprivation as a control procedure, and animals thus NREM sleep deprived have shown substantial learning deficits. But obviously, further work is necessary to determine whether NREM sleep has a role in memory consolidation, although clearly NREM sleep has a role in performance while awake.

Memory consolidation is a time-dependent process in which labile memory traces are converted into more permanent and/or enhanced forms (119). Under duress, humans can go for 40 hours or more without sleep and still be able to retain information acquired at the beginning of the sleepless period, even when faced with many distractions. Thus, what is being considered is the role of sleep in longer-term memory consolidation, or longer-term encoding of information and optimization of its recall, not a requirement of sleep for recalling events of the prior day (short-term recall) (120–122). The information acquired while awake would then be actively altered, restructured and reinforced during sleep. The subsequent robust memory trace would influence behavioral responses to environmental changes and thus expand or alter the organism's or individual's range of behaviors (119,123,124). However, this view becomes more complex with the realization that both sleep and memory are each multifaceted phenomena. While sleep is divided into NREM and REM components, the acquisition of long-term memory requires multiple memory systems, at least in humans; these are mainly delineated between declarative (or explicit) and non-declarative (or implicit or procedural) memory (125).

There has been a mix of positive and negative results in human studies which has led many researchers to suggest that REM sleep may not be important for certain kinds of memory—specifically, declarative memory. This includes rote memory, language memory, and (depending on the precise definition) certain aspects of conceptual memory. REM sleep would thus be excluded from having any substantial role in much of what is considered to be unique in human intellectual capacity. It is "procedural" memory, defined as performance on perceptual and associated motor skills, that is claimed to be impaired by sleep disruption (126–128). However, others suggest that REM sleep has a key role in language or emotional learning (129–131). On balance, studies in humans and animals suggest that both REM and NREM sleep could have memory-related functions; however, not all types of memories seem to rely on the same stage of sleep for consolidation. Accordingly, the role of sleep in memory has been interpreted in two major ways. The "dual process hypothesis" states that REM and NREM sleep act differently on memory traces, depending on the memory system to which they belong; for example, it is hypothesized that SWS facilitates consolidation of declarative memory (132,133). An alternative hypothesis is that a succession of brain processes consolidates memories (134), and thus, NREM sleep (SWS) and REM sleep work together in a serial, double-step process (135).

Furthermore, while animal models have been used to study the possible role of sleep in memory systems, there has been some controversy as to whether such systems in humans are adequately modeled in animals, such as the rat (hippocampus) (11). Perhaps the most well studied aspect of memory is that pertaining to declarative memory, which in humans, consists of episodic memory (autobiographical memory for events that occur in specific spatial and temporal contexts), and semantic memory, which pertains to general knowledge about the world (11). While some believe that only humans are capable of declarative memory, others argue that elements of episodic memory should exist in animals as well, in terms of spatial learning (which is dependent on the hippocampal and medial temporal formation) (136–138). Therefore, hippocampal-dependent spatial memory tasks could represent a relevant model, at least in rats, for human spatial episodic memory (139). If so, the surrounding entorhinal, perirhinal and parahippocampal cortices may play important roles in the semantic aspects of declarative memory (140). Non-declarative memory, which manifests as habits, priming, and simple conditioning, has been attributed to several distinct neuroanatomical structures in both humans and animals (141,142). For example, the striatum is important for habit formation (143) and interacts with the cerebellum in motor-based skill learning (144). In contrast, modality-specific neocortical regions mediate perceptual priming (142), while the amygdala plays a large role in unconscious emotional learning (145). However, these correlations have neither been extensively nor systematically studied in the context of sleep deprivation.

Individuals taking antidepressants have provided a rather unique model for chronic REM sleep deprivation; this has afforded researchers an opportunity to examine the long-term effects of such "deprivation" on learning and memory. Monamine oxidase inhibitors (MAOIs) such as phenelzine (Nardil), administered at therapeutic doses for depression, can completely suppress REM sleep and reported dreaming. Similar, tricyclic antidepressants (TCA) have been associated with less complete suppression of REM sleep (146). Used for more than 30 years and with millions having taken or currently taking these medications, to date there has been no clear evidence that these medications impair memory; instead, there is some evidence that MAOIs may actually improve memory (147–149). One way of explaining this is that these and other similar medications, may actually substitute for REM sleep. However, monoamines are known to suppress ponto-geniculo-occipital (PGO) spikes, which is the exact opposite of what occurs during REM sleep. Indeed, it is thought that one major function of REM is to prevent monoamine release (150). Alternatively, MAOIs may simply mask the polygraphic signs of REM sleep, while some essential aspect of REM persists, and allows for continued memory consolidation. Specifically, PGO spikes and hippocampal theta waves have been hypothesized to be involved in memory and learning (151–153). However, although PGO spikes have not been recorded in humans (as doing so would require depth electrodes), suppression of such spikes has been observed in a cat study in which an MAOI was administered (154). Finally, as withdrawal of MAOIs results in a massive REM rebound, this suggests that these drugs do indeed cause a significant REM sleep debt (146); thus at the neurotransmitter level, it seems apparent that MAOIs do not substitute for, or mask REM sleep (115).

Finally, another interesting model of chronic REM sleep-depression in humans derives from anatomic brain lesions. In animal models, lesions of the pontine tegmentum have been shown to result in a significant reduction, if not elimination, of REM sleep (155). Similarly lesions in humans have revealed normal intellectual function despite severely impaired motor deficits (147). In one individual who suffered a shrapnel injury to the brainstem, careful follow-up for more than 10 years has confirmed the presence of little or no REM sleep on repeated polysomnographic testing; despite this, he was able to graduate from law school. Therefore, the above examples suggest that REM sleep may not be critically important in learning—with the previously discussed caveats kept in mind.

C. Neuronal Plasticity and Synaptic Consolidation

Indeed, a better way of viewing memory consolidation may be in terms of the neurochemical changes in the brain that occur, rather than REM or NREM sleep per se. Specifically, *in vitro* and *in vivo* studies have shown that hippocampal post-tetanic potentiation is critically dependent upon norepinephrine (156), the release of which is a key feature of REM sleep. Furthermore, this cessation has been linked to reduced expression of phosphorylated CREB (cyclic adenosine monophosphate response element-binding protein), Arc (a growth factor- and activity-related gene), and BDNF (brain-derived neurotrophic factor); the phosphorylation of CREB and the upregulation of Arc and BDNF are often associated with synaptic plasticity (157). Indeed, the concept of neuronal plasticity may be the key in understanding the basis of learning and memory, with which noradrenergic systems are closely integrated. Specifically, the expression of some wake-related genes may be modulated by noradrenergic mechanisms; for example, in rats with unilateral lesions of the locus coeruleus (LC), the lesioned hemisphere fails to show marked increases in expression of genes such as immediate early genes (IEGs) and plasticity-related genes (such as CREB) during the waking state, despite normal EEG activity and behavior. It is believed that this finding links a known wake-related ascending arousal system with the expression of genes that are associated with a wake-related cognitive function—that of learning (13).

Intracellular second-messenger systems and their down-stream nuclear/genomic effects may therefore represent early stages of the neuroplastic changes that are initiated by the waking experience, which are then consolidated during sleep (13). For example, it has been shown (158) that changes in the activity of the PKA (protein kinase A) second-messenger system and its third messenger, CREB, are associated with both state-dependent neuromodulatory changes in the hippocampus and performance of hippocampus-dependent learning tasks (13). Consolidation of hippocampus-based learning in rats is disrupted at specific times after training by both REM sleep deprivation and the intraventricular injection of inhibitors of PKA or inhibitors of protein synthesis; it has been postulated (13) that such manipulations may disrupt a PKA-CREB-gene transcription-protein synthesis pathway necessary for consolidation of learning, which is specifically facilitated by REM sleep. REM-related enhanced cholinergic and decreased serotonergic modulation of adenylyl cyclase activity [linked to acetylcholine (Ach) and membrane receptors] may determine the activity of the PKA signaling pathway (13). In addition, it should be noted that rats exposed to rich sensorimotor experiences during the waking state, are found to have increased levels of the plasticity-associated IEG *zif-268* (also known as early growth response 1, *Egr 1*) during subsequent sleep (13).

Therefore, several investigators (87,159,160) have concluded that sleep is essentially a distributed process of the brain, which is organized into highly interconnected groups of neurons. However, these fundamental units are neither small nor are they discrete (87), and no specific neuronal circuit necessary for sleep, has been identified (8). Indeed, there has been numerous examples, as in post-stroke lesions, where the ability to sleep remains intact; in fact, it has been stated that if an animal or human survives an injury, no matter how severe, sleep persists. Other examples in nature include dolphins, which display high-amplitude EEG slow-wave activity characteristic of deep NREM sleep only in one half of the brain at a time (161), and in which unihemispheric sleep deprivation results in a sleep rebound only in the half that is sleep deprived (162). In addition, birds can detect predators during unihemispheric NREM sleep, the occurrence of which appears to vary with predation risk (162).

Accordingly, the distribution of brain activation during sleep, as measured by EEG or functional imaging, is dependent upon the distribution of activity during prior wakefulness. Therefore, unilateral stimulation of the somatosensory cortex during the awake state, results in enhanced SWA in the stimulated area during subsequent NREM sleep (163). Furthermore, it has been postulated based on functional magnetic resonance imaging (fMRI) studies (164,165) that the localized effects of sleep loss are dependent in part, on the specific cognitive tasks performed during wakefulness. As it pertains to memory, these effects of sleep manipulation are directly applicable to the concept of neuronal plasticity. More specifically, in 1949, Hebb proposed that synaptic efficacy (or in Hebbian terminology, synaptic weights, which can be positive or negative) is enhanced by synaptic use, thus forming the physical substrates of memory. Studies conducted since then have generally confirmed this theory, that the dynamic microcircuitry of the brain is largely determined by use and disuse of synapses. Thus, some mechanism is required to maintain such synaptic integrity, or provide synaptic activation for what has been called a "synaptic superstructure" (87). It has therefore been proposed that this is a possible function of sleep; sleep may augment the efficacy of synapses that are intensely utilized or newly formed during wakefulness, which may help with memory consolidation. As articulated by Krueger (8), when neurons are activated, associated changes occur in membrane potentials, neurotransmitter release, and in ionic conductance. Regulatory substances are also released, including growth factors, which alter expression of specific genes involved in synaptic function and thus affect the microcircuitry of the brain. Other substances may affect other cellular functions, such as intracellular calcium concentrations of nearby neurons, which alter their input-output relationships with each other. Therefore, synapses that were not activated by the initial train of events may be secondarily activated. It has been hypothesized that when neuronal groups in this state are disconnected in time from any environmental inputs, they are asleep (87). As such, the loss of environmental stimuli (sleep-associated unconsciousness) may be a graded function of the number of neuronal groups in this "sleep state".

VI. A Look to the Future

It has been stated that there is a vast contrast between our growing experimental refinement in the field of sleep medicine and our ignorance of the fundamental issues, including that pertaining to the function of sleep (2). We are indeed in the midst of an exciting time in the field of sleep research. While the search for the function of sleep continues, new and powerful integrative approaches have been developed, which have allowed researchers to address this question in novel and exciting ways (18). The use of genetics—specifically, functional genomics—will undoubtedly play a large role in this endeavor, where function is defined not simply at a cellular level, but at a more macroscopic level (i.e., with respect to system and/or integrated complex behavior) (18). As such, the approach taken will shift from a predominantly hypothesis-drive approach, to larger-scale strategies in which the potential role of thousands of genes will be studied simultaneously, through for example, array-based gene expression monitoring (18). Since so many different neuronal groups are involved in the regulation of sleep and wakefulness, uncovering the spatial patterns of gene expression in the brain and their relationship to behavioral state, is essential to the understanding of gene function in sleep (18). While the functional genomics of the rat (the key animal model in sleep research) is still in the early stages of development, the ongoing Rat Genome Project will undoubtedly encourage further research using this model. Yet, while the use of sleep deprivation would seem ideal in such a gene-driven approach, sleep deprivation in this setting would again provide only correlative information, since gene expression in the brain may be modified by sleep or wakefulness. However, in combination with other experimental technologies, such as quantitative EEG and functional imaging, this information may prove invaluable (18). A number of candidate genes have already been studied in terms of their possible roles in sleep and wakefulness, and the transcripts of many genes have been shown to change as a function of behavioral state. Upregulation of the synaptic plasticity genes, such as BDNF, is suggestive of plastic remodeling in the brain during sleep (18).

Yet at the most basic level, these experimental techniques have stimulated a paradigm shift in how sleep is defined. The study of other non-human models has allowed sleep researchers to "look outside of the box"; specifically, much of sleep research has been historically based on the EEG, but because such electroencephalographic patterns are mainly interpretable only in mammals, the definition of sleep defined this way, has limited studies mainly to these species. However, studies suggest that non-mammals may also display sleep and wakefulness equivalents, which may be utilized for more efficient screening phenotyping strategies (18). Simpler animal models of sleep may then be developed, as in the field of circadian biology, in which the study of organisms such as *Neurospora, Drosophila,* and *Danio reiro* (zebrafish) have been essential in arriving at our current understanding of the circadian clock (18). Similar models may do the same with regard to the function of sleep.

References

1. Kosik K. Beyond phrenology, at last [Opinion]. Nature Rev 2003; 4:234–239.
2. Tononi G, Cirelli C. The frontiers of sleep [Meeting Report]. TINS 1999; 22:417–418.
3. Marks G, Shaffery J, Oksenberg A, Speciale S, Roffwarg H. A functional rol for REM sleep in brain maturation. Behav Brain Res 1995; 69:1–11.
4. Rechtschaffen A, Bergmann B. Sleep deprivation in the rat: an update of the 1989 paper. Sleep 2002; 25:18–24.
5. Rechtschaffen A. Current perspectives on the function of sleep. Perspect Biol Med 1998; 41:359–390.
6. Giuditta A. The Function of Sleep: Preface. Behavioural Brain Research 1995; 69:ix-x.
7. Kavanau J. Memory, sleep, and dynamic stabilization of neural circuitry: Evolutionary perspectives. Neurosci Biobehav Rev 1996; 20:289–311.
8. Krueger J, Obal F, Fang J, Kubota T, Taishi P. The role of cytokines in physiologic sleep regulation. Ann N.Y. Acad Sci 2001; 933:211–221.
9. Hobson J, Pace-Schott E. The cognitive neuroscience of sleep: neuronal systems, consciousness and learning. Nat Rev Neurosci 2002; 3:679–93.
10. Hobson J, Pace-Schott E. Deaming and the brain: toward a cognitive neuroscience of conscious states. Behav Brain Sci 2000; 23:793–842.
11. Peigneux P, Laureys S, Delbeuck X, Maquet P. Sleeping brain, learning brain. The role of sleep for memory systems. Neuroreport 2001; 12:A111–A124.
12. Maquet P. Functional neuroimaging of normal human sleep by positron emission tomography. J Sleep Res 2000; 9:207–231.
13. Pace-Schott E, Hobson J. The neurobiology of sleep: genetics, cellular physiology and subcortical networks. Nat Rev Neurosci 2002; 3:591–605.
14. De Manaceine M. Quelques observations experimentales sur l'influence de l'insomnie absolue. Arch Ital Biol 1894; 21:322–325.
15. Patrick G, Gilbert J. On the effects of loss of sleep. Pscyhol Rev 1896; 3:469–483.
16. Aserinsky E, Kleitman N. Regularly occurring periods of eye motility, and concomitant phenomena, during sleep. Science 1953; 118:273–274.
17. Dement W. The effect of dream deprivation. Science 1960; 131:1705–1707.
18. Mackiewicz M, Pack A. Functional genomics of sleep. Respir Physiol Neurobiol 2003; 135:207–220.
19. Rechtschaffen A, Bergmann B, Gilliland M, Bauer K. Effects of Method, Duration, and Sleep Stage on Rebounds from Sleep Deprivation in the Rat. Sleep 1999; 22:11–31.
20. Mistlberger R, Bergmann B, Rechtschaffen A. Period-amplitude analysis of rat encephalogram: effects of sleep deprivation and exercise. Sleep 1987; 10:508–522.
21. Feinberg I, Campbell I. Total sleep deprivation in the rat transiently abolishes the delta amplitude response to darkness. Implications for the mechanism of the 'negative delta rebound'. J Neurophysiol 1993; 70:2695–2699.

22. Franken P, Tobler I, Borbély A. Effects of 12–h sleep deprviation and of 12–h cold exposure on sleep regualtion and cortical tempeature in the rat. Physiol Behav 1993; 54:885–894.
23. Tobler I, Franken P, Gao B, Jaggi K, Borbély A. Sleep deprivation inteh rat at different ambient termperatures: effect on sleep, EEG spectra and brain temperature. Arch Ital Biol 1994; 132:39–52.
24. Hanagasiolglu M, Borbély A. Effect of voluntary motor activity on sleep in the rat. Behav Brain Res 1982; 4:359–368.
25. Franken P, Dijk D, Tobler I, Borbély A. Sleep deprivation in the rat: effects on elecroencephalogram power spectra, vigilance states, and cortical temperature. Am J Physiol 1991a; 261:R198–208.
26. Sternthal H, Web W. Sleep deprivation of rats by punitive and nonpunitive procedures. Physiol Behav 1986; 37:249–252.
27. Rechtschaffen A, Gilliland M, Mergmann M, Winter J. Physiologic correlates of prolonged sleep deprivation in rats. Science 1983; 221:182–4.
28. Bergmann B, Kushida C, Everson A, Gilliland M, Obermeyer W, Rechtschaffen A. Sleep deprivation in the rat: II. methodology. Sleep 1989; 12:5–12.
29. Horne J. A review of the biological effects of total sleep deprivation in man. Biol Psychol 1978; 7:55–102.
30. Wilkinson R, Edwards R, Haines E. Performance following a night of reduced sleep. Psychonomic Sci 1966; 5:471–472.
31. Hobson J, Pettitt A. High incentive effects on vigilance perrformance during 72 h of total sleep deprivation. Acta Phsychol 1985; 58:123–139.
32. Sampson H. Psychological effects of deprivation of dreaming sleep. J Nerv Ment Dis 1966; 143:305–317.
33. Rechtschaffen A, Bergemann B, Everson C. Sleep deprivation in the rat, X: integration and discussion of the findings. Sleep 1989; 12:68–87.
34. Franken P. Long-term vs. short-term processes regulating REM sleep. J Sleep Res 2002; 11:17–28.
35. Borbély A, Achermann P. Concepts and models of sleep regulation: an overview. J Sleep Res 1992; 1:63–79.
36. Borbély A. A two process model of sleep regulation. Human Nurobiol 1982; 1:195–204.
37. Franken P, Chollet D, Tafti M. The homeostatic regulation of sleep need is under genetic control. J Neurosci 2001; 21:2610–2621.
38. Steriade M, McCormick D, Sejnowski T. Thalamocortical oscillations inthe sleeping and aroused brain. Science 1993; 262:679–682.
39. McCormick D, Bal T. Sleep and arousal: thalamocortical mechanisms. Annu Rev Neurosci 1997; 20:185–215.
40. Steriade M. Coherent oscillations andshort-term plasticity in corticothalamic networks. 1999 1999; Trends Neurosci.
41. Neckelmann D, Ursin D. Sleep stages and EEG power spectrum inrelation to acoustical stimulus arousal threshold in the rat. Sleep 1993; 16:467–477.
42. Borbély A, Baumann F, Brandeis D, Strauch I, Lehemann D. Sleep deprivation: effects on sleep stages and EEG power density in man. Electroencephalogr Clin Neurophysiol 1981; 51:484–493.
43. Dijk D, Beersma D, Daan S. EEG power density during nap sleep: reflection of an hourglass measuring the duration of prior wakefulness. J Biol Rhythms 1987; 2:207–219.

44. Tobler I, Borbély A. Sleep EEG in the rat as a function of prior waking. Electroencephalogr Clin Neurophysiol 1986; 64:74–76.

45. Werth E, Dijk D, Achermann P, Borbély A. Dynamics of the sleep EEG after an early evening nap: experimental data and simulations. Am J Physiol 1996; 271:R501–510.

46. Feinberg I, March J, Floyd T, Jimison R, Bossom-Demitrack L, Katz P. Homeostatic changes during post-nap sleep maintain baseline levels of delta EEG. Electroencephalogr Clin Neurophysiol 1985; 61:134–137.

47. Brunner D, Dijk D, Tobler I, Borbély A. Effect of partial sleep deprivation on sleep stages and EEGpower spectra: evidence for non-REMS and REMS homeostasis. Electroencephalogr Clin Neurophysiol 1990; 75:492–499.

48. Dijk D, Brunner D, Borbély A. EEG power density during recovery sleep in the morning. Electroencephalogr Clin Neurophysiol 1991; 78:203–214.

49. Ferrara M, De Gennaro L, Curcio G, Cristiani R, Corvasce C, Bertini M. Regional Differences of the Human Sleep Electroencephalogram in Response to Selective Slow-wave Sleep Deprivation. Cerebral Cortex 2002; 12:737–748.

50. Werth E, Achermann P, Borbély A. Brain topography of the human sleep EEG: antero-posterior shifts of spectral power. Neuroreport 1996a; 8:123–127.

51. Werth E, Achermann P, Borbély A. Fronto-occipital EEG power gradients on human sleep. J Sleep Res 1997; 6:102–112.

52. Finelli L, Borbély A, Acherman P. Functional topography of the human nonREM sleep electroencephalogram. Eur J Neurosci 2001; 13:2282–2290.

53. Cajochen C, Foy R, Dijk D. Frontal predominance of relative increase in sleep delta and theta EEG activity after sleep loss in humans. Sleep Res Online 1999; 2:65–69.

54. Beebe D, Gozal D. Obstructive sleep apnea and the prefrontal cortex: towards a comprehensive model liking nocturnal upper airway obstruction to daytime cognitive and behavioral deficits. J Sleep Res 2002; 11:1–16.

55. Harrison Y, Horne J. The impact of sleep deprivation on decision making: a review. J Exp Psychol Appl 2000; 6:236–249.

56. Balkin T, AL E. Bidirectional changes in regional cerebral blood flow across the first 20 minutes of wakefulness. Sleep Res Online [online] <http://www.sro.org/cftemplate/wfsrscongress/indiv.cfm?ID=19998006> 1999.

57. Acherman P, Werth E, Dijk D, Borbély A. Time course of sleep inertia after nighttime and daytime sleep episodes. Arch Ital Biol 1995; 134:109–119.

58. Dijk D, Brunner D, Borbély A. Quantiative analysis of the effect of slow wave sleep deprivation during the first 3 hours of sleep on subsequent EEG power density. Eur Arch Psychiatry Neurol Sci 1987a; 236:293–297.

59. Dijk D, Beersma D. Effects of SWS deprivation on suseqeunt EEG power density and sponttaneous sleep duration. Electroencephalogr Clin Neurophysiol 1989; 72:312–320.

60. Beersma D, Dijk D, Blok C, Everhardus I. REMS deprivation during 5 hours leads to an immedite REMS rebound and to suppression of non-REMS intensity. Electroencephalogr Clin Neurophysiol 1990; 76:114–122.

61. Benington J, Woudenberg M, Heller H. REMS propensity accumulates during 2–h REMS deprivation in the rest period in rats. Neurosci Lett 1994b; 180:76–80.

62. Brunner D, Dijk D, Borbély A. Repated partial sleep deprivation progressively changes in EEG during sleep and wakefulness. Sleep 1993; 16.

63. Endo T, Schwierin B, Borbély A, Tobler I. Selective and total sleep deprivation: effect on the sleep EEG in the rat. Psychiatry 1997; 66:97–110.

64. Barbato G, Wehr T. Homeostatic regualtion of REMSin humns during extended sleep. Sleep 1998; 21:267–276.
65. Benington J, Heller H. REMS timingi is controlled homeostatically by accumulation of REMS propensity in non-REMS. Am J Physiol 1994a; 266:R1992–2000.
66. Brezinova V. Sleep cycle content and sleep cycle duration. Electroencephalogr Clin Neurophysiol 1974; 36:275–282.
67. Endo T, Roth C, Landolt H, et al. Effect of frequent brief awakenings from nonREMS on the nonREM-REMS cycle. Psychiatry Clin Neurosci 1998b; 52:129–130.
68. Gaillard J, Tuglular I. Theorthodox-paradoxical sleep cyclein the rat. Experientia 1976; 32:718–719.
69. Johnson L. The REMScycleis a sleep-dependent rhythm. Sleep 1980; 2:299–307.
70. Miyasita A, Fukuda K, Inugami M. Effects of sleep interruption on REM-NREMS cycle in nocturnal human sleep. Electroencephalogr Clin Neurophysiol 1989; 73:107–116.
71. Moses J, Naitoh P, Johnson L. The REMS cyclein altered sleep/wake schedules. Pscyhophysiology 1978; 15:569–575.
72. Vivaldi E, Ocampo A, Wyneken U, Roncagliolo M, Zapata A. Short-term homeostasis of active sleep and the architecture of sleep in the rat. J Neurophysiol 1994; 72:1745–1755.
73. Whitehead W, Ronbinson T, Wincor M, Reschtschaffen A. The accumulation of REMS need during sleep and wakefulness. Common Behav Biol 1969; 4:195–201.
74. Mistlberger R, Bergemann B, Waldenar W, Rechtschaffen A. Recovery sleep following sleep deprivation in intacta nd suprachiasmatic nuclei lesioned rats. Sleep 1983; 6:217–233.
75. Tobler I, Borbély A, Groos G. The effect of sleep deprivation onsleep in rats with suprachiasmatic lesions. Neurosci Lett 1983; 42:49–54.
76. Trachsel L, Edgar D, Seidel W, Heller H, Dement W. Sleep homeostasis in suprachiasmatic nuclei-lesioned rats: effects of sleep deprivation and triazolam administration. Brain Res 1992; 589:253–261.
77. Dijk D, Czeisler C. Contribution of the circadian pacemaker and the sleep homeostat to sleep propensity, sleep structure, electroencephalographic slow waves, and sleep spindle activity in humans. J Neurosci 1995; 15:3526–3538.
78. Amici R, Zamboni G, Perez E, et al. Pattern of desynchronized sleep during depirvation and recvoery induced inthe rat by changes in ambient temperature. J Sleep Res 1994; 3:250–256.
79. Franken P, Tobler I, Borbély A. Varying photoperiod in the laboratory rat. profound effect on 24–h sleep pattern but no effect on sleep homeostasis. Am J Physiol 1995; 269:R691–701.
80. Jouvet M. The role of monoamines and acetylcholine containing neurons in the regulation ofthe sleep waking cycle. Ergebn Physiol 1972; 64:166–307.
81. Katihama K, Valatx J. Instrumental and pharmacological paradoxical sleep deprivation in mice: strain differences. Neuropharmacology 1980; 19:529–535.
82. Parmeggiani P, Ciani T, Calasso M, Zamboni G, Perez E. Quantitative analysis of short term deprivation and recovery of desynchronized sleep in cats. Electroencephalogr Clin Neurophysiol 1980; 50:293–302.
83. Perez E, Zamboni G, Amici R, Toni I, Parmeggiani P. Low ambient temperatures decrease the amoung of desynchronized sleep in the rat and elicits a rebound which is related to the degree of deprivation. J Sleep Res 1992; 1(Suppl 1):177.

84. Rechtschaffen A, Bergmann B. Sleep Rebounds and Their Implications for Sleep Stage Substrates: A Response to Benington and Heller. Sleep 1999; 22:1038–1043.

85. Benington J. Debating how REM sleep is regulated (and by what) [Comment]. J Sleep Res 2002; 11:29–33.

86. Benington J, Heller H. Does the function of REM sleep concern non REM sleep or waking? Prog Neurobiol 1994; 44:433–449.

87. Krueger J, Obal F. A neural group theory of sleep function. J Sleep Res 1993; 2:63–69.

88. Rechtschaffen A, Bergmann B. Sleep deprivation in the rat by the disk-over-water method. Behav Brain Res 1995; 69:55–63.

89. Shaw P, Kushida C, Rechtschaffen A. Hypothermia is probably not the proximal cause of death in sleep deprived rats. Sleep Res 1993; 22:345.

90. Horne J. Sleep Function, With Particular Reference to Sleep Deprivation. Ann Clin Res 1985; 17:199–208.

91. Akerstedt T. Altered sleep/wake patterns and circadian rhythms. Acta Physiol Scand 1979; suppl:469.

92. Horne J. Human sleep and tissue restitution: some qualifications and doubts. Clin Sci 1983; 65:569–578.

93. Kant G, Genser S, Thorne D, Pfalser J, Mougey E. Effect of 72 hour sleep deprivation on urinary cortisol and indices of metabolism. Sleep 1984; 7:142–146.

94. Vondura K, Brodan V, Bass A, et al. Effects of sleep deprivation on the activity of selected metabolic enzyme in skeletal muscle. Eur J Appl Physiol 1981; 47:41–46.

95. Scrimshaw N, Hubicht J, Pellet P, Piche M, Cholakos B. Effects of sleep deprivaiton and reversal of diurnal activity on protein metabolism of young men. Am J Clin Nutrition 1966; 19:313–318.

96. Martin B, Gaddis G. Effects of sleep deprivation on tolerance of prolonged exercise. Eur J Appl Physiol 1981; 47:345–354.

97. Martin B, Gaddis G. Exercise after sleep deprivation. Med Sci Sports Exerc 1981; 13:220–223.

98. Horne J, Pettitt A. Sleep deprivation and the physiological response to exercise under steady-state conditions in untrained subjects. Sleep 1984; 7:168–179.

99. Martin B, Haney R. Self-selected exercise intensity is unchanged by sleep loss. Eur J Appl Physiol 1982; 49:79–86.

100. Sawka M, Gonzalez R, Pandolf K. Effects of sleep deprivation on thermoregulation during exercise. Am J Physiol 1984; 246:R72–77.

101. Benca R, Quintas J. Sleep and host defenses: a review. Sleep 1997; 20:1027–1037.

102. Brown R, Pang G, Husband A, King M. Suppression of immunity to influenza virus infection in the respiratory tract following sleep disturbance. Reg Immunol. Vol. 2, 1989:321–325.

103. Everson C. Sustained sleep deprivation impairs host defense. Am J Physiol 1993; 265:R1148–54.

104. Bergmann B, Gilliland M, Feng P. Sleep deprivation and sleep extension: are physiological effects of sleep deprivation in the rat mediated by bacterial invasion? Sleep 1996; 19:554–62.

105. Bergmann B, Rechtschaffen A, Gilliland M, Quintans J. Effect of extended sleep deprivaiton on tumor growth in rats. Am J Physiol 1996; 271:R1460–4.

106. Dinges D, Douglas S, Hamarman S. Sleep deprivation and human immune function. Adv Neuroimmunol 1995; 5:97.

107. Pollmacher T, Mullington J, Korth C, Heinz-Selch D. Influence of host defense activation on sleep in humans. Adv Neuroimmunology 1995; 5:155–169.

108. Buguet A, Bert J, Tapie P. Sleep-wake cycle in human African trypanosomiasis. J Clin Neurophysiol 1993; 10:190–196.

109. Ishimori K. True cause of sleep: a hypnogenic substance as evidnced in the brain of sleep-deprived animals. Tokyo Igakkai Zasshi 1909; 23:429–457.

110. Legendre R, Pieron H. Recherches sur le besoin de sommeil consecutif a une veille prlongee. Z. Allgem. Physiol 1913; 14:235–262.

111. Schoenenberger G, Maier P, Tobler H, Monnier M. A naturally occurring delta-EEG enhancing nonapeptide in rabbits. X. Final isolation, characterization and activity test. Pflugers Arch. 1977; 369:99–109.

112. Inoue S. Sleep-promoting substnace (SPS) and physiological sleep regulation. Zool. Sci. 1993; 10:557–576.

113. Borbély A, Tobler I. Endogenous sleep-promoting substacnes and sleep regulation. Physiol Rev 1989; 69:605.

114. Oksenberg A, Shaffery J. Rapid eye movement sleep deprivaiton in kittens amplifies LGN cell-size disparity induced by monocular deprivation. Devel Brain Res 1996; 97:51–61.

115. Siegel J. The REM sleep-memory consolidation hypothesis. Science 2001; 294:1058–63.

116. Crick F, Mitchison G. The function of dream sleep [Commentary]. Nature 1983; 304:111–114.

117. Sutherland G, McNaughton B. Curr Opin Neurobiol 2000; 10:180.

118. Pavlides C, Winson J. Influences of hippoxampal place cell firing in the awake state on the activity of these cells during subsequent sleep episodes. J Neurosci 1989; 9:2907–2918.

119. McGaugh J. Time-dependent processes in memory storage. Science 1966; 153:1351–1358.

120. Spieler D, Balota D. Psychol Aging 1996; 11:607.

121. Martasian P, Smith N, Neill S, Rieg T. Pscyhol Rep 1992; 70:339.

122. Rider R, Abdulahad D. Percept Mot Skills 1991; 73:219.

123. Gaarder K. A conceptual model of sleep. Arch Gen Psychiatry 1966; 14:253–260.

124. Feinberg I, Evarts E. Changing concepts of the function of sleep: discovery of intense brain activity during sleep calls for revision of hypotheses as to its function. Biol psychiatry 1969; 1:331–348.

125. Tulving E. Multiple memory systems and consciousness. Hum Neurobiol 1987; 6:67–80.

126. Stickgold R, James L, Hobson J. Visual discrimination learned requires sleep after training. Nat Neurosci 2000; 3:1237–1238.

127. Karni A, Tanne D, Rubenstein B. Dependence on REM sleep of overnight improvement of a perceptual skill. Science 1994; 265:679–682.

128. Smith C, Rose G. Behav Brain Sci 2000; 23:1007.

129. De Koninck J, Prevost F, Lorti-Lussler M. J Sleep Res 1996; 5:16.

130. Wagner U, Gais S, Born J. Learn Mem 2001; 8:112–119.

131. Smith C, Lapp L. Sleep 1991; 14:325–330.

132. Pilhal W, Born J. Effects of early and late nocturnal sleep on declarative and procedural memory. J Cogn Neurosci 1997; 9:534–547.

133. Smith C. Sleep states and memory processes. Behav Brain Res 1995; 69:137–145.

134. Giuditta A, Ambrosini M, MOntagnese P, et al. The sequential hypothesis of the function of sleep. Behav Brain Res 1995; 69:157–166.

135. Stickgold R, Whidbee D, Schirmer B, Patel V, Hobson J. Visual discrimination task improvement: a multi-step process occurring during sleep. J Cogn Neurosci 2000; 12:246–254.

136. Eichenbaum H. Declarative memory: insights from cognitive neurobiology. Annu Rev Psychol 1997; 48:547–572.

137. O'Keefe J, Burgess N, Donnett J. Place cells, navigational accuracy, and the human hippocampus. Philos Trans R Soc Lond B Biol Sci 1998; 353:1333–1340.

138. Clayton N, Dickinson A. Episodic-like memory during cache recovery by scrub jays. Nature 1998; 395:272–274.

139. Kandel ER, Pittenger C. The past, the future and the biology of memory storage. Philos Trans R Soc Lond B Biol Sci 1999; 354(1352):2027–2052.

140. VarghaKhadem F, Gadian D, Watkins K. Differential effects of early hippocampal pathlogy on episodic and semantic memory. Science 1997; 277:376–380.

141. Squire L, Knowlton B, Musen G. The structure and organization of memory. Annu Rev Psychol 1993; 44:453–495.

142. Gabrieli J. Cognitive neuroscience of human memory. Annu Rev Psychol 1998; 49:87–115.

143. Graybiel A. Building action repertoires: memory and learning functions of the basal ganglia. Curr Opin Neurobiol 1995; 5:733–741.

144. Doyon J, Laforce R, Bouchard J. Role of the striatum, cerebellum and frontal lobes in the automization of a repeated visuomotor sequence of movements. Neuropsychologia 1998; 36:625–641.

145. Morris J, Ohman A, Dolan R. Conscious and unconscious emotional learning in the human amygdala. Nature 1998; 393:467–470.

146. Wyatt R, Fram D, Kupfer D, Snyder F. Total prolonged drug-induced REM sleep suppression in anxious depressed patients. Arch Gen Psychiatry 1971; 24:145–155.

147. Vertes e. The case against memory consolidation in REM sleep. Behav Brain Sci 2000; 23:867–876.

148. Parent M, Habib M, Baker G. Task-dependent effects of the antidepressant/antipani drug phenelzine on memory. Psychopharmacology (Berl.) 1999; 142:280–288.

149. Georgotas A, Reisberg B, Ferris S. First results on the effects of MAO inhibition on cognitive functioning inelderly depressed patients. Arch Gerontol Geriatr 1983; 2:249–254.

150. Siegel J, Rogawski M. A function for REM sleep: regulation of noradrenergic receptor sensitivity. Brain Res Rev 1988; 13:213–233.

151. Poe G, Nitz D, McNaughton B, Barnes C. Experience dependent phase reversal of hiippocampal neuron firing during REM sleep. Brain Res 2000; 855:176–180.

152. Louie K, Wilson M. Temporally structured replay of awake hippocampal ensemble activity during rapid eye movement sleep. Neuron 2001; 29:145–156.

153. Datta S. Avoidance task training potentiates phasic pontine-wave density in the rat: A mechanism for sleep-dependent plasticity. J Neurosci 2000; 20:8607–8613.

154. Oniani T, Akhvlediani G. Influence of some monoamine oxidase inhibitors on the sleep-wakefulness cycle of the cat. Neurosci Behav Physiol 1988; 18:301–306.

155. Jouvet M. Research on the neural structures and responsible mechanisms in different phases of physiological sleep. Arch Ital Biol 1962; 100:125–206.

156. Izumi Y, Zorumski C. Norepinephrine promotes long-term potentiation in the adult rat hippocampus in vitro. Synapse 1999; 31:196–202.

157. Cirelli C, Tononi G. Gene expression in the brain across the sleep waking cycle. Brain Res 2000; 885:303–321.
158. Graves L, Pack A, Abel T. Sleep and memory: a molecular perspective. Trends Neurosci 2001; 24:237–243.
159. Kavanau J. Sleep and dynamic stabilization of neural circuitry: a reivew and synthesis. Behav Brain Res 1994; 63:111–126.
160. Benington J, Heller H. Restoration of Brain Energy Metabolism asthe Function of Sleep. Progr Neurobiology 1995; 45:347–360.
161. Mukhametov L, AL E. Interhemispheric asymmetry of hte electroencephalographic sleep patters in dolphins. Brain Res 1977; 134:581–584.
162. Oleksenko A, AL E. Unihemispheric sleep deprivation in bottlenose dolphins. J Sleep Res 1992; 1:40–44.
163. Kattler H, AL E. Effectof unilateral somatosensory stimulation proir to sleep on the sleep EEG in humans. J Sleep Res 1994; 3:159–164.
164. Drummond S, AL E. Sleep deprivation-induced reduction in cortical functional response to serial subtraction. Neuroreport 1999; 10:3745–3748.
165. Drummond S, Brown G, Gillin J, Stricker J, Wong E, Buxton R. Altered brain response to verbal learning following sleep deprivation. Nature 2000; 403:655–657.

2

History of Sleep Deprivation

WILLIAM C. DEMENT, CLETE A. KUSHIDA, AND JUDY CHANG
Stanford University, Stanford, California, U.S.A.

I. Introduction

Why do we sleep? What happens when we sleep? Do we need to sleep? People have pondered such questions about sleep since ancient times. Aristotle addressed the issue of sleep in his essay "On Sleep and Sleeplessness," in which he wrote that sleep and waking originate in the heart and are regulated by a primary sense organ. He proposed that after food is eaten, evaporation from it rises to the brain, condenses, and sinks down to the heart, causing sleep (1).

Even before Aristotle, it is likely that people realized there were consequences if they did not sleep. In ancient times such consequences may not have been labeled under the single word "sleepy." Over the years, we have learned that there are wide-ranging complaints about sleep loss and substantial individual differences. The symptoms of sleep loss may include tiredness, nausea, headache, burning eyes, blurred vision, joint pain, and diminished libido. Because of the general misery of these symptoms, it was an almost inevitable assumption that the purpose of sleep was to get rid of a hypnotoxin or fatigue product, which accumulated during wakefulness and, if allowed to continue accumulating, resulted in these symptoms.

Many people considered sleep to represent a total shutdown of brain function along with marked quiescence of the body; a state of near death. Carried to the extreme, sleep was viewed as a short death and death as a long sleep. The phenomenon of dreaming was sometimes conceptualized along these lines with the notion that some extracorporeal being or soul of the dreamer left the body temporarily at night and left the body permanently at death. There already was a large body of literature on the phenomenon of dreaming, elegantly reviewed by Freud in his influential book "The Interpretation of Dreams" (2), by the time of the first reported sleep deprivation experiment in the late 1800s.

II. Early Studies of Sleep Deprivation

Sleep research in general has a relatively short history in comparison with other areas of medicine (Table 1). Sleep deprivation has been the major approach in

Table 1   Major Milestones in Sleep Deprivation Research

Year	Milestone
1894	Marie De Manacéine showed that puppies and adult dogs died after a few days of sleep deprivation
1896	George Thomas White Patrick and J. Allen Gilbert conducted the first reported human experimental sleep deprivation study; subjects kept awake for 88–90 hr had impairments in reaction time, voluntary motor ability, and the ability to memorize
1898	Lamberto Daddi showed that the brains of totally sleep-deprived dogs had neuronal degeneration in their central nervous system
1898	Cesare Agostini, based on experiments with totally sleep-deprived dogs, concluded that total sleep deprivation induced a "progressive exhaustion of psychic activity."
1899	Giulio Tarozzi found that elimination of nitrous compounds increased late in the deprivation period of sleep-deprived dogs and was accompanied by hyperthermia
1909	Kuniomi Ishimori initiated the search for hypnogenic substances in the central nervous system
1910	René Legendre and Henri Piéron proposed the hypnotoxin theory
1927	Nathaniel Kleitman found only red blood cell count decrements and neuron abnormalities that were also detected in control littermates of totally sleep-deprived dogs
1953	Eugene Aserinsky and Nathaniel Kleitman described rapid-eye-movement (REM) sleep
1959	Investigators at the Walter Reed Army Institute of Research studying sleep-deprived enlisted men concluded that acute severe sleep loss consistently impairs performance
1959	Researchers from the University of Oklahoma monitored the prolonged wakefulness of New York disc jockey Peter Tripp
1960	William C. Dement conducted the first selective REM sleep deprivation experiment; REM sleep rebound was discovered.
1964	Randy Gardner, a 17–year-old high school senior, stayed awake for 264 hours
1976	Mary Carskadon and William C. Dement described the Multiple Sleep Latency Test (MSLT)
1989	Allan Rechtschaffen reported that sleep deprivation in rats is associated with death, increased energy expenditure, a debilitated appearance, impaired thermoregulation, and REM rebound

studies aimed at understanding the function of sleep. There were very few sleep researchers at the level of Henri Piéron, Frederick Bremer, and Walter Hess in the early years of the field. Nathaniel Kleitman (Fig. 1) was the first investigator to devote his entire career to the study of sleep.

Sleep deprivation research commenced by first keeping animals and people awake to see what would happen, and then inferring the function or functions of sleep from these deprivation periods. Bentivoglio and Grassi-Zucconi elegantly described this early research (3); the key studies described in their review are summarized below. In 1894, Marie De Manacéine (Fig. 2) showed that puppies and adult dogs deprived of sleep died after a few days and that the most severe lesions observed were found in the central nervous systems of these animals (4). In order to prevent sleep, the puppies and adult dogs were pulled about on leashes. Lamberto Daddi (5) in 1898 showed that the brains of three totally sleep-deprived dogs (one of which had also been starved) had neuronal degeneration in the spinal ganglia and cerebellar and cerebral cortices. However, Daddi concluded that these changes were not specific in light of comparisons with the effects of toxins or infectious agents. Cesare Agostini (Fig. 3) used a metal cage with bells to sleep deprive two dogs until their death at 12 and 17 days. He concluded in 1898 (6) that total sleep deprivation induced a "progressive exhaustion of psychic activity." Giulio Tarozzi (7) in 1899 investigated the metabolic effects of sleep deprivation in four sleep-deprived dogs (one of which was starved), and found that elimination of nitrous compounds increased late in the deprivation period and was accompanied by hyperthermia; the body temperature then declined prior to death.

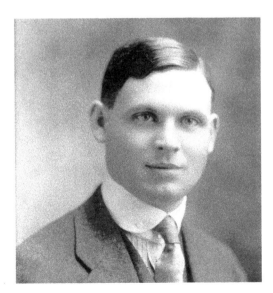

Figure 1   Nathaniel Kleitman.

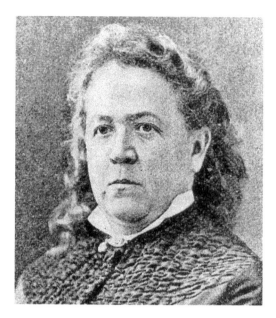

Figure 2 Marie De Manacéine.

Nathaniel Kleitman in 1927 kept puppies awake for 2–7 days by gentle stimulation and walking, and found only red blood cell count decrements and neuron abnormalities that were also detected in control littermates (8). Other sleep deprivation experiments in the 1920s in rabbits revealed central nervous sys-

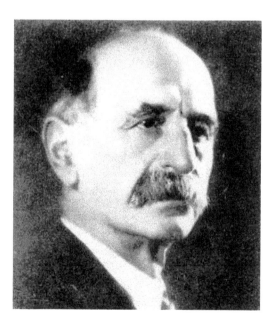

Figure 3 Cesare Agostini.

tem (CNS) abnormalities ranging from chromatolytic changes in neurons to actual lesions (9–11).

Some have questioned the results of these early studies because the method of sleep deprivation used to keep the animals continuously awake may have independently stressed or injured the animals. Since the animals must be forced to stay awake and maintaining wakefulness becomes progressively more difficult, adequate controls for the independent effects of the methodology are important.

Although there were several published case reports on the physical and psychological effects of sleep deprivation (6,12–14), George Thomas White Patrick and J. Allen Gilbert conducted the first reported human experimental sleep deprivation study in 1896. They kept three young subjects awake for 88–90 hr, during which time the subjects were administered a variety of physiological and psychological tests. As controls, the investigators used the performance of the same subjects on the day following the first sleep period that terminated the sleep deprivation. They found impairments in reaction time, voluntary motor ability, and ability to memorize. They also observed visual hallucinations in one subject and a gradual overall decrease in body temperature, although the circadian rhythm of the temperature curve was preserved. The subjects actually gained weight. They slept for 10.5–12 hr at the conclusion of the experiment and seemed to completely recover to their normal baseline upon awakening (15).

In 1909, Kuniomi Ishimori initiated the search for hypnogenic substances in the CNS (16). In 1910, following their observation that blood from sleep-deprived dogs caused sleep in normal dogs, René Legendre and Henri Piéron proposed the hypnotoxin theory (17). However, Kleitman observed in the 1920s that sleep-deprived subjects were less sleepy the next morning than during the middle of the sleep-deprived night (18). This suggested that either there were other influences that held the effects of hypnotoxin at bay in the morning or the steady buildup of hypnotoxin could not completely explain the waxing and waning nature of sleepiness. Kleitman also pointed out that in reaction time tests during prolonged wakefulness, the fastest reaction times did not change, suggesting that no hypnotoxic damage to the neural circuitry had occurred.

The so-called "germ warfare" confessions are purported to have been elicited from captives who underwent sleep deprivation torture during the Korean War. These reports initiated concerns that prolonged sleep loss could lead to mental breakdown in addition to physical deterioration. In 1959, Hal Williams, Artie Lubin, and Jacqueline Goodnow reported their studies of Army enlisted men at Walter Reed Army Institute of Research, concluding that acute severe sleep loss consistently impairs performance. They further concluded that the performance deficits were mainly due to lapses that they described as "brief periods of no response accompanied by extreme drowsiness and a decline in EEG alpha amplitude" (19). They did not observe unambiguous signs of psychosis either during or following the deprivation period.

In 1959, researchers from the University of Oklahoma monitored the prolonged wakefulness of a New York disc jockey, Peter Tripp (Fig. 4). He stayed

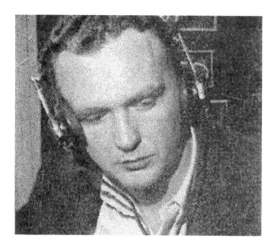

Figure 4 New York disc jockey Peter Tripp, who stayed awake for 201 hours in 1959.

awake for 201 hr to benefit the March of Dimes (20) and was observed the entire time. He was also given large doses of stimulants. "After a few days, he began to hallucinate, seeing kittens, mice and cobwebs. He also became paranoid, insisting that an electrician had dropped a hot electrode into his shoe" (21). It is unclear whether the paranoia and delusions were due to amphetamine psychosis, a pre-existing condition, or sleep deprivation.

At around this time, the *Guinness Book of World Records* stated that 260 hr was the record for staying awake, although the careful monitoring that would be necessary to verify continuous wakefulness had not been documented. In 1964, a 17-year-old high school senior named Randy Gardner decided to sleep deprive himself to study the effects of sleep loss as his high school science fair project. An important goal of his project was to break the world's record for sleep deprivation by staying awake for 264 hr (exactly 11 days). One of us (WCD) read about him in the newspaper and recognized that he presented a unique opportunity to observe very prolonged wakefulness and to be sure he was indeed continuously awake.

Aside from very brief periods of sleep, probably always less than a minute when he was "resting his eyes," Gardner stayed awake for 264 hours. At the end of his very prolonged period of wakefulness, Gardner held a press conference, handled many questions from reporters, and appeared to be quite unimpaired. He went to bed at the U.S Naval Hospital where his sleep was continuously monitored by means of electroencephalography (EEG), electrooculography (EOG), and electromyography (EMG) (22). His first recovery sleep, which lasted 14 hr and 40 min, was continuously recorded, and three additional nights—1 week, 6 weeks, and 10 weeks later—were also recorded. Given the state of our knowledge in 1964, quantifying the exact amount of extra sleep during recovery was unfortunately not considered important at the time. Over the years, there was occasional contact with Gardner to observe any ill effects; none was noted. Gardner visited Stanford in 1999 (Fig. 5). He appeared to be in excellent health, and once again no ill effects from the experience were noted. In marked contrast to Tripp, Gardner did not show any signs of psychosis (23).

III. Psychiatric Consequences of Selective REM Sleep Deprivation

In the past, the methods utilized to study human sleep were relatively crude. The first real departure from earlier approaches began with the electrooculographic observations of the occurrence of rapid, binocularly synchronous eye movements during sleep reported by Eugene Aserinsky and Nathaniel Kleitman in 1953 (24). Continuous all-night recording of EEG, EOG, and EMG potentials soon became the standard, and initiated the so-called "modern era of sleep research." Studies during the ensuing years both at the University of Chicago and in Lyons, France firmly established that there are two distinct organismic states of sleep: non-REM (NREM) sleep with slow waves and spindles and rapid-eye-movement (REM) sleep in which rapid eye movements are ineluctably associated with low-amplitude, high-frequency EEG and absence of EMG potentials. Both states occur as part of a very regular and stable sleep cycle in both humans and animals (25–27).

With the dominance of psychoanalytic thinking at this time, the universality of REM periods, and the link between REM sleep and dreaming, it was hypothesized that REM sleep was a kind of safety valve of the mind and REM sleep deprivation would lead to psychosis. William C. Dement (Fig. 6) performed the first selective REM sleep deprivation experiment in 1960. He found that REM sleep

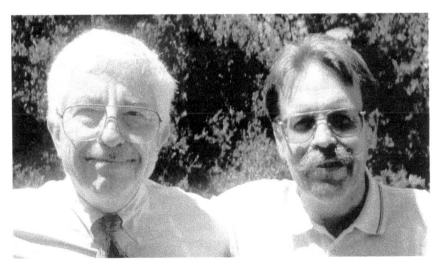

Figure 5 Randy Gardner, the 17–year-old high school student who stayed awake for 264 hours in 1964. (Photograph was taken with Dr. William C. Dement in 1999.)

deprivation is associated with more frequent attempts to enter into REM sleep, that the percentage of REM sleep rebounds after deprivation, and that psychological disturbances occur. These include anxiety, irritability, and difficulties in concentration. Dement concluded: "It is possible that if the dream suppression were carried on long enough, a serious disruption of the personality would result" (28).

Tripp's experience and these early observations triggered a long series of additional selective "REM sleep deprivation" studies during the 1960s in cats,

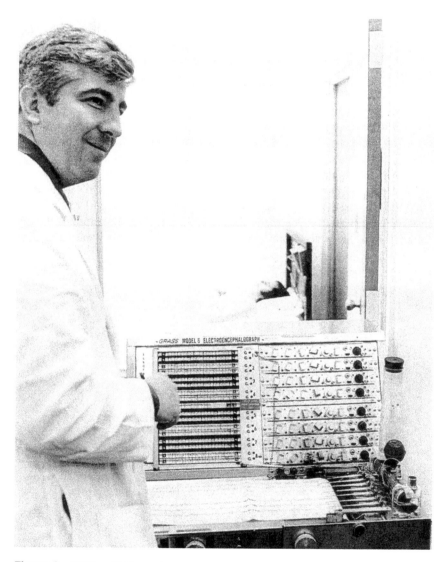

Figure 6   William C. Dement.

rats, and mice, as well as humans (29). An absolutely vital function for REM sleep was not revealed, although it was demonstrated that REM sleep had independent homeostatic regulation with a markedly increasing frequency of REM onsets during deprivation and robust REM rebounds during recovery. No negative changes suggesting the development of psychosis were observed in humans or animals. On the other hand, various brain excitability and behavioral changes were reported (29–31). Finally, Gerald Vogel reviewed the literature in 1975 and concluded REM sleep deprivation is relatively harmless to schizophrenic, depressed, and healthy people, and suggested it might actually improve depression (32).

IV. Sleep Loss and Daytime Sleepiness

Some of the early researchers conducting partial sleep deprivation studies included M. Smith (33), D. A. Laird (34), G. L. Freeman (35), Laverne Johnson (22), and Wilse Webb (36). Partial sleep deprivation involves both REM and NREM sleep deprivation, and may disproportionately deprive humans or animals of REM sleep. Amazingly, the issue that sleep loss results in daytime sleepiness was largely ignored during all these years. This important issue was finally brought to center stage by clinicians because sleepiness is such a prominent symptom of several sleep disorders.

The Multiple Sleep Latency Test (MSLT) was first described in 1975 by Mary Carskadon and William C. Dement, as an objective measure of sleep loss. They sleep deprived six normal college students and every 2 hr provided 20-min opportunities for the students to fall asleep. They found that sleep latency was markedly shortened with sleep deprivation and that it returned to baseline levels after the second recovery night (37). Gary Richardson and colleagues later validated (1978) the MSLT as a method to demonstrate pathological sleepiness (38).

Around this time, sleep researchers began to recognize the consequences of daytime sleepiness on safety and productivity. Investigators realized that the symptom of the drive to sleep, i.e., sleepiness, has its own significance. Sleepiness can be compared to thirst. Thirst in and of itself is neither dangerous nor damaging; it is the dehydration, of which thirst is a symptom, that is important. Given a valid objective method for the study of the nocturnal determinants of daytime sleepiness, investigators began to explore the connection between partial sleep loss and daytime sleepiness and other behavioral impairments, independent of searching for a vital function or functions of sleep.

V. The Function(s) of Sleep

We will briefly review selected theories of the function(s) of sleep that have received attention in the past but have not received conclusive exploration. These theories are still relevant today.

A. Body Restitution Hypothesis

In 1969, Ian Oswald proposed the body restitution hypothesis, postulating that "REM sleep rebound may indicate increased protein synthesis in the brain." He believed that brain repair occurs during REM sleep and that NREM sleep exists for bodily restitution (39). Kristin Adam concurred with Oswald's theory citing the observation that "rates of protein synthesis or of mitotic division are higher during the time of rest and sleep" as evidence for restitution (40). In 1978, Jim Horne reviewed the biological effects of total sleep deprivation in humans and discounted the body restitution hypothesis. However, he proposed a CNS or cerebral restitutional role for human sleep (41). In 1985, Horne revisited the effects of total sleep deprivation in humans again and concluded that it results in impaired homeostatic control, especially thermoregulation, which is significant in small mammals but has a minor role in humans. He proposed that only a certain portion of a night's sleep is essential to the brain, with the remainder being optional (42).

Ray Meddis also disagreed with the restitution hypothesis, proposing instead the immobilization theory, i.e., sleep keeps the sleeper out of harm's way, in 1975. He wrote that sleep "does not supply any unique physiological benefit. The major benefits gained from sleeping would then accrue only indirectly through the advantages of increasing the efficiency of rest-activity cycles" (43). As evidence for his theory, he cited several short sleepers reported by H. S. Jones and Ian Oswald in 1968 (44) as well as several others he identified who claimed to need only 15 min of sleep per day.

The most extreme short sleepers were described by Meddis. One of us (WCD) journeyed to London and met two of these individuals in the middle of the night when they seemed to be wide awake and fully alert. However, a stringent set of observations that would prove this very short sleep requirement beyond the shadow of a doubt was not performed. Most sleep researchers have a somewhat cynical attitude about people who claim they almost never sleep, or sleep a very short time (1 or 2 hr). The claims are usually unverifiable or prove to be false or exaggerated. Nonetheless, this is an area that has not been thoroughly investigated.

Noteworthy is the report of Jones and Oswald that describes people who slept fewer than 3 hr a night. In contrast to Meddis, for the Jones and Oswald subjects all-night EEGs were obtained for at least seven consecutive nights. They tended to be very busy people who were not particularly disturbed by their sleeping habits. They were quite productive with the extra time they had and did not seem to suffer any deleterious consequences of their diminished sleep times. Meddis interpreted this as evidence against the restitution theory of sleep (45). However, comprehensive testing of daytime functioning was not performed, so it is not known if there was a negative impact on daytime functioning. Therefore, if other short sleepers are encountered, every effort should be made to perform a thorough assessment of daytime functioning in the context of a number of consecutive 24-hr days of continuous monitoring.

B. Vital Physiological Function

Different researchers have discovered that total sleep deprivation is associated with death, raising the question of whether sleep fulfills a critical function necessary to sustain life. Walle J. H. Nauta reported that in rats hypothalamic lesions rostral to the mammillary bodies induced sleeplessness. Of note, the sleepless rats died (46).

Allan Rechtschaffen (Fig. 7) surmised that sleep serves a vital physiological function, based on his prodigious program of experiments on chronic sleep deprivation in rats (47). *However, if we assume that sleep has a vital function or functions, can we also assume that these function(s) are the same across species?*

In 1985, James Krueger hypothesized that "sleep acting through the immune system aids in the recovery from pathological states and from environmental challenges normally encountered in daily waking activity" (48). In 1989, Ruth Benca and her colleagues disagreed with the idea that sleep deprivation results in immunosuppression. Their conclusions were based on immune function studies on splenic lymphocytes obtained from sleep-deprived rats (49). In 1989 and 2002, Rechtschaffen reviewed the effects of total sleep deprivation in rats and concluded that it caused impaired thermoregulation, REM rebound, and increased energy expenditure with the rats also becoming scrawny and debilitated (50). If sleep deprivation is continued, the consistent final outcome is death. However, the cause of death has been debated, with Carol Everson proposing that total sleep deprivation induces failure of host defense via a hyper-catabolic state and secondary malnutrition. She concluded that death resulted from "breakdown of host defense against indigenous and pathogenic microorganisms" (51). In contrast, Bernard Bergmann and colleagues have argued that the physiological effects of sleep deprivation are not mediated by bacterial invasion (52).

C. Homeostatic Model (See Chap. 24)

In the 1960s, H. D. Ephron and Patricia Carrington speculated that homeostasis exists between REM and NREM sleep, with a decrease in cerebral vigilance occurring during NREM sleep, which is then countered by cortical activation during REM sleep (53). Joel Benington (54) agreed with these investigators, contending that "REM sleep may be homeostatically regulated in relation to prior NREM sleep rather than prior waking." This means that REM sleep deprivation could have more important consequences for NREM sleep than for the waking state.

D. Learning and Memory (see Chapter 12) (See Chap. 11)

Several researchers have proposed a learning and memory function for REM sleep, including Giuseppe Moruzzi and E. M. Dewan. Moruzzi suggested that

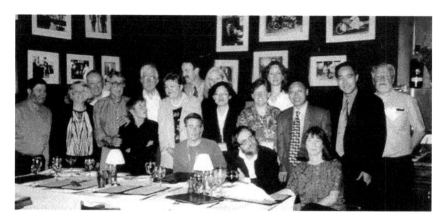

Figure 7a Allan Rechtschaffen with some members of his research team, family, and colleagues. (Photograph was taken at the Associated Professional Sleep Societies Meeting in Chicago, Illinois in June 2001.)

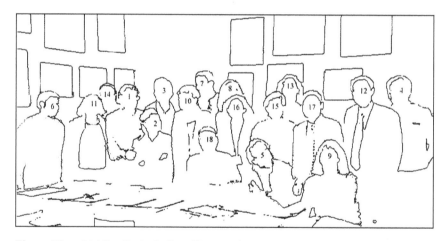

Figure 7b (1) Allan Rechtshaffen, (2) Karen Rechtschaffen, (3) William C. Dement, (4) James Horne, (5) Bernard M. Bergmann, (6) John Metz, (7) Donald Bliwise, (8) Jacqueline Winter, (9) Charmane Eastman, (10) Kristyna Hartse, (11) Marcia Gilliland, (12) Clete A. Kushida, (13) Carol A. Everson, (14) William Obermeyer, (15) June Pilcher, (16) Ling-Ling Tsai, (17) Pingfu Feng, (18) Paul Shaw

sleep is involved in recovery from plastic activities associated with learning and conditioning (55). Dewan created the programming hypothesis in which he drew an analogy between the brain and a computer, and suggested that REM sleep is involved in programming the brain (56). Gerald Vogel (32) and Ira Albert (57) independently reviewed the behavioral effects of REM sleep deprivation and concluded that it increases central neural excitability and motivational behavior but has unclear or inconclusive effects on learning.

E. Central Nervous System Development

Given the inconclusive results of selective REM sleep deprivation and the large percentage of REM sleep seen in both newborn human infants and other infant mammals, Roffwarg and colleagues (58) proposed that REM sleep provides crucial stimulation for brain activity in the fetus and newborn. They marshaled evidence supporting the general role of stimulation for optimal CNS development. Nearly four decades has passed and the issue remains inconclusive because selectively eliminating REM sleep in newborns is extremely difficult.

VI. Confounds of Experimental Methodology

It is possible that the changes reported in sleep deprivation experiments are confounded by disruption of circadian rhythm and stress, rather than being solely due to sleep deprivation. Rechtschaffen controlled for circadian rhythm effects by repeating the basic total sleep deprivation disk-over-water experiment under 12:12 light/dark conditions, and he obtained the same results in this control study as in his original experiments. He controlled for the physical stress of the deprivation technique by equally subjecting the yoked control rats to the same degree of disk rotation in the deprivation apparatus. Separate control rats were subjected to food deprivation and the same degree of water exposure as the experimental rats in the deprivation apparatus; however, none of these control rats exhibited the changes observed in the sleep-deprived rats. In order to evaluate the possibility that the observed changes were due to stress responses rather than due to sleep deprivation, Rechtschaffen also examined "stress" indicators observed by other researchers, such as stomach ulcers, adrenal hypertrophy, and elevated adrenocorticotropic hormone and corticosteroids. However, none of these indicators explained the proximal cause of death in these rats (50).

VII. Conclusions

Despite all the sleep deprivation studies that have been performed, the function of sleep remains elusive. As Rechtschaffen wrote: "The effects of sleep deprivation alone will not tell us the function of sleep" and "a simple deficit equals function equation is sadly naïve" (50). Even so, sleep deprivation is the best available method to study the function of sleep. Questions that remain to be answered include why there are two totally different kinds of sleep, why these two kinds of sleep alternate rhythmically, why their homeostatic regulation is independent, and whether they have completely different functions.

References

1. Aristotle. 1994–2000, On sleep and sleeplessness. In: Stevenson, DC, ed. The Internet Classics Archive [Online]. Available: http://classics.mit.edu/Aristotle/sleep.1b.txt [Accessed 10 Dec. 02].
2. Freud S. The Interpretation of Dreams. New York: Basic Books, 1955.
3. Bentivoglio M, Grassi-Zucconi G. The pioneering experimental studies on sleep deprivation. Sleep 1997; 20(7):570–576.
4. De Manacéine M. Quelques observations expérimentales sur l'influence de l'insomnie absolue. Arch Ital Biol 1894; 21:322–325.
5. Daddi L. Sulle alterazioni degli elementi del sistema nervoso centrale nell'insonnia sperimentale. Rivista di Patologia Nervosa e Mentale 1898; 3:1–12.
6. Agostini C. Sui disturbi psichici e sulle alterazioni del sistema nervoso centrale per insomnia assoluta. Rivista Sperimentale di Freniatria 1898; 24:113–125.
7. Tarozzi G. Sull'influenza dell'insonnio sperimentale sul ricambio materiale. Rivista di Patologia Nervosa e Mentale 1899; 4:1–23.
8. Kleitman N. Studies on the physiology of sleep. V. Some experiments on puppies. Am J Physiol 1927; 84:386–395.
9. Crile GW. Studies on exhaustion. Arch Surg 1921; 2:196–220.
10. Bast TH, Schacht F, Vanderkamp H. Studies in experimental exhaustion due to lack of sleep. III. Effect on the nerve cells of the spinal cord. Am J Physiol 1927; 82:131–139.
11. Bast TH, Bloemendal WB. Studies in experimental exhaustion due to lack of sleep. IV. Effect on the nerve cells in the medulla. Am J Physiol 1927; 82:140–146.
12. Renaudin E. Observations sur l'influence pathogénique de l'insomnie. Ann Méd Psych 1857; 3:384–397.
13. Hammond W. On sleep and insomnia. NY Med J 1865; 1:89–101.
14. Baillarger M. Des hallucinations psycho-sensorielles. Ann Méd Psych 1846; 7:1–12.
15. Patrick GTW, Gilbert JA. On the effects of loss of sleep. Psychol Rev 1896; 3:469–483.
16. Ishimori K. True cause of sleep: a hypnogenic substance as evidenced in the brain of sleep-deprived animals. Tokyo Igakkai Zasshi 1909; 23:429–457.
17. Legendre R, Pieron H. Le probleme des facteurs du sommeil. Resultats d'injections vasculaires et intra-cerebrales de liquids insomniques. Compt Rend de la Soc de Biol 1910; 68:1077–1079.
18. Kleitman N. Deprivation of sleep. In: Kleitman N, ed. Sleep and Wakefulness. Chicago: University of Chicago Press, 1963:215–229.
19. Williams HL, Lubin A, Goodnow JJ. Impaired performance in acute sleep loss. Psychol Monographs: General and Applied 1959; 73:1–26.
20. Man From Mars Productions: Peter Tripp Marathon [Online], 2002. Available: http://manfrommars.com/tripp.html [Accessed 15 Dec. 2002].
21. Sleep Deprivation: It's More than Dark Circles Under the Eyes [Online]. Available: http://www.pbs.org/livelyhood/nightshift/sleep_deprivation.html [Accessed 15 Dec. 2002].
22. Johnson LC, Slye ES, Dement W. Electroencephalographic and autonomic activity during and after prolonged sleep deprivation. Psychosomatic Med 1965; 27:415–423.
23. Gulevich G, Dement W, Johnson L. Psychiatric and EEG observations on a case of prolonged (264 hours) wakefulness. Arch Gen Psychiatry 1966; 15:29–35.

24. Aserinsky E, Kleitman N. Regularly occurring periods of eye motility, and concomitant phenomena, during sleep. Science 1953; 118:273–274.
25. Dement W, Kleitman N. Cyclic variations in EEG during sleep and their relation to eye movements, body motility, and dreaming. Electroencphalogr Clin Neurophysiol 1957; 9:673–690.
26. Dement W. The occurrence of low voltage, fast electroencephalogram patterns during behavioral sleep in the cat. Electroencphalogr Clin Neurophysiol 1958; 10:291–296.
27. Jouvet M. Paradoxical sleep—a study of its nature and mechanisms. Prog Brain Res 1965; 18.
28. Dement W. The effect of dream deprivation. Science 1960; 131:1705–1707.
29. Dement W, Henry P, Cohen H, Ferguson J. Studies on the effect of REM deprivation in humans and in animals. In: Kety S, Evarts E, Williams H, eds. Sleep and Altered States of Consciousness. Baltimore: Williams and Wilkins, 1967:456–468.
30. Dewson J, Dement W, Wagener T, Nobel K. Rapid eye movement sleep deprivation: a central-neural change during wakefulness. Science 1967; 156:403–406.
31. Cohen H, Duncan R, Dement W. Sleep: the effects of electroconvulsive shock in cats deprived of REM sleep. Science 1967; 156:1646–1648.
32. Vogel GW. A review of REM sleep deprivation. Arch Gen Psychiatry 1975; 32:749–761.)
33. Smith M. A contribution to the study of fatigue. Br J Psychol 1916; 8:327–50.
34. Laird DA. Effects of loss of sleep on mental work. Indust Psychol 1926; 1:427–428.
35. Freeman GL. Compensatory reinforcements of muscular tension subsequent to sleep loss. J Exp Pyschol 1932; 15:267–283.
36. Webb WB. Partial and differential sleep deprivation. In: Kales A, ed.. Sleep: Pathology and Physiology. Philadelphia: Lippincott, 1969:221–230.
37. Carskadon M, Dement W. Sleep tendency: an objective measure of sleep loss. Electroenceph Clin Neurophysiol 1975; 39:145–155.
38. Richardson GS, Carskadon MA, Flagg W, Van den Hoed J, Dement WC, Mitler MM. Excessive daytime sleepiness in man: multiple sleep latency measurement in narcoleptic and control subjects. Electroencephalogr Clin Neurophysiol 1978; 45(5):621–627.
39. Oswald I. Human brain protein, drugs and dreams. Nature 1969; 223:893–897.
40. Adam K. Sleep as a restorative process and a theory to explain why. Progr Brain Res 1980; 53:289–306.
41. Horne JA. A review of the biological effects of total sleep deprivation in man. Biol Psychol 1978; 7:55–102.
42. Horne JA. Sleep function, with particular reference to sleep deprivation. Ann Clin Res 1985; 17:199–208.
43. Meddis R. On the function of sleep. Anim Behav 1975; 23:676–691.
44. Jones HS, Oswald I. Two cases of healthy insomnia. Electroenceph clin Neurophysiol 1968; 24:378–80.
45. Meddis R. Very short sleepers. In: Meddis R. The Sleep Instinct. Boston: Routledge & Kegan Paul, 1977:31–52.
46. Nauta WJH. Hypothalamic regulation of sleep in rats. An experimental study. J Neurophysiol 1946; 9:285–316.
47. Rechtschaffen A, Gilliland MA, Bergmann BM, Winter JB. Physiological correlates of prolonged sleep deprivation in rats. Science 1983; 221:182–184.

48. Krueger J, Walter J, Levin C. In: McGinty DJ, Drucker-Colin R, Morrison A, Parmeggiani L, eds. Brain Mechanisms of Sleep. New York: Raven Press, 1985:253–275.
49. Benca RM, Kushida CA, Everson CA, Kalski R, Bergmann BM, Rechtschaffen A. Sleep deprivation in the rat: VII. Immune function. Sleep 1989; 12(1):47–52.
50. Rechtschaffen A, Bergmann BM. Sleep deprivation in the rat: an update of the 1989 paper. Sleep 2002; 25:18–24.
51. Everson CA. Sustained sleep deprivation impairs host defense. Am J Physiol 1993; 265:R1148–R1154.
52. Bergmann BM, Gilliland MA, Feng PF, Russell DR, Shaw P, Wright M, Rechtschaffen A, Alverdy JC. Are physiological effects of sleep deprivation in the rat mediated by bacterial invasion? Sleep 1996; 19(7):554–562.
53. Ephron HS, Carrington P. Rapid eye movement sleep and cortical homeostasis. Psychol Rev 1966; 73:500–526.
54. Benington JH, Heller HC. Implications of sleep deprivation experiments for our understanding of sleep homeostasis. Sleep 1999; 22(8):1033–1037.
55. Moruzzi G. The functional significance of sleep with particular regard to the brain mechanisms underlying consciousness. In: Eccles JC, ed. Brain and Conscious Experience. Berlin: Springer-Verlag, 1966:345–388.
56. Dewan EM. The programming (P) hypothesis for REM sleep. Int Psychiatry Clin 1970; 7(2):295–307.
57. Albert IB. REM sleep deprivation. Biol Psychiatry 1975; 10(3):341–351.
58. Roffwarg H, Muzio J, Dement W. Ontogenetic development of the human sleep–dream cycle. Science 1966; 152:604–619.

3

Animal Models of Sleep Deprivation

JOAN C. HENDRICKS

4041 Ryan Veterinary Hospital of the University of Pennsylvania, Philadelphia, Pennsylvania, U.S.A.

I. Introduction

In studies of any complex behavior the choice of model system influences the results and their interpretation. Generally, of course, the major interest of the human experimenter is to shed light on humans. The shortest route to this goal would seem to be either to study humans themselves or, to take advantage of the ease of manipulating and controlling experimental variables, to study animals that closely resemble humans. The findings in such animals would intuitively seem to be more directly relevant to humans than studies of organisms that are not as obviously close to us. It would be common sense to expect results from studying closely related mammals to lead more quickly to clinical application than studies of animals that are evolutionarily remote from humans (e.g., invertebrates such as flies and worms). However, historically, pragmatic issues such as ease and cost of obtaining and maintaining animals have often dictated that simpler animals be used. Furthermore, in order to reduce the complexity of the system, some fields have sacrificed resemblance to humans and have used reduced preparations, ranging from anesthetized or decerebrate mammals to slice preparations and the study of cells in culture. As an example, it is obviously impossible to assert that a small group of cells or a brain slice learns and remembers in a fashion that strictly resembles the process that occurs in a human learner. Nonetheless, the field of learning and memory has long accepted the limits of such systems. For example, they have drawn cautious parallels between the electrophysiological phenomenon of long-term potentiation in brain slices or simple reflex behaviors in the sea slug *Aplysia* and the process of human learning and memory (1,2).

Interestingly, the field of sleep research has been particularly late to accept reduced or "simple" models to study sleep. Not only is sleep nearly always studied in whole animals, but the use of anesthesia and even of restraint has been eschewed. My personal speculation is that this is in part because of the enormous interest occasioned by the discovery that rapid-eye-movement (REM) sleep was associated with dream mentation in humans. Thus, until recently, sleep studies were conducted almost entirely in intact mammals and birds, in whom the behavioral and electrophysiological (electroencephalographic, EEG) manifestations of two distinct REM and non-REM (NREM) stages of sleep are present, although features of sleep have long been identified in other species (3). In addition to relevance and economics, the interests and orientation of the investigators have influenced the choice of models. As detailed further below, an overview of the models mentioned in studies of sleep deprivation suggest a shift away from larger vertebrates toward smaller vertebrates, especially mice, as well as the emergence of interest in simpler models. Recent influences beyond relevance and economics have begun to shift the choice of models used to study sleep, as by other students of complex behavior. These and possible future models are reviewed briefly. Lastly, some difficult methodological and interpretive issues that are raised in considering sleep deprivation in different models are discussed.

II. Historical Overview: What Models Have Been Used to Study Sleep Deprivation?

To get a general sense of the use of the animal models used to study sleep deprivation we queried the Medline database in September 2003 for individual species of laboratory animals and "sleep deprivation." This method will not of course detect studies not included in Medline, such as those prior to the mid-1960s or in journals not included in the database. Furthermore, if no species is mentioned we would not identify the publication, and we do not account for the possibility that multiple species might be used in a single publication. Nonetheless, some trends are suggested by the results shown in Table 1. There were 3947 total publications identified in a search for "sleep deprivation;" this is 7.3% of the total of 53,782 publications found on "sleep." For both "sleep" and "sleep deprivation" searches, approximately 20% of the references were published in this millennium (2000 and later). Since sleep deprivation is a relatively innocuous procedure and, as mentioned above, the focus on humans is a rather natural tendency for humans who do research, it should not be surprising that 76% of sleep deprivation reports involved humans. Together with humans, seven other species were mentioned in 94% of the studies. The largest number of nonhuman studies was in rats, followed by mice. Together rodents accounted for almost 15% of all sleep deprivation pub-

Table 1 Results of a Series of Searches of the Medline Publications Database.

Search keywords	Total no. references (% of all sleep deprivation studies)	Published ≥ 2000 (% of total)
sleep	53,782	9729 (18)
sleep deprivation	3,947	785 (20)
"and human	3,012 (76% of sleep deprivation studies)	604 (20)
"and primate or monkey	10 (0.3%)	1 (10)
"and mouse or mice	133 (4.4%)	52 (39)
"and rabbit	11 (0.4%)	0 (0)
"and feline or cat	44 (1.4%)	5 (11)
"and canine or dog	9 (0.3%)	3 (33)
"and hamster	13 (0.4%)	4 (13)

See text for further information.

lications. Other mammals accounted for only approximately 4% of all sleep deprivation studies. Furthermore, by looking at the proportion of studies conducted more recently (2000 to present), it is apparent that there has been a trend toward mice and away from nonhuman primates, cats, and rabbits in studies of sleep deprivation. The use of rats has remained steady: as for sleep deprivation studies in general, the proportion of publications using rats since 2000 is 20%. Both dogs and hamsters, while relatively rarely studied overall (totaling less than 1% of all studies between them), have also shown a proportional increase since 2000 (more than 30% of the studies have been conducted in 2000 or later). The possible reasons for these apparent shifts are discussed further below.

III. Influences on the Use of Higher Vertebrates for Sleep Research

In recent decades two emerging forces have shaped the choice of animal models for neuroscience generally, and sleep research is no exception. One is the great advance in sequencing the genomes of multiple species, and the other is the set of regulatory and financial burdens imposed by the upsurge in public interest in animal welfare.

(1) As more genomes have been sequenced, the data have indicated that, whereas an enormous array of phenotypic manifestations of genes produce the wild proliferation of fauna that populate the earth, at the level of the molecular gene sequencing remarkable conservation is found even between such widely divergent species as flies and people (4). Together with the ease of conducting genetic studies in smaller laboratory models such as invertebrates, these studies have provided a great impetus for studying simpler models. Convincing parallels in molecular mechanisms have been established, such as in learning and memory

and circadian rhythms [reviewed in (5)]. Thus, the historical importance of studying species whose anatomy and behavior resembles that of the human is now counterbalanced by evidence that genetic mechanisms are often well conserved among animals that are not superficially similar.

(2) The animal rights movement and the acceptance by major federal funding bodies of many regulations to ensure humane and appropriate attention to animal welfare in the conduct of research has undoubtedly affected the choice of animals used in research [for a thoughtful review and commentary, see (6)]. Many if not most researchers are content to ensure the well-being of their subjects and even to fill out the paperwork necessary to document this care. However, another (not necessarily unintended) consequence has also been to dramatically increase the cost and time delays involved in studying mammals and thus to prompt researchers to think about avoiding these burdens. The psychological burden of performing research that is routinely attacked is impossible to quantify, but subjectively it seems that this is a very real deterrent to the use of large vertebrate species in research.

Perhaps in part because of both of these forces, recent efforts to identify a sleeplike state in *Drosophila melanogaster* in order to take advantage of the advances in genomics have prompted a reevaluation of the traditional exclusion of nonmammalian species for sleep studies. Although the use of *Drosophila* is relatively recent, it appears that the fly is already demonstrating conservation of molecular mechanisms. As in other fields, the hope is that such models will be very useful in refining the use of mammalian models (5,7,8), directing attention at molecular pathways that have already been shown to be important in simpler animals. Although, as for any complex behavior, the full array of behavioral and physiological manifestations seen in humans is present in only a fragmentary form in invertebrates and older vertebrate phyla such as reptiles, it now appears that even such incomplete forms may have shared molecular underpinnings. Thus, the choices available for studies of the effects of sleep deprivation have been broadened, and it is now possible to conceive of a future in which even slices and cells might be useful in the effort to understand sleep mechanisms.

IV. Cost-Benefit Analysis: Choosing a Model

A speculative summary of the costs and benefits of selected models for sleep research is presented in Table 2. Literally, some animals cost more than others to obtain, house, and study. As a reference, compensation for normal human subjects is about $200/day at the University of Pennsylvania. Per-diem costs to house vertebrates commonly used for sleep studies range from $1 for rats and mice to $5-10/day for cats and dogs. The cost for housing a nonhuman primate is almost $10/day. In addition to these direct housing costs, genetically modified mice or specific strains of rats (e.g., Zucker rats) are valuable scientific resources. Furthermore, to maintain the health and psychological well-being of complex

Table 2 A Speculative View of the Utility of Established, New, and Possible Future Animal Models to Study Particular Aspects of Sleep[a]

History of use in sleep research	Model (approximate per diem cost)	Area where model has been/could be useful						
		Pathophysiology	Pharmacology	Neuroanatomy	Neurophysiology	Natural gene variation and genetic diseases	Gene alterations: mutants, transgenics	CR and sleep
20th century	Human ($200)	+++	+++	++	++	+++		++
	Nonhuman primates ($10)	++		++	++			++
	Dogs ($10)					++		
	Cats ($5)		++		++			
	Rats ($1)		++		++			
	Mice ($1)					++	+++	++
21st century	Zebrafish		+	?	?		+++	++
	Drosophila		+	?	?		+++	++
	Honeybees			?	+	Sociogenomics?		?
Future?	*C. elegans*			?	?			
	Large insects: locust, cockroach			?	?			

[a]The literal "cost" for humans who are compensated for each day of volunteering and for housing experimental animals are approximate costs at the University of Pennsylvania in 2003. Invertebrates and zebrafish are not housed within lab animal facilities and thus there is no specific cost for their housing, although labor and supplies are involved; in addition, as noted, the maintenance of honeybees requires special care and precautions. The number of plus (+) signs for each area of study is intended to reflect the author's view of how useful this model has been to date, where the possibility of a contribution is only speculative. This ranges from a proven and extensive contribution (+++) to the speculation that a contribution could be made in the future (+ or ?).

animals such as nonhuman primates and dogs dramatically increases labor costs in maintaining the animals. If they are genetic models of human diseases, there may also be additional costs related to maintaining the health and reproductive status of individual animals. There are also scientific costs to studying animals that are difficult or expensive to obtain. Animals that are difficult to obtain and maintain will be used sparingly and judiciously to maximize the scientific gain from studying each individual. As a personal example, the largest number of animals I ever used in a study of the English bulldog was eight individuals (9), and no animals were ever sacrificed in those studies. This obviously limits the kinds of questions that can be asked and answered. Even in healthy mammals, studies can be long and labor intensive. The duration of studies of reproduction, maturity, or aging is necessarily long in animals whose development and aging takes months and years, respectively. Sample size may also be reduced because of animal welfare concerns, time, and expense. That is, to maximize the use and statistical validity of valuable animals that are laboriously instrumented, each individual is extensively studied but the ability to survey large numbers or populations is forfeited. By contrast, either small vertebrates (zebrafish) or invertebrates (flies, worms) are inexpensive to maintain, short lived, and rapidly reproducing. These animals are routinely maintained easily in the lab, and the delays inherent in regulatory oversight are minimal. Some invertebrate models that might be very valuable are nonetheless difficult to obtain (*Aplysia*) or to house (honeybees).

V. Use of Mammalian Models

The use of lab animal models throughout history seems to reflect not only changing attitudes toward the use of animals in research (and thus their costs) but also species-specific scientific advantages. As noted above, the relevance to humans is the most obvious benefit for the larger vertebrates, especially primates. In examining the data shown in Table 1, it is obvious that primate studies have always been unusual, and are decreasing rather than increasing (only one study since 2000). This suggests that the costs as described above outweigh the benefit of relevance to humans. The primate studies focus largely on endocrinology. The one recent study examined hypocretin (10), identified as important for narcolepsy (11,12).

Similarly, whereas cats were the most commonly used model for many pioneering studies of sleep, only 3 of the 41 studies found in a search using the key words "cats and sleep deprivation" were conducted after 2000. The use of rodents is increasing. Rats, whose use remains steady, have been used to study almost every facet of sleep, including neuroanatomy, neurophysiology, neurochemistry, interactions with learning, and gene expression (13–16). To a limited extent, abnormal rats (e.g., the Zucker rat) have also served as models of human disease. The utility of mice for studying genetic features has long been obvious, but the ease of instrumenting larger animals to obtain the electroencephalogram has certainly led to a preference for the use of rats.

Mice were early used to study pharmacology, infectious diseases, and the interaction of circadian rhythms with sleep need. In 1997, a mouse knockout was first used to study sleep, when mice lacking prion were studied and found to have abnormal recovery from sleep deprivation (17,18). With their increasing use in investigating the genetic basis of disease and behavior, mice are likely to soon rival rats, despite the challenge of surgically instrumenting these small animals. The discovery of narcolepsy in mouse hypocretin/orexin knockouts has helped to impress the relevance of the mouse knockout model on the sleep community (11). Use of the ob/ob mouse to study the role of leptin in sleep seems likely to increase, with its relevance to sleep apnea and obesity and sleep (19). Of course, specific molecular hypotheses can be studied in mice, as the cyclic adenosine monophosphate (cAMP) response element-binding protein (CREB) has been (20). A disadvantage for mice is the relative paucity of normative data about sleep. This is being remedied with careful studies of strain differences in sleep patterns and regulation (21, 22).

A useful feature of mice is that exercise and wheel running has been extensively studied, so that the interaction of circadian activity and locomotion with sleep is relatively readily investigated (23–26). The availability of mouse mutants in the central clock (clock mouse, BMAL, period mutant mice) has also begun to foster a field examining the role of the clock in regulating the quality and propensity for sleep, in addition to the obvious role for the clock in timing the onset of sleep bouts (27–29). Sophisticated studies to test specific mechanistic theories of sleep physiology can be designed [for example, see (30)]. Technical advances to allow telemetry (to avoid the complications of a cable), to miniaturize and reduce the surgical implants, and eventually to develop a noninvasive method for monitoring sleep (e.g., video analysis by computer and/or breathing, electromyography alone, etc.) are underway and would dramatically increase the utility of mice, allowing the sleep community to exploit the extensive genetic database and knockouts in mice by rapidly phenotyping the sleep patterns and regulation of large numbers of animals. Several efforts to conduct screens of large-scale mutagenized mice are underway using a variety of strategies.

Relatively speaking, published studies of dogs and hamsters have also increased, although the numbers are so small (fewer than 25 total) that the increase may be spurious. It may be that dogs will increasingly be recognized as useful in serving as models of human sleep disorders. Spontaneous canine models of narcolepsy (12) and sleep apnea (31) have had utility for understanding the pathophysiology of these conditions shared with humans. In the case of hamsters, recent studies have generally investigated the interaction of circadian behavior and sleep patterns. Given that hamsters have long been used to study circadian locomotion, the likely reason for an increase in such studies is the recent explosion in information about the molecular basis of these endogenous rhythms (32,33).

Among the 6% of sleep deprivation studies that do not use the eight species described earlier, some are used because of species-specific behaviors such as hibernation, where squirrels (34) and bears (35) are being studied. As in all human endeavors, individual preference may account for the choice of, for example, ferrets for brain slice studies of serotonin in the thalamus (36). There is, of course, also a wealth of studies that specifically focus on comparative aspects of sleep in animals, but these do not appear to use sleep deprivation as a tool.

VI. Newer "Simple" Models

A. Drosophila

Sleep studies have long focused on mammals, at least in part because electroencephalographic measures of sleep structure readily reveal states that parallel the two major states of human sleep: REM and NREM (37). However, surveys of behavioral sleep have strongly suggested that sleep is a more global feature in evolution (3). The limits of mammalian models for investigating molecular mechanisms (5) were cited by two groups that investigated whether the laboratory fruit fly, *Drosophila*, could serve as a useful model for the study of sleep, with encouraging results (38,39). The specific contribution of this model to sleep research has recently been reviewed [for example, see (8)] and will not be reexplored here. In brief, it appears that at least two conserved transcription factors (*cycle*/BMAL1 and CREB) (40–42) are involved in regulating fly sleep. For one of these, CREB, the role in sleep regulation has also been established to be conserved in mice (43). Studies of state-dependent changes in gene expression also reveal considerable although not perfect conservation from flies to mammals (39, 44, and unpublished observations). Some obvious areas where flies are likely to permit relatively rapid understanding of molecular mechanisms are the links between the circadian clock and homeostatic mechanisms (40,42) and the link between sleep deprivation and cellular stress (42,44, and unpublished observations). One intriguing area where short-lived models could make an enormous contribution is in understanding the role of sleep in aging. Several fly mutants with altered lifespans (45) have been identified, and the relevance of flies to normal human aging and as models of neurodegenerative disease (4,46,47) is generating great excitement. Surprisingly, it even appears that drug mechanisms may be conserved. Not only caffeine (38,39) but also the novel wake-promoting agent modafinil (48) appear to have the same effect on *Drosophila* behavioral sleep as they do on mammalian sleep. An unexpected finding in *Drosophila* was that at least one gene (*cycle*) appears to function differently in males and females (40,42); gender influences on sleep have not been extensively studied in humans, but what data there are suggest that there may be important differences (49–51).

Arguably, the greatest historical contribution of *Drosophila* to science has been the ease of conducting unbiased mutagenesis screens. Extensive efforts to identify genes involved in regulating sleep are underway using a variety of mutagenesis strategies in at least four laboratories both in the United States and abroad.

B. Zebrafish

A sleeplike state has been established in *Danio rerio*, the laboratory model used extensively to study development (52). Not only behavioral similarities but also a response to modafinil was established (52). A second study examining circadian gene expression has already begun to build on the initial description of sleep in this model (53). I have proposed that the zebrafish might be useful for its utility in neuroanatomical and electrophysiological studies because the nervous system is visible in the intact animal (5).

C. Other Insects

Two species of cockroach (54,55) and honeybees (56–58) have been shown to have sleeplike behavior and correlated changes in neurophysiology. Studying anatomy and neurophysiology is technically easier in these relatively large insects yet the central nervous system (CNS) is still relatively simple; these larger insects might be very interesting to study in depth. The locust has been used for sophisticated computer-assisted analyses of its electrophysiological responses to sensory stimuli; a 40-Hz oscillation has been identified as critical for olfactory sensory processing (59). In addition to the general advantage of studying a larger insect, honeybees have particular interest because of a long history of studying learning and plasticity, and their fascinating social organization. The bee genome has been sequenced (V.1.2 released July 2004; www.hgsc.bcm.tmc.edu./projects/honeybee), and extensive information already exists about genes expressed in the bee brain. A particularly fascinating story is that of the developmental switch from nurse to forager behavior. This is accompanied by the manifestation of a circadian rhythm (60–65). The idea that the developmental program and the social environment interact to influence gene expression and thus behavior has been dubbed "sociogenomics" (64). The fascinating observation that honeybees acquire and can also be induced to lose a circadian rhythm in order to adapt to the need of the hive for nurses (arrhythmic) or foragers (rhythmic) (61,62) leads to obvious questions about a possible function for sleep in these animals.

D. Other Invertebrates

C. elegans has long been thought to have no circadian rhythm [for example, see (5)], but recent studies indicate that both physiological and behavioral circadian rhythms can be demonstrated in particular conditions (66,67). Given the extraordinary value of *C. elegans* for investigating molecular regulation of behavior in a set of identified neurons, and the ability to ablate individual identified neurons, investigating sleep in such an organism would have specific advantages beyond those of simply identifying another simple organism. The tools available to manipulate the genome of course rival those in *Drosophila*, and the relevance for aging also offers enormous potential.

VII. Even Simpler Models?

Is there a possibility that sleep studies could eventually be conducted in vitro or even in silico? It would seem that "ex vivo" studies as in brain slices, where tissue is explanted or rapidly dissected and then studied, could become increasingly useful. Study of brain slices has already begun [e.g., (68)]. If specific genetic markers or fingerprints are identified that distinguish waking from sleeping states, it seems possible to at least speculate that cultured explants or even cells could be used to investigate molecular mechanisms related to state. Also, as mutants that have grossly abnormal sleep patterns are identified, these could be useful to study at the cellular as well as at the organismal level.

While they are obviously not the same as human brains in their information processing (69), computer models have been developed that manifest some of the basic features of sleep, namely, the oscillating patterns that underlie slow waves and spindles in single cells (70) and networks (71). In complex artificial intelligence programs a period of downtime benefits the operation of the system, and this has been called "sleep" by some computer and artificial intelligence theoreticians. Investigators have also described roles for this "sleep" such as "unlearning" spurious memories that they see as parallel to dreaming (72). This idea, which has some similarities to the hypothesis put forth by Crick (69), has reached the general culture in the form of popular scientific publications (73).

VIII. Interpretive and Methodological Issues Raised in Comparative Studies of Sleep Deprivation

As well as their specific contributions to specific studies, a strength of comparative biology is that the use of diverse models generates some new questions and refocuses attention on others. Some questions that occur at this time are: *What constitutes deprivation and rebound? How shall we define sleep in diverse models? Is the effect of sleep deprivation species variable?* Unless and until we identify one or more accepted, conserved molecular markers for sleep, we are currently faced with some issues that affect the design and interpretation of studies of sleep deprivation in diverse models.

A. Temporal Issues and the Definition of Recovery from Sleep Deprivation

How can we compare sleep deprivation in animals that have naturally polyphasic sleep (e.g., small mammals) with those that have consolidated sleep (e.g., humans, primates)? Is there a conserved or species-specific requirement for some minimal duration of continuous sleep ("consolidation")? Does this apply to recovery as well? A related question is whether sleep changes in quality as its duration is extended. *In the absence of recorded delta waves (nonmammalian models), what consititutes depth of sleep? Can we use consolidation as a proxy for depth?* In bees, small versus large antennal movements appear to reflect changes in state (74), but no behavioral (38) or electrophysiological (75) stages of sleep in *Drosophila* have been found.

B. Competing Homeostatic Drives?

Does sleep deprivation have species-variable effects because of other mechanisms unintentionally altered by the deprivation? Wheel running, the timing of which is regulated by the clock, has been found to have features of an "appetitive drive" in rats (26) and mice (Sigrid Veasey, personal communication). Since sleep deprivation usually also includes "exercise deprivation" if a wheel is not provided, a mouse will show both wheel-running "rebound" and also sleep rebound, which obviously cannot be accomplished simultaneously. The strength of this need might vary with species. When the procedure of sleep deprivation also unintentionally deprives animals of other needs such as food or sex, we must consider that these competing drives may change the response to sleep deprivation.

C. The Question of "Stress" and Sleep Deprivation Methodology

Stress, in the general sense of an unpleasant unavoidable situation that increases cortisol and adrenaline levels, was a concomitant of some older methods of sleep deprivation such as restraint or the "flower pot" method. It has been argued that such stressful methods invalidate many studies (76). More recent studies include appropriate controls and deprivation with "gentle handling" or presenting novel stimuli, greatly reducing this obvious form of stress. A general issue for experimental animals is that whatever the stimuli involved in sleep deprivation, they are unavoidable. It has been theorized that learned helplessness (a model of depression) and sleep deprivation paradigms share some fundamental features (77). Indeed, if sleep has a vital function, it is probably nonsensical to believe that we can prevent the organism from obtaining sleep without any resultant stress. Even for volunteer humans, "arousal" is an unavoidable concomitant of sleep deprivation (78,79), since by definition the failure to maintain arousal would lead the subjects to succumb to their increasing sleepiness. The subjective experience is that this arousal is increasingly unpleasant with prolonged sleep deprivation; it seems merely a semantic distinction between the feeling of misery that accompanies prolonged sleep loss and stress.

Are there individual and species differences in the effects of such arousing stimuli, even if they are intrinsic? The issue of concomitant stress is of more than theoretical interest, as gene expression studies of the effects of sleep deprivation have consistently revealed changes in expression of genes related to cellular stress

(16,42,44, Mackiewicz et al., personal communication; Naidoo et al., personal communication; and unpublished observations). *Are these truly wake related or are they byproducts of the methods used to cause sleep deprivation?* One approach is to use a variety of methods to deprive animals or human subjects of sleep, and look for overlap in the results. Multiple methodologies and species comparisons should help with such questions. The question of stress has also arisen in studies of insect sleep states [cockroach (54,55); *Drosophila*, personal observations]. For flies, mechanical methods are in general use (38,39), but there is the possibility of drug-induced sleep loss (48) as perhaps in mice (80), and perhaps of other modalities such as sound, electrical stimulation, and olfactory input. The specific modality of sensory stimulation may itself have effects on the organism (and these might be species variable).

IX. Concluding Thoughts

Sleep and sleep deprivation studies have benefited from research in multiple species; the expansion of sleep studies into invertebrates and the potential to identify genetic markers seem likely to provide a quantum leap in understanding molecular mechanisms of sleep and its function. Using data from multiple models to interrogate mammalian models should improve both the efficiency and the efficacy of studies in the future.

References

1. Bailey CH, Kandel ER. Structural changes underlying long-term-memory in aplysia: a molecular perspective. Semin Neurosci 6: 35–44, 1994.
2. Baron A, Alancon JM, Kandel ER. Expression of constitutively active CREB protein facilitates the late phase of long-term potentiation by enhancing synaptic capture. Cell 108: 689–703, 2002.
3. Campbell S, Tobler I. Animal sleep: a review of sleep duration across phylogeny. Neurosci Biobehav Rev 8: 269–300., 1984.
4. Kornberg TB, Krasnow MA. The Drosophila genome sequence: implications for biology and medicine. Science 287: 2218–2220, 2000.
5. Hendricks JC, Sehgal A, Pack AI. The need for a simple animal model to understand sleep. Prog Neurobiol 61: 339–351, 2000.
6. Morrison AR. Understanding the effect of animal-rights activism on biomedical research. Actas de fisiologica 8: 9–22, 2002.
7. Kilduff TS. What rest in flies can tell us about sleep in mammals. Neuron 26: 295–298, 2000.
8. Hendricks JC. Sleeping flies don't lie: the use of *Drosophila melanogaster* to study sleep and circadian rhythms. J Appl Physiol 94: 1650–1659, 2003.
9. Schotland HM, Insko EK, Panckeri KA, Leigh JS, Pack AI, Hendricks JC. Quantitative magnetic resonance imaging of upper airway musculature in an animal model of sleep apnea. J Appl Physiol 81: 1339–1346, 1996.

10. Zeitzer JM, Buckmaster CL, Parker KJ, Hauck CM, Lyons DM, Mignot E. Circadian and homeostatic regulation of hypocretin in a primate model: implications for the consolidation of wakefulness. J Neurosci 23: 3555–3560, 2003.

11. Chemelli RM, Willie JT, Sinton CM, Elmquist Jk, Scammell T, Lee C, Richardson JA, Williams SC, Xiong Y, Kisanuki Y, Fitch TE, Nakazato M, Hammer RE, Saper CB, Yanagisawa M. Narcolepsy in orexin knockout mice: molecular genetics of sleep regulation. Cell 98: 437–451, 1999.

12. Lin L, Faraco J, Li R, Kadotani H, Rogers W, Lin X, Qiu X, de Jong PJ, Nishino S, Mignot. E. The sleep disorder canine narcolepsy is caused by a mutation in the hypocretin (orexin) receptor 2 gene. Cell 98: 365–, 1999.

13. Rechtschaffen A, Bergmann BM. Sleep deprivation in the rat: an update of the 1989 paper. Sleep 25: 18–24, 2002.

14. Rechtschaffen A. Current perspectives on the function of sleep. Perspect Biol Med 41: 359–390., 1998.

15. Everson CA, Toth LA. Systemic bacterial invasion induced by sleep deprivation. Am J Physiol 278: R905–R916, 2000.

16. Cirelli C. How sleep deprivation affects gene expression in the brain: a review of recent findings. J Appl Physiol 92: 394–400, 2002.

17. Tobler I, Deboer T and M. F. Sleep and sleep regulation in normal and prion protein-deficient mice. J Neurosci 17: 1869–1879, 1997.

18. Huber R, T. D, Tobler I. Effects of sleep deprivation on sleep and sleep EEG in three mouse strains: empirical data and simulations. Brain Res 857: 8–19, 2000.

19. O'Donnell CP, Tankersley CG, Polotsky VP, Schwartz AR, Smith PL. Leptin, obesity, and respiratory function. Respir Physiol 119: 163–170, 2000.

20. Graves L, Hellman K, Veasey S, Blendy JA, Pack AI, Abel TA. Genetic evidence for a role of CREB in sustained cortical arousal. J Neurophysiol epub ahead of print, 2003.

21. Huber R, Deboer T, Tobler I. Prion protein: a role in sleep regulation? J Sleep Res 8 (suppl 1): 30–36, 1999.

22. Franken P, Chollet D, Tafti M. The homeostatic regulation of sleep need is under genetic control. J Neurosci 21: 2610–2621, 2001.

23. Werme M, Messer C, Olson L, Gilden L, Thoren P, Nestler EJ, Brene S. Delta FosB regulates wheel running. J Neurosci 22: 8133–8138, 2002.

24. Deboer T, Tobler I. Running wheel size influences circadian rhythm period and its phase shift in mice. J Comp Physiol A Sensory Neural Behav Physiol 186: 969–973, 2000.

25. Mistlberger RE, Holmes MM. Behavioral feedback regulation of circadian rhythm phase angle in light-dark entrained mice. Am J Physiol Regul Integr Comp Physiol 279: R813–821, 2000.

26. Mueller DT, Herman G, Eikelboom R. Effects of short- and long-term wheel deprivation on running. Physiol Behav 66: 101–107, 1999.

27. Kopp C, Albrecht U, B. Z, Tobler I. Homeostatic sleep regulation is preserved in mPer1 and mPer2 mutant mice. Eur J Neurosci 16: 1099–1106, 2002.

28. Naylor E, Bergmann kM, Krauski K, Zee PC, Takahashi JS, Vitaterna MH, Turek FW. The circadian clock mutation alters sleep homeostasis in the mouse. J Neurosci 20: 8138–8143, 2000.

29. Bunger MK, Wilsbacher LD, Moran SM, Clendenin C, Radcliffe LA, Hogenesch JB, Simon MC, Takahashi JS, Bradfield CA. Mop3 is an essential component of the master circadian pacemaker in mammals. Cell 103: 1009–1018, 2000.

30. Kopp C, Rudolph U, Keist R, I. T. Diazepam-induced changes on sleep and the EEG spectrum in mice: role of the alpha3–GABA(A) receptor subtype. Eur J Neurosci 17: 2226–2230, 2003.

31. Hendricks JC, Kline LR, Kovalski JA, O'Brien JA, Morrison AR, Pack AI. The English bulldog: a natural model of sleep-disordered breathing. J Appl Physiol 53: 1344–1350, 1987.

32. Dunlap JC. Molecular bases for circadian clocks. Cell 96: 271–290., 1999.

33. Reppert SM. A clockwork explosion! Neuron 21: 1–4, 1998.

34. Larkin JE, Franken P, Heller HC. Loss of circadian organization of sleep and wakefulness during hibernation. Am J Physiol Regul Integr Comp Physiol 282: R1086–R1095, 2002.

35. Prunescu C, Serban-Parau N, Brock JH, Vaughan DM, Prunescu P. Liver and kidney structure and iron content in romanian brown bears (*Ursus arctos*) before and after hibernation. Comp Biochem Physiol. A Mol Integr Physiol 134: 21–26, 2003.

36. Monckton JE, McCormick DA. Neuromodulatory role of serotonin in the ferret thalamus. J Neurophysiol 87: 2124–2136, 2002.

37. Siegel JM. Phylogeny and the function of sleep. Behav Brain Res 69: 29–34, 1995.

38. Hendricks JC, Finn SM, Panckeri KA, Chavkin J, Williams JA, Sehgal A, Pack AI. Rest in Drosophila is a sleep-like state. Neuron 25: 129–138, 2000.

39. Shaw PJ, Cirelli C, Greenspan RJ, Tononi G. Correlates of sleep and waking in *Drosophila melanogaster*. Science 287: 1834–1837, 2000.

40. Hendricks JC, Lu S, Kume K, Yin JC-P, Yang Z, Sehgal A. Gender dimorphism in the role of cycle (BMAL1) in rest, rest regulation, and longevity in *Drosophila melanogaster*. J Biol Rhythms 18: 12–25, 2003.

41. Hendricks JC, Williams JA, Panckeri K, Kirk D, Yin JC-P, Sehgal A. A non-circadian role for cAMP signaling and CREB activity in waking and rest homeostasis in *Drosophila melanogaster*. Nat Neurosci 4: 1108–1115, 2001.

42. Shaw PJ, Tononi G, Greenspan RJ, Robinson DF. Stress response genes protect against lethal effects of sleep deprivation in *Drosophila*. Nature 417: 287–291, 2002.

43. Graves L, Dalvi A, Lucki I, Blendy JA, Abel E. Behavioral analysis of the CREB alpha delta mutation on a B6/129. Hippocampus (in press).

44. Terao A, Steininger TL, Hyder K, Apte-Deshpande A, Ding J, Rishipathak D, Davis RW, Heller HC, TS. K. Differential increase in the expression of heat shock protein family members during sleep deprivation and during sleep. Neuroscience 116: 187–200, 2003.

45. Helfand SL and Rogina B. From genes to aging in *Drosophila*. [Review] Adv Genet 49: 67–109, 2003.

46. Feany MB. Studying human neurodegenerative diseases in flies and worms. J Neuropathol Exp Neurol 59: 847–856, 2000.

47. Chan HY, Bonini NM. *Drosophila* models of polyglutamine diseases. Meth Mol Biol 217: 241–251, 2003.

48. Hendricks JC, Kirk D, Panckeri K, Miller MS, Pack AI. Modafinil maintains waking in the fruit fly *Drosophila melanogaster*. Sleep 26: 139–146, 2003.

49. Reyner LA, Horne JA, Reyner A. Gender- and age-related differences in sleep determined by home-recorded sleep logs and actimetry from 400 adults. Sleep 18: 127–134, 1995.

50. Armitage R, Hoffmann R, Trivedi M, Rush AJ. Slow-wave activity in NREM sleep: sex and age effects in depressed outpatients and healthy controls. Psychiatry Res 95: 201–213, 2000.

51. Armitage R, Smith C, Thompson S, Hoffman R. Sex differences in slow-wave activity in response to sleep deprivation. Sleep Res Online 4: 33–41, 2001.

52. Zhdanova IV, Wang SY, Leclai OJ, Danilova NP. Melatonin promotes sleep-like state in zebrafish. Brain Res 903: 263–268, 2001.

53. Gamse JT, Shen YC, Thisse C, Thisse B, Raymond PA, Halpern ME, Liang JO. Otx5 regulates genes that show circadian expression in the zebrafish pineal complex. Nat Genet 30: 117–121, 2002.

54. Tobler I. The effect of forced locomotion on the rest-activity cycle of the cockroach. .Behav Brain Res.8: 351–360, 1983.

55. Tobler I, Neuner-Jehle M. 24–h variation of vigilance in the cockroach *Blaberus giganteus.* J Sleep Res 1: 231–239, 1992.

56. Kaiser WJ. Busy bees need rest, too. Comp Physiol A:163: 565–584, 1988.

57. Kaiser W, Faltin T, Bayer G. Sleep in a temperature gradient—behavioural recordings from forager honey bees. J Sleep Res 11 (suppl): 115–116, 2002.

58. Kaiser K. Honey bee sleep is different from chill coma—behavioural and electrophysiological recordings in forager honey bees. J Sleep Res 115 (suppl 1): 115, 2002.

59. Wehr M, Laurent G. Odour encoding by temporal sequences of firing in oscillating neural assemblies. Nature 384: 162–166, 1996.

60. Ben-Shahar Y, Robichon A, Sokolowski MB, Robinson GE. Influence of gene action across different time scales on behavior. Science 296: 741–744, 2002.

61. Bloch G, Toma DP, Robinson GE. Behavioral rhythmicity, age, division of labor and period expression in the honey bee brain. J Biol Rhythms 16: 444–457, 2001.

62. Bloch G, Robinson GE. Reversal of honeybee behavioural rhythms. Nature 410: 1048, 2001.

63. Madison RD, Robinson G. lambda RNA internal standards quantify sensitivity and amplification efficiency of mammalian gene expression profiling. Biotechniques 25: 504–508, 510, 512, passim, 1998.

64. Robinson GE. Sociogenomics takes flight. Science 297: 204–205, 2002.

65. Toma DP, Bloch G, Moore D, Robinson GE. Changes in period mRNA levels in the brain and division of labor in honey bee colonies. Proc Natl Acad Sci USA 97: 6914–6919, 2000.

66. Kippert F, Saunders DS, Blaxter ML. *Caenorhabditis elegans* has a circadian clock. Curr Biol 12: R47–49, 2002.

67. Saigusa T, Ishizaki S, Watabiki S, Ishii N, Tanakadate A, Tamai Y, K. H. Circadian behavioural rhythm in *Caenorhabditis elegans.* Curr Biol 12: R46–47, 2002.

68. Borg-Graham LJ. Systems neuroscience: the slowly sleeping slab and slice. Curr Biol 11: R140–R143, 2001.

69. Crick F, Mitchison G. REM sleep and neural nets. Behav Brain Res 69: 147–155, 1995.

70. Lytton WW, Destexhe A, Sejnowski TJ. Control of slow oscillations in the thalamocortical neuron: a computer model. Neuroscience 70: 673–684., 1996.

71. Kostopoulos GK. Spike-and-wave discharges of absence seizures as a transformation of sleep spindles: the continuing development of a hypothesis. Clin Neurophysiol 111 (suppl 2): S27–S38, 2000.

72. Hopfield JJ, Feinstein DI, Palmer RG. Unlearning' has a stabilizing effect in collective memories. Nature 304: 158–159, 1983.
73. Kaku M. Machines that think. In: Visions. New York: Anchor Books, 1997, p. 85–87.
74. Sauer S, Kinkelin M, Herrmann E, Kaiser W. The dynamics of sleep-like behaviour in honey bees. J Comp Physiol A 189: 599–607, 2003.
75. Nitz DA, van Swinderen B, Tononi G, Greenspan RJ. Electrophysiological correlates of rest and activity in Drosophila melanogaster. Curr Biol 12: 1934–1940, 2002.
76. Vertes RP, Eastman KE. The case against memory consolidation in REM sleep. Behav Brain Sci 23: 867–876.
77. Rotenberg VS. Sleep after immobilization stress and sleep deprivation: common features and theoretical integration. Crit Rev Neurobiol 14: 225–231, 2000.
78. Horne JA. Sleep function, with particular reference to sleep deprivation. Ann Clin Res. 17:199–208, 1985.
79. Horne JA, McGrath MJ. The consolidation hypothesis for REM sleep function: stress and other confounding factors—a review. Biol Psychol 18: 165–184, 1984.
80. Kopp C, Petit J-M, Magistretti P, Borbely AA, Tobler I. Comparison of the effects of modafinil and sleep deprivation on sleep and cortical EEG spectra in mice. Neuropharmacology 43: 110–118, 2002.

4

Total Sleep Deprivation

CHIARA CIRELLI AND GIULIO TONONI

University of Wisconsin–Madison, Madison, Wisconsin, U.S.A.

I. Introduction

Two main procedures have been used to enforce total sleep deprivation (TSD) in animals: gentle handling and forced locomotion with continuously rotating wheels or with the disk-over-water method. Brain electrical stimulation and pharmacological stimulation have also been used. Perhaps not surprisingly, some of these techniques have also been popular in human studies, where effective awakening stimuli include physical activity and taking cold showers. Below, we will briefly describe the most common methods used to enforce TSD in animals, their relative efficacy, and their disadvantages. We will also discuss whether some aspects of the TSD syndrome depend on the method used to enforce continuous wakefulness. Furthermore, we will address what is probably the most problematic issue in any sleep deprivation experiment, namely, whether the effects of TSD can be ascribed to sleep loss per se rather than to nonspecific factors. As we shall see, the "perfect control" experiment in a sleep deprivation study is, if not impossible, certainly very difficult to design.

II. TSD Methods: Advantages and Disadvantages

A. "Gentle Handling" Technique

With the "gentle handling" technique, also called "hand deprivation" or "novel objects exposure," the subjects—mainly rats and mice, but also rabbits [e.g.,

(1,2)], cats (3) and dogs [e.g., (4,5)]—receive tactile, olfactory, or visual stimulation whenever they enter the forbidden state [rapid-eye-movement (REM) or non-REM (NREM) sleep] as detected by polygraphic recording or behavioral observation. Stimuli may be complex, e.g., novel objects introduced in the cage. This method requires constant monitoring and a score of dedicated investigators. In one study in which sleep deprivation was enforced in rats for 3 hr at the beginning of the light period [animals were kept in 12:12 light/dark (LD) schedule], the number of required stimuli (tactile and/or acoustic stimuli lasting 1–2 sec) was 23 ± 11 [mean ± standard deviation (SD), $n = 5$ animals], 44 ± 13, and 75 ± 34 in the first, second, and third hour, respectively (Cirelli, unpublished data, 2003). The method is completely effective only for a few hours. For instance, in a study in which TSD was enforced in rats for 6 hr during either the dark or the light phase, NREM sleep represented only 0.5% of total recording time during the deprivation period (6). However, in another study in rats in which TSD continued for the entire dark period (12 hr), short NREM sleep episodes that could not be avoided accounted for about 4% of total recording time (7). REM sleep, by contrast, was completely suppressed in these two studies. In a study in cats in which TSD was enforced for 24 hr it was noted that short mild stimuli such as noise or displacement of the cage were only effective for the first few hours and then failed to prevent the appearance of spindles after the fifth hour. At the end of the experiment, strong and even painful stimuli were presented every 20–30 sec, yet spindle activity accounted for at least 3% of the total recording time (8). One study used gentle handling for up to 15 days, but rats were often immersed in shallow water to maintain wakefulness (9). In that study, the estimated sleep time per day during the deprivation was 3–5% of total recording time and did not change from the second to the last day of deprivation. Similarly, sleep pressure as measured by change in sleep latency increased progressively during the first 3 days but then stabilized for the rest of the experiment.

A mixture of gentle handling and forced locomotion (walking) was used in the first documented long-term sleep deprivation study in animals, which was performed by Marie de Manacéine in 1894 (4). She sleep deprived 10 young dogs (2–4 months old) for 92–146 hr. Four animals died at the end of the experiment, while in the other six cases the experiment was ended after 96–120 hr when death appeared imminent. Thus, gentle handling has been used both for short-term and long-term sleep deprivation experiments in different animal species, but this method can prevent NREM sleep completely for only a few hours. By the end of the first day, NREM sleep already represents 3–5% of total recording time, a percentage that does not seem to increase significantly if TSD is prolonged for several days.

B. Forced Locomotion Techniques

A common way to keep animals awake is to use forced locomotion in slowly rotating cylinders. In one study in which rats were polygraphically recorded during the deprivation, it was shown that this technique could reduce total sleep to one-tenth of baseline values for the first 24 hr of TSD [(10); see also (11)]. The method affects NREM sleep and REM sleep equally, and therefore differs from the "platform" or "flower pot "methods (see Chap. 5), which affect primarily, although not exclusively, REM sleep (12–14). One study (15) documented with electroencephalography the presence of microsleeps (slow waves in the electroencephalogram (EEG) associated with behavioral immobility) of 1–4 sec every time rats on a treadmill "ride to the rear." In this study microsleeping was already present within the first 24 hr and accounted for up to 20% of total time after 32 hr of TSD. In another TSD study (16), total sleep accounted for about 5% of total recording time in the first 12 hr of the experiment, and for 10–20% by the end of 24 hr. Tobler and Jaggi found in Syrian hamsters that 24–hr TSD enforced by forced locomotion or by gentle handling gave very similar results (17). However, the loss of muscle tone at the end of the deprivation period and a shortened sleep latency suggested that gentle handling was more effective than forced locomotion. Constantly moving wheels have also been used to enforce long-term sleep deprivation. For instance, some of the early TSD experiments used revolving cages set in continuous revolution to sleep deprive rabbits for several days (8–31 days) until the animals reached or were close to exhaustion (18,19). In a variant of the technique, two-thirds of the rotating wheel is submerged into the water. When exhausted, the subjects would fall into the water and would be unable to remount the wheel. In one case (20), the experiment was terminated when the rats fell into the water after being replaced on the wheel three times during a 15–min period. This occurred within 80 to about 200 hr, depending in part on the age of the rat. "Gentle shaking" has also been used to sleep deprive insects such as cockroaches (21), scorpions (22), honeybees (23), and fruit flies (24,25). Thus, methods based on slowly rotating or gently shaking cages can enforce wakefulness for several days, but microsleeping is already substantial (about 20% of total recording time) within the first 24–36 hr.

Another method based on forced locomotion is the *disk-over-water (DOW) method* introduced by Rechtschaffen and colleagues in 1983 [(26); see also Chap. 5]. This method uses minimal stimulation to enforce chronic sleep deprivation in the sleep-deprived rat, while it simultaneously applies to the control rat the same stimulation, but without severely limiting its sleep. The sleep-deprived and the control rat are housed each on one side of a divided 46–cm horizontal disk suspended over a shallow tray of 2– to 3–cm-deep water (Fig. 1). Electroencephalographic and electromyographic data are continuously recorded to detect sleep states. When the experimental rat starts to sleep or enters the "forbidden" state (e.g., REM sleep), the disk is automatically rotated at a low speed (3.33 rpm), awakening the rat and forcing it to walk opposite to disk rotation to avoid being carried into the water. The yoked control rat receives the same physical stimulation because it is on the same disk. However, while sleep is severely reduced in the sleep-deprived rat, the control rat can sleep *ad libitum* whenever the sleep-deprived rat is spontaneously awake and eating, drinking, or grooming and therefore the disk is still. Typically,

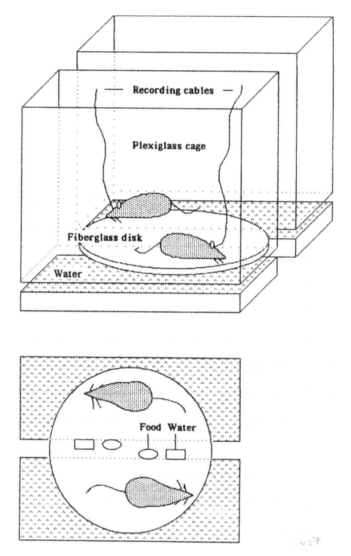

Figure 1 Schematic diagram of disk-over-water apparatus used by Rechtschaffen and colleagues. An experimental rat and a control rat are placed on either side of a divided 46-cm horizontal disk suspended over a shallow tray of 2–3 cm deep water. Each rat is housed in separate Plexiglas® cages with separate food and water containers. Electroencephalographic and electromyographic data are continuously recorded to detect sleep states via implanted electrodes, and recording cables transfer the data from these electrodes to the monitoring equipment. When the experimental rat starts to sleep or enters the "forbidden" state (e.g., REM sleep), the disk is automatically rotated at a low speed (3.33 rpm). This stimulus awakens the rat and forces it to walk opposite to the direction of the disk rotation to avoid being carried into the water. The yoked control rat receives the same physical stimulation as the experimental rat because it is on the same disk. (Courtesy of Clete A. Kushida, M.D., Ph.D., Stanford, CA.)

control rats show modest to moderate sleep restriction. For instance, in a TSD study by Rechtschaffen et al. (27), total sleep was reduced by 91% in sleep deprivation rats versus 28% in yoked controls, and disk rotation occupied 20% of the total time. In a more recent study, sleep-deprived rats lost 78 ± 2% of their total sleep whereas controls lost 29 ± 3% (28). In another recent study, sleep-deprived rats lost 72 ± 7% of their total sleep, whereas yoked controls lost 39 ± 5% (29). In yet another study in which the DOW method was used to enforce relatively short periods of sleep deprivation (1–4 days), NREM sleep accounted for about 5–10% of total recording time by the end of the first day of sleep deprivation and was maintained at that level for the subsequent 3 days. REM sleep, by contrast, was totally suppressed (30). It should be mentioned that because of the fragmented nature of sleep episodes during TSD, sleep percentages such as those given above are significantly affected by the duration of the epochs used to score behavioral states. For instance, in our experience, during a TSD experiment with the DOW method NREM sleep accounts for less than 10% of total recording time when using a 30–sec epoch scoring system, and up to 20–25% when using 4–sec epochs (Cirelli and Tononi, unpublished results). Thus, like any other method discussed so far, the DOW method can totally prevent NREM sleep for only a few hours. After the first day, NREM may account for up to 10–20% of total recording time.

It has been argued that one reason to prefer gentle handling over forced locomotion paradigms is the potential confounding effect of locomotor activity on the recovery sleep after sleep loss. This issue is still controversial. Some studies in rats have shown no evidence that locomotor activity per se significantly affects the amount of sleep and of sleep rebound after sleep deprivation, but other studies have found an effect. For instance, sleep rebound was similar at different cylinder rotation rates in two studies (11–16) but slow-wave incidence (but not slow-wave amplitude) was greater at higher rotation rates in another study (31). Moreover, neither the amount of total sleep [e.g., (32)] nor that of NREM sleep (33) was affected by free access to a running wheel. However, the increase in slow-wave activity (mean power density 0.75–4 Hz) in NREM sleep after TSD by gentle handling was not as significant and/or as prolonged as after a TSD of similar duration performed by forced locomotion (34,35). A recent meta-analysis of the acute effects of exercise on human sleep found very little (if any) effect of motor activity on slow-wave sleep (36). Thus, whether locomotor activity per se has any consistent effect on sleep is still a matter of debate, but if it does such effect appears to be small.

C. Punitive Methods

Punitive methods have also been used to enforce sleep deprivation, but they have been surprisingly ineffective. In one study rats received an inescapable foot shock whenever slow-wave sleep was detected electroencephalographically (9). The number of shocks rose progressively as a function of the number of hours of sleep deprivation. It was noted that even with the highest level of shock slow-wave sleep eventually appeared almost immediately after the cessation of the shock. When slow-wave sleep occurred within 20 sec after 10 consecutive shocks, the experiment was ended. Even with the highest intensity of shock, the experiment had to be terminated within 24 hr. In the same study, 24–hr TSD by punitive (foot shock) and nonpunitive (gentle handling) methods gave similar results in terms of sleep rebound (total amount of sleep, NREM and REM sleep). Thus, sleep cannot be prevented for more than 24 hr even when using a punitive method such as foot shocks.

D. Brain Electrical or Chemical Stimulation

Brain electrical stimulation methods have been used, especially for larger animals such as cats and dogs. For instance, an electroencephalographically controlled system was designed to prevent sleep in cats by stimulating the hypothalamic predatory area (37). More recently, the anterolateral hypothalamus of rats was stimulated to produce TSD for 8 hr (38). In one of the best documented studies using this approach, Lucas (39) directly stimulated the midbrain reticular formation of cats to prevent sleep for up to 7 days. Electrical stimulation was delivered either continuously or intermittently whenever slow activity appeared in the EEG. The continuous-stimulation paradigm prevented sleep completely for up to 3 days, during which the animals ate regularly and showed sustained polygraphic and behavioral signs of wakefulness (sphinx-like posture, eyes open or closed halfway). At the beginning of the fourth day, however, stimuli were less effective, and their locus, duration, and intensity needed to be changed almost every hour. By contrast, with the intermittent stimulation paradigm cats started assuming a sleeplike posture and had their eyes already closed at the end of the first day. Thus, continuous (but not intermittent) electrical stimulation of the midbrain reticular formation seems to be able to totally prevent sleep for up to 3 days.

Levitt (40) used repetitive injections of dextroamphetamine sulfate (10 mg/kg) to prevent sleep for 5 days in rats. The method appeared to be effective in keeping the animals awake. However, since animals were monitored with an ultrasound system rather than with EEG, the author could only calculate total sleep time after the deprivation, which was increased. In a later study (15), in which rats were monitored electroencephalographically, the same author could document that dextroamphetamine (10 mg/kg) totally prevented slow-wave sleep for 24 hr, but longer periods of TSD were not attempted. In another study, a lower dose of methylamphetamine (5 mg/kg) was given twice 5 hr apart to prevent sleep for 10 hr (41). In the cat, amphetamine (1 mg/kg) completely suppressed cortical slow-wave activity for 6–8 hr (42). In humans, dextroamphetamine given 3 times a night on two consecutive days suppressed slow-wave activity for 55–59 hr (43). Thus, repetitive doses of amphetamine can totally prevent sleep for at least 1 day in animals and for more than 2 days in humans.

E. Summary

All TSD methods discussed here, with the exception of the continuous electrical stimulation of the reticular formation and amphetamines, failed to elicit complete and uninterrupted wakefulness after the first 24 hr. Evidently, sleep pressure over-comes whatever method is used to maintain wakefulness. Electrical stimulation of the reticular formation, by contrast, can apparently maintain electroencephalo-graphic and behavioral signs of wakefulness for up to 3 days. However, this method is invasive, and the continuous direct stimulation of brain tissue at quite high intensity (2–7 V, 70–120 cycles/sec, 0.1 msec pulse duration) may have long-lasting effects that are not well characterized at the present time. For short-term TSD, gentle handling and DOW have similar efficacy, and both are prefer-able to the treadmill, which is less effective and has the potential confounding factor of locomotor activity (this confounding factor is not present in gentle han-dling and is controlled for by the yoked control in the DOW method). To obtain TSD for less than 24 hr, gentle handling should probably be considered the method of choice. In our experience, the yoked control (see below) offered by the DOW method constitutes a key asset but only after 2–3 days of sleep deprivation rather than for the first 24 hr. This is because the yoked control needs some time to learn how and when to sleep when the disk starts moving, and therefore its sleep is significantly reduced for the first day of the experiment. In addition, the DOW requires a dedicated apparatus including a sophisticated computer-based controller. When using gentle handling for TSD, however, investigators should apply gentle handling to the control animals when they are spontaneously awake. Note that even when sleep pressure is highest, e.g., at the beginning of the light period in rats, control animals are still spontaneously awake 20–30% of the time. After 24 hr, the gentle handling method becomes impractical. In addition, the availability of the DOW yoked control becomes essential. Thus, the DOW is the method of choice for long-term TSD.

III. Effects of Total Sleep Deprivation

The most comprehensive series of TSD experiments have been performed using the DOW method. Long-term TSD in rats with the DOW method produces a series of dramatic physiological changes that culminate invariably in death after 2–3 weeks (26,27). Initially (within the first 1–2 days) long-term sleep-deprived rats develop a syndrome characterized by an increase in food intake, energy expenditure, and heart rate, followed by a decrease in body weight, and a decline in body and brain temperature. The sleep deprivation syndrome and its lethal con-sequences have also been observed after selective REM sleep deprivation, although the pathological process associated with the loss of sleep takes longer to appear, the survival time is longer (4–5 weeks instead of 2–3 weeks), and body and brain temperature are not significantly decreased (27,44). Despite a long series of studies, the DOW sleep deprivation syndrome has not been fully explained (45). As discussed in Rechtschaffen et al. (27), the long-term TSD syn-drome produced by the DOW method is not unique, and other methods of chronic sleep deprivation in other animal species have resulted in similar effects. In exper-iments in dogs, rabbits, and, to a lesser extent, cats, chronic (several days) TSD by gentle handling and/or forced locomotion by a treadmill causes increases in food intake and in heart rate, weight loss, and death. Fruit flies prevented from sleeping for several days also die of sleep deprivation (46). Interestingly, survival time in DOW sleep-deprived rats is negatively correlated with the rate of increase of energy expenditure and with the percentage of REM sleep loss, but not with the amount of disk rotation. Interestingly, the effects of sleep restriction in yoked controls also correlate with the partial loss of REM sleep but not with the amount of disk rotation.

IV. Yoked Control

A "yoked" stimulation was used early on in state-selective sleep deprivation. For instance, Siegel and Gordon prevented REM sleep in cats for 3–10 days by using high-frequency stimulation of the reticular formation (47). The same amount of stimulation was given to control animals during NREM sleep. However, as was discussed above, most methods to enforce TSD do not involve yoked controls. The "control" in gentle handling or forced locomotion experiments is usually a cage control, which is not gently handled or forced to move when awake. With the DOW method, by contrast, the amount of stimulation (forced locomotor activity) is the same in experimental and control rats. Thus, the effects of sleep deprivation are more likely to depend on sleep loss per se. When compared with the treadmill-type design for long-term sleep deprivation, the DOW method has also other advantages, such as the larger range of free movement, the brief duration of arousal stimuli (≤ 6 sec), the minimal behavioral requirements to avoid the water, and the minimal amount of forced locomotion (about 1 mile/day; when given free access to a running wheel, rats may run up to 30 miles/day).

The yoked control in the DOW method may be the best possible control, but it is still not the perfect control as we shall discuss. First, the sleep of the yoked control in a TSD experiment is restricted. Chronic sleep restriction in the yoked control is inevitable due to the fact that the disk rotates at least 20% of the time (by contrast, in REM-selective sleep deprivation, the yoked control can maintain a normal amount of sleep because the disk rotates only 5% of the time). In fact, on most variables, yoked controls in a TSD experiment with the DOW method show changes from the baseline in the same direction as the respective sleep-deprived rats. Second, while the amount of stimulation is the same between the sleep-deprived rat and its yoked control, the quality of the stimulation differs. In fact, the totally sleep-deprived rat in the DOW method always receives the stimulus at the transition from waking to NREM sleep, while the yoked control is aroused in any behavioral state—waking, NREM sleep, and REM sleep. This difference is potentially important because at least some aspects of the TSD syndrome could be due not so much to the fact that the sleep-deprived rat does not sleep but rather to the fact that it is constantly been disturbed when trying to go to sleep. However, an informative comparison can be done between the yoked control of a TSD experiment and a rat selectively deprived of REM sleep with the DOW method. Based on Rechtschaffen et al. (27) and on our own data, it appears that while the REM-deprived rat is only aroused 5% of the time (always at the transition between NREM and REM), the control yoked to a TSD rat is actually aroused while asleep 10–15% of the time. This calculation is based on the facts that sleep on the DOW accounts for 50–60% of total time during baseline and that during the TSD the disk rotates about 20% of the time. Since only the REM-deprived animal develops a sleep deprivation syndrome and eventually dies, sleep loss appears to be more important than repetitive arousals in determining the sleep deprivation syndrome.

V. Sleep Deprivation and Stress

A. Acute Stress

Stress is generically defined as "a mentally or emotionally disrupting, upsetting condition occurring in response to adverse external influences and capable of affecting physical health" (48). In a more scientific context, stress is defined as "a perceived threat to homeostasis" (49). Thus, there is little doubt that enforced wakefulness is stressful. The very fact that sleep is homeostatically regulated implies that any attempt to prevent sleep will trigger a stressful (disrupting and upsetting) condition. It thus seems that completely eliminating the "stress of being awake" during a TSD experiment is impossible by definition. It is possible, however, to reduce and to control for the stress related to the specific awakening stimulus that is being used. This goal can be achieved by choosing particularly mild stimuli (e.g., a food reward is likely to be less stressful than a foot shock) and/or by having a yoked control receiving the same stimulation. Acute stress is characterized by activation of the hypothalamic-pituitary-adrenal (HPA) axis. Short periods of sleep deprivation (less than 24 hr), whether with gentle handling, rotating cylinders, or the DOW method, are generally associated with increased plasma levels of corticosterone (30,50–54). If there is no yoked control, the only way to limit the effects due to the stimulus is to keep the duration of sleep deprivation as short as possible and to use the most gentle method. In our experience, novel objects work quite well as awakening stimuli for a few hours (4–6 hr from lights on in a rat), but the rats need to be habituated in advance to the stress of being exposed to new objects [e.g., (55)]. In our experiments, for instance, animals are exposed to new objects for 0.5–1 hr every day during the baseline period.

The best indication that the stress of being awake can be distinguished from the stress of being stimulated comes from the DOW studies (27). At the beginning (first 1–3 days) of a TSD experiment, adrenocorticotropic hormone (ACTH) and corticosterone levels are increased to a similar extent in the sleep-deprived rat and its yoked control. However, the sleep-deprived rat shows early signs that are either absent (increase in food intake) or significantly less pronounced (increase in energy expenditure) in the yoked control. Thus, activation of the HPA axis is due to the stress of being stimulated by disk rotation (common to the two rats), while the increase in energy expenditure and in food intake is mainly due to the stress of being awake.

B. Chronic Stress

As discussed above and recently summarized by Rechtschaffen and others (30,52), the issue is not so much whether sleep deprivation is stressful but whether the signs and symptoms observed in sleep-deprived animals are specifically due to the stress of being awake. The alternative is that such signs and symptoms are indistinguishable from those produced by other forms of stress, such as food deprivation or repetitive foot shock, and are therefore nonspecific. We have already observed that some of the early signs of sleep deprivation with the DOW method cannot be explained by the acute activation of the HPA axis.

Extensive studies of chronic stress have been performed by Kant et al. (56), who subjected rats to a foot-shock (either escapable or inescapable) every 5 min for 1–14 days. During the first week of stress rats showed an increase in plasma levels of corticosterone, a decrease in lever pressing for food pellets, and weight loss. However, by the end of the second week rats adapted to the stressful procedure, and hormonal levels, food intake, and body weight returned to normal. Sleep parameters also normalized in these animals by the second day of stress, which is remarkable considering the very high number of daily stimulations they received (about 280 trials/day). Most importantly for the present purposes, chronically shocked animals never showed an increase in energy expenditure or in food intake in any phase of the experiment. In another study (57), rats were chronically stressed with shocks paired with warning tones every 5 min for 23 days. Animals suffered from weight loss associated with a decrease in food intake and showed significant hypertrophy of the adrenal glands. They never showed an increase in energy expenditure or skin lesions, nor did they die at the end of the experiment. Most importantly, other studies in rats reviewed by McCarty (58) showed that chronic exposure to a familiar stressor—either restraint stress or intermittent shock or swim stress—results in a reduced plasma catecholamine response.

Thus, rats chronically stressed by a repetitive foot shock or other stressors shared with chronically sleep-deprived rats only the increase in corticosterone and the decrease in body weight during the first week of the experiment. Specifically, chronically stressed animals never showed an increase in energy expenditure, and they resumed their normal appearance and behavior within the first week of persistent stress. By contrast, chronically sleep-deprived rats showed a persistent increase in energy expenditure and a decrease in body weight, as well as progressively higher levels of plasma catecholamines. Finally, other canonical signs of chronic stress may include stomach ulcers, shrinking of the spleen, and hypertrophy of the adrenal glands. The first two were not present in rats chronically sleep deprived with the DOW method, and the third was only present when death was imminent (27,30,52). Thus, chronic inescapable stress or chronic mild stress does not explain the sleep deprivation syndrome.

Chronic exposure to painful inescapable stress or to mild chronic stress can also cause a general loss of interest in rats, such as interest in exploring their environment or in palatable food [see references in (59)]. Behavior has not been extensively studied in long-term sleep-deprived animals. However, we have observed that rats totally sleep deprived with the DOW method for 7–10 days and their yoked controls show a similarly intense exploratory behavior when exposed to novel objects for 1 hr (Cirelli and Tononi, unpublished results, 2003). Moreover, if allowed to do so once a day, they avidly consume palatable food (e.g., Cheetos). Acute or chronic exposure to a painful and inescapable foot shock can also produce learned helplessness, a well-studied animal model of unipolar depression. Learned helplessness refers to the fact that after exposure to uncontrollable shock training, some rats do not learn to escape from a new stressor even if it is avoidable. Because one can think of sleep deprivation methods as imposing a form of inescapable punishment (loss of sleep), it has been suggested that the sleep deprivation syndrome may be a form of learned helplessness [e.g., (60)]. However, in learned-helplessness paradigms energy expenditure, heart rate, and central catecholamine levels are normal (61), body temperature and the sleep/waking cycle are unaltered (62), and animals do not die. Moreover, avoidance learning can be restored by specific noradrenergic agonists, suggesting a deficit in catecholaminergic function [e.g., (63)]. Thus, all available evidence indicates that the physiological changes after sleep deprivation are completely unlike those in learned helplessness.

VI. Sleep Deprivation and the Noradrenergic System

As mentioned before, long-term total or REM-selective sleep deprivation with the DOW produces the same syndrome, but such a syndrome takes significantly longer to develop when only REM sleep is prevented. This suggests that both NREM and REM sleep are important. NREM sleep and REM sleep differ radically in terms of electroencephalographic and single-unit activity, metabolic parameters, and the level of firing of the cholinergic system. However, they are both characterized by a reduced activity of neuromodulatory systems with diffuse projections, such as the noradrenergic and the serotonergic systems. These observations suggest that at least some of the detrimental effects of sustained enforced wakefulness may be due to the continuous activity of these systems, although why this is the case and who are the victims of their damaging action remain to be identified. Consistent with this possibility, there is strong evidence that DOW sleep-deprived rats show a significant and chronic activation of catecholaminergic systems, both peripherally—increase in plasma catecholamine levels, increase in resting energy expenditure and heart rate (45)—as well as in the brain—increase in brain arylsulfotransferase (64). The enzyme arylsulfotransferase is responsible for the sulfonation of norepinephrine, dopamine, and, to a lesser extent, serotonin, and the extent of its induction during TSD is related to the duration of sleep loss. Arylsulfotransferase induction during TSD may therefore represent an attempt of the brain to counterbalance the uninterrupted activity of the central noradrenergic system.

We are currently investigating whether the DOW syndrome is at least partly due to chronic catecholaminergic hyperactivity. It is important to remember here that several factors that could potentially explain the syndrome and its final outcome, such as a decrease in body temperature or infections, have already been ruled out (27,45). Moreover, as mentioned before, energy expenditure increases early in long-term sleep deprivation, and this increase is correlated with survival time. However, as shown by Rechtschaffen et al. (27), an increase in energy expenditure per se without sleep loss does not cause the DOW syndrome. An attempt to block the increase in plasma catecholamines with the peripheral sympathetic blocking agent guanethidine was previously unsuccessful because an increase in epinephrine levels compensated for the missed increase in norepinephrine levels (65). In our experiments, a central block of the noradrenergic system is achieved by treating rats with DSP-4, a neurotoxin specific for the noradrenergic fibers of the locus coeruleus. If the hypothesis is correct, after central noradrenergic lesions the TSD syndrome should be reduced in intensity and its fatal consequences perhaps delayed or prevented.

VII.   NREM vs. REM Rebound After Sleep Deprivation

Studies in rats and other species show that short-term sleep deprivation (less than 24 hr) produces a rebound of both NREM sleep and REM sleep, whereas long-term sleep deprivation (several days) produces mainly a rebound of REM sleep [(30,52) and references therein; see also (66)]. At face value, this observation could suggest that REM sleep is more restorative than NREM sleep—the more sleep an animal has lost, the more urgent it becomes to recover REM sleep. A plausible biological interpretation of the preeminence of REM sleep rebound after long-term sleep deprivation could be the following. As reviewed above, long-term sleep deprivation is associated with a chronic activation of catecholaminergic systems. It is well established that the activity of the noradrenergic and serotonergic systems, which is high in waking, is reduced during NREM sleep. During REM sleep, however, it is completely abolished. If a fundamental function of sleep were to interrupt the activity of catecholaminergic systems, REM sleep would offer more relief than NREM sleep, especially after extreme waking.

There are, however, alternative explanations. The animal studies of long-term sleep deprivation that produce a preferential rebound of REM sleep were characterized, as reviewed above, by a significant and unavoidable amount of NREM sleep during the deprivation procedure, typically around 10–20% of the recording time with the DOW method (30,52). Such "leakage" of slow-wave activity in the form of microsleep episodes could account for the much reduced NREM rebound observed after long-term sleep deprivation. Additional leakage may occur in the form of local sleep in circumscribed neuronal populations in the context of waking-like behavior and electroencephalography ("piecemeal sleep"). The latter possibility is consistent with the increased levels of power in the delta frequency band in animals kept awake for 24 hr (16,34,67). The "leakage" hypothesis is also consistent with the few studies in which NREM sleep could be completely prevented; NREM then constituted a significant portion of rebound sleep.

The previously mentioned study by Lucas (39) provides a direct comparison of a nonleakage versus a leakage condition. Continuous electrical stimulation of the reticular formation, which kept cats uninterruptedly awake for 3 days, produced a strong rebound of NREM sleep followed by REM sleep. By contrast, intermittent stimulation that allowed microsleeps produced mainly REM sleep rebound. Another example is provided by the study by Levitt (15), in which sleep deprivation was enforced for 24 hr using either *d*-amphetamine or a treadmill. Behavioral observation and electroencephalographic recording confirmed that the first method totally prevented microsleeps, whereas the second did not. Recovery sleep was characterized by a rebound of both NREM and REM sleep with *d*-amphetamine, and of REM sleep only with the treadmill. Additional evidence comes from human studies (68–71), where the methods used to enforce sleep deprivation (motivational factors, social interactions, resort to demanding tasks) may be effective at avoiding substantial microsleep episodes for a longer time, consistent with the longer time constant of the buildup of slow-wave activity compared to other species (67). In all such studies in which recovery sleep was studied, chronic TSD was followed by a sleep rebound of both NREM and REM sleep, though unfortunately the EEG was not consistently recorded during the sleep deprivation period.

VIII. Conclusions

The most popular methods of short-term TSD in animals include gentle handling and forced locomotion by treadmill-type systems. Gentle handing is probably the preferred method, but an effort should be made to also stimulate the control animals when using this technique. For TSD longer than 24 hr, DOW is the method of choice because of its efficacy and the presence of a yoked control. Controls are essential to rule out nonspecific effects due to the stimulation used to enforce wakefulness. Sleep deprivation is inherently stressful, and the specific "stress of being awake" cannot be eliminated from a sleep deprivation experiment. Perhaps the most important lesson derived from hundreds of sleep deprivation experiments using the most elaborate and ingenious techniques is that sleep can only be prevented for a few hours. No matter which arousing stimulus is used, it is soon overcome by the synchronization of the thalamocortical system. This view was taken by Dement (72) as an indication of the serious limits of any experimental sleep deprivation method. Before that, however, this view should be taken as an indication of the paramount importance of sleep.

References

1. Crile GW. Studies in exhaustion. Arch Surg 1921; 2:196–220.
2. Tobler I, Franken P, Scherschlicht R. Sleep and EEG spectra in the rabbit under baseline conditions and following sleep deprivation. Physiol Behav 1990; 48:121–129.
3. Tobler I, Scherschlicht R. Sleep and EEG slow-wave activity in the domestic cat: effect of sleep deprivation. Behav Brain Res 1990; 37:109–118.
4. Manaceine M. Quelques observations experimentales sur l'influence de l'insomnie absolue. Arch Ital Biol 1894; XXI: 322–325.
5. Tobler I, Sigg H. Long-term motor activity recording of dogs and the effect of sleep deprivation. Experientia 1986; 42:987–991.
6. Vyazovskiy VV, Borbely A, Tobler I. Interemispheric sleep EEG asymmetry in the rat is enhanced by sleep deprivation. J Neurophysiol 2002; 88:2280–2286.
7. Franken P, Tobler I, Borbély AA. Effects of 12–h sleep deprivation and of 12-h cold exposure on sleep regulation and cortical temperature in the rat. Physiol Behav 1993; 54:885–894.
8. Vimont-Vicary P, Jouvet-Mounier D, Delorme F. Effects EEG et comportementaux des privations de sommeil paradoxal chez le chat. EEG Clin Neurophysiol 1966; 20:439–449.
9. Sternthal HS, Webb WB. Sleep deprivation of rats by punitive and non punitive procedures. Physiol Behav 1986; 37:249–252.
10. Stefurak SJ, Stefurak ML, Mendelson WB, Gillin JC, Wyatt RJ. A method for sleep depriving rats. Pharmacol Biochem Behav 1977; 6:137–139.
11. Borbély AA, Neuhaus HU. Sleep deprivation: effects on sleep and EEG in the rat. J Comp Physiol 1979; 133:71-87.
12. Jouvet D, Vimont P, Delorme F, Jouvet M. Etude de la privation selective de la phase paradoxale de sommeil chez le chat. C R Soc Biol Lyon 1964; 158:756–759.
13. Mendelson WB, Guthrie RD, Frederick G, Wyatt RJ. The flower pot technique of rapid eye movement (REM) sleep deprivation. Pharmacol Biochem Behav 1974; 2:553–556.
14. Porkka-Heiskanen T, Smith SE, Taira T, Urban JH, Levine JE, Turek FW, Stenberg D. Noradrenergic activity in rat brain during rapid eye movement sleep deprivation and rebound sleep. Am J Physiol 1995; 268: R1456–1463.
15. Levitt RA. Paradoxical sleep: activation by sleep deprivation. J Comp Physiol Psychol 1967; 63: 505–509.
16. Friedman L, Bergmann BM, Rechtschaffen A. Effects of sleep deprivation on sleepiness, sleep intensity, and subsequent sleep in the rat. Sleep 1979; 1:369–391.
17. Tobler I, Jaggi K. Sleep and EEG spectra in the Syrian hamster (*Mesocricetus auratus*) under baseline conditions and following sleep deprivation. J Comp Physiol A 1987; 161: 449–459.
18. Bast TH. Morphological changes in fatigue. Wisconsin Med J 1925; 24:371-372.

19. Leake C, Grab JA, Senn MJ. Studies in exhaustion due to lack of sleep. Am J Physiol 1927; 92; 127–130.

20. Webb WB, Agnew HW. Sleep deprivation, age, and exhaustion time in the rat. Science 1962; 136: 1122.

21. Tobler I, Neuner-Jehle M. 24-h variation of vigilance in the cockroach *Blaberus giganteus*. J Sleep Res 1991; 1:231-239.

22. Tobler I, Stalder J. Rest in the scorpion—a sleep-like state? J Comp Physiol A 1988; 163:227–235.

23. Sauer S, Herrmann E, Kaiser W. The effect of forced activity on a behavioral sleep sign in honey bees. Sleep Res Online 1999; 2 (suppl. 1): 217.

24. Hendricks JC, Finn SM, Panckeri KA, Chavkin J, Williams JA, Sehgal A, Pack AI. Rest in *Drosophila* is a sleep-like state. Neuron 2000; 25:129–38.

25. Shaw PJ, Cirelli C, Greenspan RJ, Tononi G. Correlates of sleep and waking in *Drosophila melanogaster*. Science 2000; 287:1834–1837.

26. Rechtschaffen A, Gilliland MA, Bergmann BM, Winter JB. Physiological correlates of prolonged sleep deprivation in rats. Science 1983; 221:182–184.

27. Rechtschaffen A, Bergmann BM, Everson CA, Kushida CA, Gilliland MA. Sleep deprivation in the rat: X. Integration and discussion of the findings. Sleep 1989; 12:68–87.

28. Cirelli C, Shaw PJ, Rechtschaffen A, Tononi G. No evidence of brain cell degeneration after long-term sleep deprivation in rats. Brain Res 1999; 840:184–193.

29. Ramanathan L, Gulyani S, Nienhuis R, Siegel JM. Sleep deprivation decreases superoxide dismutase activity in rat hippocampus and brainstem. Neuroreport 2002; 13:1387–1390.

30. Rechtschaffen A, Bergmann BM, Gilliland MA, Bauer K. Effects of method, duration, and sleep stage on rebounds from sleep deprivation in the rat. Sleep 1999; 22:11-31.

31. Mistlberger R, Bergmann B, Rechtschaffen A. Period-amplitude analysis of rat electroencephalogram: effects of sleep deprivation and exercise. Sleep 1987; 10:508–522.

32. Webb WB, Friedmann J. Activity as a determinant of sleep in rats. Psychophysiology 1969; 6:272.

33. Hanagasioglu M, Borbély AA. Effect of voluntary locomotor activity on sleep in the rat. Behav Brain Res 1982; 4:359–368.

34. Franken P, Dijk DJ, Tobler I, Borbely AA. Sleep deprivation in rats: effects on EEG power spectra, vigilance states, and cortical temperature. Am J Physiol 1991; 261:R198–208.

35. Feinberg I, Campbell IG. Total sleep deprivation in the rat transiently abolishes the delta amplitude response to darkness: implications for the mechanism of the "negative delta rebound." J Neurophysiol 1993; 70:2695–2699.

36. Youngstedt SD, O'Connor PJ, Dishman RK. The effects of acute exercise on sleep: a quantitative synthesis. Sleep 1997; 20:203–214.

37. Detari L, Kukorelli T, Hajnik T. Long-term sleep deprivation by hypothalamic stimulation in cats. J Neurosci Meth 1993; 49:225–230.

38. Gvilia I, Darchia N, Oniani T. Ethological analysis of sleep deprivation effects in the rats. J Sleep Res 2002; 11(S1):89.

39. Lucas EA. Effects of five to seven days of sleep deprivation produced by electrical stimulation of the midbrain reticular formation. Exp Neurol 1975; 49:554–568.

40. Levitt RA. Sleep deprivation in the rat. Science 1966; 153:85–87.

41. Gonzalez MM, Valatx JL, Debilly G. Role of the locus coeruleus in the sleep rebound following two different sleep deprivation methods in the rat. Brain Res 1996; 740:215–226.

42. Lin JS, Gervasoni D, Hou Y, Vanni-Mercier G, Rambert F, Frydman A, Jouvet M. Effects of amphetamine and modafinil on the sleep/wake cycle during experimental hypersomnia induced by sleep deprivation in the cat. J Sleep Res 2000; 9:89–96.

43. Caldwell JA, Smythe NK, Leduc PA, Caldwell JL. Efficacy of Dexedrine for maintaining aviator performance during 64 hours of sustained wakefulness: a simulator study.Aviat Space Environ Med 2000; 71:7–18.

44. Shaw PJ, Bergmann BM, Rechtschaffen A. Effects of paradoxical sleep deprivation on thermoregulation in the rat. Sleep 1998; 21:7–17.

45. Rechtschaffen A, Bergmann BM. Sleep deprivation in the rat: an update of the 1989 paper. Sleep 2002; 25:18–24.

46. Shaw PJ, Tononi G, Greenspan RJ, Robinson DF. Stress response genes protect against lethal effects of sleep deprivation in *Drosophila*. Nature 2002; 417:287–291.

47. Siegel J, Gordon TP. Paradoxical sleep: deprivation in the cat. Science 1965; 148:978–980.

48. Pickett JP, ed. The American Heritage Dictonary of the English Language. 4th ed. Boston: Houghton Mifflin, 2000.

49. McEwen B. Introduction: stress and the nervous system. Semin Neurosci 1994; 6:195–196.

50. Takahashi Y, Ebihara S, Nakamura Y, Takahashi K. A model of human sleep-related growth hormone secretion in dogs: effects of 3, 6, and 12 hours of forced wakefulness on plasma growth hormone, cortisol, and sleep stages. Endocrinology 1981; 109: 262–272.

51. Tobler I, Murison R, Ursin R, Ursin H, Borbely AA. The effect of sleep deprivation and recovery sleep on plasma corticosterone in the rat. Neurosci Lett 1983; 35:297–300.

52. Rechtschaffen A, Bergmann BM. Sleep stage priorities in rebound from sleep deprivation: a response to Feinberg. Sleep 1999; 22:1025–1030.

53. Hairston IS, Ruby NF, Brooke S, Peyron C, Denning DP, Heller HC, Sapolsky RM. Sleep deprivation elevates plasma corticosterone levels in neonatal rats.Neurosci Lett 2001; 315: 29–32.

54. Campbell IG, Guinan MJ, Horowitz JM. Sleep deprivation impairs long-term potentiation in rat hippocampal slices. J Neurophysiol 2002; 88:1073–1076.

55. Dallman MF, Akana SF, Bradbury MJ, Strack AM, Hanson ES, Scribner KA. Regulation of the hypothalamo-pituitary-adrenal axis during stress: feedback, facilitation and feeding. Semin Neurosci 1994; 6:205–213.

56. Kant GJ, Pastel RH, Bauman RA, Meininger GR, Maughan KR, Robinson TN 3rd, Wright WL, Covington PS. Effects of chronic stress on sleep in rats. Physiol Behav 1995; 57:359–365.

57. Paré WP. The effect of chronic environmental stress on stomach ulceration, adrenal function, and consummatory behavior in the rat. J Psychol 1964; 57:143–151.

58. McCarty R. Regulation of plasma catecholamine responses to stress. Semin Neurosci 1994; 6:197–204.

59. Cheeta S, Ruigt G, van Proosdij J, Willner P. Changes in sleep architecture following chronic mild stress. Biol Psychiatry 1997; 41:419–427.
60. Rial RV, Nicolau MC, Gamundi A, Akaarir M, Pereda E, Gonzalez J. Sleep deprivation and learned helplessness: are they different? J Sleep Res 2002; 11(S1):191.
61. Petty F, Chae Y, Kramer G, Jordan S, Wilson L. Learned helplessness sensitizes hippocampal norepinephrine to mild restress. Biol Psychiatry 1994; 35:903–908.
62. Adrien J, Dugovic C, Martin P. Sleep-wakefulness patterns in the helpless rat.Physiol Behav 1991; 49:257–262.
63. Martin P, Soubrie P, Simon P. Shuttle-box deficits induced by inescapable shocks in rats: reversal by the beta-adrenoreceptor stimulants clenbuterol and salbutamol. Pharmacol Biochem Behav 1986; 24:177–181.
64. Cirelli C, Tononi G. Changes in gene expression in the cerebral cortex of rats after short-term and long-term sleep deprivation. Sleep 1999; 22(S1):113.
65. Pilcher JJ, Bergmann BM, Fang VS, Refetoff S, Rechtschaffen A. Sleep deprivation in the rat: XI. The effect of guanethidine-induced sympathetic blockade on the sleep deprivation syndrome. Sleep 1990;13:218–231.
66. Kiyono S, Kawamoto T, Sakakura H, Iwama K. Effects of sleep deprivation upon the paradoxical phase of sleep in cats. EEG Clin Neurophysiol 1965; 19: 34–40.
67. Huber R, Deboer T, Tobler I. Effects of sleep deprivation on sleep and sleep EEG in three mouse strains: empirical data and simulations. Brain Res 2000; 857:8–19.
68. Berger RJ, Oswald I. Effects of sleep deprivation on behavior, subsequent sleep, and dreaming. J Mental Sci 1962; 108: 457–465.
69. Gulevich G, Dement W, Johnson L. Psychiatric and EEG observations on a case of prolonged (264 hours) wakefulness. Arch Gen Psychiatry 1966; 15:29–35.
70. Kales A, Tan TL, Kollar EJ, Naitoh P, Preston TA, Malmstrom EJ. Sleep patterns following 205 hours of sleep deprivation. Psychosom Med 1970; 32:189–200.
71. Naitoh P, Kales A, Kollar EJ, Smith JC, Jacobson A. Electroencephalographic activity after prolonged sleep loss. Electroencephalogr Clin Neurophysiol 1969; 27:2–11.
72. Dement WC. Sleep deprivation and the organization of behavioral states. In: Clemente CD, Purpura DP, Mayer FE, eds. Sleep and the Maturing Nervous System. New York: Academic Press, 1972:319–355.

5

Partial and Sleep-State Selective Deprivation

CAROL A. LANDIS

University of Washington, Seattle, Washington, U.S.A.

I. Introduction

This chapter provides an overview of methods and procedures used to experimentally induce partial or sleep-state selective deprivation (SSSD) in humans and in animals. The chapter describes limitations of the various deprivation methods as well as potential confounding variables and threats to validity in the interpretation and generalizability of study findings. Instrumental methods rather than pharmacological methods and procedures for partial and SSSD are described. Psychoactive stimulants enhance waking and have been used to restrict sleep. Similarly, hypnotics, analgesics, and antidepressant medications reduce non-REM (NREM) stages 3 and 4; dose dependently reduce rapid-eye-movement (REM) sleep (1); and could be used to induce a relative SSSD. However, the interpretation of findings is rendered far more complex when drugs are used. Drug dose, pharmacokinetic properties, an individual's sensitivity and reactivity, as well as side effects must be taken into consideration in the interpretation of the findings.

II. Definitions of Partial Sleep and Sleep-State Selective Deprivation

The definition of partial sleep deprivation (SD) usually refers to preventing individuals from obtaining their usual amount of daily sleep (2,3). This is typically accomplished in humans by restricting time in bed at night and prohibiting day-time naps. Partial SD is analogous to a restricted sleep schedule in which sleep is limited to 3–5 rather than 7–8 hr. SSSD refers to depriving subjects of a specific sleep stage. NREM stages 3 and/or 4 (slow-wave sleep in humans or its equivalent in animals) or REM sleep are the usual target stages in SSSD experiments.

III. Experimental Studies in Humans

A. Partial Sleep Deprivation

Partial SD is considered the easiest method of restricting sleep and can be accomplished in several ways. Sleep time is reduced by advancing sleep offset time (early partial SD), delaying sleep onset time (late partial SD), both advancing sleep offset and delaying sleep onset, or permitting a daily brief sleep episode during an experiment that extends over several consecutive days. Partial SD is most analogous to every day experience when sleep is restricted because of work or school schedules, travel, and social activities. Partial SD can be used to simulate daily life situations or those during extreme or unusual circumstances (e.g., war, space flight, or natural disasters), when individuals must be alert and are prohibited from obtaining their usual amount of sleep (4). Classic partial SD studies focused on describing changes in sleep architecture during the restricted sleep period and in comparing performance outcomes to those of total sleep deprivation (2,5). Health consequences of partial SD have been systematically investigated in controlled experiments only in recent years (6–10).

Partial SD experiments vary with respect to duration, time of night, and number of consecutive nights of sleep restriction. Typically, time in bed is limited to 4 hr or less in laboratory-based studies extended over several consecutive days. Partial SD protocols have been continued for a week to several weeks (11,12). Because in humans most slow-wave sleep (SWS) occurs in the first third of a night and most REM sleep occurs in the latter third of the night, partial SD of 4 hr or less will differentially reduce REM sleep with minimal effects on the amount of SWS obtained during the restricted sleep period. Results from a classic study showed that REM sleep was reduced by more than 60% compared to baseline with time in bed limited to 3 hr/night for eight consecutive nights (5). In this study, during the restricted sleep period, the percentage of NREM stage 4 was greater and the percentages of other sleep stages were reduced relative to baseline nights, regardless of whether sleep was permitted in the first third or the middle third of the night. Early partial SD differentially reduces REM sleep with minimal effects on SWS or delta activity as a measure of NREM sleep intensity (13). However, when sleep onset time is delayed by several hours (late partial SD), there is an immediate rebound of SWS and of delta activity when sleep is permitted. Greater amounts of REM sleep with shorter onset latencies also have been reported after late partial SD (14). The actual amount of delta activity or REM sleep obtained following sleep delay is dependent, in part, on the strength of the homeostatic sleep drive, the timing of the protocol with respect to the subject's circadian sleep-wake rhythm, and the duration of time in bed permitted.

Partial SD is relatively easy to implement in clinical studies. Since it differentially reduces REM sleep, and since REM sleep deprivation has been associated with clinical improvement in depression, investigators have assessed effects of early partial SD on elevating mood in depression (15) and relieving symptoms in premenstrual dysphoric disorder (16). Sleep delay protocols have been used in clinical populations to assess the integrity and responsiveness of homeostatic processes involved in sleep state regulation (17).

B. Sleep-State Selective Deprivation

SSSD experiments must be carried out in a laboratory setting and are both arduous and time consuming. The removal of REM or stages 4 and/or 3 sleep requires the recognition of electrophysiological state indicators. With careful monitoring, an individual can be deprived almost completely of either stage for a few consecutive nights. Total sleep time is well preserved in human SSSD as subjects obtain more stages 1 and 2 sleep with the loss of REM or SWS. As the deprivation duration is increased, REM or SWS processes intensify and small amounts of these sleep stages are obtained.

Selective REM Sleep Deprivation

Dement (18) conducted the first selective REM sleep deprivation study in humans. The investigator awakened the subjects after the onset of each REM period. Following baseline nights most subjects were subjected to five consecutive nights of REM deprivation followed by recovery. In this classic study (18) and in a more recent study (19), subjects also participated in a subsequent series of control experiments in which NREM sleep was interrupted an equal number of times and for the same number of nights as in the REM deprivation protocol. Techniques such as acoustic devices or electric foot shock have been developed to disrupt REM sleep automatically based on electrophysiological signals of REM sleep onset (20–22). However, these techniques are less effective in removing REM sleep than human monitoring of polysomnograhic REM sleep indicators and manual arousal (e.g., calling the subject's name or gently shaking the subject) (19,23,24).

Classic studies of REM sleep deprivation relied on the identification of rapid eye movements as an indication of REM sleep onset (18,25). When rapid eye movements are used as the sole criteria for the identification of epochs of REM sleep, subjects will be deprived of phasic but not tonic [desynchronized electroencephalogram (EEG), low electromyogram (EMG) amplitude, absent eye movements] REM sleep. Recently, investigators used the presence of a desynchronized EEG with absence of spindles and K complexes along with a reduction in EMG amplitude with or without rapid eye movements to identify the onset of REM sleep episodes (19). These investigators argued that standard criteria require retroactive, not prospective, identification of rapid eye movements to identify REM sleep.

Selective REM deprivation has been compared to selective deprivation of stage 4 sleep (20). Stage 4 sleep was interrupted by brief (200-msec) strong foot shock (5–15 ma) whenever five delta waves appeared in a 1-min epoch. The number (not specified) and intensity of shocks were delivered to change the EEG toward stage 2 or stage 1 sleep. REM deprivation was carried out in a similar manner based on muscle tone, eye movements, and desynchronized EEGs. The stimulation requirements to remove either REM sleep or SWS differ by time of night and increase as the number of deprivation nights is increased. For example, the mean number of 1-min epochs required to reduce stage 4 was four times that of REM, but the stimulation intensity requirements also differed by thirds of the night and in opposite directions (20). Subjects required more stimulation to remove stage 4 in the first and second thirds of the night, and more stimulation to reduce REM sleep in the last third of the night. The number required to interrupt REM sleep was fivefold higher in the last third than in the first third of the night.

Selective SWS Deprivation

In SWS deprivation studies, a noise stimulus is most often used to disrupt stage 4 and/or stage 3 sleep based on visual recognition of electroencephalographic delta wave activity during a designated recording interval. The type, frequency (e.g., 1000–2000 Hz) and intensity (e.g., 40–110 dB) of the noise stimulus vary among studies (26–30). Some investigators simply call the subject's name (31). The number of delta waves and the epoch duration required prior to stimulus delivery varies among studies depending on whether deprivation of stage 4 or SWS is the goal (21,26,28,29,31,32). The duration of the stimulus usually is maintained until evidence of stage 2 or stage 1 sleep is obvious in the EEG. In some studies signs of movement arousal were needed to terminate the stimulus (26). In other studies, actual awakening was desired in order for subjects to carry out various tasks to avoid falling immediately back to sleep (19,31).

Automated computer systems have been developed for the selective SWS deprivation (28,33). In one study, the detection and summation of low (0.5–2 Hz) and high (8–11.5 and 14.5–35 Hz) frequency electroencephalographic activity (power) was used to turn a buzzer (2000-Hz tone) on and off, respectively (28). The threshold for detecting low-frequency activity (3/sec) was established on adaptation and baseline nights. As expected, increasingly louder tones were needed as time in deprivation increased. If low-frequency waves were still present in the EEG 15 sec after delivery of the maximal tone, the technician called the subject's name or tapped on the wall between the control room and the bedroom until the low-frequency activity disappeared. By the third night of selective SWS deprivation, the technicians occasionally had to go into the subject's room and gently shake the subject's shoulder. Although automated systems are capable of disrupting SWS, they still require human monitoring and intervention to induce SSSD.

C. Research Design and Procedures in Human Studies

A within-subject design is used in most partial and state-selective sleep deprivation studies. Outcomes of interest are not routinely assessed in a separate control group. On rare occasions the same subjects have been studied in a separate sleep disruption condition as a control for state-selective deprivation in a counterbalanced crossover design (14,31,34). The number of subjects in most studies is small. Except in clinical populations, healthy young men, ages 20–30 years, with presumably stable sleep patterns have been studied. Although young women also have been subjects, the timing of the study with respect to the phase of the menstrual cycle has not been controlled consistently (14,35). The extent of subject screening about medical and psychiatric history as well as habitual sleep habits varies considerably among studies (6,9,11,12,18,19,23,24,36). In some studies, the hours of sleep restriction were established and standardized across subjects without regard to the individual's usual circadian sleep-wake schedule. With increased recognition of the contribution of circadian regulation of sleep and wake states, protocols have been based on prestudy assessments of habitual sleep onset time and duration (13). In laboratory-based studies, sleep is usually monitored throughout baseline, experimental, and recovery nights. Subjects have been supervised to ensure adherence to the sleep restriction protocol throughout all experimental days (5,14) or they have been permitted to carry out their daily routines only being monitored in the laboratory at night (11,25). Some investigators use actigraphy combined with daily self-report sleep logs, or rely only on questionnaires to monitor adherence to sleep restriction (7,12,13,19,36,37). In a few studies, activity levels and dietary intake have been standardized. Most often, subjects are permitted to carry out their normal activities and to consume their usual diet. However, subjects are usually asked to refrain from consuming food and beverages containing caffeine or alcohol during all experimental days, but adherence to these instructions is only rarely confirmed by laboratory blood or urine analysis (19). Investigators sometimes control ambient temperature, activity levels, and light exposure in order to avoid shifts in circadian rhythm phase (37).

IV. Experimental Studies in Animals

A. Partial Sleep Deprivation

Compared to humans, there have been far fewer partial SD studies in animals. Sleep in animals is polyphasic, and the sleep cycle duration is shorter such that partial SD experiments require 24-hr monitoring and frequent awakenings to prevent or disrupt sleep. Gentle handling of animals housed in standard recording cages has been used to study short-term (e.g., 3 and 6 hr) sleep deprivation effects on subsequent intensity of NREM sleep in rats during the light (inactive) period of the diurnal cycle (38). Partial SD in rats has been induced by walking on a slowly rotating wheel (one rotation/min) or a wheel placed in an environment in which walking was necessary to avoid being submerged in water with sleep time in home cages restricted to 4 of 24 hr (39–40). Most sleep deprivation studies for ≤6 to 12 hours are considered short-term total sleep deprivation, and the animals often are sacrificed without undergoing recovery sleep. The platform method of selective REM deprivation (see below) has been used to induce sleep loss for 10 hr during the light period (41). When rats were maintained in constant lighting conditions, placed on small platforms surrounded by water for 11.5 hr, and put in standard recording cages for the next 11.5 hr, almost complete total SD occurred during the period on small platforms, followed by an immediate rebound and recovery sleep. In this situation, total sleep time was not different from that obtained during a 24-hr recording in standard cages (pilot studies, unpublished observations). It is nearly impossible to instrumentally restrict total sleep time and induce partial sleep loss in animals without constant monitoring and stimulation.

B.   Sleep-State Selective Deprivation

REM sleep deprivation has been the most common type of SSSD in animals. The term REM sleep will be used although many investigators use the term paradoxical sleep for animals. An ideal REM deprivation experiment in animals would be similar to that in humans; REM sleep would be interrupted selectively, total sleep time would be preserved, and adequate controls would be established for the non-specific effects from stimuli used to disrupt sleep. Based on electrophysiological criteria, experimental animals would be aroused at the onset of each REM episode, and NREM sleep in a control group would be interrupted randomly an equal number of times. One of the first selective REM deprivation experiments combined forced walking on a treadmill with manual stimulation ("hand" awakenings) by investigators to interrupt REM sleep (42). Cats were forced to walk on or next to a slowly moving treadmill (1 m/min) and ride for short intervals (20 sec) on the belt for 15–16 hr to maintain wakefulness. For the remaining 8 hr, the cats were housed in recording cages with access to food and water, and the investigators monitored and manually aroused the cats each time electrophysiological signs of REM sleep appeared in the recording. Similar procedures were carried out in controls, except the cats were aroused from NREM sleep and permitted REM sleep. Investigators considered that these procedures controlled for the stimuli used to disrupt sleep, but the experiments were laborious and time consuming, often involving hundreds of arousals during the recording period (42). This protocol actually combined total SD with selective REM deprivation, thus leading to effects that could result from their interaction (43).

Platform Techniques of REM Sleep Deprivation

Classic Single Platform

Jouvet and colleagues introduced the classic single-platform technique for selective REM sleep deprivation in the cat (44). This technique is also called the pedestal or water tank procedure and was adapted to deprive mice and rats of

REM sleep (43,45,46). The single-platform technique is the most popular method of selective REM sleep deprivation and has been used extensively in rats. In this technique, a rat is placed in an apparatus or chamber, such as a plastic bucket (e.g., 25 cm diameter), containing a small platform; often an inverted flower pot fitted with a round plexiglas top (e.g., 4.5–8 cm diameter). During adaptation, the container is filled with wood shavings. At the start of deprivation, the shavings are replaced with water, either to within 1 cm of the platform or 1 cm deep in the bottom of the bucket. The rat sits or crouches on the platform to avoid the water. At the start of each REM period, as muscle tone decreases, the animal arouses itself briefly when its nose hits the water or it loses its balance, occasionally falling off the platform. As the deprivation period is prolonged, the rat may fall into the water more frequently. The typical control is to place an animal in a similar environment on a large platform (e.g., 10–18 cm diameter) that is considered sufficient space for it to obtain sleep.

Electrophysiological recordings of animals on small platforms have shown a greater loss of REM sleep than animals on large platforms, but NREM sleep was also reduced (47–49). Rats on either size platform obtained the least amount of REM sleep during the first 24 hr of deprivation. In one study from day 1 to day 2 and from day 3 to day 4, rats on small platforms showed increasing amounts of REM sleep but decreasing amounts of HS2 (analogous to human SWS) (49). Although decreased from baseline, rats on large platforms showed stable amounts of both REM and HS2 sleep from days 2–4. It is commonly assumed that animals on large platforms obtain near-normal amounts of sleep. However, during the first 24–48 hr of deprivation, rats were often observed sleeping near the edge of the large platform underneath the feeder (48). In this position, the rat would be aroused at the onset of REM sleep in a similar fashion as rats on small platforms. The size of the platform with respect to the weight of the animal is important in terms of the extent of REM sleep lost for animals on small and large platforms (50-51). That is, the ratio of surface area of the small platform to the animal's body weight was suggested to be 14 $cm^2/100$ g for maximal REM sleep deprivation. For the large platform, the suggested ratio was 58 $cm^2/100$ g (47). It is assumed that animals on small platforms experience more arousals and water exposure than animals on large platforms, although some investigators have reported no group differences between animals on small compared to large platforms (43). Animals exposed to swimming for 1 hr/day have been used and advocated as a control group for water exposure (47). Other investigators used additional controls with animals placed on small platforms but removed from the apparatus for 6 hr/day, and NREM sleep was disrupted with the same frequency as the animals on small platforms (45).

The platform technique is simple to implement and is less intrusive in that external stimuli are not required to arouse the animal. The animal is placed in an environment in which it cannot nest and curl up in a corner of the cage. The animal quickly learns to self-arouse at REM sleep onset and rarely falls into the water. With other REM deprivation techniques an animal is forced to walk on a slowly rotating wheel or treadmill, shaken, or manually disturbed by an investigator at the onset of a REM episode. The platform method is effective for removing most of REM sleep for approximately 72 hr (48). If water depth is limited to 1 cm in the bottom of the bucket, the animal gets minimal water exposure. However, it learns to sleep stretched out over the top of the small platform such that by the fourth day REM sleep episodes of several minutes duration can be obtained. As more REM sleep is obtained, the amount of NREM sleep, especially SWS, is reduced. For practical purposes, this technique is popular because a number of animals can be deprived of REM sleep simultaneously but electrophysiological recordings are not routinely done.

Despite practical considerations, from the earliest studies, investigators were unsatisfied with the platform technique because there were no adequate controls for confounding variables—water exposure, damp humid environment, stress response [hypothalamic-pituitary-adrenal (HPA) activation], restricted movement, and social isolation. Large platforms have been considered adequate controls for water exposure and increased humidity, and animals on both small and large platforms showed similar weight loss and signs of the stress response (adrenal enlargement, thymus involution, corticosterone concentration in plasma) (43). A control used by some investigators for the damp, humid environment involved fitting a small platform with a cuff or lip that allowed the animal to curl up and sleep on top of the small platform but restricted movement (52).

Multiple Platform Technique

Multiple small platforms in a single apparatus with one rat (52) or multiple small platforms and multiple rats have been used with the intent to control confounding variables of immobility and social isolation (53–55). A modification of the multiple-platform method has also been used to deprive individual kittens of REM sleep (56). The multiple-platform/multiple-rat technique has been used with 5 rats and 7 platforms or 10 rats and 18 platforms. Control rats were placed in similar conditions with large platforms. Validation of the extent of lost REM sleep has been carried out with the multiple-platform/multiple-rat technique but the apparatus was modified so that wire mesh separated the animals, effectively creating the single-platform condition with restricted movement and social isolation (54). The multiple-platform/multiple-rat technique is associated with increased social conflict and greater HPA axis activity compared to animals on single platforms (57). Thus, social isolation was replaced by social conflict, a new confounding variable that investigators have tried to control (58).

Other Methods of REM Sleep Deprivation

Methods in Adult Animals

Direct brain stimulation, the pendulum or swing technique, and a cold ambient environment are examples of methods that have been used to induce REM deprivation in adult animals.

Electrical Stimulation. Electrical stimulation of the midbrain reticular formation at the onset of REM episodes was found to be less effective in removing REM sleep than the small-platform technique in rats (59). Direct brain stimulation was carried out in those animals that showed a two to three times higher threshold for emotional responses compared to raising the head, which was the typical arousal response. The arousal stimulus (0.1 msec, 100 Hz, amplitude 2–12 V, duration 0.5–2 sec) was activated when the EEG showed cortical desynchronization, a hippocampal theta rhythm, and reduced EMG. The animals usually obtained 3–8 sec of REM sleep prior to arousal. If the animals failed to arouse the amplitude of the stimulation was increased. Unlike other REM deprivation methods, direct brain stimulation led to lower adrenal gland weight.

Pendulum or Swing Technique. The pendulum technique involved a slowly rotating apparatus (divided into three separate compartments) that resembled a swing (60). During deprivation the apparatus continuously oscillated back and forth between two extremes (a 42-degree angle from the horizontal plane) producing awakenings. Postural balance was lost at the extremes, and the rat quickly learned to walk toward the other side of the cage to avoid exerting effort to maintain balance or tumbling about the cage. The bottom of the cage was covered with a rough surface to prevent the rats from sliding and the top was covered with wire mesh to prevent escape. The speed of the cage oscillations was adjusted to increase the number of awakenings, thereby presumably permitting NREM sleep but preventing REM sleep. The control condition involved a continuously moving swing without extreme tilts. The pendulum technique avoided exposing animals to a wet and humid environment. Although sleep was only assessed during the light period, the pendulum technique was effective in reducing REM sleep, but decreased amounts of SWS were also observed over a 3-day deprivation period (60). When the pendulum technique was compared to the single small-platform technique and to the single-rat/multiple-platform technique, REM sleep was reduced equally by all three methods (61).

Cold Ambient Environment. Cold and hot ambient temperatures reduce REM sleep. Recently exposure to cold ambient temperatures of 0°C and –10°C for 1–2 days has been used to study the physiological regulation of REM sleep episodes (62–63). The loss of REM sleep is much higher and nearly complete at –10°C compared to 0°C. The use of extreme ambient temperatures to selectively REM deprive an animal is confounded by physiological thermoregulatory defenses and acclimation processes.

Methods in Neonatal Animals

Antidepressant drugs (e.g., clomipramine) have been administered to neonatal rats to reduce REM sleep. Recently, a new automated instrumental method has been developed for selective REM deprivation of neonatal rats by a mechanical apparatus (64). The method relies on electrophysiological recognition of electroencephalographic and electromyographic signs of REM sleep onset and the activation of a laboratory shaker device. A small Plexiglas® recording chamber that was divided in half to house a neonatal experimental rat and its yoked neonatal control rat was mounted on top of the shaker. At the onset of REM sleep in the experimental rat the computer activated the shaker, which moved in a horizontal direction, for 5 sec. Similar to the disk-over-water method (see below), the yoked control rat could sleep whenever the experimental rat was spontaneously awake. The 5-sec shaking interval "usually" was sufficient to shift the neonatal rat from REM to NREM sleep or awake. To prevent the rats from sliding about the cage floor, small screws were implanted in the cage floor. The extent of REM deprivation was affected by the oscillation speed of the shaker such that at higher speeds fewer stimulations were required and more REM sleep was lost compared with that at slower speeds. An additional control group consisted of maternally separated neonates recorded in their home cages. Maternal separation is an unavoidable confound for long-term recordings and deprivation of REM sleep in neonates.

Disk-Over-Water Method of Sleep-State Selective Deprivation

The automated computer-based disk-over-water (DOW) method for total and state-selective deprivation controlled many of the confounds introduced by other deprivation techniques (65,66; see also Chap. 4). Disk rotation (3.33 RPM), a relatively mild stimulus, was delivered equally to the experimental and control rat. In this method, the experimental rat was housed with its yoked control rat on top of a shared horizontal disk (46 cm diameter), in separate Plexiglas® square cages, each with a removable plastic cage floor. Square metal pans several centimeters deep with the same dimensions as the plastic cages were placed under the disk. The space between the two plastic cages was just large enough to hold the motor that drives disk rotation, a feeder, and a water bottle for each animal. Heat lamps were mounted above each cage to maintain cage temperature at 29°C. During recovery from surgery and adaptation to the cages, newspaper and shavings covered the plastic cage floor. At the start of baseline recordings, the metal pans were filled with water and the plastic cage floors were removed. During baseline, the disk was automatically rotated at a slow speed once each hour for 6 sec in order for the animals to become accustomed to disk movement. Baseline recordings were carried out for varying lengths of time, usually at least 5–6 days. At the start of deprivation, each time the experimental rat showed signs of sleep onset (based on 2-sec floating averages of EMG and EEG amplitude for total sleep deprivation), or the "target" stage for either high-amplitude sleep (HS2) or REM sleep deprivation, the computer automatically started disk rotation (67). The animals walked opposite to disk rotation to avoid being carried into the water. To minimize the animals' ability to ride the disk, its rotation was programmed randomly to move in either direction. The control rat could obtain sleep whenever the experimental rat was awake (e.g., grooming, eating, or rearing) and the disk was still. From arrival in the laboratory and throughout the duration of an experimental run, the rats were maintained continuously in constant light to minimize circadian fluctuations. Typically, the deprivation was halted each day for 1 hr to clean cages, weigh the animals, and weigh and replace food and water. Various control experiments were conducted to examine effects of water exposure (67), light-dark schedules (68), and chronic partial sleep loss in the selective REM (69) and NREM high-amplitude sleep deprivation (70) studies on sleep deprivation outcomes. The DOW method was found to be particularly useful for studying the effects of chronic long-term sleep deprivation but it was not completely effective or selective (66).

REM Deprivation with Disk-Over-Water Method

For REM selective deprivation, animals were implanted with depth electrodes to record ponto-geniculo-occipital (PGO) waves as well as electroencephalographic and electromyographic activity. An increase in the amplitude of the PGO wave signal combined with a drop in electroencephalographic and electromyographic activity, along with increased electroencephalographic theta activity, were used as criteria for the identification of REM (i.e., paradoxical) sleep (67,71). The use of PGO recordings permitted the almost complete removal of REM sleep episodes since an increase in PGO wave activity often preceded a drop in muscle tone. However, NREM high-amplitude sleep (HS2) was reduced 57% (69) and 30% (71). The DOW has been used to study effects of REM sleep loss over 24 hr with minimal effects on the amount of NREM sleep but substantial reductions of REM sleep (72).

SWS Deprivation with Disk-Over-Water Method

For NREM HS2 deprivation (analogous to SWS), sustained increased EEG amplitude combined with a drop in EMG amplitude was used as criteria. This is the only known report of selective SWS deprivation in animals. Because experimental rats lost much REM sleep, the rats were permitted short naps in which they obtained some HS2 and REM sleep (70). Compared to selective REM deprivation, selective deprivation of SWS in animals was quite difficult to achieve, and an interaction of the loss of both SWS and REM sleep stages could explain the results.

C. Research Design and Procedures in Animal Studies

Experimental designs with separate control groups are consistently used, although the type of control varies with the specific deprivation method. A home cage control group may be used but is not always considered in the analysis if the major comparison is between experimental and yoked control rats (67). Various animal species have been used, but male, albino rats of the Sprague-Dawley and Wistar strains have been used most frequently. Female rats and, more recently, female mice (73) have been used in SSSD studies, but estrous cycles have not been monitored. Female rats have been observed to be more active in single-platform REM deprivation cages and escaped more frequently than male rats (74). Rats of various ages and sizes have been used in REM platform studies. However, the size of the platform has been more consistent across studies than the age and weight of the animals (51). Large platforms are considered adequate control for small platforms (43). For the DOW method, rats at least 4–6 months of age were considered optimal for operation of the experimental apparatus (67). Studies vary considerably as to whether the animals are adapted to experimental cages prior to the start of deprivation and thus differ with respect to controlling for novelty effects (50). Most studies house animals in standard 12-hr light-dark cycles, with temperatures around 23°C to 25°C, with the exception of studies using the DOW method in which animals were housed in constant light and cages were maintained at 29°C. For most studies, the actual cage temperature or temperature of the water in the cage was not monitored except when necessary to prevent the rat from sleeping if the water became warm (75).

Electrophysiological recordings of sleep were consistently obtained in studies in which the timing of the deprivation stimulus was based on recognition of a particular state (42,45,64,66). Most investigators have conducted validation studies in a separate group of rats for the SSSD method selected (47–50,53–55), although the duration of the recordings varies among studies. Only a few studies have used continuous 24-hr recordings throughout the deprivation period (47,48), but some investigators limited recordings to a few hours or only report findings for the light period (54). At the present time there are no suitable techniques to validate the extent of sleep loss using multiple platforms and multiple animals with multiple platforms. Gentle handling as a means of arousing an animal is minimally described in studies that reported findings based on this method (38,42,45). Frequency of stimulation, similar to the number of arousals in the platform method, is not documented except in studies with automated computer-based systems, which quantify stimulation time.

The duration of SSSD varies from less than 24 hr to months. Most REM deprivation experiments using the platform or pendulum methods were conducted for 72 to 96 hr. However, there are reports on chronic deprivation by the platform method for as long as a week to 10 days in mice (73) and rats (76,77). Clearly some of the longest chronic SSSD experiments were carried out in rats with the DOW method (69–71).

V.   Perspectives and Limitations for Interpretation of Findings

Most methods of partial SD and SSSD lack specificity and adequate controls such that potential threats to the validity and generalizability of the study findings are ever present. Especially in animal studies it is a challenge to control confounding variables from the effects of the procedures used to disrupt sleep. Among the various methodological issues in partial SD and SSSD studies, the effectiveness of the intervention to restrict or remove sleep, subject selection bias, and the extent of stress response activation are perhaps of greatest concern. These are discussed below.

A. Effectiveness and Specificity of Sleep Deprivation Procedures

In human partial SD studies, individuals could lose disproportionately more SWS or REM depending on whether sleep offset time is advanced or sleep onset is delayed. Studies that limit both sleep offset and onset equally may reduce both SWS and REM sleep, although SWS is usually preserved at the expense of REM sleep. Objective measures of sleep are not always obtained but are required to ensure adherence to sleep restriction. In animal studies, partial SD protocols are more challenging to implement without constant stimulation and monitoring over a 24-hr period. Nevertheless, various methods such as hand arousal for short periods of time and walking on slowly rotating devices have been used to simulate sleep delay or restriction over 24 hr or longer periods of time (38–40). The DOW method in adult rats (66) and the shaker method in neonates (64) are examples of other methods that could be used to address questions of morbidity effects from chronic partial sleep loss in animals.

SSSD procedures are never complete in removing all REM or SWS; nor are they completely selective in human and in animal studies. Arousal thresholds and time to return to sleep are variables that are not controlled well in SSSD studies. Separate control groups are not routinely used to assess study outcomes. Only on rare occasions have the same subjects participated in selective deprivation and in a separate random sleep disruption protocol. In both human and animal SSSD experiments, transitional sleep stages increase and sleep continuity is disrupted. Compared to human studies, animals deprived of REM sleep often lose large amounts of high-amplitude sleep (HS2), the NREM sleep equivalent of SWS. In the only reported NREM HS2 deprivation study, rats were permitted naps in order to avoid almost complete loss of REM sleep (70). All methods of REM sleep deprivation produce reductions in NREM sleep in experimental animals, although the extent of the loss of SWS-equivalent reported varies across studies (43,47–49,54,69,71). However, the amount of NREM sleep lost was similar in the one study that compared the small- and multiple-platform technique to the pendulum technique (61).

In both partial SD and SSSD protocols, there is a potential interaction between sleep loss and circadian regulation in the timing and distribution of sleep and wake. In human studies, the status of the individual's sleep system and habitual sleep duration have not been assessed and controlled consistently before the start of the deprivation period. Novelty effects are almost impossible to eliminate in human studies. In animal studies, to avoid novelty effects, animals ought to be adapted to experimental cages and exposed to deprivation procedures during a baseline period prior to SSSD.

B. Subject Selection Bias

Subject selection bias is an important issue in partial SD and SSSD studies. Individual subject characteristics (e.g., age, sex, ethnicity, race, species) likely influence outcomes. However, mostly men and male albino rats have been the subjects in a majority of partial SD and SSSD studies. This severely limits the generalizability of findings to the greater population of interest. It has only been in the last decade that investigators have studied increased numbers of females and individuals of different racial and ethnic groups. Of necessity, volunteers are used in human studies. Personal beliefs about sleep and sleep loss and the *willingness* to undergo procedures for sleep restriction or disruption likely influences the motivation of volunteers to participate and to adhere to partial SD and SSSD protocols. In all likelihood individuals who consider themselves resistant to sleep loss effects will volunteer more readily than those who consider themselves vulnerable. Subjects are not blind to their sleep status and neither are the investigators, such that "expected" outcomes may be observed. Subject and investigator interactions may also influence the outcomes of the study. The question of bias in assessing outcomes of partial SD and SSSD experiments has to be taken into consideration in the interpretation of the findings.

C. Stress Reactivity and Responses

Sleep scientists generally admit that methods of sleep deprivation activate the stress response but debate the extent to which such activation affects the interpretation of outcomes (43,50,78–80). Although the goal has been to eliminate confounding variables (43,66), including stress response effects, such that outcomes can be attributable to sleep loss, this may be unrealistic given the inevitable interaction that occurs between sleep loss and stress response activation (80). The nature, intensity, quantity, timing, and duration of the stimulus to remove sleep have the potential to elicit a stress response. Individual reactivity to sleep loss also influences activation of the stress response (81). There is evidence that the HPA axis is centrally activated in humans after several days of partial SD (82) and in animals after several days of REM deprivation (83). Most partial SD and SSSD paradigms in animals are associated with increased plasma concentrations of adrenocorticotropic hormone (ACTH) and corticosterone (39,57,66,74,76,77,82–86). The multiple-platform/multiple-animal technique of REM deprivation has reported even higher levels of cortisocosterone in tested animals compared to those subjected to the single-platform technique (57). The small-platform and pendulum techniques of REM deprivation produce similar effects on various indicators of the stress response (87). The plasma concentration of catecholamines, indicating activation of the sympathetic nervous system, is increased also by SSSD in animals (66,76), but these indicators have not been measured very often. An interaction between sleep loss and some degree of stress response activation is unavoidable in partial SD and SSSD.

Large individual variations in outcomes are a common finding from sleep deprivation studies and could be explained by differences in stress response activation. Age and sex influence the extent of stress response activation. REM-deprived 6-month-old male rats showed higher concentrations of corticosterone compared to 3-month-old male rats (85). Female REM-deprived rats showed considerably elevated concentrations of corticosterone compared to values typically found in male rats (74). Although large variability in outcomes may be related to individual vulnerability factors, e.g., genetic predisposition, prior sleep history, age, sex, personal characteristics, and psychological status, individual differences in the reactivity of the stress system to sleep loss procedures are possible yet are rarely studied.

Sleep deprivation effects could contribute or actually lead to HPA axis activation (66,72,88). Recent evidence has shown that partial sleep loss in animals was associated with a small increase in ACTH and corticosterone (39). In chronic SSSD by the DOW method it is likely that as the animals developed greater energy expenditure needs, thermoregulatory system impairments, and decubitus ulcers, the stress system would become activated. However, the syndrome produced by chronic total and SSSD in rats is unique and has distinctive features that are not typical of other stress paradigms (72,79,88–90). The lack of large increases in ACTH and in corticosterone could be related to sleep pressure that dampens central activation of the neuroendocrine stress response. When the deprivation procedures were halted, neuroendocrine indices of stress response activation fell quite rapidly, to levels throughout recovery that were below those of baseline (91). Interactions between stress and sleep are further complicated by the emerging evidence that 1–2 hr of restraint is associated with increased sleep in rats (92–94) and that sleep loss may alter the HPA response to subsequent stressors (39,95,96).

The shaker method in neonates (64) and the DOW method in adult rats (65,66,72) are probably the best paradigms available for the experimental manipulation of sleep in small mammals. In these paradigms, both experimental and yoked control animals are exposed to the same environment and sleep disruption stimulus. Even with these more sophisticated paradigms, yoked control adult rats lose sleep and show similar sleep deprivation effects as the experimental rats, albeit to a lessor extent. The question is not "are sleep deprived animals stressed more than controls?"; rather, it is important to address the extent of stress response activation, the similarity of the response in experimental and control animals, and the degree to which the response is correlated with the outcomes in the study.

VI. Conclusions

In human studies, great care is taken to avoid exposing subjects to "stressors." Yet, to remain awake can take considerable effort on the part of an individual, and inevitably more intense stimuli are required to restrict sleep as the duration of the sleep loss period is extended or continued over several days or weeks. Nonetheless the goal has been to control confounding variables introduced by experimental procedures in order to "unequivocally" attribute outcomes to sleep loss. This is an overwhelming challenge given the number of potential confounding variables, as well as the inability to blind subjects to their sleep state or to control their individual reactivity to experimental manipulations. It is extremely difficult to separate effects of sleep loss *per se* from methods used to disrupt sleep in sleep deprivation experiments. Yet, attempts to control or reduce confounding variables in sleep deprivation experiments or to differentiate effects are important concerns of sleep scientists interested in using these methods.

References

1. Vogel GW, Buffenstein A, Minter K, Hennessey A. Drug effects on REM sleep and on endogenous depression. Neurosci Biobehav Rev 1990; 14:49–63.
2. Webb WB. Partial and differential sleep deprivation. In Kales A, ed. Sleep Physiology and Pathology: A Symposium. Philadelphia: JB Lippincott, 1969:221-231.
3. Naitoh P. Sleep deprivation in humans. In Venables PH, Christie MJ, eds. Research in Psychophysiology. London: John Wiley & Sons, 1975:153–180.
4. Naitoh P, Kelly TL, Englund C. Health effects of sleep deprivation. Occup Med 1990, 5:209–237.
5. Webb WB, Agnew HW. Sleep: Effects of a restricted regime. Science 1965, 150:1745–47.
6. Irwin M, Mascovich A, Gillin JC, Willoughby R, Pike J, Smith TL. Partial sleep deprivation reduces natural killer cell activity in humans. Psychosom Med 1994; 56:493–498.
7. Spiegel K, Leproult R, Van Cauter E. Impact of sleep debt on metabolic and endocrine function. Lancet 1999; 354:1435–1439.
8. Speigel K, Sheridan JF, Van Cauter E. Effect of sleep deprivation on response to immunization. JAMA 2002; 288:1471-1472.
9. Redwine L, Hauger RL, Gillin JC, Irwin M. Effects of sleep and sleep deprivation on interleukin-6, growth hormone, cortisol, and melatonin levels in humans. J Clin Endocrinol Metab 2000; 85:3597–3603.
10. Shearer WT, Rueben JM, Mullington JM, Price NJ, Lee BN, Smith EO, Szuba MP, Van Dongen HP, Dinges DF. Soluble TNF-alpha receptor 1 and IL-6 plasma levels in humans subjected to the sleep deprivation model of space flight. J Allergy Clin Immunol 2001; 107:165–170.
11. Sampson H. Deprivation of dreaming sleep by two methods. Arch Gen Psychiatry 1965; 13:79–86.
12. Dinges DF, Pack F, Williams K, Gillen KA, Powell JW, Ott GE, Aptowicz C, Pack AI. Cumulative sleepiness, mood disturbance, and psychomotor vigilance performance decrements during a week of sleep restricted to 4–5 hours per night. Sleep 1997; 20:267–277.
13. Brunner DP, Dijk DJ, Tobler I, Borbeby AA. Effect of partial sleep deprivation on sleep stages and EEG power spectra: evidence for non-REM and REM sleep homeostasis. Electroenceph Clin Neurophysiol 1990; 75:492–499.
14. Tilley AJ, Wilkinson RT. The effects of a restricted sleep regime on the composition of sleep and on performance. Psychophysiology 1984; 21:406–412.

15. Schilgen B, Tolle R. Partial sleep deprivation as therapy for depression. Arch Gen Psychiatry 1980; 37:267–271.

16. Parry BL, Hauger R, LeVeau B, Mostofi N, Cover H, Clopton P, Gillin JC. Circadian rhythms of prolactin and thyroid-stimulating hormone during the menstrual cycle and early versus late sleep deprivation in premenstrual dysphoric disorder. Psychiatry Res 1996; 62:147–160.

17. Irwin M, Gillin JC, Dang J, Weissman J, Phillips E, Ehlers C. Sleep deprivation as a probe of homeostatic sleep regulation in primary alcoholics. Biol Psychiatry 2002; 51:632–641.

18. Dement W. The effect of dream deprivation. Science 1960; 131:1705–1707.

19. Endo T, Roth C, Landolt H, Werth E, Aeschbach D, Achermann P, Borbely AA. Selective REM sleep deprivation in humans: effects on sleep and sleep EEG. Am J Physiol 1998; 274:R1186–R1194.

20. Agnew HW, Webb WB, Williams RL. Comparison of stage four and 1-REM sleep deprivation. Percept Mot Skills 1967; 24:851-858.

21. Lubin A, Moses JM, Johnson LC, Naitoh P. The recuperative effects of REM sleep and stage 4 sleep on human performance after complete sleep loss: experiment 1. Psychophysiology 1974; 11:133–158.

22. Kawahara R, Miyazaki I, Takata S, Kuwai T, Arai, H, Imaoka K, Tanaka Y, Hazama H, Okuma T, Ozaki C. A trial production of REM sleep depriver. Jpn J Psychiatry Neurol 1988; 42:127.

23. Reynolds CF, Buysse DJ, Kupfer DJ, Hoch CC, Houck PR, Matzzie J, George CJ. Rapid eye movement sleep deprivation as a probe in elderly subjects. Arch Gen Psychiatry 1990; 47:1128–1136.

24. Brandenberger G, Charifi C, Muzet A, Saini J, Simon C, Follenius M. Renin as a biological marker of the NREM-REM sleep cycle: effect of REM sleep suppression. J Sleep Res 1994; 3:30–35.

25. Dement W, Greenberg S, Klein R. The effect of partial REM sleep deprivation and delayed recovery. J Psychiat Res 1966; 4:141-152.

26. Moldofsky H, Scarisbrick P, England R, Smythe H. Musculoskeletal symptoms and non-REM sleep disturbance in patients with "fibrositis syndrome" and healthy subjects. Psychosom Med 1975;37:341-351.

27. Moldofsky H, Scarisbrick P. Induction of neurasthenic musculoskeletal pain syndrome by selective sleep stage deprivation. Psychosom Med 1976;38:35–44.

28. Lentz MJ, Landis CA, Rothermel J, Shaver JLF. Effects of selective slow wave sleep disruption on musculoskeletal pain and fatigue in middle-aged women. J Rheumatol 1999; 26:1586–1592.

29. Ferrara M, De Gennaro L, Bertini M. Selective slow-wave sleep (SWS) deprivation and SWS rebound? Do we need a fixed SWS amount per night? Sleep Res Online 1999; 2:15–19.

30. Arima T, Svensson P, Rasmussen C, Nielsen KD, Drewes AM, Arendt-Nielsen L. The relationship between selective sleep deprivation, nocturnal jaw-muscle activity and pain in healthy men. J Oral Rehab 2001; 28:140–148.

31. Walsh JK, Hartman PG, Schweitzer PK. Slow-wave sleep deprivation and waking function. J Sleep Res 1994; 3:16–25.

32. Dijk DJ, Beersma DGM, Daan S, Bloem GM, Van den Hoofdakker RH. Quantitative analysis of the effects of slow wave deprivation during the first 3 h of subsequent EEG power density. Eur Arch Psychiatry Neurol Sci 1987; 236:323–328.

33. Rasmussen C, Nielson KD, Arima T, Svensson P, Rossel P, Drewes AM, Arendt-Nielsen L. An automatic system for selective and standardized sleep deprivation. J Sleep Res 1998; 7:221.

34. Parry BL, Cover H, Mostofi N, LeVeau B, Sependa PA, Resnick A, Gillin JC. Early versus late partial deprivation in patients with premenstrual dysphoric disorder and normal comparison subjects. Am J Psychiatry 1995; 152:401-412.

35. Baumgartner A, Dietzel M, Saletu B, Wolf R, Campos-Barros A, Graf K, Kurten I, Mannsmann U. Influence of partial sleep deprivation on the secretion of thyrotropin, thyroid hormones, growth hormone, prolactin, luteinizing hormone, follicle stimulating hormone, and estradiol in healthy young women. Psychiatry Res 1993; 48:153–178.

36. Tanabe K, Osada N, Suzuki N, Nakayma M, Yokoyama Y, Yamamoto A, Murabayashi T, Yamamoto M, Omiya K, Itoh H, Murayama M. Erythrocyte magnesium and prostaglandin dynamics in chronic sleep restriction. Clin Cardiol 1997; 20:265–268.

37. Brunner DP, Dijk D, Borbely AA. Repeated partial sleep deprivation progressively changes the EEG during sleep and wakefulness. Sleep 1993; 16:100–113.

38. Tobler I, Borbely AA. The effect of 3–h and 6–h sleep deprivation on sleep and EEG spectra of the rat. Behav Brain Res 1990; 36:73–78.

39. Meerlo P, Koehl M, van der Borght K, Turek FW. Sleep restriction alters the hypothalamic-pituitary-adrenal response to stress. J Neuroendocrinol 2002; 14:397–402.

40. Licklider JCR, Bunch ME. Effects of enforced wakefulness upon the growth and maze-learning performance of white rats. J Comp Psychol 1946; 39:339–350.

41. del Gonzalez MM, Valatx JL, Debilly G. Role of the locus coeruleus in the sleep rebound following two different sleep deprivation methods in the rat. Brain Res 1996; 740:215–226.

42. Dewson JH, Dement WC, Wagener TE, Nobel K. Rapid eye movement sleep deprivation: a central neural change during wakefulness. Science 1967; 156:403–406.

43. Vogel GW. A review of REM sleep deprivation. Arch Gen Psychiatry 1975; 32:749–761.

44. Jouvet D, Vimont P, Delorme F, Jouvet M. Etude de la privation selective de la phase paradoxale de sommeil chez le chat. C R Soc Biol Lyon 1964; 158:756–759.

45. Cohen HB, Dement WC. Sleep: Changes in threshold to electroconvulsive shock in rats after deprivation of 'paradoxical' phase. Science 1965; 150:1318–1319.

46. Morden B, Mitchell G, Dement W. Selective REM sleep deprivation and compensation phenomena in the rat. Brain Res 1967; 5:339–359.

47. Mendelson WB, Guthrie RD, Frederick G, Wyatt RJ. The flower pot technique of rapid eye movement (REM) deprivation. Pharm Biochem Behav 1974; 2:553–556.

48. Landis CA. Altered sleep patterns with the platform method of REM sleep deprivation in rats. Sleep Res 1996; 25:469.

49. Grahnstedt S, Ursin R. Platform sleep deprivation affects deep slow wave sleep in addition to REM sleep. Behav Brain Res 1985; 18:233–239.

50. Ellman SJ, Spielman AJ, Luck D, Steiner SS, Halperin R. REM deprivation: a review. In Arkin AM, Antrobus JS, Ellman SJ, eds. The Mind in Sleep: Psychology and Psychophysiology. Hillsdale, NJ: Lawrence Erlbaum Associates, 1978:419–457.

51. Hicks RA, Okuda A, Thomsen D. Depriving rats of REM sleep: The identification of a methodological problem. Am J Psych 1977; 90:95–102.

52. Van Hulzen ZJM, Coenen AML. Paradoxical sleep deprivation and locomotor activity in rats. Physiol Behav 1981; 27:741-744.

53 Nunes GP Jr, Tufik S. Validation of the modified multiple platform method (MMP) of paradoxical sleep deprivation in rats. Sleep Res 1994; 22:339.

54. Porkka-Heiskanen T, Smith SE, Taira T, Urban JH, Levine JE, Turek FW, Stenberg D. Noradrenergic activity in rat brain during rapid eye movement sleep deprivation and rebound sleep. Am J Physiol 1995; 268:R1456–R1463.

55. Suchecki D, Palma BD, Tufik S. Sleep rebound in animals deprived of paradoxical sleep by the modified multiple platform method. Brain Res 2000; 875:14–22.

56. Oksenberg A, Shaffery JP, Marks GA, Speciale SG, Mihailoff, Roffwarg HP. Rapid eye movement sleep deprivation in kittens amplifies LGN cell-size disparity induced by monocular deprivation. Dev Brain Res 1996; 97:51-61.

57. Suchecki D, Lobo LL, Hipolide DC, Tufik S. Increased ACTH and cortiscosterone secretion induced by different methods of paradoxical sleep deprivation. J Sleep Res 1998; 7:276–281.

58. Suchecki D, Tufik S. Social stability attenuates the stress in the modified multiple platform method for paradoxical sleep deprivation in the rat. Physiol Behav 2000; 68:309–316.

59. Kovalzon VM, Tsibulsky VL. REM-sleep deprivation, stress and emotional behavior in rats. Behav Brain Res 1984; 14:235–245.

60. Van Hulzen ZJM, Coenen AML. The pendulum technique for paradoxical sleep deprivation in rats. Physiol Behav 1980; 25:807–811.

61. Van Luijtellaar ELJM, Coenen AML. Electrophysiological evaluation of three paradoxical sleep deprivation techniques in rats. Physiol Behav 1986; 36:603–609.

62. Amici R, Zamboni G, Perez E, Jones CA, Parmeggiani PL. The influence of heavy thermal load on REM sleep in the rat. Brain Res 1998; 781:252–258.

63. Zamboni G, Perez E, Amici R, Jones CA, Parmeggiani PL. Control of REM sleep: an aspect of the regulation of physiological homeostasis. Arch Ital Biol 1999; 137:249–262.

64. Feng P, Vogel GW, Obermeyer W, Kinney GG. An instrumental method for long-term continuous REM sleep deprivation of neonatal rats. Sleep 2000; 23:175–183.

65. Rechtschaffen A, Gilliland M, Bergmann BM, Winter JB. Physiological correlates of prolonged sleep deprivation in the rat. Science 1983; 221:182–184.

66. Rechtschaffen A, Bergmann BM. Sleep deprivation in the rat by the disk-over-water method. Behav Brain Res 1995; 69:55–63.

67. Bergmann BM, Kushida CA, Everson CA, Gilliland MA, Obermeyer W, Rechtschaffen A. Sleep Deprivation in the rat: II. Methodology. Sleep 1989; 12:5–12.

68. Tsai LL, Bergmann BM, Rechtschaffen A. Sleep deprivation in the rat. XIV. Effects in a light/dark cycle. Sleep 1992; 15:537–544.

69. Kushida CA, Bergmann BM, Rechtschaffen A. Sleep deprivation in the rat: IV. Paradoxical sleep deprivation. Sleep 1989; 12:22–30.

70. Gilliland MA, Bergmann BM, Rechtschaffen A. Sleep deprivation in the rat: VIII. High EEG amplitude sleep deprivation. Sleep 1989; 12:53–59.

71. Landis CA, Bergmann BM, Ismail MM, Rechtschaffen A. Sleep deprivation in the rat: XV. Ambient temperature choice in paradoxical sleep-deprived rats. Sleep 1992; 15:13–20.

72. Rechtschaffen A, Bergmann BM, Gilliland MA, Bauer K. Effects of method, duration, and sleep stage on rebounds from sleep deprivation in the rat. Sleep 1999; 22:11-31.

73. Moussard C, Alber J, Mozer JL, Henry JC. Effect of chronic REM sleep deprivation on pituitary, hypothalamus and hippocampus PGE2 and PGD2 biosynthesis in the mouse. Prostag Leukot Essen Fatty Acids 1994; 51:369–372.

74. Landis CA, Pollack SB, Helton WS. Microbial translocation and NK cell cytotoxicity in female rats sleep deprived on small platforms. Sleep Res 1997; 26:619.

75. Shaw PJ, Bergmann BM, Rechtschaffen A. Operant control of ambient temperature during sleep deprivation. Am J Physiol 1997; 272:R682–R690.

76. Patchev V, Felszeghy K, Koranyi L. Neuroendocrine and neurochemical consequences of long-term sleep deprivation in rats: similarities to some features of depression. Homeostasis 1991; 33:97–108.

77. Morden B, Conner R, Mitchell G, Dement W, Levine S. Effects of rapid eye movement (REM) sleep deprivation on shock-induced fighting. Physiol Behav 1968; 3:425–432.

78. Feinberg I. Delta homeostasis, stress, and sleep deprivation in the rat: a comment on Rechtschaffen et al. Sleep 1999; 22:1021-1024.

79. Rechtschaffen A, Bergmann BM. Sleep stage priorities in rebounds from sleep deprivation: a response to Feinberg. Sleep 1999; 22:1025–1030.

80. Toth LA. Sleep, sleep deprivation and infectious disease: studies in animals. Adv Neuroimmunol 1995; 5:79–92.

81. Bouyer JJ, Vallee M, Deminiere JM, Le Moal M, Mayo W. Reaction of sleep-wakefulness cycle to stress is related to differences in hypothalamo-pituitary-adrenal axis reactivity in rat. Brain Res 1998; 804:114–124.

82. Leproult R, Copinschi G, Buxton O, Van Cauter E. Sleep loss results in an elevation of cortisol levels the next evening. Sleep 1997; 20:865–870.

83. Fradda P, Fratta W. Stress-induced sleep deprivation modifies corticotropin releasing factor (CRF) levels and CRF binding in rat brain and pituitary. Pharamcol Res 1997; 35:443–446.

84. Tobler I, Murison R, Ursin R, Ursin H, Borbely AA. The effect of sleep deprivation and recovery sleep on plasma cortisosterone in the rat. Neurosci Lett 1983; 35:297–300.

85. Landis CA, Reeder D, Tsuji J. REM sleep deprivation effects on natural killer cell activity, corticosterone and norepinephrine in 80 and 160 day old F344 male rats. Sleep 1999; 22: Supplement, S234.

86. Hairston IS, Ruby NF, Brooke S, Peyron C, Denning DP, Heller HC, Sapolsky RM. Sleep deprivation elevates plasma corticosterone levels in neonatal rats. Neurosci Lett 2001; 315:29–32.

87. Coenen AML, Van Luijtellaar ELJM. Stress induced by three procedures of deprivation of paradoxical sleep. Physiol Behav 1985; 35:501-504.

88. Rechtschaffen A, Bergmann BM, Everson CA, Kushida CA, Gilliland MA. Sleep deprivation in the rat: X. Integration and discussion of the findings. Sleep 1989; 12:68–87.

89. Rechtschaffen A, Bergmann BM. Sleep deprivation in the rat: an update of the 1989 paper. Sleep 2002; 25:18–24.

90. Everson CA. Functional consequences of sustained sleep deprivation in the rat. Behav Brain Res 1995; 69:43–54.

91. Everson CA, Gilliland MA, Kushida CA, Pilcher JJ, Fang VS, Refetoff S, Bergmann BM, Rechtschaffen A. Sleep deprivation in the rat: IX. Recovery. Sleep 1989; 12:60–67.

92. Koehl M, Bouyer JJ, Darnaudery M, Le Moal M, Mayo W. The effect of restraint stress on paradoxical sleep is influenced by the circadian cycle. Brain Res 2002; 937:45–50.

93. Cespuglio R, Marinesco S, Baudet V, Bonnet C, Kafi BE. Evidence for a sleep-promoting influence of stress. Adv Neuroimmunol 1995; 5:145–154.

94. del Gonzalez MM, Valatx JL. Involvement of stress in the sleep rebound mechanism induced by sleep deprivation in the rat: use of alpha-helical CRH (9–41). Behav Pharmacol 1998; 9:655–662.

95. Palma BD, Suchecki D, Tufik S. Differential effects of acute cold and footshock on the sleep of rats. Brain Res 2000; 861:97–104.

96. Suchecki D, Tiba PA, Tufik S. Paradoxical sleep deprivation facilitates subsequent corticosterone response to a mild stressor in rats. Neurosci Lett 2002; 320:45–48.

6

Sleep Fragmentation

MICHAEL H. BONNET

Dayton Department of Veterans Affairs Medical Center, Wright State University,
Kettering Medical Center, and the Wallace-Kettering Neuroscience Institute,
Dayton, Ohio, U.S.A.

I. Introduction

Traditional sleep stage scoring (1) has provided an effective means to summarize nightly sleep. However, traditional sleep stage scoring has been less sensitive to the relationship between brief events and the sleep process. As sleep deprivation has improved the understanding of the role of total sleep time in preserving alertness and function, sleep fragmentation has allowed the description and examination of the microstructure of sleep and the relationship of such brief events to sleep restoration. Sleep fragmentation is the result of these increases in electroencephalographic frequency, called arousals, that are frequently associated with extrinsic or intrinsic events (e.g., noise or apnea) but which may not be scored using the traditional Rechtschaffen and Kales rules (1). A working definition of electroencephalographic arousals has been published as an American Sleep Disorders Association (ASDA) report (2), although research continues to refine the parameters of arousal events. Most studies have defined an electroencephalographic arousal as "an abrupt shift in electroencephalographic frequency, which may include theta, alpha and/or frequencies greater than 16 Hz but not

Supported by the Dayton Department of Veterans Affairs Medical Center, Wright State University School of Medicine, and the Sleep-Wake Disorders Research Institute spindles" with several additional criteria. The most contentious of the additional criteria proposed by the ASDA report was that the electroencephalographic frequency shift be at least 3 sec in duration.

Early studies of sleep fragmentation in animals (3,4) documented that arousals produced by 30 sec of noise turned on after each 2.5 min for two or three consecutive nights were sufficient to make dogs both appear sleepy and fall asleep more rapidly when given the chance (4). In addition, arousal responses to hypoxia and hypercapnia were impaired, and responses to laryngeal stimulation were reduced (3,4). Early studies of sleep fragmentation in humans (5) demonstrated that arousals produced by an audiometer after each minute of accumulated sleep resulted in significantly increased auditory thresholds (Fig. 1) along with

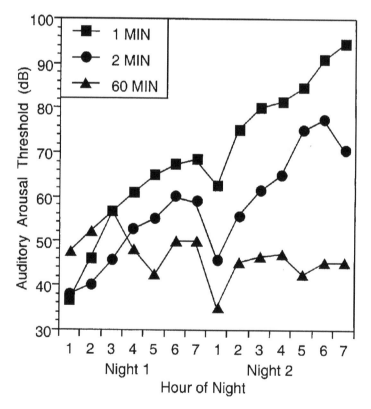

Figure 1 Auditory arousal threshold during two nights with arousals performed after each minute, each 2 min, or each 60 min of accumulated sleep. (Data from Refs. 5, 7, and 16.)

decreased psychomotor performance and increased subjective sleepiness on the day that followed. A following study (6) directly compared the effects of three sleep fragmentation paradigms with total sleep deprivation for 64 hr to determine the similarity and degree of deficits produced in a within-subjects design. The data showed that performance on addition, vigilance, and reaction time tasks and nap latency decreased as the rate of sleep fragmentation increased from once after each 10 min of sleep to once after each minute of sleep. On vigilance and nap latency tests, values were similar after two nights of sleep fragmentation at the once-per-minute rate to those seen after two nights of total sleep loss. These data can be criticized because total sleep time was reduced to about 4.5 hr in the 1-min condition, and the results therefore reflect both partial sleep deprivation and sleep fragmentation effects. However, the magnitude and direction of the effects associated with the sleep fragmentation established the fragmentation procedure as a potential analog to sleep deprivation.

About 20 additional empirical studies of sleep fragmentation and a number of clinical studies of sleep fragmentation were published in the years that followed. The empirical papers can be broadly grouped in five categories: papers replicating and extending the relationship between various schedules of sleep fragmentation and daytime alertness; papers with improved experimental control for parameters not completely controlled in early studies (such as total sleep time during the fragmentation conditions); papers showing the impact of the sleep fragmentation procedure on a range of physiological and behavioral variables; papers comparing sleep fragmentation with sleep deprivation; and papers exploring different types of arousal. Each of these topics will be examined in the sections that follow.

II. Relationship Between Various Schedules of Sleep Fragmentation and Daytime Alertness

In sleep fragmentation studies, it is common to find increased objective and subjective sleepiness and decreased psychomotor performance on days following disturbed sleep. Thirteen of 14 studies that measured objective sleepiness on the day after various sleep fragmentation paradigms found significant increases in sleepiness. Change in the Multiple Sleep Latency Test (MSLT) as a function of rate of sleep fragmentation is plotted in Figure 2 for a group of eight studies (some with multiple conditions) that produced a consistent and identified rate of fragmentation for one night and measured MSLT as an outcome variable on the next day (6–13). As can be seen from the figure, sleepiness increased as the rate of fragmentation was increased (the Pearson correlation between rate of fragmentation and percent decrease in sleep latency across the studies was $r = 0.775$, $p < 0.01$). A best-fit logarithmic curve has been added to the data plot in the figure.

An excellent review including a tabular summary of 15 major studies of the relationship of experimental sleep fragmentation to daytime impairment in humans was published in 2002 (14). In addition to findings of increased objective sleepiness, decrements on several psychomotor performance tests, including vigilance (6–8,13,15–17), reaction time (5,13,17), addition (6,15), divided attention (18), trail making (10), and digit symbol substitution task (5), have been commonly reported.

The impact of sleep fragmentation on mood was also measured in many of these studies. Measures including the Profile of Mood States, the Clyde Mood Scale, and the University of Wales Institute of Science and Technology (UWIST) mood adjective checklist have been used. Typical findings have included increased subjective sleepiness (5), inability to think clearly (5), or decreased vigor (8,10). Mood and subjective report measures are affected more by fragmentation paradigms that require a conscious response from subjects, but MSLT results were similar regardless of type of response as long as the rate of sleep fragmentation was the same (16).

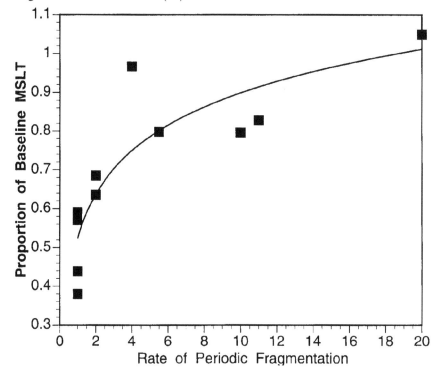

Figure 2   Proportion of baseline multiple sleep latency test value (i.e., sleep latency after fragmentation nights divided by sleep latency after baseline) in eight (two separate fragmentation conditions were identified in three of the eight studies) sleep fragmentation studies plotted as a function of rate of sleep fragmentation during the night. Rate of fragmentation is defined as the interval, in minutes, between the onset of sleep and disturbance. (From Ref. 68.)

III. Experimental Control for Sleep Fragmentation Parameters

Sleep deprivation is commonly used to measure the restorative function of sleep. Subjects deprived of sleep will demonstrate increasing sleepiness. When sleep is allowed, normal alertness returns. Sleep fragmentation is an analogous procedure that makes it possible for the investigator to vary a number of parameters such as the amount of time allowed between disturbances, the type of sleep allowed, or the total amount of sleep that is allowed to accumulate during the night. The sleep fragmentation procedure also produces large changes in sleep stage parameters including a decrease in slow-wave-sleep (SWS) and rapid-eye-movement (REM) sleep and an increase in stage 1 sleep. This led some investigators (19) to speculate that the effects of sleep fragmentation are mediated through changes in sleep stage parameters rather than through the fragmentation itself. Empirical studies have examined these issues either by minimizing disturbance of ongoing electroencephalography (13,20) or by manipulating fragmentation parameters (6). One study (13) has shown significant increases in sleepiness following empirical sleep fragmentation as measured by the MSLT with no significant change in any nocturnal sleep stage parameter. A second study has shown significant increases in sleepiness as measured by the MSLT and Maintenance of Wakefulness Test (MWT) (20), with the only sleep stage change being an 18% decrease in SWS on the sleep fragmentation nights. Two other studies have shown that similar small changes in SWS do not have any additional impact above the effect of sleep fragmentation alone (15,21). In general, an 18% decrease in SWS is less than that seen in normal males as they progress from the third to the fourth decade of life (22).

In a different type of study, Bonnet (6) compared sleep staging, daytime sleepiness, and psychomotor performance after three patterns of disturbance: after each minute of sleep; after each 10 min of sleep; and at each sleep onset following 2.5 hr of undisturbed sleep. These patterns were chosen to look at frequent periodic disturbance versus less frequent periodic disturbance versus frequent but not periodic disturbance. As expected, SWS and REM were greatly decreased after disturbance at a rate of once per minute. SWS was about 50% of baseline in the 10-min condition and about 75% of baseline in the 2.5-hr condition. REM was about 70% of baseline in the 10-min condition and 40% of baseline in the 2.5-hr condition. There were about 158 experimental arousals per night in the 1-min condition and about 29 and 110, respectively, in the 10-min and 2.5-hr conditions. This wide range of sleep stage amounts and arousal frequencies along with data from a total sleep deprivation condition allowed predictions to be made concerning the degree of deficits relative to the degree of sleep fragmentation, sleep loss, or sleep stage loss. Because performance and sleepiness values were known after baseline and total sleep deprivation, specific performance predictions could be made based on a number of specific hypotheses. For example, if SWS were the determiner of sleep restoration, then performance and alertness would be predicted to be: (a) midway between the base-line and total sleep deprivation values in the 10-min condition where SWS was 50% of baseline; and (b) midway between the 10-min condition values and the baseline value for the 2.5-hr sleep condition where it was 75% of baseline. In the paper (6), predictions were made between sleep and performance from three psychomotor tests (Wilkinson vigilance, Wilkinson additions, and simple reaction time) and a nap latency value for four sleep stage values: total sleep time, total sleep time minus stage 1 sleep time, total SWS, and total SWS plus REM. For each test, a predicted value, based on the sleep variables listed above, was compared with the actual observed performance score. The major finding from these analyses was that subjects in the 2.5-hr condition consistently performed better than predicted based on all of the sleep variables: total sleep time (80% of scores better than predicted); total sleep time excluding stage 1 (100% of scores better than predicted); SWS plus REM (100% of scores better than predicted); and SWS (80% of scores better than predicted). Conversely, subjects in the 10-min condition performed worse than predicted based on their total sleep time (75% worse than predicted), based on their total sleep time excluding stage 1 (62% of scores worse than predicted), and based on their SWS plus REM (62% of scores worse than predicted), but not based on their SWS (38% of scores worse than predicted).

The differences in these conditions were (a) more total arousals in the 2.5-hr condition and (b) a 2.5-hr period of consolidated sleep (i.e., no experimental arousals) in the 2.5-hr condition. These data imply that it is the periodicity of arousals rather than the total number of arousals that is important for sleep restoration and that, with sleep fragmentation at significant levels, neither total sleep nor total sleep excluding stage 1 sleep is a good predictor of sleep restoration. In this study, however, total amounts of SWS were related to daytime performance and alertness values, and SWS therefore could not be eliminated as a possible predictor of sleep restoration. The specific role of SWS in sleep restoration was addressed in a separate experiment (15). In that study, subjects were assigned to have their sleep fragmented after each 10 min of sleep. However, in one condition, subjects had additional arousals whenever they reached stage 3 sleep. In another condition, subjects had the same number of additional arousals during stage 2 sleep. Experimental arousals averaged 59 per night in both conditions; SWS averaged 9% in the SWS condition and 3% in the no-SWS condition. As expected, significant performance and sleepiness effects were found secondary to the sleep fragmentation but there was no significant interaction with SWS amount. These results are consistent with those found in human sleep deprivation studies that also have not shown differences in daytime psychomotor performance secondary to SWS or REM sleep stage deprivation (23–25).

Such studies provide evidence that it is the disturbance of sleep continuity rather than changes in sleep stages per se that produce the effects of sleep fragmentation. However, sleep fragmentation protocols are difficult, and additional work to replicate and extend these findings is needed.

IV. Sleep Fragmentation and Other Physiological and Behavioral Measures

A. Hormonal Effects

Spath-Schwalbe (26) examined profiles of cortisol and ACTH during baseline and sleep fragmentation nights (fragmentation at a rate of once after each minute of sleep). They found that plasma cortisol increased significantly when the experimental sleep fragmentation began. However, this burst of secretion was inhibited after about 80 min and cortisol secretion dropped below baseline sleep levels before returning to normal. A similar but less pronounced effect was found for ACTH.

Patients with sleep apnea show decreased growth hormone and prolactin secretion at night (27,28). Although this decrease is probably secondary to sleep fragmentation and reverses after sleep is normalized, changes in these hormones have not been studied after simple sleep fragmentation.

B. Pulmonary and Cardiovascular Effects

In an elegant series of animal studies, Phillipson's group first demonstrated the impact of sleep fragmentation on increasing sleepiness in dogs and showed that the fragmentation procedure resulted in impaired arousal responses to hypercapnia and hypoxia during sleep (4). More recently, the group developed a model to allow normal sleep in dogs followed by a period of experimentally produced sleep apnea lasting up to 133 days followed by recovery and a period of experimental sleep fragmentation without apnea lasting up to 60 days (29). The results of this study showed that both the sleep fragmentation procedure and the experimentally produced sleep apnea resulted in lengthening of the time to arousal in response to airway occlusion (see also ref. 30) and to greater tolerated oxygen desaturation, greater peak inspiratory pressure, and greater tolerated surges in blood pressure during airway conclusion. As a result, these authors concluded that simple sleep fragmentation was responsible not only for the sleepiness symptoms associated with sleep apnea but also that "the changes in the acute responses to airway occlusion resulting from obstructive sleep apnea are primarily the result of the associated sleep fragmentation" (29, p. 1609).

One study has found an increase in upper airway collapsibility and apnea/hypopnea index in normal subjects after sleep fragmentation (31). However, other studies have not found changes in hypercapnic ventilatory responsiveness or in arousal responses to external inspiratory resistive loading after sleep fragmentation (32,33).

Davies et al. (34) examined blood pressure responses following arousal produced by a combined auditory and vibrating stimulus. Arousals were associated with significant increases in both systolic and diastolic pressure that were about 75% as large as the blood pressure increases seen after periods of obstructive apnea in patients with sleep apnea.

C. Metabolic Effects

A study recording continuous VO_2 and VCO_2 during separate nights of baseline sleep, experimental sleep fragmentation, and recovery after the sleep fragmentation showed that average VO_2 across the night was significantly elevated on the disturbance night as compared to the baseline night and significantly decreased on the recovery night as compared to baseline (95% vs. 85% vs. 78%, respectively, of baseline waking values). As expected, metabolic rate increased in conjunction with arousals and remained elevated for as long as 6–9 min depending on the length of the arousal (8). VO_2 is also increased in patients with sleep apnea. In patients with mild sleep apnea, the increase in VO_2 is about 5% during periods of the night with apneas compared to periods without apnea (35). In patients with severe obstructive sleep apnea, decreases in VO_2 of up to 35% were seen on continuous positive airway pressure (CPAP) therapy nights as compared to untreated nights. It was estimated that about half of the decrease in VO_2 on the recovery nights was related to the sleep effects [reduction in arousals and recovery from fragmented sleep (35)].

D. Auditory Arousal Threshold

A majority of the empirical sleep fragmentation experiments have used auditory stimuli to produce sleep fragmentation. Figure 1 provides a comparison of auditory arousal threshold during two nights with arousals placed after each 1 min, 2 min, or 60 min of sleep (5,7,16). The increase in arousal threshold across the 1-min and 2-min night was significant. One study (5) used occasional novel tones to measure the extent to which the increase in auditory threshold was secondary to sleep fragmentation as compared to habituation and concluded that about two-thirds of the increase in arousal threshold was related to the fragmentation procedure. Increases in arousal threshold of a similar magnitude are found during recovery sleep following total sleep deprivation (36). It has been hypothesized that increased arousal threshold is an adaptive mechanism to ensure sleep continuity (i.e., to reduce the probability of repetitive arousals) as a means of preserving the sleep restoration process (6).

E. Electroencephalographic Effects

A recent study has examined the effect of one night of sleep fragmentation on cortical function in humans by the use of topographic brain mapping. It was reported that visual evoked responses had decreased amplitude at several sites (frontal, central, and temporal) after fragmentation, but no significant increases in latency were found (37). One previous study has shown significantly decreased amplitude and increased latencies for visual evoked responses from a central site after one night of total sleep loss (38).

V. Sleep Fragmentation Compared with Sleep Deprivation

Sleep fragmentation may be conceptualized as different from sleep deprivation because subjects are allowed to sleep. However, this may be more a theoretical difference than an actual difference. Studies of total sleep deprivation in humans and animals attempt to maintain the wake state for extended periods. Unfortunately, studies of total sleep loss in humans do not proceed for very long before the appearance of microsleeps when subjects sit down. Eventually, slow waves may appear in the electroencephalogram (EEG) of subjects who are inter- acting or moving (39). In rats, sleep deprivation is frequently monitored by com- puter analysis of brain activity; when brain activity consistent with sleep onset appears, this starts a platform in motion. This motion eventually awakens a sleep- ing animal by knocking it into water. However, the model is more properly a sleep fragmentation model; sleep onset occurs and the animal is aroused after a short period of sleep. In general, sleep fragmentation studies differ from the total sleep deprivation model primarily in that the periods of sleep are carefully monitored to be the same based on the fragmentation design. As an extension of this con- cept, several studies of sleep fragmentation have also contained a total sleep loss comparison group.

A few empirical studies have directly compared the impact of total sleep deprivation and sleep fragmentation within the same experiment (6,18,26,31). All four studies compared total sleep loss for one or two nights (6) with similar peri- ods of sleep fragmentation. Sleep fragmentation was produced following each minute of sleep in three studies and at each onset of stage 2 in the fourth. In the Spath-Schwalbe study (26), profiles of cortisol and ACTH peaked shortly after the initiation of sleep deprivation or sleep fragmentation and then showed the same pattern of inhibition followed by a later peak in both sleep deprivation and sleep fragmentation conditions. This pattern was different from the normal sleep condition. In the Levine et al. study (18), MSLT was reduced after both total sleep deprivation and 1-min sleep fragmentation, and these conditions did not differ statistically (the actual latencies were 2.2 and 4.1 min, respectively). In the Bonnet study (6), performance deficits were significantly greater following total sleep deprivation than following 1-min sleep fragmentation on number of addi- tion problems completed and simple reaction time. However, deficits were simi- lar on vigilance hit rate (25% vs. 25%) and on nap latency (2.2 vs. 3.7 min.) after total sleep deprivation as compared to sleep fragmentation. At least two studies have shown an increase in apnea/hypopnea events following sleep fragmentation

(31,32), and in one of these (31) a significant increase in the apnea/hypopnea index was found after sleep fragmentation in comparison with a similar period of total sleep deprivation. This latter finding is the single instance where the effects of sleep fragmentation have been reported to be more extreme than a comparable period of total sleep loss.

These comparison studies are important because they establish direct links between the effects of sleep fragmentation and sleep deprivation. The demonstration of similar effects on hormones, respiratory parameters, psychomotor performance, and objective sleepiness provides evidence that the high-frequency sleep fragmentation procedure is effectively the same as total sleep deprivation.

VI. Different Types of Arousal

Many clinical studies have examined the correlation between arousal parameters and residual sleepiness. In an early study, Carskadon et al. (40) reported significant correlations between the MSLT and the number of brief arousals ($r = -0.47$), the arousal index ($r = 0.42$), the number of respiratory events ($r = 0.49$) and the respiratory index ($r = 0.41$). Similar low but usually statistically significant correlations have been reported in other studies (41–44). Inability to explain large amounts of variance in daytime sleepiness by traditional arousal scoring techniques has resulted in a number of investigations of alternative electroencephalographic and respiratory scoring paradigms that might be more predictive.

Several studies have recently published comparisons of different scoring paradigms in normals and patients with sleep apnea. Catcheside et al. (45) examined electroencephalographic arousals and a number of cardiovascular measures including heart rate, pulse arrival time (PAT), pulse transit time (PTT), pulse wave amplitude (PWA), pulse wave velocity (PWV), and skin blood flow (SBF). All of these measures changed significantly with arousals, but the changes in finger PWA and SBF were largest. Martin et al. (46) compared ASDA arousal scoring (2) with a similar technique based on 1.5-sec or longer events with or without a required increase in electromyographic activity and 15-sec events (the standard used to score wake in traditional Rechtschaffen and Kales scoring). In this study, as in earlier studies, the respiratory index was significantly correlated with MSLT (Spearman correlation = -0.30, $p < 0.05$). All arousal scoring methods except the Rechtschaffen and Kales wake scoring method were significantly correlated with MSLT values, and the correlations were very similar (range: -0.22 to -0.24; $p < 0.04$). Pitson and Stradling (47) compared ASDA arousals with respiratory index, SaO_2 dips, and changes in heart rate and blood pressure as forms of autonomic arousal. Unfortunately, MSLT was not recorded in this study, and the subjective sleepiness variable used (Epworth Sleepiness Scale, ESS) may not be highly correlated with MSLT. However, in agreement with previous results, low correlations ranging from $r = 0.21$ to $r = 0.36$ were found between each of the arousal measures (except the heart rate increase measure, which had a correlation of $r = 0.06$) and the ESS score. Only the relationship to SaO_2 dips ($r = 0.36$) was statistically significant. In a third study, Bennett et al. (48) scored ASDA arousals; 1.5-sec arousals; two "neural network" digitized EEG variables; pulse transit time; and a video movement index in a group of patients with sleep apnea. Instead of the MSLT, a test of visual vigilance (OSLER test) was used to assess sleepiness. Again, results from the many tests of brief arousals were similar. All of the scored arousal variables were found to be weakly but significantly correlated with the alertness measure. The range of Spearman correlations was -0.38 to -0.53 (all significant). The correlation for traditional ASDA arousals was -0.51. In a 2002 study, Poyares et al. (49) compared visually scored arousals with PTT (see also Ref. 50) responses and spectral electroencephalographic changes in groups of upper airway resistance and mild sleep apnea patients. Abnormal breathing events were associated with both visual electroencephalographic arousals and PTT responses 59% of the time. Abnormal breathing events were associated with electroencephalographic arousals but no PTT response 2.5% of the time and PTT but no electroencephalographic arousal 14% of the time. However, 15% of PTT responses occurred when there was no respiratory event (and two-thirds of those had no electroencephalographic arousal either). Unfortunately, the electroencephalographic spectral analysis data were not presented on an event-by-event basis (we are only told that there were significant increases in delta, alpha, and beta following respiratory events in NREM and that these changes were the same regardless of the presence of visual electroencephalographic changes or PTT). It is well known that patients with sleep apnea have electroencephalographic arousals following some but not all apnea events. A recent examination of respiratory events not followed by scorable arousals compared to arousal events using spectral analysis of the EEG (51) also found significant increases in alpha, beta, theta, and delta activity in patients with upper airway resistance syndrome. It is reported that changes in delta activity were found in 95–97% of events. Unfortunately, the percentage of events showing shifts toward faster frequencies in the EEG was not given. However, the finding that spectral analysis techniques were successful in showing changes in the EEG associated with a high percentage of respiratory events suggests that some electroencephalographic arousals may not be visually scorable. This could explain why the correlation between visually scored arousals and measures of sleepiness is not always high. On the other hand, the Black et al. study (51) also showed that those events that produced more alpha (i.e., visually scored arousals) resulted in a greater drop in pressure. The implication from all of these data is that there may not be a single arousal response but rather a spectrum of responses producing different outcomes.

The major conclusions that can be drawn from these studies are as follows: (a) there are many independent physiological ways to measure brief arousals during sleep; (b) these methods tend to be highly correlated with each other; and (c) these variables are typically weakly but significantly correlated with daytime sleepiness in these clinical studies. A number of reasons have been presented for the lack of higher correlations. It was observed by Stepanski (41) that correlations were much lower when patients with similar pathologic conditions were grouped because the variance in MSLT was greatly reduced. As a result, most recent studies have examined apnea patients with a wide range of pathologic conditions. Martin et al. speculated that the lack of higher correlations might be secondary to: (a) an inability to observe arousals visually because of background electroencephalographic activity; (b) traditional electroencephalographic scoring from central and occipital brain areas (as opposed to frontal areas); or (c) the use of the MSLT as compared to the MWT. Alternatively, the lack of agreement could also be secondary to variable patterns or frequency of arousal in patients with positional apnea where position is not controlled either on sleep evaluation nights or preceding nights of sleep at home. Other recent research also suggests that both state and trait levels of central nervous system activation have a significant independent impact on the MSLT result (52,53).

The other important question is the extent to which all of these different types of arousal are equivalent in terms of impact on the sleep process. For example, some investigators hypothesize the K complexes are indicators of arousal because they are reliably associated with an increase in heart rate (54). However, Johnson showed that K complexes "occur with considerable regularity at a rate of 1.21 per minute" (54, p. 444). This means that if K complexes were as disruptive of sleep as electroencephalographic arousals, then everyone would be overwhelmingly sleepy based simply on the disturbance related to K complexes. In an empirical study, Townsend et al. (55) produced 80- to 90-dB tones every 22 sec for 30 consecutive days and nights. The investigators reported that they did not find changes in sleep parameters, including sleep stages, sleep stage changes, or number of arousal episodes during the course of the experiment. However, they did find that heart rate, finger pulse volume, and electroencephalographic (typically a K complex in this literature) responses to the auditory stimuli continued without habituation throughout the 30 days and nights. Despite 30 nights of physiological arousal at a rate of more than two events per minute, subjects did not have any change in sleep latency throughout the study, did not have any changes in recovery sleep parameters at the end of the study, and had no apparent changes in mood or performance. Such findings indicate that, while it is important to understand the broad range of physiological changes that occur during sleep, all of the responses are not equivalent even if they often occur at the same time. If cardiovascular measures are to become common measures of arousal in lieu of electroencephalographic measures, empirical work must establish the impact of elevation of those measures in limiting sleep restoration when produced with no concurrent electroencephalographic arousals.

VII.   Clinical Effects of Sleep Fragmentation: Sleep Apnea and Periodic Limb Movements

Many clinical studies have examined the relationship between sleep fragmentation variables and daytime function. In an early study of the determinants of daytime sleepiness, Carskadon et al. (40) looked at many sleep-related variables but found that only measures of arousal and measures of sleep-related respiratory events correlated significantly with daytime sleepiness (with correlation values ranging from 0.41 to 0.49). In the years that followed, several studies attempted to differentiate the effects of sleep fragmentation from the effects of apnea-associated oxygen desaturation in producing the daytime sleepiness. For example, Colt et al. (56) treated sleep apnea patients with CPAP to reduce sleep fragmentation and daytime sleepiness before experimentally adding periods of oxygen desaturation while on CPAP to document that daytime sleepiness did not return from periods of oxygen reduction alone. Results from the many studies that have empirically produced fragmentation independent of apnea (and a study independently producing fragmentation and apnea in dogs) have been very clear in differentiating sleep fragmentation effects from desaturation effects (29). Finally, patients with upper airway resistance syndrome are defined as having minimal oxygen desaturation and apnea but nonetheless suffering from significant daytime sleepiness. Despite the absence of clear apnea, these patients show periodic increases in airway resistance followed by arousal (51). These several types of studies, in agreement with the empirical fragmentation studies, support the idea that it is the fragmentation rather than the oxygen desaturation in apnea patients that produces the sleepiness symptoms.

A few studies have examined the relationship between sleep fragmentation and hypertension. One study found that the incidence of hypertension was higher in a group of snorers with fragmented sleep (but no apnea or hypopnea) than in a group of snorers without fragmented sleep (57). The second, a population-based study of individuals with a respiratory disturbance index (RDI) of less than 1, reported a correlation of 0.54 ($p = 0.005$) between blood pressure and a sleep fragmentation index (58). Unfortunately, these studies did not control for the possible incidence of upper airway resistance syndrome. However, one single case study also has reported increases in blood pressure in conjunction with periodic limb movements (59). Therefore, further research is needed to more firmly link sleep fragmentation with hypertension.

A few studies have examined airway collapsibility and gas challenge responses in patients and normals. Gleadhill et al. (60) demonstrated that patients with obstructive apnea had a more easily collapsible upper airway than patients with obstructive hypopneas and patients who snored. Series et al. then demonstrated that sleep fragmentation by itself significantly increased collapsibility in the upper airway in normals to levels seen in some patients who snored (31). In one study, sleep fragmentation was significantly related to a reduced vasodilation response to a hypercapnic challenge in the morning in a mixed group of normal and apnea patients (61), whereas in another study the hyperoxic hypercapnic ventilatory response was not altered after nights of fragmented sleep (32).

A final group of studies examined sleep fragmentation variables in patients with periodic limb movements. An initial study split patients with periodic limb movements into groups based on their primary complaint of either insomnia or excessive daytime sleepiness (62). Measures of brief arousals were not reported in this study, but patients with excessive daytime sleepiness did have significantly increased shifts to stage 1 sleep and more (but shorter) awakenings. More recently, three studies have examined sleep fragmentation in sleepy patients with periodic limb movements with the hypothesis that medications should decrease arousals during sleep and improve daytime alertness. Doghramji et al. (63) found that short-term administration of triazolam at doses of 0.25 or 0.5 mg had no effect on the periodic limb movement index but decreased total arousals significantly. Sleep latency on the MSLT was significantly longer following the final medication night. However, total sleep time was also increased by the medication. Two studies by Bonnet and Arand in a similar patient group also showed that triazolam increased total sleep at night and alertness during the day but showed no reduction in limb movements or arousals (64,65). However, a study in which triazolam was administered to patients with central sleep apnea showed a reduction in central apnea, a reduction in arousals, an increase in total sleep, and improvement in daytime psychomotor performance (66). Together these studies provide mild evidence that reduction of arousals in patients with fragmenting sleep disorders can improve alertness and function on the day that follows.

VIII. Future Research

Despite the fact that the initial studies examined sleep fragmentation in animals, very little animal work on the physiology or neurophysiology of arousals has followed. One study has suggested that brief periods of wakefulness arising from sleep are neurophysiologically different from later wakefulness (67), but basic neurophysiological questions remain unexplored: *(a) What is the interaction of the sleep and arousal systems? (b) How does sleep fragmentation limit sleep restoration? (c) What is the timing of sleep restoration at the neurophysiological level?*

Much recent work has shown that arousal can be measured in many physiological systems. Even in the EEG, spectral analysis procedures suggest that changes consistent with arousal occur at times when visible arousals cannot be identified. However, identification of a new measure is only the first research step. To the extent that such measures are highly correlated with traditional measures of arousal, they may provide a more convenient measure. However, if such measures are not highly correlated with traditional arousals (or are proposed as more elemental or sensitive measures), empirical work is needed to show that this type of arousal actually has an impact on sleep restoration. For example, K complexes are sometimes described as arousals because there is evidence of an associated small increase in heart rate. As K complexes are frequently seen in normal sleep, however, they will not be accepted as arousals until empirical data can support the hypothesis that increased K complexes reduce the restorative function of sleep.

For both human and animal studies, sleep fragmentation also presents a convenient "control" situation ("sham" sleep). Because participants in sleep fragmentation studies actually go to bed, remain in a reclining position all night, and sleep, sleep fragmentation is actually a better control condition to use than total sleep deprivation because it controls for body position, light exposure, and amount of physical activity while sleep deprivation conditions typically do not. For example, a good deal is known about hormone excretion during sleep deprivation but some of those changes might be the result of activity, posture, light, social interaction, eating, or other behavioral interventions that occur during sleep deprivation but that do not occur during sleep or sleep fragmentation. Sleep fragmentation, like sleep deprivation, can be a powerful tool in understanding both the function of sleep and the time-based process through which restoration occurs during sleep.

References

1. Rechtschaffen A, Kales A. A manual of standardized terminology, techniques, and scoring systems for sleep stages of human subjects. Washington, DC: Public Health Service, U.S. Government Printing Office, 1968.
2. Bonnet MH, Carley D, Guilleminault CG, Harper R, Hayes B, Hirshkowitz M, Ktonas P, Keenan S, Roehrs T, Smith J, Walsh J, Weber S, Westbrook P. ASDA report EEG arousals: scoring rules and examples. Sleep 1992; 15: 173–184.
3. Bowes G, Woolf GM, Sullivan CE, Phillipson EA. Effect of sleep fragmentation on ventilatory and arousal responses of sleeping dogs to respiratory stimuli. Am Rev Respir Dis 1980; 122:899–908.
4. Phillipson EA, Bowes G, Sullivan CE, Woolf GM. The influence of sleep fragmentation on arousal and ventilatory responses to respiratory stimuli. Sleep 1980; 3:281–288.
5. Bonnet MH. Effect of sleep disruption on sleep, performance, and mood. Sleep 1985; 8:11–19.
6. Bonnet MH. Performance and sleepiness as a function of frequency and placement of sleep disruption. Psychophysiology 1986; 23:263–271.
7. Bonnet MH. Infrequent periodic sleep disruption: effects on sleep, performance and mood. Physiology and Behavior 1989; 45:1049–1055.
8. Bonnet MH, Berry RB, Arand DL. Metabolism during normal sleep, fragmented sleep, and recovery sleep. J Appl Physiol 1991; 71:1112–1118.
9. Magee J, Harsh J, Badia P. Effects of experimentally-induced sleep fragmentation on sleep and sleepiness. Psychophysiology 1987; 24:528–534.
10. Martin SE, Engleman HM, Deary JJ, Douglas NJ. The effect of sleep fragmentation on daytime function. Am J Respir Crit Care Med 1996; 153:1328–1332.

11. Philip P, Stoohs R, Guilleminault C. Sleep fragmentation in normals: a model for sleepiness associated with upper airway resistance syndrome. Sleep 1994; 17:242–247.

12. Roehrs T, Merlotti L, Petrucelli N, Stepanski E, Roth T. Experimental sleep fragmentation. Sleep 1994; 17:438–443.

13. Stepanski E, Lamphere J, Roehrs T, Zorick F, Roth T. Experimental sleep fragmentation in normal subjects. Int J Neurosci 1987; 33:207–214.

14. Stepanski E. The effect of sleep fragmentation on daytime function. Sleep 2002; 25:268–276.

15. Bonnet MH. Performance and sleepiness following moderate sleep disruption and slow wave sleep deprivation. Physiol Behav 1986; 37:915–918.

16. Bonnet MH. Sleep restoration as a function of periodic awakening, movement, or electroencephalographic change. Sleep 1987; 10:364–373.

17. Bonnet MH. The effect of sleep fragmentation on sleep and performance in younger and older people. Neurobiol Aging 1989; 10:21–25.

18. Levine B, Roehrs T, Stepanski E, Zorick F, Roth T. Fragmenting sleep diminishes its recuperative value. Sleep 1987; 10:590–599.

19. Wesensten NJ, Balkin TJ, Belenky G. Does sleep fragmentation impact recuperation? A review and reanalysis. J Sleep Res 1999; 8:237–245.

20. Martin SE, Wraith PK, Deary IJ, Douglas NJ. The effect of nonvisible sleep fragmentation on daytime function. Am J Respir Crit Care Med 1997; 155:1596–1601.

21. Martin SE, Brander PE, Deary IJ, Douglas NJ. The effect of clustered versus regular sleep fragmentation on daytime function. J Sleep Res 1999; 8:305–12.

22. Williams L, Karacan I, Hursch C. Electroencephalography of Human Sleep: Clinical Applications. New York: John Wiley & Sons, 1974:169.

23. Johnson LC. Are stages of sleep related to waking behavior? Am Scientist 1973; 61:326–338.

24. Lubin A, Moses JM, Johnson LC, Naitoh P. The recuperative effects of REM sleep and stage 4 sleep on human performance after complete sleep loss: experiment 1. Psychophysiology 1974; 11:133–146.

25. Johnson LC, Naitoh P, Moses JM, Lubin A. Interaction of REM deprivation and stage 4 deprivation with total sleep loss: experiment 2. Psychophysiology 1974; 11:147–159.

26. Spath-Schwalbe E, Gofferje M, Kern W, Born J, Fehm HL. Sleep disruption alters nocturnal ACTH and cortisol secretory patterns. Biol Psychiatry 1991; 29:575–584.

27. Cooper BC, White JES, Ashworth LA, Alberti KG, Gibson GJ. Hormonal and metabolic profiles in subjects with obstructive sleep apnea syndrome and the effects of nasal continuous positive airway pressure (CPAP) treatment. Sleep 1995; 18:172–179.

28. Spiegel K, Follenius M, Krieger J, Sforza E, Brandenberger G. Prolactin secretion during sleep in obstructive sleep apnea patients. J Sleep Res 1995; 4:56–62.

29. Brooks D, Horner RL, Kimoff RJ, Kozar LF, Render-Teixeira C, Phillipson EA. Effect of obstructive sleep apnea versus sleep fragmentation on responses to airway occlusion. Am J Respir Crit Care Med 1997; 155:1609–1617.

30. Fewell JE. The effect of short-term sleep fragmentation produced by intense auditory stimuli on the arousal response to upper airway obstruction in lambs. J Dev Physiol 1987; 9:409–417.

31. Series F, Roy N, Marc I. Effects of sleep deprivation and sleep fragmentation on upper airway collapsibility in normal subjects. Am J Respir Cri Care Med 1994; 150:481–485.

32. Espinoza H, Thornton AT, Sharp D, Antic R, Mcevoy RD. Sleep fragmentation and ventilatory responsiveness to hypercapnia. Am Rev Respir Dis 1991; 144:1121–1124.

33. Gugger M, Keller U, Mathis J. Arousal responses to inspiratory resistive loading during REM and non-REM sleep in normal men after short-term sleep fragmentation/deprivation. Schweiz Med Wochenschr 1998; 128:696–702.

34. Davies RJ, Belt PJ, Roberts SJ, Ali NJ, Stradling JR. Arterial blood pressure responses to graded transient arousal from sleep in normal humans. J Appl Physiol 1993; 74:1123–1130.

35. Bonnet MH. Metabolic rate during sleep, sleep fragmentation, and apnea. J Sleep Res 1994; 3 (suppl 1):28 (abstract).

36. Williams HL, Hammack JT, Daly RL, Dement WC, Lubin AL. Responses to auditory stimulation, sleep loss, and the EEG stages of sleep. Electroencephal Clin Neurophysiol 1964; 16:269–279.

37. Kingshott RN, Cosway RJ, Deary I, Douglas NJ. The effect of sleep fragmentation on cognitive processing using computerized topographic brain mapping. J Sleep Res 2000; 9:353–357.

38. Corsi-Cabrera M, Arce C, Del Rio-Portilla IY, Perez-Garci E, Guevara MA. Amplitude reduction in visual event-related potentials as a function of sleep deprivation. Sleep 1999; 22:181–189.

39. Blake H, Gerard RW, Kleitman N. Factors influencing brain potentials during sleep. J Neurophysiol 1939; 2:48–60.

40. Carskadon MA, Brown ED, Dement WC. Sleep fragmentation in the elderly: relationship to daytime sleep tendency. Neurobiol Aging 1982; 3:321–327.

41. Stepanski E, Lamphere J, Badia P, Zorick F, Roth T. Sleep fragmentation and daytime sleepiness. Sleep 1984; 7:18–26.

42. Roehrs T, Zorick F, Wittig R, Conway W, Roth T. Predictors of objective level of daytime sleepiness in patients with sleep-related breathing disorders. Chest 1989; 95:1202–1206.

43. Cheshire K, Engleman H, Deary I, Shapiro C, Douglas NJ. Factors impairing daytime performance in patients with sleep apnea/hypopnea syndrome. Arch Intern Med 1992; 152:538–541.

44. Kribbs NB, Getsy JE, Dinges DF. Investigation and management of daytime sleepiness in sleep apnea. In: Saunders NA, Sullivan CE, eds. Sleep and Breathing. New York: Marcel Dekker, 1994:575–604.

45. Catcheside PG, Orr RS, Chiong SC, Mercer J, Saunders NA, McEvoy RD. Noninvasive cardiovascular markers of acoustically induced arousal from non-rapid-eye-movement sleep. Sleep 2002; 25:797–804.

46. Martin SE, Engleman HM, Kingshott RN, Douglas NJ. Microarousals in patients with sleep apnoea/hypopnoea syndrome. J Sleep Res 1997; 6:276–280.

47. Pitson DJ, Stradling JR. Autonomic markers of arousal during sleep in patients undergoing investigation for obstructive sleep apnea, their relationship to EEG arousals, respiratory events and subjective sleepiness. J Sleep Res 1998; 7:53–59.

48. Bennett LS, Langford BA, Stradling JR, Davies RJ. Sleep fragmentation indices as predictors of daytime sleepiness and nCPAP response in obstructive sleep apnea. Am J Respir Crit Care Med 1998; 158:778–786.

49. Poyares D, Guilleminault C, Rosa A, Ohayon M, Koester U. Arousal, EEG spectral power and pulse transit time in UARS and mild OSAS subjects. Clin Neurophysiol 2002; 113:1598–1606.

50. Pitson DJ, Chhina N, Knijn S, vanHerwaaden M, Stradling JR. Changes in pulse transit time and pulse rate as markers of arousal from sleep in normal subjects. Clin Sci 1994; 87:269–273.

51. Black JE, Guilleminault C, Colrain IM, Carrillo O. Upper airway resistance syndrome. Central electroencephalographic power and changes in breathing effort. Am J Respir Crit Care Med 2000; 162:406–411.

52. Bonnet MH, Arand DL. Activity, arousal, and the MSLT in patients with insomnia. Sleep 2000; 23:205–212.

53. Bonnet MH, Arand DL. Level of arousal and the ability to maintain wakefulness. J Sleep Res 1999; 8:247–254.

54. Johnson LC, Karpan WE. Autonomic correlates of the spontaneous K-complex. Psychophysiology 1968; 4:444–452.

55. Townsend RE, Johnson LC, Muzet A. Effects of long term exposure to tone pulse noise on human sleep. Psychophysiology 1973; 10:369–375.

56. Colt HG, Haas H, Rich GB. Hypoxemia vs sleep fragmentation as cause of excessive daytime sleepiness in obstructive sleep apnea. Chest 1991; 100:1542–1548.

57. Lofaso F, Coste A, Gilain L, Harf A, Guilleminault C, Goldenberg F. Sleep fragmentation as a risk factor for hypertension in middle-aged nonapneic snorers. Chest 1996; 109:896–900.

58. Morrell MJ, Finn L, Kim H, Peppard PE, Safwan Badr M, Young T. Sleep fragmentation, awake blood pressure, and sleep-disordered breathing in a population-based study. Am J Respir Crit Care Med 2000; 162:2091–2096.

59. Ali NJ, Davies RJ, Fleetham JA, Stradling JR. Periodic movements of the legs during sleep associated with rises in systemic blood pressure. Sleep 1991; 14:163–165.

60. Gleadhill IC, Schwartz AR, Schubert N, Wise RA, Permutt S, Smith PL. Upper airway collapsibility in snorers and in patients with obstructive hypopnea and apnea. Am Rev Respir Dis 1991; 143:1300–1303.

61. Qureshi Al, W. CW, Bliwise DL. Sleep fragmentation and morning cerebrovasomotor reactivity to hypercapnia. Am J Respir Crit Care Med 1999; 160:1244–1247.

62. Rosenthal L, Roehrs T, Sicklesteel J, Zorick F, Wittig R, Roth T. Periodic movements during sleep, sleep fragmentation, and sleep-wake complaints. Sleep 1984; 7:326–330.

63. Doghramji K, Browman CP, Gaddy JR, Walsh JK. Triazolam diminishes daytime sleepiness and sleep fragmentation in patients with periodic leg movements in sleep. J Clin Psychopharmacol 1991; 11:284–290.

64. Bonnet MH, Arand DL. The use of triazolam in older patients with periodic leg movements, fragmented sleep, and daytime sleepiness. J Gerontol 1990; 45:M139–M144.

65. Bonnet MH, Arand DL. The chronic use of triazolam in older patients with periodic leg movements, fragmented sleep, and daytime sleepiness. Aging Clin Exp Res 1991; 3:313–324.

66. Bonnet MH, Dexter JR, Arand DL. The effect of triazolam on arousal and respiration in central sleep apnea patients. Sleep 1990; 13:31–41.

67. Homer R, Sanford L, Pack A, Morrison A. Activation of a distinct arousal state immediately after spontaneous awakening from sleep. Brain Res 1997; 778:127–134.

68. Bonnet MH, Arand DL. Clinical effects of sleep fragmentation versus sleep deprivation. Sleep Med Rev 2003, 7:297–310.

7

Environmental Influences on Sleep and Sleep Deprivation

KENNETH P. WRIGHT, JR.

University of Colorado, Boulder, Colorado, U.S.A.

I. Introduction

Human sleep across the 24-hr day and human performance during sleep deprivation are sensitive to the effects of environmental conditions. Scientific evidence demonstrates that the brain sensory systems are active during sleep. Environmental factors such as noise, odors, temperature, and bed partners can negatively influence sleep. Exposure to altered or extreme environments such as urban noise, medical intensive care units, altitude, and space flight also disrupt sleep and may lead to chronic sleep loss. Ambient light levels influence human performance during sleep deprivation, but the influence of other environmental factors on human performance during sleep deprivation has not been well characterized. Humans have gone to great lengths to improve the sleeping environment. There is often an environmentally controlled room in the home with a bed surface dedicated to sleep. It has been recommended that the optimal sleep environment is a quiet and dark room that is well ventilated and temperature controlled. The mattress should not be too soft or too firm, and the pillow should be at a comfortable height and firmness. Pets or the need to care for other people should not interrupt sleep. These recommendations form the basis of sleep hygiene, a basic tool used in clinical sleep medicine. Currently, there is experimental evidence to support some but not all of these recommendations.

II. Assessment of Human Sleep and Performance

Accurate assessment of sleep and performance is essential for making inferences about the influence of environmental factors on human brain function and behavior. Common measures of sleep include behavioral responsiveness to stimuli, patterns of brain wave activity, and levels of motility. Research studies have commonly used microswitch button pressing, deep breathing, and memory as behavioral measures of responsiveness to stimuli during sleep. Since the 1950s the electroencephalogram (EEG) has been the gold standard measure of sleep (see Chap. 12). Research studies have primarily focused on sleep staging and evoked responses as electroencephalographic measures of responsiveness to stimuli during sleep. Technological advances in ambulatory electroencephalographic recording equipment have increased the number of studies that have assessed the sleep EEG outside of the laboratory. Another technique that has been widely used to assess sleep (but not sleep stages) has been estimation of the amount of time at which activity/motility levels are below a defined threshold. Changes in motility are most commonly measured via wrist actigraphy recordings but also have been measured via electromyographic recordings. Actigraphic measures are a cost effective tool that can be used to assess sleep under conditions where electroencephalographic recordings would be prohibitive. However, since activity levels are low if the person is lying quietly but awake, actigraphic measures can overestimate sleep (1).

There are many types of human performance tasks that have been used to assess neurobehavioral and cognitive function in humans during sleep deprivation (see Chaps. 11–13). In general, vigilance performance tasks tend to be the most sensitive to sleep deprivation, whereas cognitive tasks are less sensitive because they are influenced by learning curves.

III. Sensory Neurophysiology and Behavioral Responsiveness During Sleep

Neurophysiological studies have demonstrated that sensory processing occurs during sleep (2). Steriade (3) reviewed the evidence showing that the transmission of sensory information from the thalamus to the cortex is enhanced during wakefulness and rapid-eye-movement (REM) sleep compared to non-REM (NREM) sleep. In humans, a number of studies have demonstrated that behavioral responsiveness to stimuli can occur in all stages of sleep. In the 1930s, Loomis and colleagues first described electroencephalographic activation (4,5) and the K-complex electroencephalographic response to environmental stimuli during sleep (6,7). More recent studies have reported that a meaningful stimulus, such as a person's name, produces more K complexes than an unimportant stimulus (8,9).

A. Auditory Processing During Sleep

Kleitman (10) and Bonnet (11) reviewed early research examining auditory arousal thresholds prior to the use of the EEG to define sleep. They discussed the pioneering work of Kohlschütter in 1862 that demonstrated higher arousal thresholds during sleep than during wakefulness. Kohlschütter and other investigators also characterized time-of-night differences in auditory arousal thresholds during sleep. It has since been demonstrated, by electroencephalographic studies of sleep, that auditory arousal thresholds progressively increase from stage 1 through stage 4 of NREM sleep. Auditory arousal thresholds during REM sleep have been reported to be similar to those observed during deep NREM sleep or stage 2 sleep (11–15). Time of night and/or internal circadian phase is also reported to influence auditory arousal thresholds within stage 2 sleep and REM sleep (14,16–18). Auditory arousal thresholds have been reported to decrease with age (18–20), and increase following sleep deprivation (15) and the use of hypnotics (21–23).

Behavioral responsiveness to tones can occur in all stages of sleep, however, the likelihood of a behavioral response is greatest in stages 1 and 2 sleep (6,15,24–30). In addition, evidence from sleep deprivation studies indicates that behavioral responsiveness to tones during recovery sleep is reduced by increased homeostatic sleep drive (15,31). Interindividual differences in behavioral responsiveness during sleep have also been reported, especially during stage 1 sleep (32). In 1938 Loomis et al. (6) reported that abortive attempts to squeeze a bulb in response to a stimulus during EEG-defined sleep appeared in the forearm electromyogram, without a successful bulb press. Taken together, these data indicate that responsiveness to stimuli during sleep is dependent on changes in sensory thresholds as well as the ability to perform and complete the behavioral response. For example, a button press is less likely during the muscle atonia of REM sleep. To overcome the influence of muscle atonia on button press responding during REM sleep, Badia and colleagues conducted a series of studies that examined breathing as a behavioral response to stimuli presented during sleep (25,28,30,33–35). In those studies, subjects were instructed to respond to auditory tones by taking a deep breath. A successful behavioral response occurred when the magnitude of the breathing response increased 50% more than the background signal. Following two consecutive failures to respond, the decibel level of the tone was raised. Figure 1 shows the breathing response to a 30-sec beeping tone (0.5 sec on and 0.5 sec off) during slow-wave sleep. Similar to the results from studies that examined button press responses to tones, they found that the rate of breathing responses to tones varied as a function of sleep stage and tone intensity. However, the rate of breathing responses to tones was higher than the rate reported for button press responses to tones. Subjects usually responded to 50–100 tones per night but in the morning subjects reported that they remembered responding to only a small number of the tones. These results demonstrate that

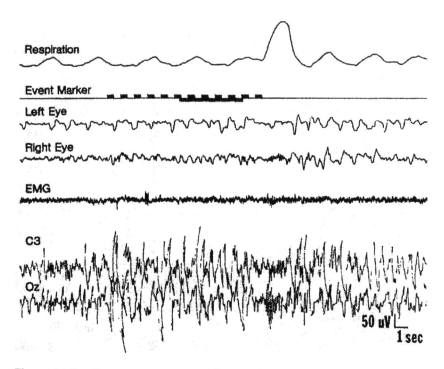

Figure 1 Respiratory response to tone stimuli during slow-wave sleep. Respiration was measured with a strain gauge abdominal belt. The event marker indicates the number of 0.5–sec tone pips prior to the deep breathing response. Also shown are left and right electrooculogram, chin EMG, and central (C3) and occipital (Oz) electroencephalographic brain recordings. Note the brief electroencephalographic activation during the deep breathing response and the return to slow wave activity following the response. (Reproduced from Ref. 25 with permission.)

while humans maintain the capability to process information during sleep, the transfer of these behavioral responses into long-term memory appears to be altered by sleep [see also (36–41)].

The finding that auditory information can be processed during sleep is also supported by findings from evoked or event-related potential studies. Early components of the evoked potential are linked to the sensory processing of stimuli and later components are linked to higher-order cognitive processing of stimuli (42). Campbell et al. (43) reviewed evidence for the maintenance of auditory evoked potentials during sleep. In general, the early brainstem components of the evoked potential are similar between sleep and wakefulness whereas the later cognitive components are altered by sleep. During wakefulness the cognitive evoked potential known as the P300 is elicited when targeted infrequent stimuli are both detected and attended. It has been reported that the P300 in response to auditory

name vs beep during WAKEFULNESS   name vs beep during SLEEP

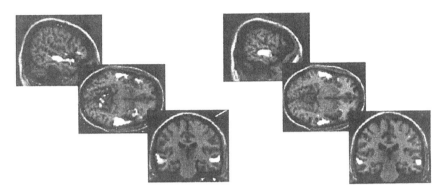

Figure 2 Functional magnetic resonance imaging differential brain activation for name and beeps stimuli during wakefulness (left panel) and during sleep (right panel). Views from left to right: sagittal, horizontal, and coronal. Tone beeps and the subject's name were presented during wakefulness and NREM sleep. Brain activation was higher for name compared to beep presentations. The middle temporal gyrus and the orbitofrontal cortex were bilaterally more activated in both sleep and wakefulness to name stimuli, suggesting that auditory processing of meaningful stimuli is preserved during sleep. (Reproduced from Ref. 51 with permission.)

stimuli is present during sleep but that the latency of the P300 is delayed and the amplitude is reduced (42,44–48). Other auditory evoked components such as the N1 and P2 are altered during sleep as opposed to wakefulness (43,44,49,50). Portas et al. (51) used functional magnetic resonance imaging to examine brain responses to auditory stimuli presented during NREM sleep and reported bilateral activation of the auditory cortex, the thalamus, and the caudate nucleus (Fig. 2). These brain structures have been shown to be important for the sensory and higher order processing of auditory stimuli.

B. Olfactory Processing During Sleep

In 1990, Badia et al. (52) were among the first to examine the influence of odors on the sleep EEG in humans. They reported transient electroencephalographic arousals and heart rate increases in response to brief exposures to peppermint odor during stage 2 sleep. Behavioral responsiveness during sleep also occurred more frequently to odors than to filtered air. In another study, Badia et al. (53) reported that continuous exposure to jasmine and peppermint odors during daytime naps increased stage 1 sleep, the number of spontaneous electroencephalographic awakenings and the number of stage shifts. Carskadon et al. (54) reported a greater number of electroencephalographic and behavioral arousals during stage

2 than in REM or stage 4 sleep in response to nighttime exposure to peppermint and pyridine odors. The latter data suggest that the sleep stage sensitivity to olfactory stimuli is similar to the sleep stage variation in auditory arousal thresholds. Badia et al. (55) examined the influence of heliotropin on sleep, an odor judged to be relaxing during wakefulness. They reported more stage shifts during continuous exposure to the odor than to filtered air. They also examined the influence of two musky odors androstenone (16,5–∝androsten-3-one) and galaxolide on sleep. Some individuals report the odor of androstenone as pleasant and musky, whereas others report it as unpleasant, resembling the smell of strong sweat (56). In addition, approximately 47% of people are reported to be unable to detect the odor during wakefulness. When subjects were exposed to androstenone during sleep, total sleep time and sleep efficiency were decreased and the latency to sleep and number of electroencephalographic awakenings were increased regardless of the pleasant or unpleasant rating of the odor during wakefulness. Thus, the hedonic rating of the odor did not influence the negative impact of androstenone on sleep. Sleep was also disturbed in subjects who reported not being able to smell the odor during wakefulness. These data are consistent with the reported finding that odors below detection threshold can influence brain electroencephalographic activity during wakefulness (57). Unlike most other odors, exposure to galaxolide did not significantly influence sleep. Although the aforementioned studies suggest that the olfactory system is active during sleep and that exposure to most odors disrupts sleep, the influence of trigeminal chemoreception on the reported findings remains to be determined. Currently, there is no evidence that odors can enhance or improve sleep.

C. Somatosensory Processing During Sleep

Davis et al. (7) were among the first to examine somatosensory processing during sleep and they reported electroencephalographic activation and K-complex electroencephalographic responses following electric shocks to the finger. Shagass and Trusty (58) reported that the latency of most peaks and the amplitude of the early components of the somatosensory evoked potential were increased during sleep and that the latency of the peaks during REM sleep were more similar to stage 1 than deep NREM sleep or wakefulness. Saier et al. (59) also reported that the latency and amplitude of the somatosensory evoked potentials were increased during NREM sleep but that evoked potentials were similar between wakefulness and REM sleep. More recent studies have reported that somatosensory evoked potentials during NREM sleep are slower and of higher amplitude than during wakefulness (60–62) whereas evoked potentials during REM sleep are more similar to those observed during wakefulness (61,62).

Other studies have applied nociceptive stimuli to assess somatosensory responsiveness during sleep. Drewes et al. (63) examined responsiveness to saline infusion into the right anterior quadriceps muscle, pneumatic stimulator pressure on the second right proximal interphalangeal joint and cutaneous thermal stimulation with a laser beam applied to the dorsal part of the hand. They reported electroencephalographic arousals during slow-wave sleep in response to the muscle and joint pain stimuli but not in response to the cutaneous thermal pain stimuli. Lavigne et al. (64,65) reported that cold and hot water stimuli applied to the shoulder resulted in a greater number of electroencephalographic arousals and increased heart rate response during stage 2 than in REM sleep or stage 4 sleep, although the criteria for electroencephalographic arousals were different for the sleep stages.

D. Visual Processing During Sleep

In 1939, Davis et al. (7) reported the K-complex electroencephalographic response following room lights being turned on while subjects slept. Fischgold and Schwartz (66) reported that behavioral responses, consisting of two presses of a microswitch, occurred to a flash of light from a stroboscope during pentobarbitone sodium-induced NREM sleep. They reported behavioral responses to the photic stimulus occurred in stages 1 and 2 sleep, but not in slow-wave sleep. However, electroencephalographic activation responses occurred in all stages of sleep. Okuma et al. (67) reported behavioral button switch press responses to photic flash stimuli during stages 1 and 2 sleep and also REM sleep. Shagass and Trusty (58) and Saier et al. (59) reported that the latency of most peaks and the amplitude of the early components of the visual evoked potential were increased during sleep but that the amplitude of the later components was decreased during sleep. The latencies of the visual evoked potential during REM sleep were reported to be more similar to the latency during stage 1 sleep than deep NREM sleep or wakefulness in one study (58) and more similar to wakefulness in another study (59). Sleep-wakefulness state has also been reported to influence late visual evoked potentials in human neonates (68–70). Pena et al. (71) reported that the electroretinogram response to light stimuli was greater during REM sleep compared to NREM sleep in human infants.

IV. Environmental Factors that Influence Sleep

A. Effects of Noise Masking Stimuli on Sleep: White Noise, Pink Noise, and Music

Noise masking stimuli such as white noise, fans, music, and radio static have been used to help patients with sleep disorders sleep in noisy environments (72–74). White noise is a combination of sound frequencies in equal amounts whereas pink noise, fans, music, and radio static are combinations of noises in unequal amounts. At present, there is no scientific evidence to support that such noise-masking stimuli improve sleep in noisy environments. However, the influence of these noise-masking stimuli on sleep compared to exposure to a quiet room has been examined. Scott (75) reported that nighttime exposure to 93-dB white noise reduced REM sleep and increased the percentage of stage 1 and 2 sleep as well as the latency to REM sleep compared to exposure to a quiet room. Similarly, Kawada and Suzuki (76) reported that continuous exposure to 60-dB pink noise decreased the amount of REM sleep and increased the amount of stage 2 sleep. In contrast, Sanchez and Bootzin (77) reported that exposure to 63-dB white noise increased sleep efficiency and reduced the latency to stage 2 sleep and wakefulness after sleep onset compared to exposure to a quiet room. The latter study examined sleep during a 2-hr nap scheduled during the wake maintenance zone of the circadian rhythm of sleep propensity (78,79). Thus, it is unclear whether the inconsistent findings for the effect of white noise on sleep are dependent on circadian phase or other factors that differed among the studies such as the decibel level of the white noise.

While conflicting results have been reported for the effects of white noise on sleep, results from studies that have examined the effect of music on sleep indicate that music disturbs sleep. Sanchez and Bootzin (77) reported that exposure to 71 dB of self-selected radio music played during a 2-hr nap reduced sleep efficiency, reduced stages 3 and 4 sleep and increased wakefulness after sleep onset. Bonnet and Arand (80) reported that self-selected music played during Multiple Sleep Latency Tests (MSLTs) increased the latency to sleep.

B. Effects of Simulated Traffic and Aircraft Noise on Sleep

Findings from early research studies that examined the influence of simulated traffic noise and simulated aircraft noise on sleep indicated that higher intensity noises resulted in a higher probability of arousal from sleep [reviewed in (81)]. Thiessen (82) reported that exposure to seven 65 dB truck passing noises per night increased awakenings and shifts to lighter stages of sleep. Furthermore, after 12 days of exposure to the truck noises there was no evidence of adaptation for the increased number of stage shifts to lighter sleep. However, the number of behavioral awakenings tended to decrease across days. Di Nisi et al. (83) exposed subjects to simulated truck, jet plane, motorcycle, and phone ring noises of approximately 76–88 dB during sleep and reported increased numbers of transient electroencephalographic arousals during sleep, especially during REM and stage 2 sleep. They also reported that heart rate and finger pulse responses to the noises were two to four times as large during sleep than those observed during wakefulness. Libert et al. (84) presented traffic noises of 64–71 dB at a frequency of 9 per hr and reported that traffic noise increased the number of stage changes and amount of stage 1 sleep. Continuous nighttime exposure to 32-, 47-, or 60-dB traffic noise was reported to increase stage 2 "spindle" sleep (85). The increased stage 2 sleep continued across 24 nights of noise presentation without evidence of adaptation to the noise.

Le Vere et al. (86) reported that exposure to simulated aircraft noise disrupted sleep and that reducing the decibel of noise from 80 to 65 reduced the number of electroencephalographic arousals from REM sleep. Carter et al. (87)

reported that aircraft noise of 65 to 72 dB increased the likelihood of electroencephalographic arousal responses and sympathetic activation during sleep. Griefahn and Jansen (88) reported that simulated sonic booms of 80–85 dB increased the number of arousals from sleep. They also reported that there was no evidence of habituation to the arousing effects of the sonic booms presented nightly for one month. Taken together, findings from the above laboratory studies indicate that urban noises disrupt sleep and that there is little evidence for habituation to the sleep-disruptive effects of urban noise.

C. Effects of Light Exposure on Sleep

In nocturnal rodents, exposure to light has been reported to disturb sleep (2,89). In humans, environmental light has been reported to disrupt the subjective sleep quality of intensive care patients (90). However, additional experiments will be required to quantify the degree to which ambient light levels influence objective measures of sleep in humans. Characterization of the sleep response to light stimuli is important for quantifying environmental factors that disrupt the daytime sleep of nightshift workers and the sleep of people living in northern and southern extreme latitudes during the summer when sunlight is present 24 hr/day because of the Earth's tilt on its axis toward the sun.

The influence of morning light exposure during sleep and of evening light exposure on subsequent sleep has been examined. Avery et al. (91) reported that exposure to a dawn simulator with increasing light levels from 0400 to 0600 hr during scheduled sleep episodes resulted in an easier time of awakening and higher subjective alertness upon awakening in adolescents with hypersomnia associated with seasonal affective disorder. Dijk et al. (92) and Cajochen et al. (93) reported that exposure to bright light for 3 hr prior to bedtime increased sleep latency but did not affect sleep staging. However, changes in spectral electroencephalographic power and temperature during sleep were observed after exposure to bright light. Carrier and Dumont (94) reported that exposure to 3 days of 5 hr of bright light in the morning decreased sleep latency at night and exposure to bright light in the evening increased sleep latency at night. Bunnell et al. (95) reported that a single 2 hr episode of bright light prior to bedtime delayed REM sleep, changed spectral electroencephalographic power, and increased temperature levels during sleep. These data indicate that bright light exposure during the daytime can affect sleep propensity without a large change in sleep structure. The effect of daytime light exposure on sleep propensity might be related to a shift in circadian phase. Daurat et al. (96) reported that following exposure to 36 hr of bright light during sleep deprivation, wakefulness after sleep onset and stage 2 sleep were increased and stage 4 sleep was reduced during the first night of recovery sleep. Stage 4 sleep was increased in the bright light condition on the second recovery night, suggesting that the extended exposure to bright light delayed recovery from sleep deprivation.

D. Effects of Ambient Temperature on Sleep

It is well established that extremes in environmental temperature disrupt sleep. Experiments in cats and rats have identified a thermoneutral zone where total sleep time is maximal (97–99). However, thermoregulatory processes are altered during REM sleep (100) making REM sleep more sensitive than NREM to variations in ambient temperature (97,99).

The observation that humans habitually go to sleep on the downward slope of the circadian rhythm of body temperature has led to the suggestion that heat loss plays an important role in the sleep process (79,101–106). Findings from studies that examined the influence of passive heating in the afternoon or evening have indicated that exposure to a sauna (107) or a hot bath (108–112) increased the amount of slow-wave sleep later that night.

While body heating prior to sleep has been reported to improve sleep, nighttime exposure to hot ambient temperature has been reported to disrupt sleep in humans. Libert et al. (84,113) reported that exposure to a hot 35°C ambient temperature increased the latency to sleep, wakefulness after sleep onset, stage 1 sleep, and number of stage changes. Moreover, total sleep time, stage 2 sleep, REM cycle length, and REM duration length decreased. There was no evidence for adaptation to the hot ambient temperature across the 5 days of the study (113). Okamoto-Mizuno et al. (114) reported that a hot 35°C and humid (75% humidity) environment increased wakefulness and reduced slow-wave sleep, REM sleep, and sleep efficiency. However, a 35°C ambient temperature with 50% humidity did not significantly change sleep compared to a 29°C environment at 50% or 75% humidity. These data suggest that humidity alters the sleep disruptive effects of hot ambient temperature. Bach et al. (115) examined the influence of exposure to a hot 35°C ambient temperature combined with sleep restriction and reported that the amount of wakefulness and stage 2 as well as the latencies to sleep and to stage 4 sleep were increased in the hot environment. It is well established that sleep restriction produces effects on sleep that are opposite of the above (i.e., sleep restriction reduces the amounts of wakefulness and stage 2 sleep as well as the latencies to sleep and to stage 4 sleep). Therefore, these data suggest that the effect of ambient temperature on sleep was stronger than was the effect of sleep restriction.

Electric blankets are used in far northern and southern latitudes during sleep in the winter months. At present, it is unknown whether electric blankets improve sleep in cold winter bedroom environments. However, results from several studies indicate that heated blankets that are set to a hot temperature disturb sleep. Karacan et al. (116) reported that an electric blanket that raised bed temperature to 39°C increased the frequency and duration of awakenings and the number of stage shifts, reduced total sleep time, reduced the amount of REM sleep and stages 3 and 4 sleep, and delayed the onset of deep sleep. Fletcher et al. (117) reported that increased bed and body temperature as a result of laying on an electric blanket increased the amount of wakefulness, stage 1, stage changes, and arousals, and decreased sleep efficiency. Baker et al. (118) reported that exposure to a hot 38.1°C microclimate controlled by an air-perfused porous quilt increased stage 2 sleep and reduced REM sleep, especially in women.

Exposure to cold ambient environments has also been reported to disrupt sleep in humans. Haskell et al. (119,120) reported that sleep was disturbed and that subjects shivered during stage 1 and stage 2 sleep, but not stages 3 and 4 sleep or REM sleep when exposed to a cold 21°C ambient temperature environment. Berger et al. (121) and Palca et al. (122) reported that exposure to a cold 21°C environment increased wakefulness and stage 1 sleep, and decreased stage 2 and REM sleep. Sewitch et al. (123) reported decreased sleep efficiency and increased wakefulness in subjects who slept naked, without bed covers, in rooms at 26.7–28.3°C. Muzet et al. (124,125) examined the sleep of 5 subjects at 13, 16, 19, 22, and 25°C and reported that a 9°C decrease in ambient temperature resulted in only a 2.3°C decrease in bed temperature and a lengthening of the average REM cycle length. They concluded that heat dissipation from the body could build a microclimate in the bed that may protect sleep [see also Muzet et al. (126) for a discussion of thermoregulation and human sleep]. Research has also been conducted on the sleep disturbing influence of cold exposure on sleep in human neonates (127,128).

Taken together, the data indicate that environments that are too hot or too cold disturb sleep in humans. In particular, REM sleep and stages 1 and 2 sleep appear to be most sensitive to ambient temperature. Stages 3 and 4 were reduced in some hot exposure studies but not cold exposure studies. Additional studies are needed to quantify a thermoneutral zone for sleep in humans (126) and to examine individual (121) and gender (118) differences in the thermosensitivity of sleep. The disruptive effect of cold and hot ambient temperatures on sleep has been reported to be greater in older than in younger cats (129). Whether older humans are more sensitive than younger humans to the effect of cold and hot ambient temperatures on sleep is unknown. Also, whether time of day and/or circadian phase alters the influence of environmental temperature on sleep in humans is unknown.

E. Effects of Bed Surfaces on Sleep

Kleitman (10) discussed the work by Bowers who "traced the evolution of the bed from a pile of leaves, skins of beasts, framework interlaced with thongs, through the ornate beds of Cleopatra and the Roman emperors, the couch, the bedstead, the twelfth-century high-post canopy-top beds, down to the iron beds of the eighteenth century and the modern folding cot" (p. 309). He also discussed the improvement of bedding with the vertical coil spring and mattress of the early twentieth century. Sullivan (130) reviewed the evolution of the bed from Egyptian to present time. McKennah (131) reviewed cross-cultural differences of infant bed surfaces, such as the wood beds of the Bemba in central Africa, the scooped-out earthen hut of the Maori in New Zealand, the bamboo mattress of the Semang in Malaysia, and the mats of leather or bark of the Tzeltul in Central America. The history of the mattress from sacks filled with cotton felt to foam has been reviewed by Wagner (132), and the history of the pillow from the wood head rests of ancient Egypt (Fig. 3A) to the polyester fiber fill (Fig. 3B) of the present time has been reviewed by Siegel (133). Although there is a rich history on the development of bed surfaces, few studies have investigated the influence of bed surfaces on sleep.

Suckling et al. (134) compared sleep on three bed surfaces—a spring mattress, a feather bed, and a sheet of plywood covered by a thin carpet—and reported that auditory arousal thresholds were lowest and the numbers of movements were greatest on the hard plywood surface. Rosekind et al. (135) compared sleep on a box spring mattress to sleep on a waterbed and reported no difference in sleep architecture between the surfaces across a month-long field and laboratory pilot study of three subjects. Scharf et al. (136) compared sleep on a high-quality innerspring hospital mattress to sleep on a foam mattress and reported no difference in sleep architecture between subjects using these mattresses. However, fewer cyclic patterns of alternating states of arousal during sleep were reported for sleep on the foam surface, the significance of which remains to be determined. Bader and Engdal (137) examined the relationship between sleep quality and bed surface firmness at the homes of participants and reported that compared to the participants' own bed, body movements during sleep were similar on both softer and harder mattresses. Bed surfaces designed to reduce back pain have been reported to improve subjective sleep quality in patients with chronic back pain (134,138); however, the influence of these bed surfaces on objective measures of sleep is unknown.

There are many bed surface options currently available, including foam, flotation, air, fiber, feather, spring, and combination mattresses. Some of these

A   B

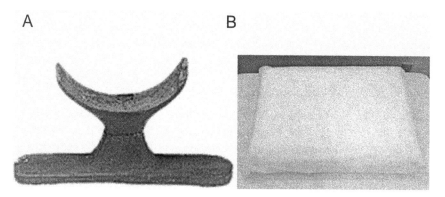

Figure 3   (A) (Courtesy of the Michael C. Carlos Museum of Emory University.) Wooden headrest dated from the New Kingdom of ancient Egypt ca. 1500–1400 BC. Royalty slept on ornate beds while most people slept on the ground or on wood planks (80). Wooden headrests such as the one pictured were used as pillows during sleep and to support the heads of mummies after death. (B) Modern polyester-filled pillow.

mattresses are available heated and others are adjustable. However, the current evidence suggests that the relative advantage of these bed surfaces for sleep is a matter of personal preference.

F. Effects of Bed Partners on Sleep (Cosleeping)

In 1969, Monroe (139) was one of the first investigators to examine the sleep of married couples. He reported that stage 4 sleep was increased by nearly 20 min when husbands and wives slept alone than when they slept together. Furthermore, REM sleep was reduced by approximately 15 min and the numbers of awakenings were reduced by 60 percent when bed partners slept alone. The large increase in slow-wave sleep that was observed when bed partners slept alone might reflect recovery from sleep deprivation since slow-wave sleep is a marker of homeostatic sleep drive (79,140). This finding suggests that the common practice of sharing a bed maybe a significant contributing factor to daytime sleepiness and chronic sleep loss. Pankhurst and Horne (141) examined the sleep of bed partners in a study designed to examine the influence of aircraft noise on sleep. They reported that approximately one-third of arousals from sleep, as measured by wrist actigraphy, were common to bed partners and that arousals decreased during temporary absence of the usual bed partner. Furthermore, arousals from sleep were greater in people who slept with a partner than matched subjects who slept alone. When sleeping with a bed partner, males had more arousals from sleep and females reported being disturbed more often by their partner. The degree to which sleep disorders contributed to the latter finding is unknown, however, treatment of sleep apnea has been reported to improve the sleep efficiency of nonapneic bed partners (142). Future research is required to characterize the degree to which other sleep disorders impact the sleep of bed partners.

McKenna (131) reviewed the history and cross-cultural practices of parent-infant cosleeping that is common in nonindustrialized cultures. Following reports that parent-infant cosleeping resulted in more awakenings and "transient" arousals in infants during sleep (131,143), there has been debate whether or not cosleeping influences the incidence of sudden infant death syndrome (144,145).

There are many other circumstances of bed sharing that are likely to disrupt sleep but have yet to be scientifically investigated. These include the influence of pets on the sleep of their human companions, the influence of sharing beds or bedrooms with siblings, the influence of sharing sleeping quarters in tents while camping, in college dorms, in military barracks, and aboard naval ships, airplanes, and spacecraft.

V. Sleep in Altered Environments

Many studies have been conducted to determine the influence of altered environments on sleep. Some of these studies have examined the influence of environmental factors on sleep in the homes of participants whereas others have examined sleep outside of the home environment. In general, most of these studies have reported that sleep is disturbed in altered environments. Sleep is also disturbed during the first night when people sleep in a new environment. This finding has been coined the "first night effect" (146). As a result of this finding, scientific studies of sleep have typically excluded the first night of sleep recording from data analysis.

A. Effect of City Traffic and Aircraft Noise on Sleep at Home

Survey studies have reported that sleep in urban environments is disturbed by nighttime traffic (147,148) and aircraft noise (148). Horne et al. (149) reported that 6.49% of aircraft noise events measured at the airport were associated with actigraphically measured arousals from sleep. However, they also reported that domestic factors produced more arousals from sleep than did aircraft events (141). Fidell et al. (150) measured the decibel level of aircraft events in the homes of participants and reported that aircraft events of greater than 60 dB lasting for at least 2 sec were associated with arousals from sleep. Wrist actigraphy arousals ranged from approximately 42% to 85% for indoor sound exposure events that ranged from 60 to 90 dB. Figure 4 shows the dose-response relationship between

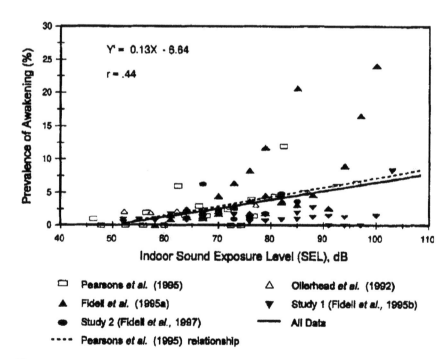

Figure 4   Combined data plot from field studies that examined the influence of aircraft noise on behavioral awakenings from sleep. (Reproduced from Ref. 150 with permission.)

indoor sound exposure levels of aircraft noise events and behavioral awakenings from six field studies. Few behavioral awakenings were reported for aircraft events below 60 dB, whereas aircraft events above 60 dB were more likely to result in a behavioral awakening. Since electroencephalographic arousals from sleep often occur without a behavioral arousal response, these data likely underestimate the influence of aircraft noise on sleep.

Stevenson and McKellar (151) reported a significant correlation between sleep disturbance and traffic noise. Vallet and Mouret (152) reviewed studies published primarily in government and technical reports that showed improvements in sleep following noise reduction by thermopane windows and air plugs. Wilkinson and Campbell (153) implemented a noise attenuation treatment program for people living in areas of high traffic in Cambridge, England. Double glazing of windows in the bedrooms of participants decreased the noise level from 46.6 to 40.8 dB, range 36–47 dB. Figure 5 shows that the intervention increased the amount of electroencephalographic slow-wave activity, improved subjective sleep quality and improved vigilance performance on the Unprepared Reaction Time Test. They also reported that the intervention increased the amount of stage 4 sleep and decreased the number of reported awakenings from sleep. Results from other field studies have also reported that reducing traffic noise by insulating home windows increased slow-wave sleep (154) and reduced the number of body movements during sleep (155).

B.   Sleep in Medical Intensive Care Units and Nursing Homes

Freedman et al. (90) reported that intensive care unit (ICU) patients perceived their sleep to be disturbed by medical treatment and environmental noise. Noise levels in ICUs have been reported to exceed U.S. Environmental Protection Agency noise level recommendations during both the daytime and the nighttime hours (156). Freedman et al. (156) reported that 11.5% of arousals from sleep followed environmental noise. Aaron et al. (157) reported a significant relationship between the number of noises 80 dB or more and the number of arousals in a respiratory care unit. Schnelle et al. (158) reported that environmental noise exceeding 60 dB from staff, residents, televisions, and medical and housekeeping equipment accounted for more than one-fourth of behavioral awakenings from sleep in the nursing home environment. Following a sleep education intervention of the nursing home staff, the average nighttime noise level decreased from 83 to 58 dB and nighttime light levels were reduced. These environmental changes decreased the number of awakenings reported to be associated with noise and light.

C.   Sleep in the Arctic

Few studies have examined sleep outside in the cold extreme of the polar regions. Buguet et al. (159) examined the sleep of two males who slept in an unheated tent for 10 nights in the Arctic where ambient temperatures ranged between −35°C and

-25°C. They reported that the latency to sleep, the number of awakenings, and wakefulness were increased relative to baseline sleep at room temperature. In a follow-up study of eight subjects, Buguet et al. (160) reported that sleeping in unheated tents for 17 nights in the Arctic with an average ambient temperature of -

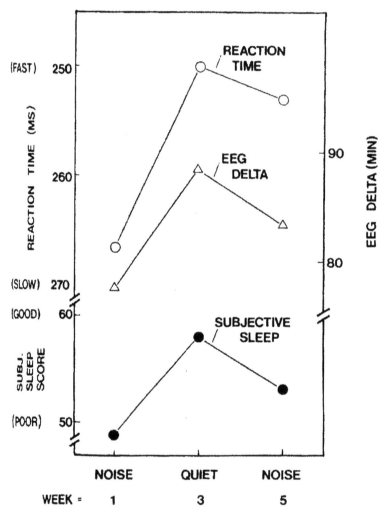

Figure 5   Data showing improvement of sleep and daytime performance following traffic noise reduction in the home. Subjective sleep quality (closed circles), slow-wave electroencephalographic activity (open triangles) and unprepared reaction time performance (open circles) during baseline week 1, during the intervention of window double glazing week 3, and following removal of window glazing during week 5. During the intervention week, reaction time was faster, delta electroencephalographic activity was higher and subjective sleep quality was better compared to baseline and following removal of window glazing. (Reproduced from Ref. 153 with permission.)

25°C decreased REM sleep. In both studies, slow-wave sleep was not significantly affected by sleeping in the extreme Arctic cold. This result is consistent with laboratory studies that did not show an effect of cold exposure on slow-wave sleep. See Buguet et al. (161) for a review of sleep inside polar base housing.

D. Sleep at Altitude

Ascent to altitude affects many physiological processes and insomnia is a common complaint at altitude. Reite (162) was one of the first to describe the influence of altitude on sleep EEG in humans. Figure 6 shows the sleep hypnogram of a subject studied first at sea level and then after a rapid ascent to 4300 m altitude atop Pikes Peak in Colorado. During sleep at sea level the subject progressed to deep NREM sleep and cycled between NREM and REM sleep across the night. However, during sleep at altitude, the amounts of stages 3 and 4 sleep were reduced and the number of awakenings and amount of stage 1 sleep were increased. This sleep fragmentation is typical for sleep at altitude (163,164). Nicholson et al. (165) reported that the sleep of six climbers during an expedition to the Himalayas was disturbed compared to sleep at sea level. Sleep efficiency

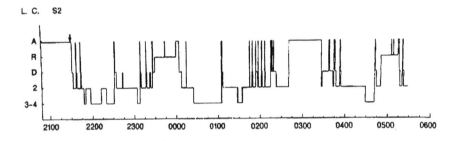

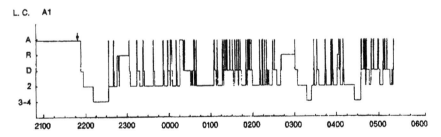

Figure 6 Sleep hypnogram for one subject during baseline sleep at sea level (top panel, S2) and the first night at altitude (bottom panel, A1). Clock hour is plotted on the *x* axis and sleep stage on the *y* axis. Lights out occurred at the small vertical arrow in each plot. Prior to lights out, the subject was being instrumented. Most prominent is the increased number of arousals at altitude. A, awake; R, REM; D, stage 1; 2, stage 2; 3–4, stages 3 and 4 sleep combined. (Reproduced from Ref. 162 with permission.)

was reduced at altitudes above 1100 m. Sleep was most disturbed above 4150 m with average sleep efficiency of 70% compared to 93% at sea level. REM sleep was also reduced above 4150 m. Half of the subjects were taking the respiratory stimulant acetazolamide, which significantly improved sleep above 2750 m. Subjects taking placebo showed nearly 80 more min of wakefulness compared to the group mean at sea level, whereas subjects taking acetazolamide showed just over 10 min more wakefulness compared to that at sea level. Finnegan et al. (163) reported reduced amounts of stage 4 sleep in British Army mountaineers sleeping at heights ranging from 4115 to 6220 m. Miller and Horvath (166) reported that stage 1 sleep and wakefulness were increased and stage 2 sleep was decreased in a hypobaric chamber simulating an altitude of 3500 m.

Sleep disturbance at altitude may be related to lower levels of oxygen, hypoxia, increased apneas and periodic breathing. However, oxygen supplementation reduced periodic breathing but did not change frequency of arousals during sleep (162). Sleep and respiratory physiology at altitude has been reviewed in detail elsewhere (164,167). Other factors such as cold ambient temperature, discomfort of sleeping surfaces, dehydration, and symptoms of acute and chronic mountain sickness may also affect sleep at altitude.

E. Sleep in Space

Graeber reviewed early research that reported the sleep of astronauts and cosmonauts to be disturbed during space flight (168,169). Santy and colleagues (170) surveyed crew members from nine shuttle missions and reported that most crew members slept an average of only 6 hr/day of flight as compared to 7.9 hr/night on the ground. Sleep was polygraphically recorded from an astronaut during a short duration space mission by Gundel et al. (171), from four astronauts aboard the 17-day STS-78 space shuttle mission by Monk et al. (172), from four astronauts aboard the 16-day STS-90 (Neurolab), and from one aboard the 10-day STS-95 space shuttle mission by Dijk et al. (173). The results from these studies confirmed prior subjective reports of reduced sleep duration during space flight. Furthermore, these studies showed that the amount of slow-wave sleep was reduced (172,173) and the amount of wakefulness was increased during space flight (173). Other indications that sleep is disturbed during space flight are the high use of sleep medications by crew members (174) and the rebound of REM sleep upon return to Earth (Fig. 7).

At present, it is unclear whether microgravity and/or other factors of the spacecraft environment are responsible for sleep disruption during space flight. Figure 8 shows the sleeping environment in space. Possible environmental causes of sleep disruption include ambient noise, ambient temperature, the excitement and novelty of the spacecraft environment, mission demands, disruption of the relationship between the internal circadian clock and sleep related to weak synchronizing time cues and/or exposure to bright sunlight at inappropriate circadian times (175,176). In addition, physiological changes associated with microgravity

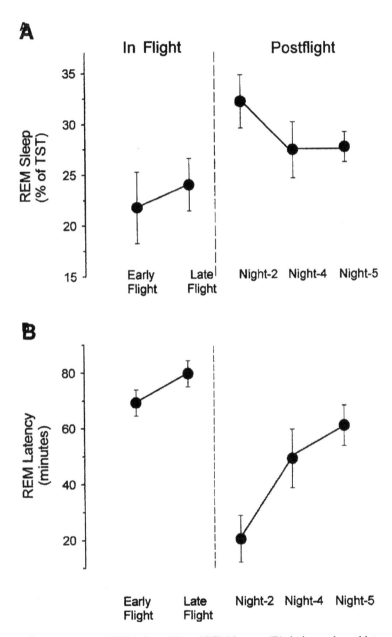

Figure 7 Percentage of REM sleep (A) and REM latency (B) during early and late space flight and the second, fourth, and fifth nights following return to Earth. Sleep EEG was recorded from brain sites C3, C4, O1, and O2 using a sensor array and ambulatory digital sleep recorder (see Fig. 8, middle left panel). On return from space, REM sleep was increased and REM latency was shortened especially on the first postflight recording night perhaps due to an influence of space flight on REM sleep. (Reproduced from Ref. 173 with permission.)

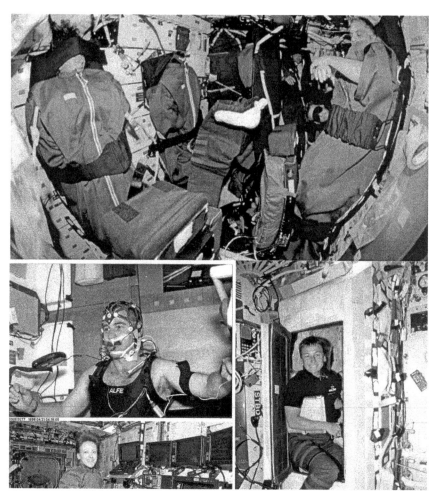

Figure 8 Space environment. Space shuttle (STS-112) crew members sleep on the middeck of Space Shuttle Atlantis (top panel). Pictured are astronauts Sandra H. Magnus, David A. Wolf, Piers J. Sellers, and Jeffrey S. Ashby. Astronauts sometime sleep in sleeping bags that are anchored to the shuttle wall, whereas others have reported sleeping while free floating. Some astronauts restrain their arms and heads whereas others let them free float. Some astronauts wear eyeshades to block light exposure from the shuttle environment while sleeping, especially if they are sleeping in areas of the shuttle with windows. During Earth orbit, the shuttle is exposed to a 90–min light-dark cycle composed of about 45 min of bright sunlight and about 45 min of solar darkness. Sleep stations have been developed to improve the sleeping environment in space (lower right panel). Astronaut Peggy A. Whitson in the doorway of a temporary sleep station in the Destiny laboratory on the International Space Station. Sleep has been recorded in space via polysomnography (middle left panel) and via wrist actigraphy (lower left panel). Astronaut Dave Williams (middle left panel) wears recording equipment that measured electroencephalographic, electromyographic, electrooculographic, and electrocardiographic and respiratory activity during the Neurolab STS-90 sleep study aboard Space Shuttle Columbia. Astronaut Janet L. Kavandi (lower left panel) wears a wrist actilight watch that recorded sleep-wakefulness activity levels throughout the STS-104 space mission. (Courtesy of NASA.)

may influence sleep. In microgravity there is no postural change or vestibular change prior to sleep. There is also a fluid shift from the lower extremities to the chest and head that is maintained throughout the duration of exposure to microgravity. Therefore, the change in sympathetic tone associated with lying down on Earth does not occur in space nor is there a sensation of lying down and placing the head on a pillow in space. The microgravity environment may also influence the activity of brain regions that are important regulators of sleep-wakefulness states (177,178). Additional studies are needed to improve our knowledge of the influence that the space environment has on sleep in humans to prevent chronic sleep loss on long-duration space missions.

VI. Effects of Environmental Factors on Performance During Sleep Deprivation

A. Effects of Noise on Human Performance During Sleep Deprivation

Early research examining the influence of stimuli on performance during sleep deprivation resulted in the hypothesis that arousing stimuli would improve performance (179); however, the available data are conflicting with respect to the influence of noise on performance during sleep deprivation. Corcoran (179) reported that 90 dB white noise increased correct responses on a serial reaction time performance task compared to a no noise condition during total sleep deprivation. In addition, worse performance associated with time-on-task was observed for the no-noise but not the noise condition. However, white noise did not improve visual vigilance performance. Wilkinson (180) reported that continuous exposure to 100-dB white noise with and without exposure to 32 hr of sleep deprivation impaired choice serial reaction time performance. Tassi et al. (181) reported that exposure to 75-dB pink noise improved response times on a spatial memory test when sleep time was delayed to 0100 hr but no performance-enhancing effect was observed when sleep was delayed to 0200 hr following a short nap. Bonnet and Arand (80) exposed subjects to music during MSLT and Maintenance of Wakefulness (MWT) tests after 1 night of total sleep deprivation and reported that music had no effect on sleep onset latency. Thus far, the experiments that have examined the influence of noise on performance during sleep deprivation have tested different measures of performance. Additional experiments will be required to assess whether the influence of noise on performance during sleep deprivation is dependent on the type of brain function examined.

B. Acute Effects of Nocturnal Bright Light on Human Physiology and Performance During Sleep Deprivation

It is well established that exposure to bright light during the biological night can reduce melatonin levels and increase body temperature levels. It has been reported that when melatonin is suppressed and temperature increased, that cognitive performance is enhanced by exposure to bright light during the nighttime work hours and across sleep deprivation (182-189). Figure 9 shows the effects of nighttime exposure to about 2000 lux of bright light versus dim room light of less than 100 lux on melatonin, body temperature, and performance across two nights of sleep deprivation. During continuous exposure to all-night bright light, melatonin levels are lower and temperature and performance levels are higher than during dim light. The effects of bright light on temperature and performance appear to be limited to the nighttime hours; exposure to bright light outside of the biological night has little effect on temperature and performance (185,190). Some studies have also shown bright light exposure to produce signs of electroencephalographic arousal (185,190) whereas others report no effect of bright light on electroencephalographic signs of alertness (184,188,191). In addition to improving performance during the biological night, exposure to bright light can phase shift internal biological time [reviewed in Czeisler and Wright (192)].

C. Effects of Temperature on Human Performance

Extreme body cooling and heating have been reported to impair human performance under non-sleep-deprived conditions (193–199). Figure 10 shows that human performance is better when body temperature is higher regardless of internal circadian phase or time awake.

One study has examined the influence of ambient temperature on performance during sleep deprivation. Pepler (201) examined tracking and serial-choice reaction time performance following one night of total sleep deprivation in a 21°C versus 38°C ambient temperature. He reported that the number of tracking errors and number of lapses increased in the hot room regardless of sleep loss but that the worst performance occurred in the hot room-sleep loss combined condition. These data suggest that ambient temperature and sleep deprivation can interact to influence human performance. The findings from studies of body cooling under non-sleep-deprived conditions suggest that a cold environment combined with sleep deprivation may also impair performance more than either cold or sleep deprivation alone, but such an effect remains to be demonstrated.

VII. Conclusions and Future Directions

Research has shown that the brain senses exposure to auditory, visual, olfactory and somatosensory stimuli during sleep. Environmental factors such as urban noise, cold and hot ambient temperature, odors, bed partners, altitude, and microgravity disturb sleep. Additional research on other factors such as light exposure and bed surfaces is required to characterize their impact on sleep. Environmental sleep disruption is often characterized by increased wakefulness after sleep onset, increased number of electroencephalographic arousals, greater number of stage shifts, and more stage 1 or 2 sleep. REM sleep is reduced by many environmental factors whereas deep slow-wave sleep tends to be less impacted by most envi-

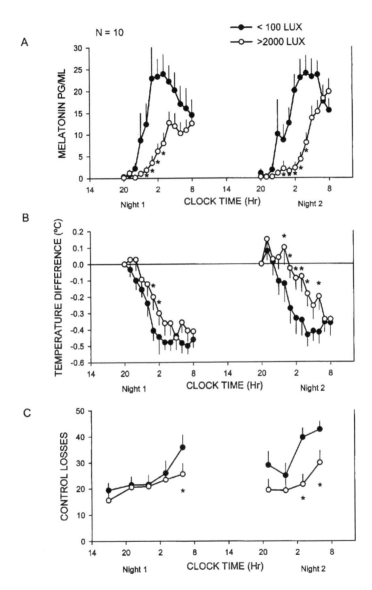

Figure 9 Salivary melatonin (A), tympanic temperature (B), and dual-task control loss performance (C) during two nights of sleep deprivation. Melatonin and temperature data were collected in hourly intervals from 2000 to 0800 hr each night. Temperature data are presented as a difference score from 2000 hr baseline on night 1. Cognitive performance was assessed every 3 hr each night. Higher scores on the dual-task control loss performance task represent worse performance. During the daytime hours all subjects were exposed to less than 100 lux. Between 2000 and 0800 hr, subjects in the bright light condition were exposed to more than 2000 lux. Error bars represent standard error of the mean. Asterisk represents significant difference between dim and bright light exposure. (Reproduced from Ref. 192 with permission.)

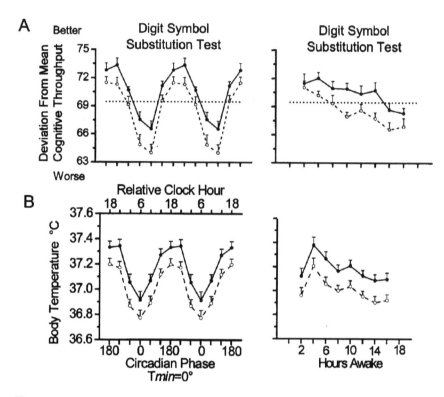

Figure 10 Circadian phase-dependent (left panel; data double plotted) and hours awake-dependent variation (right panel) of cognitive throughput/working memory performance associated with high versus low body temperature. Performance was better when body temperature was high even after controlling for circadian phase and hours awake. Neurobehavioral data are expressed in deviation from individual subject's mean. Scores in the upward direction represent better performance. The group mean (*N* = 14) is added to the high-low deviation scores to indicate the amount of change in performance. Error bars represent ± SEM. The dotted line represents the group mean. (Reproduced from Ref. 200 with permission.)

ronmental stimuli. However, exposures to bed partners, hot ambient temperature, altitude, and space flight have resulted in reduced slow-wave sleep. There is little evidence to suggest that people habituate to environmental factors that disturb sleep. While much is known about the effects of environmental stimuli on sleep, little is known about the consequences of environmental sleep disturbance on physiological and psychological health. Environmental factors that disturb sleep may contribute to chronic sleep loss and daytime sleepiness and fatigue. Future research is required for quantifying the influence of environmental sleep disruption on human brain function and behavior during subsequent wakefulness. Additional studies are also needed to examine factors such as age, gender, and individual differences that may interact with environmental factors that disturb sleep. For example, while it is generally accepted that auditory arousal thresholds are lower with increasing age, little is known about age-related sensitivity to other environmental factors that influence sleep.

Noise reduction interventions have improved sleep in urban environments and the improved sleep was associated with improved performance during wakefulness, although little research has been conducted on developing measures to improve sleep in other altered environments. Additional intervention studies are needed to test strategies for improving sleep in hospital and related environments and to look at the influence of these interventions on health recovery time. Future studies are needed to understand the mechanisms that influence sleep in extreme environments and to develop measures to improve sleep under those conditions. Additional studies are also needed to examine the influence of environmental factors on recovery sleep following sleep deprivation and on performance during sleep deprivation.

Acknowledgments

This chapter is dedicated in honor of the contributions of Pietro Badia to the field of sleep research. Some of the work described in this chapter was supported in part by General Clinical Research Center grant NCRR-GCRC-M01-RR02635 from the National Center for Research Resources; by a Non-Service Fellowship Award of Bowling Green State University and NIH T32-DK07529 Institutional National Research Service Award; by Army Research Institute MDA 903-93-K-002, U.S. Army Medical Research Acquisition and Activity DAMD17-95-2-5015; by NASA Cooperative Agreement NCC9-58 with the National Space Biomedical Research Institute and NASA; and by the Ohio Board of Regents Selective Excellence Program, the Medical Foundation and The Harold Whitworth Pierce Charitable Trust, the Brigham and Women's Hospital, Boston, MA, and the University of Colorado at Boulder.

References

1. Pollak CP, Tryon WW, Nagaraja H, Dzwonczyk R. How accurately does wrist actigraphy identify the states of sleep and wakefulness? Sleep 2001;24:957–965.
2. Velluti RA. Interactions between sleep and sensory physiology. J Sleep Res 1997;6:61–77.
3. Steriade M. Brain electrical activity and sensory processing during waking and sleep states. In: Chase MH, ed. Sleep Mechanisms. Philadelphia: WB Saunders, 2000:93–111.
4. Loomis AL, Harvey EN, Hobart G. Potential rhythms of the cerebral cortex during sleep. Science 1935;81:597–598.
5. Loomis AL, Harvey EN, Hobart G. Further observations on the potential rythms of the cerebral cortex during sleep. Science 1935;82:198–200.

6. Loomis AL, Harvey EN, Hobart G. Distribution of disturbance-patterns in the human electroencephalogram with special reference to sleep. J Neurophysiol 1938;1:413–430.

7. Davis H, Davis PA, Loomis AL, Harvey EN, Hobart G. Electrical reactions of the human brain to auditory stimulation during sleep. J Neurophysiol 1939;2:500–514.

8. Oswald I, Taylor AM, Treisman M. Discrimination responses to stimulation during human sleep. Brain 1960;83:440–452. 1960.

9. Voss U, Harsh J. Information processing and coping style during the wake/sleep transition. J Sleep Res 1998;7:225–232.

10. Kleitman N. Sleep and Wakefulness. Chicago: University of Chicago Press, 1963.

11. Bonnet MH. Depth of sleep. In: Carskadon MA, ed. Encyclopedia of Sleep and Dreaming. New York: Macmillan, 1993:186–188.

12. Rechtschaffen A, Hauri P, Zeitlin M. Auditory awakening thresholds in REM and NREM sleep stages. Percept Mot Skills 1966;22:927–942.

13. Blake H, Gerard RW. Brain potentials during sleep. Am J Physiol 1937; 119:692–703. 1937.

14. Roehrs T, Merlotti L, Petrucelli N, Stepanski E, Roth T. Experimental sleep fragmentation. Sleep 1994;17:438–443.

15. Williams HL, Hammack JT, Daly RL, Dement WC, Lubin A. Responses to auditory stimulation, sleep loss and the EEG stages of sleep. Electroencephalogr Clin Neurophysiol 1964;16:269–279.

16. Lammers WJ, Badia P. Motor responsiveness to stimuli presented during sleep: the influence of time-of-testing on sleep stage analyses. Physiol Behav 1991;50:867–868.

17. Lammers WJ, Badia P, Hughes R, Harsh J. Temperature, time-of-night of testing, and responsiveness to stimuli presented while sleeping. Psychophysiology 1991;28:463–467.

18. Pivik RT, Joncas S, Busby KA. Sleep spindles and arousal: the effects of age and sensory stimulation. Sleep Res Online 1999;2:89–100.

19. Zepelin H, McDonald CS, Zammit GK. Effects of age on auditory awakening thresholds. J Gerontol 1984;39:294–300.

20. Busby K, Pivik RT. Failure of high intensity auditory stimuli to affect behavioral arousal in children during the first sleep cycle. Pediatr Res 1983;17:802–805.

21. Bonnet MH, Webb WB, Barnard G. Effect of flurazepam, pentobarbital, and caffeine on arousal threshold. Sleep 1979;1:271–279.

22. Hartse KM, Thornby JI, Karacan I, Williams RL. Effects of brotizolam, flurazepam and placebo upon nocturnal auditory arousal thresholds. Br J Clin Pharmacol 1983;16 Suppl 2:355S-364S.

23. Mendelson WB, Martin JV, Stephens H, Giesen H, James SP. Effects of flurazepam on sleep, arousal threshold, and the perception of being asleep. Psychopharmacology (Berl) 1988;95:258–262.

24. Williams HL, Morlock HC Jr, Morlock,JV. Instrumental behavior during sleep. Psychophysiology 1966;2:208–216.

25. Badia P, Harsh J, Balkin T, Cantrell P, Klempert A, O'Rourke D, Schoen L. Behavioral control of respiration in sleep. Psychophysiology 1984;21:494–500.

26. Bonnet MH. Auditory thresholds during continuing sleep. Biol Psychol 1986;22:3–10.

27. Kennedy WA, Czeisler CA, Richardson GS. Electroencephalographic recordings at the transition from wakefulness to sleep do not precisely cooerelate with the ability to respond to auditory stimuli. Sleep Res 1985;14:119.

28. Harsh J, Badia P, O'Rourke D, Burton S, Revis C, Magee J. Factors related to behavioral control by stimuli presented during sleep. Psychophysiology 1987;24:535–541.

29. Ogilvie RD, Wilkinson RT. Behavioral versus EEG-based monitoring of all-night sleep/wake patterns. Sleep 1988;11:139–155.

30. Burton SA, Harsh JR, Badia P. Cognitive activity in sleep and responsiveness to external stimuli. Sleep 1988;11:61–68.

31. Balkin T, Badia P, Harsh J, Klempert A. Behavioral responsivity during recovery sleep. Biol Psychol 1985;20:17–20.

32. Ogilvie RD, Wilkinson RT, Allison S. The detection of sleep onset: behavioral, physiological, and subjective convergence. Sleep 1989;12:458–474.

33. Badia P, Harsh J, Balkin T, O'Rourke D, Burton S. Behavioral control of respiration in sleep and sleepiness due to signal-induced sleep fragmentation. Psychophysiology 1985;22:517–524.

34. Badia P, Harsh J, Balkin T. Behavioral control over sleeping respiration in normals for ten consecutive nights. Psychophysiology 1986;23:409–411.

35. Harsh J, Purvis B, Badia P, Magee J. Behavioral responsiveness in sleeping older adults. Biol Psychol 1990;30:51–60.

36. Loomis AL, Harvey EN, Hobart G. Cerebral states during sleep, as studied by human brain potentials. J Exp Psychol 1937;21:127–144.

37. Badia P. Memories in sleep: Old and new. In: Bootzin RR, Kihlstrom JF, Schacter DL, eds. Sleep and Cognition. Washington, DC: American Psychological Association, 1990:67–76.

38. Guilleminault C, Dement,WC. Amnesia and disorders of excessive daytime sleepiness. In: Drucker-Colin RR, McGaugh JL, eds. Neurobiology of Sleep and Memory. New York: Academic Press, 1977:439–456.

39. Wyatt JK, Bootzin RR, Allen JJ, Anthony JL. Mesograde amnesia during the sleep onset transition: replication and electrophysiological correlates. Sleep 1997;20:512–522.

40. Wyatt JK, Bootzin RR, Anthony J, Bazant S. Sleep onset is associated with retrograde and anterograde amnesia. Sleep 1994;17:502–511.

41. Roehrs T, Roth T. Sleep-wake state and memory function. Sleep 2000;23 Suppl 3:S64–S68.

42. Wesensten NJ, Badia P. The P300 component in sleep. Physiol Behav 1988;44:215–220.

43. Campbell K, Bell I, Bastien C. Evoked potential measures of information processing during natural sleep. In: Broughton RJ, Ogilvie RD, eds. Sleep, Arousal, and Performance. Boston: Birkhäuser, 1992:88–116.

44. Harsh J, Voss U, Hull J, Schrepfer S, Badia P. ERP and behavioral changes during the wake/sleep transition. Psychophysiology 1994;31:244–252.

45. Atienza M, Cantero JL, Escera C. Auditory information processing during human sleep as revealed by event-related brain potentials. Clin Neurophysiol 2001;112:2031–2045.

46. Cote KA, Etienne L, Campbell KB. Neurophysiological evidence for the detection of external stimuli during sleep. Sleep 2001;24:791–803.

47. Cote KA, Campbell KB. P300 to high intensity stimuli during REM sleep. Clin Neurophysiol 1999;110:1345–1350.
48. Nashida T, Yabe H, Sato Y, Hiruma T, Sutoh T, Shinozaki N, Kaneko S. Automatic auditory information processing in sleep. Sleep 2000;23:821–828.
49. Williams HL, Tepas DI, Morlock HC. Evoked responses to clicks and electroencephalographic stages of sleep in man. Science 1962;138:685–686.
50. Ornitz EM, Ritvo ER, Carr EM, La Franchi S, Walter RD. The effect of sleep onset on the auditory averaged evoked response. Electroencephalogr Clin Neurophysiol 1967;23:335–341.
51. Portas CM, Krakow K, Allen P, Josephs O, Armony JL, Frith CD. Auditory processing across the sleep-wake cycle: simultaneous EEG and fMRI monitoring in humans. Neuron 2000;28:991–999.
52. Badia P, Wesensten N, Lammers W, Culpepper J, Harsh J. Responsiveness to olfactory stimuli presented in sleep. Physiol Behav 1990;48:87–90.
53. Badia P, Boecker M, Lammers,W. Some effects of different olfactory stimuli on sleep. Sleep Res 1990;19:145.
54. Carskadon MA, Bigler P, Carr J, Gelin J, Etgen G, Davis SS, Herman KB. Olfactory arousal thresholds during sleep. Sleep Res 1990;19:147.
55. Badia P, Boecker MR, Wright KP Jr. Some effects of fragrances on sleep. Compendium of Olfactory Research 1982–1994: Explorations in Aroma-Chology: Investigating the Sense of Smell and Human Response to Odors. Dubuque: Kendall/Hunt, 1994:31–37.
56. Wysocki CJ, Beauchamp GK. Ability to smell androstenone is genetically determined. Proc Natl Acad Sci U S A 1984;81:4899–4902.
57. Schwartz GE, Bell IR, Dikman ZV, Fernandez M, Kline JP, Peterson JM, Wright KP. EEG responses to low-level chemicals in normals and cacosmics. Toxicol Ind Health 1994;10:633–643.
58. Shagass C, Trusty DM. Somatosensory and visual cerebral evoked response changes during sleep. Rec Adv Biol Psychiatry 1965;8:321–334.
59. Saier J, Regis H, Mano T, Gastaut H. Visual and somatosensory evoked potentials, during sleep, in man. Brain Res 1968;10:431–440.
60. Addy RO, Dinner DS, Luders H, Lesser RP, Morris HH, Wyllie E. The effects of sleep on median nerve short latency somatosensory evoked potentials. Electroencephalogr Clin Neurophysiol 1989;74:105–111.
61. Noguchi Y, Yamada T, Yeh M, Matsubara M, Kokubun Y, Kawada J, Shiraishi G, Kajimoto S. Dissociated changes of frontal and parietal somatosensory evoked potentials in sleep. Neurology 1995;45:154–160.
62. Nakano S, Tsuji S, Matsunaga K, Murai Y. Effect of sleep stage on somatosensory evoked potentials by median nerve stimulation. Electroencephalogr Clin Neurophysiol 1995;96:385–389.
63. Drewes AM, Nielsen KD, Arendt-Nielsen L, Birket-Smith L, Hansen LM. The effect of cutaneous and deep pain on the electroencephalogram during sleep—an experimental study. Sleep 1997;20:632–640.
64. Lavigne G, Zucconi M, Castronovo C, Manzini C, Marchettini P, Smirne S. Sleep arousal response to experimental thermal stimulation during sleep in human subjects free of pain and sleep problems. Pain 2000;84:283–290.
65. Lavigne GJ, Zucconi M, Castronovo V, Manzini C, Veglia F, Smirne S, Ferini-Strambi L. Heart rate changes during sleep in response to experimental thermal

(nociceptive) stimulations in healthy subjects. Clin Neurophysiol 2001;112:532–535.

66. Fischgold H, Schwartz BA. A clinical, electroencephalographic and polygraphic study of sleep in the human adult. In: Wolstenholme GEW, O'Connor M, eds. Nature of Sleep. Boston: Little, Brown, 1960:209–236.

67. Okuma T, Nakamura K, Hayashi A, Fujimori M. Psychophysiological study on the depth of sleep in normal human subjects. Electroencephalogr Clin Neurophysiol 1966; 21:140–147.

68. Whyte HE, Pearce JM, Taylor MJ. Changes in the VEP in preterm neonates with arousal states, as assessed by EEG monitoring. Electroencephalogr Clin Neurophysiol 1987;68:223–225.

69. Apkarian P, Mirmiran M, Tijssen R. Effects of behavioural state on visual processing in neonates. Neuropediatrics 1991;22:85–91.

70. Mercuri E, von Siebenthal K, Tutuncuoglu S, Guzzetta F, Casaer P. The effect of behavioural states on visual evoked responses in preterm and full-term newborns. Neuropediatrics 1995;26:211–213.

71. Pena M, Birch D, Uauy R, Peirano P. The effect of sleep state on electroretinographic (ERG) activity during early human development. Early Hum Dev 1999;55:51–62.

72. Hauri P. Current Concepts: Sleep Disorders. Kalamazoo, MI: The Upjohn Company, 1992.

73. Culebras A. Clinical Handbook of Sleep Disorders. Boston: Butterworth-Heinemann, 1996.

74. Aldrich MS. Sleep Medicine. New York: Oxford, 1999.

75. Scott TD. The effects of continuous, high intensity, white noise on the human sleep cycle. Psychophysiology 1972;9:227–232.

76. Kawada T, Suzuki S. Change in rapid eye movement (REM) sleep in response to exposure to all- night noise and transient noise. Arch Environ Health 1999;54:336–340.

77. Sanchez R, Bootzin RR. A comparison of white noise and music: effects of predictable and unpredictable sounds on sleep. Sleep Res 1985;14:121.

78. Lavie P. Ultrashort sleep-waking schedule III. "Gates" and "forbidden zones" for sleep. Electroenceph Clin Neurophysiol 1986;63:414–425.

79. Dijk DJ, Czeisler CA. Contribution of the circadian pacemaker and the sleep homeostat to sleep propensity, sleep structure, electroencephalographic slow waves, and sleep spindle activity in humans. J Neurosci 1995;15:3526–3538.

80. Bonnet MH, Arand DL. The impact of music upon sleep tendency as measured by the multiple sleep latency test and maintenance of wakefulness test. Physiol Behav 2000;71:485–492.

81. Lukas JS. Noise and sleep: a literature review and a proposed criterion for assessing effect. J Acoust Soc Am 1975;58:1232–1242.

82. Thiessen GJ. Disturbance of sleep by noise. J Acoust Soc Am 1978;64:216–222.

83. Di Nisi J, Muzet A, Ehrhart J, Libert JP. Comparison of cardiovascular responses to noise during waking and sleeping in humans. Sleep 1990;13:108–120.

84. Libert JP, Bach V, Johnson LC, Ehrhart J, Wittersheim G, Keller D. Relative and combined effects of heat and noise exposure on sleep in humans. Sleep 1991;14:24–31.

85. Thiessen GJ. Effect of traffic noise on the cyclical nature of sleep. J Acoust Soc Am 1988;84:1741–1743.

86. LeVere TE, Bartus RT, Hart FD. Electroencephalographic and behavioral effects of nocturnally occurring jet aircraft sounds. Aerospace Med 1972;43:384–389.

87. Carter NL, Hunyor SN, Crawford G, Kelly D, Smith AJ. Environmental noise and sleep—a study of arousals, cardiac arrhythmia and urinary catecholamines. Sleep 1994;17:298–307.

88. Griefahn B, Jansen G. Disturbance of sleep by sonic booms. Sci Total Environ 1975;4:107–112.

89. Tobler I, Franken P, Alfoldi P, Borbely AA. Room light impairs sleep in the albino rat. Behav Brain Res 1994;63:205–211.

90. Freedman NS, Kotzer N, Schwab RJ. Patient perception of sleep quality and etiology of sleep disruption in the intensive care unit. Am J Respir Crit Care Med 1999;159:1155–1162.

91. Avery DH, Kouri ME, Monaghan K, Bolte MA, Hellekson C, Eder D. Is dawn simulation effective in ameliorating the difficulty awakening in seasonal affective disorder associated with hypersomnia? J Affect Disord 2002;69:231–236.

92. Dijk DJ, Cajochen C, Borbely AA. Effect of a single 3–hour exposure to bright light on core body temperature and sleep in humans. Neurosci Lett 1991;121:59–62.

93. Cajochen C, Krauchi K, Danilenko KV, Wirz-Justice A. Evening administration of melatonin and bright light: interactions on the EEG during sleep and wakefulness. J Sleep Res 1998;7:145–157.

94. Carrier J, Dumont M. Sleep propensity and sleep architecture after bright light exposure at three different times of day. J Sleep Res 1995;4:202–211.

95. Bunnell DE, Treiber SP, Phillips NH, Berger RJ. Effects of evening bright light exposure on melatonin, body temperature and sleep. J Sleep Res 1992;1:17–23.

96. Daurat A, Aguirre A, Foret J, Benoit O. Disruption of sleep recovery after 36 hours of exposure to moderately bright light. Sleep 1997;20:352–358.

97. Parmeggiani PL. Influence of the temperature signal on sleep in mammals. Biol Signals Recept 2000;9:279–282.

98. Szymusiak R, Satinoff E. Ambient temperature-dependence of sleep disturbances produced by basal forebrain damage in rats. Brain Res Bull 1984;12:295–305.

99. Glotzbach SF, Heller HC. Temperature Regulation. In: Kryger MH, Roth T, Dement WC, eds. Principles and Practice of Sleep Medicine. Philadelphia: WB Saunders, 2000:289–304.

100. Heller HC, Glotzbach SF. Arousal state influences on thermosensitivity of hypothalamic neurons. In: Koella WP, Rüther E, Schultz H, eds. Sleep '84. Stuttgart: Gustav Fischer Verlag, 1985:69–71.

101. Czeisler CA, Weitzman E, Moore-Ede MC, Zimmerman JC, Knauer RS. Human sleep: its duration and organization depend on its circadian phase. Science 1980;210:1264–1267.

102. Campbell SS, Broughton RJ. Rapid decline in body temperature before sleep: fluffing the physiological pillow? Chronobiol Int 1994;11:126–131.

103. Murphy PJ, Campbell SS. Nighttime drop in body temperature: a physiological trigger for sleep onset? Sleep 1997;20:505–511.

104. Krauchi K, Cajochen C, Werth E, Wirz-Justice A. Warm feet promote the rapid onset of sleep. Nature 1999;401:36–37.

105. Krauchi K, Cajochen C, Werth E, Wirz-Justice A. Functional link between distal vasodilation and sleep-onset latency? Am J Physiol Regul Integr Comp Physiol 2000;278:R741–R748.

106. Krauchi K, Wirz-Justice A. Circadian clues to sleep onset mechanisms. Neuropsychopharmacology 2001;25:S92–S96.

107. Putkonen PTS, Elomaa E, Kotilanen. Increase in delta (3+4) sleep after heat stress in sauna. Scand J Clin Lab Invest 1973;31:19.

108. Horne JA, Reid AJ. Night-time sleep EEG changes following body heating in a warm bath. Electroencephalogr Clin Neurophysiol 1985;60:154–157.

109. Bunnell DE, Horvath SM. Effects of body heating during sleep interruption. Sleep 1985;8:274–282.

110. Horne JA, Shackell BS. Slow wave sleep elevations after body heating: proximity to sleep and effects of aspirin. Sleep 1987;10:383–392.

111. Bunnell DE, Agnew JA, Horvath SM, Jopson L, Wills M. Passive body heating and sleep: influence of proximity to sleep. Sleep 1988;11:210–219.

112. Jordan J, Montgomery I, Trinder J. The effect of afternoon body heating on body temperature and slow wave sleep. Psychophysiology 1990;27:560–566.

113. Libert JP, Di Nisi J, Fukuda H, Muzet A, Ehrhart J, Amoros C. Effect of continuous heat exposure on sleep stages in humans. Sleep 1988;11:195–209.

114. Okamoto-Mizuno K, Mizuno K, Michie S, Maeda A, Iizuka S. Effects of humid heat exposure on human sleep stages and body temperature. Sleep 1999;22:767–773.

115. Bach V, Maingourd Y, Libert JP, Oudart H, Muzet A, Lenzi P, Johnson LC. Effect of continuous heat exposure on sleep during partial sleep deprivation. Sleep 1994;17:1–10.

116. Karacan I, Thornby JI, Anch AM, Williams RL, Perkins HM. Effects of high ambient temperature on sleep in young men. Aviat Space Environ Med 1978;49:855–860.

117. Fletcher A, van den HC, Dawson D. Sleeping with an electric blanket: effects on core temperature, sleep, and melatonin in young adults. Sleep 1999;22:313–318.

118. Baker FC, Selsick H, Driver HS, Taylor SR, Mitchell D. Different nocturnal body temperatures and sleep with forced-air warming in men and in women taking hormonal contraceptives. J Sleep Res 1998;7:175–181.

119. Haskell EH, Palca JW, Walker JM, Berger RJ, Heller HC. Metabolism and thermoregulation during stages of sleep in humans exposed to heat and cold. J Appl Physiol 1981;51:948–954.

120. Haskell EH, Palca JW, Walker JM, Berger RJ, Heller HC. The effects of high and low ambient temperatures on human sleep stages. Electroencephalogr Clin Neurophysiol 1981;51:494–501.

121. Berger RJ, Palca JW, Walker JM. Human sleep, metabolism, and thermoregulation during cold exposure. In: Koella WP, Rüther E, Schultz H, eds. Sleep '84. New York: Gustav Fischer Verlag, 1985:77–80.

122. Palca JW, Walker JM, Berger RJ. Thermoregulation, metabolism, and stages of sleep in cold-exposed men. J Appl Physiol 1986;61:940–947.

123. Sewitch DE, Kittrell EM, Kupfer DJ, Reynolds CF, III. Body temperature and sleep architecture in response to a mild cold stress in women. Physiol Behav 1986;36:951–957.

124. Muzet A, Libert JP. Effects of ambient temperature on sleep in man. In: Koella WP, Rüther E, Schultz H, eds. Sleep '84. New York: Gustav Fischer Verlag, 1985:74–76.

125. Muzet A, Ehrhart J, Candas V, Libert JP, Vogt JJ. REM sleep and ambient temperature in man. Inter J Neurosci 1983;18:117–226.

126. Muzet A, Libert JP, Candas V. Ambient temperature and human sleep. Experientia 1984;40: 425–429.

127. Telliez F, Bach V, Dewasmes G, Leke A, Libert JP. Sleep modifications during cool acclimation in human neonates. Neurosci Lett 1998;245:25–28.

128. Franco P, Scaillet S, Valente F, Chabanski S, Groswasser J, Kahn A. Ambient temperature is associated with changes in infants' arousability from sleep. Sleep 2001;24:325–329.

129. Bowersox SS, Dement WC, Glotzbach SF. The influence of ambient temperature on sleep characteristics in the aged cat. Brain Res 1988;457:200–203.

130. Sullivan J. Beds. In: Carskadon MA, ed. Encyclopedia of Sleep and Dreaming. New York: Macmillan, 1993:66–68.

131. McKenna JJ. Co-sleeping. In: Carskadon MA, ed. Encyclopedia of Sleep and Dreaming. New York: Macmillan, 1993:143–148.

132. Wagner R. Mattress. In: Carskadon MA, ed. Encyclopedia of Sleep and Dreaming. New York: Macmillan, 1993:348–249.

133. Siegel DJ. Pillows. In: Carskadon MA, ed. Encyclopedia of Sleep and Dreaming. New York: Macmillan, 1993:454–456.

134. Suckling EE, Koenig EH, Hoffman BF, Brooks C. The physiological effects of sleeping on hard or soft beds. Hum Biol 1957;29:274–288.

135. Rosekind M, Phillips R, Rappaport J, Babcock D, Dement WC. Effects of waterbed surface on sleep: a pilot study. Sleep Res 1976;5:132.

136. Scharf MB, Stover R, McDannold M, Kaye H, Berkowitz DV. Comparative effects of sleep on a standard mattress to an experimental foam surface on sleep architecture and CAP rates. Sleep 1997;20:1197–1200.

137. Bader GG, Engdal S. The influence of bed firmness on sleep quality. Appl Ergon 2000;31:487–497.

138. Jacobson BH, Gemmell HA, Hayes BM, Altena TS. Effectiveness of a selected bedding system on quality of sleep, low back pain, shoulder pain, and spine stiffness. J Manip Physiol Ther 2002;25:88–92.

139. Monroe LJ. Transient changes in EEG sleep patterns of married good sleepers: the effects of altering sleeping arrangement. Psychophysiology 1969;6:330–337.

140. Borbély AA, Achermann P. Sleep homeostasis and models of sleep regulation. J Biol Rhythms 1999;14:557–568.

141. Pankhurst FP, Horne JA. The influence of bed partners on movement during sleep. Sleep 1994;17:308–315.

142. Beninati W, Harris CD, Herold DL, Shepard JW Jr. The effect of snoring and obstructive sleep apnea on the sleep quality of bed partners. Mayo Clin Proc 1999;74:955–958.

143. Mosko S, Richard C, McKenna J. Infant arousals during mother-infant bed sharing: implications for infant sleep and sudden infant death syndrome research. Pediatrics 1997;100:841–849.

144. Gunn TR, Davis S, Tonkin S. Bed sharing as a risk factor for sudden infant death (cot death). N Z Med J 1992;105:155–156.

145. Thogmartin JR, Siebert CF Jr, Pellan WA. Sleep position and bed-sharing in sudden infant deaths: an examination of autopsy findings. J Pediatr 2001;138:212–217.

146. Agnew HW, Webb WB, Williams RL. The first night effect: an EEG study of sleep. Psychophysiology 1966;2:263–266.

147. Langdon FJ, Buller IB. Road traffic noise and disturbance to sleep. J Sound Vib 1977;50:13–28.

148. Pollak CP. Noise. In: Carskadon MA, ed. Encyclopedia of Sleep and Dreaming. New York: Macmillan, 1993:412–413.

149. Horne JA, Pankhurst FL, Reyner LA, Hume K, Diamond ID. A field study of sleep disturbance: effects of aircraft noise and other factors on 5,742 nights of actimetrically monitored sleep in a large subject sample. Sleep 1994;17:146–159.

150. Fidell S, Pearsons K, Tabachnick BG, Howe R. Effects on sleep disturbance of changes in aircraft noise near three airports. J Acoust Soc Am 2000;107:2535–2547.

151. Stevenson DC, McKellar NR. The effect of traffic noise on sleep of young adults in their homes. J Acoust Soc Am 1989;85:768–771.

152. Vallet M, Mouret J. Sleep disturbance due to transportation noise: ear plugs vs oral drugs. Experientia 1984;40:429–437.

153. Wilkinson RT, Campbell KB. Effects of traffic noise on quality of sleep: assessment by EEG, subjective report, or performance the next day. J Acoust Soc Am 1984;75:468–475.

154. Eberhardt JL, Akselsson KR. The disturbance by road traffic noise of the sleep of young male adults as recorded in the home. J Sound Vib 1987;114:417–434.

155. Ohrstrom E, Bjorkman M. Sleep disturbance before and after traffic noise attenuation in an apartment building. J Acoust Soc Am 1983;73:877–879.

156. Freedman NS, Gazendam J, Levan L, Pack AI, Schwab RJ. Abnormal sleep/wake cycles and the effect of environmental noise on sleep disruption in the intensive care unit. Am J Respir Crit Care Med 2001;163:451–457.

157. Aaron JN, Carlisle CC, Carskadon MA, Meyer TJ, Hill NS, Millman RP. Environmental noise as a cause of sleep disruption in an intermediate respiratory care unit. Sleep 1996;19:707–710.

158. Schnelle JF, Cruise PA, Alessi CA, Ludlow K, al Samarrai NR, Ouslander JG. Sleep hygiene in physically dependent nursing home residents: behavioral and environmental intervention implications. Sleep 1998;21:515–523.

159. Buguet AC, Livingstone SD, Reed LD, Limmer RE. EEG patterns and body temperatures in man during sleep in Arctic winter nights. Int J Biometeorol 1976;20:61–69.

160. Buguet A, Roussel B, Radomski MW. Sleep quality in adverse environments depends on individual stress reaction. In: Koella WP, Rüther E, Schultz H, eds. Sleep '84. Stuttgart: Gustav Fischer Verlag, 1985:72–73.

161. Buguet A, Cespuglio,R, Radomski MW. Sleep and stress in man: an approach through exercise and exposure to extreme environments. Can J Physiol Pharmacol 1998;76:553–561.

162. Reite M, Jackson D, Cahoon RL, Weil JV. Sleep physiology at high altitude. Electroencephalogr Clin Neurophysiol 1975;38:463–471.

163. Finnegan TP, Abraham P, Docherty TB. Ambulatory monitoring of the electroencephalogram in high altitude mountaineers. Electroencephalogr Clin Neurophysiol 1985;60:220–224.

164. Weil JV. Respiratory physiology: sleep at high altitudes. In: Kryger MH, Roth T, Dement WC, eds. Principles and Practice of Sleep Medicine. Philadelphia: WB Saunders, 2000:242–253.

165. Nicholson AN, Smith PA, Stone BM, Bradwell AR, Coote JH. Altitude insomnia: studies during an expedition to the himalayas. Sleep 1988;11:354–361.

166. Miller JC, Horvath SM. Sleep at altitude. Aviat Space Environ Med 1977;48:615–620.

167. Coote JH. Sleep at high altitude. In: Cooper R, ed. Sleep. London: Chapman & Hall, 1994:243–264.

168. Graeber RC. Sleep in space. In: Roussel B, Jouvet M, eds. Actes du 27eme seminaire du GRD le sommeil et ses implications militaires. Lyon: ACEML, 1988:59–69.

169. Graeber RC. Microgravity and space flight. In: Carskadon MA, ed. Encyclopedia of Sleep and Dreaming. New York: Macmillan, 1993:371–373.

170. Santy PA, Kapanka H, Davis JR, Stewart DF. Analysis of sleep on shuttle missions. Aviat Space Environ Med 1988;59:1094–1097.

171. Gundel A, Nalishiti V, Reucher E, Vejvoda M, Zulley J. Sleep and circadian rhythm during a short space mission. Clin Invest 1993;71:718–724.

172. Monk TH, Buysse DJ, Billy BD, Kennedy KS, Willrich LM. Sleep and circadian rhythms in four orbiting astronauts. J Biol Rhythms 1998;13:188–201.

173. Dijk D-J, Neri DF, Wyatt JK, Ronda JM, Riel E, Ritz-De Cecco A, Hughes RJ, Elliott AR, Prisk GK, West JB, Czeisler CA. Sleep, performance, circadian rhythms, and light-dark cycles during two space shuttle missions. Am J Physiol 2001;281:R1647–R1664.

174. Putcha L, Berens KL, Marshburn TH, Ortega HJ, Billica RD. Pharmaceutical use by U.S. astronauts on space shuttle missions. Aviat Space Environ Med 1999;70:705–708.

175. Wright KP Jr, Hughes RJ, Kronauer RE, Dijk DJ, Czeisler CA. Intrinsic near-24–h pacemaker period determines limits of circadian entrainment to a weak synchronizer in humans. Proc Natl Acad Sci U S A 2001;98:14027–14032.

176. Wright KP Jr, Czeisler CA. Entrainment of the Non-24–hour Circadian Period of the Human Biological Clock to the 24–hour Day. Dordrecht: Kluwer Academic, 2002:475–489.

177. Pompeianoa M, d'Ascaniob P, Centini C, Pompeiano O, Balaban E. Short-term (FOS) and long-term (FRA) protein expression in rat locus coeruleus neurons during the neurolab mission: contribution of altered gravitational fields, stress, and other factors. Neuroscience 2002;115:111–123.

178. Pompeiano O, d'Ascaniob P, Centini C, Pompeianoa M, Balabanc E. Gene expression in rat vestibular and reticular structures during and after space flight. Neuroscience 2002 114:135–155.

179. Corcoran DW. Noise and loss of sleep. Q J Exp Psychol 1962;14: 178–182.

180. Wilkinson RT. Interaction of noise with knowledge of results and sleep deprivation. J Exp Psychol 1963;66:332–337.

181. Tassi P, Nicolas A, Seegmuller C, Dewasmes G, Libert JP, Muzet A. Interaction of the alerting effect of noise with partial sleep deprivation and circadian rhythmicity of vigilance. Percept Mot Skills 1993;77:1239–1248.

182. Campbell SS, Dawson D. Enhancement of nighttime alertness and performance with bright ambient light. Physiol Behav 1990;48:317–320.

183. Dawson D, Campbell SS. Timed exposure to bright light improves sleep and alertness during simulated night shifts. Sleep 1991;14(6):511–516.

184. Myers BL, Badia P. Immediate effects of different light intensities on body temperature and alertness. Physiol Behav 1993;54:199–202.

185. Daurat A, Aguirre A, Foret J, Gonnet P, Keromes A, Benoit O. Bright light affects alertness and performance rhythms during a 24–h constant routine. Physiol Behav 1993;53:929–936.

186. Leproult R, Van Reeth O, Byrne MM, Sturis J, Van Cauter E. Sleepiness, performance, and neuroendocrine function during sleep deprivation: effects of exposure to bright light or exercise. J Biol Rhythms 1997;12:245–258.

187. Murphy PJ, Badia P, Wright KP Jr., Boecker M, Hakel M. Bright light and nonsteroidal anti-inflammatory drug effects on performance and alertness during extended sleep deprivation. Sleep Res 1995;24:532.

188. Wright KP Jr, Badia P, Myers BL, Plenzler SC. Combination of bright light and caffeine as a countermeasure for impaired alertness and performance during extended sleep deprivation. J Sleep Res 1997;6:26–35.

189. Wright KP, Jr., Badia P, Myers BL, Plenzler SC, Hakel M. Caffeine and light effects on nighttime melatonin and temperature levels in sleep-deprived humans. Brain Res 1997;747:78–84.

190. Badia P, Myers B, Boecker M, Culpepper J, Harsch JR. Bright light effects on body temperature, alertness, EEG and behavior. Physiol Behav 1991;50:583–588.

191. Cajochen C, Dijk D-J, Borbély AA. Dynamics of EEG slow-wave activity and core body temperature in human sleep after exposure to bright light. Sleep 1992;15:337–343.

192. Czeisler CA, Wright KP Jr. Influence of light on circadian rhythmicity in humans. In: Turek FW, Zee PC, eds. Regulation of Sleep and Circadian Rhythms. New York: Marcel Dekker, 1999:149–180.

193. Giesbrecht GG, Arnett JL, Vela E, Bristow GK. Effect of task complexity on mental performance during immersion hypothermia. Aviat Space Environ Med 1993;64:206–211.

194. Vaughan JA, Higgins EA, Funkhouser GE. Effects of body thermal state on manual performance. Aerospace Med 1968;39:1310–1315.

195. Wilkinson RT, Fox RH, Goldsmith R, Hampton IFG, Lewis HE. Psychological and physiological responses to raised body temperature. J Appl Physiol 1964;19:287–291.

196. Allnutt MF, Allan JR. The effects of core temperature elevation and thermal sensation on performance. Ergonomics 1973;16:189–196.

197. Coleshaw SRK, Van Someren RNW, Wolff AH, Davis HM, Keatinge WR. Impaired memory registration and speed of reasoning caused by low body temperature. J Appl Physiol 1983;55:27–31.

198. Fort A, Harrison MT, Mills JN. Psychometric performance: circadian rhythms and effect of raising body temperature. J Physiol (Lond) 1973;231:114P-115P.

199. Giesbrecht GG. Cold stress, near drowning and accidental hypothermia: a review. Aviat Space Environ Med 2000;71:733–752.

200. Wright KP, Jr., Hull JT, Czeisler CA. Relationship between alertness, performance, and body temperature in humans. Am J Physiol Regul Integr Comp Physiol 2002;283:R1370–R1377.

201. Pepler RD. Warmth and lack of sleep: accuracy or activity reduced. J Comp Physiol Psych 1959;52:446–450.

8

Shift Work

JUNE J. PILCHER

Clemson University, Clemson, South Carolina, U.S.A.

I. Introduction

Humans are a diurnal species, habitually awake and active during the day and sleeping at night. However, modern society has changed this normal state for many workers. A variety of shift work schedules ranging from permanent or fixed night shifts to many different types of rotating shifts are currently used in a wide range of facilities and industries that require round-the-clock operation. Not surprisingly, much research has been devoted to examining the effects of shift work on sleep, alertness, performance, health, and well-being. One major concern with shift work is the impact of working at different times of the 24-hr day on the workers' ability to sleep. As shown in the top portion of Figure 1, there are many factors that can influence the effect of shift work on sleep. In permanent shifts, the primary influence is the time of day that the shift takes place. The time of day that work is required can negatively impact endogenous circadian rhythms making it difficult for the workers to sleep during off-duty times. The ability to sleep while working rotating shifts is influenced by many factors (see bottom portion of Figure 1), one of which is the time of day. Rotating shifts are also influenced by the speed of shift rotation and the direction of shift rotation. In addition, the length of the shift may affect sleep in both permanent and rotating shifts.

Perhaps the clearest finding from the literature is that working the night shift is associated with problems in sleeping and with on-duty alertness. Given

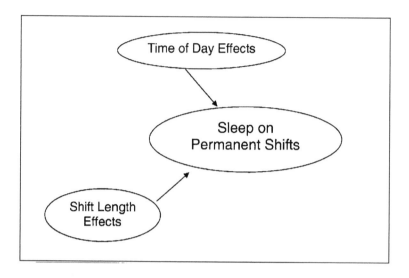

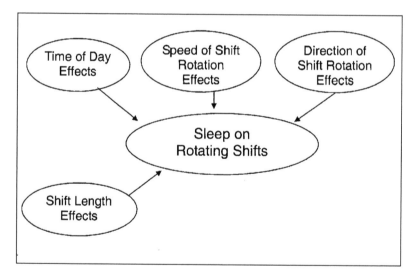

Figure 1 Models of factors influencing sleep on permanent shifts (top) and on rotating shifts (bottom).

the 24/7 needs of modern society, however, shift work including night shifts is essential. What is needed is a compromise that minimizes the negative effect of shift work on the worker. The purpose of this chapter is to review the relationship between different types of shift work systems and sleep loss to help determine the best compromise for shift work scheduling.

II. Normal Day Shifts

Day shifts, those work days that start in the morning and conclude in late afternoon (the typical 9-to-5 job), are classified as the normal work period. Day shifts allow the worker to sleep at night, go to work soon after awakening, and have free time in the evening before going to sleep again. The Omnibus Sleep in America Poll results (1) from the National Sleep Foundation found that permanent day workers in the United States reported an average sleep length of 7.0 hr/night with a standard deviation of 1.1 hr. These data were gathered from 555 participants who were selected to include all aged adults (mean age: 39.9 ± 12.4 years), approximately equal representation of each gender and all racial/ethnic groups.

III. Permanent Shifts

Permanent shifts usually refer to work schedules where employees are required to work either on shifts that take place primarily in the evening hours or shifts that take place primarily in the late night and early morning hours. The day shift is also a permanent shift but is not typically classified as part of a shift work system unless it is part of a rotating shift schedule. The sleep length data from permanent shifts discussed here were derived from the National Sleep Foundation report as indicated above or from our meta-analysis and are shown for comparison purposes in the upper left portion of Figure 2.

A. Permanent Evening Shifts

Permanent evening shifts, shifts that generally start mid- to late afternoon, seem to result in the fewest sleep-related problems of all of the shift work possibilities (2). Although the workers typically go to sleep in the early morning hours after getting off of work, they usually "sleep in" and thus obtain normal amounts of sleep. A meta-analysis examining sleep length across a wide range of shift work conditions found that workers on permanent evening shifts reported an average of 7.57 hours of sleep each night (3). This ability of workers on the evening shift to obtain adequate sleep is most likely due to their ability to take advantage of sleeping at night after getting off work and not having to get up early in the morning to report to work.

B. Permanent Night Shifts

Research has shown that working on night shifts frequently results in sleep-related problems (2,4,5). Most people who work night shifts have problems adjusting to sleeping during the day and experience some degree of chronic partial sleep deprivation. Our meta-analysis found that permanent night shift workers reported sleeping 6.6 hr/day (3). This average sleep duration was very similar to the average of 6.55 hr/day reported in Wilkinson's review of the literature (6).

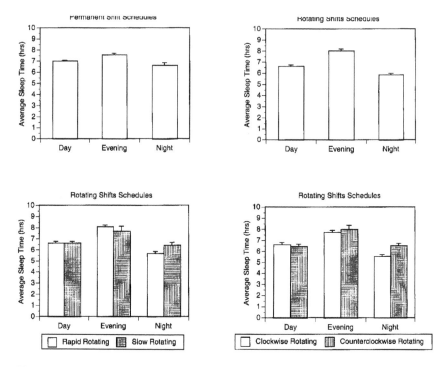

Figure 2   Average sleep length in hours for day, evening, and night shifts for permanent and rotating shift schedules. Rotating shift schedules have also been categorized by rate of rotation and by direction of rotation (bottom). Error bars represent the standard error.

In addition to less sleep, day sleep also results in a different organization to the normal sleep pattern. In an earlier review of the literature, Åkerstedt (7) concluded that the most common finding in sleep stage organization during day sleep was a decrease in rapid-eye-movement (REM) and stage 2 sleep. Thus, less sleep as well as different sleep stage organization is associated with working the night shift.

Research indicates that the problems with sleeping when working the night shift are at least in part due to problems with circadian adjustment (8–10). Several studies have found that when sleep is out of phase with the circadian rhythm in body temperature, it is often disrupted and shortened (11,12). Furthermore, experimental studies that induced a phase shift have supported this conclusion. A study that manipulated bedtimes and examined sleep duration concluded that sleep was shorter when bedtimes were out of phase with the endogenous circadian rhythm, such as with bedtimes in the late morning hours (13). A different type of circadian adjustment problem could be the normal demands from society and family to be awake and active during the day. For example, family, social, and business obligations have been shown to negatively influence workers' ability to sleep during the day (14).

In addition to the problems with the circadian adjustment of sleeping during the day, night shift workers must contend with a shift in their waking pattern. Most night workers sleep soon after getting off of work and then are awake for hours before reporting to work. Thus, night shift workers are not in the same phase of their sleep-wake cycle as most day workers when they report to work. Day workers usually go to work shortly after awakening whereas night shift workers are often awake 8 hr or more before reporting to work. This prolonged period of wakefulness experienced by most night workers before going to work combined with trying to work during the night when they naturally want to sleep often leads to increased levels of fatigue while working.

Another issue that can impact a worker's ability to adapt to working at night is the number of consecutive night shifts in a row. Prolonged exposure to night shifts can cause the workers to begin to adjust their internal circadian rhythms. However, the workers never seem to fully adapt (15,16). It seems that even a small amount of exposure to the sun is enough to prevent their internal clock from readily changing to the different time schedule. Furthermore, as soon as night shift workers have a day off, they revert to sleeping at night and being awake during the day (17). Then, when they have to go back to work, they must once again go through the process of adapting to working nights.

In summary, permanent night shifts result in less sleep whereas permanent evening shifts result in more sleep than normal day shifts (see upper left portion of Figure 2). Although workers seem to adapt to some extent to working on permanent night shifts, they never totally adapt. Thus, when considering the best shift work compromise, the question becomes what is the relative detriment of working permanent nights versus nights as part of a rotating shift system.

IV. Rotating Shifts

Rotating shifts incorporate the same problems and advantages as permanent evening and night shifts. Similar to permanent shifts, night shifts as part of a rotating shift schedule result in less sleep whereas evening shifts result in more sleep than that seen in day shifts. The studies used in our meta-analysis indicated that workers on night shifts reported sleeping 5.85 hr, workers on day shifts reported sleeping 6.62 hr, and workers on evening shifts reported sleeping 8.03 hr (3). Thus, workers on rotating shifts report less sleep on night shifts and on day shifts, but more sleep on evening shifts, than their comparable permanent shift workers (see upper right portion of Figure 2). When collapsing across all shifts (mornings, evenings, and nights), rotating shifts resulted in 6.65 hr of sleep on work days—about equal to the amount of sleep seen in permanent night shifts (3).

A. Time of Shift

The decrease in sleep in day shift workers on rotating shifts in comparison to permanent day workers is most likely due to the earlier reporting time of most day shift workers. Rotating shift systems often result in early work onset times, often as early as 6 a.m., which reduces sleep and increases fatigue during work (18). Although many people assume that day shift workers could compensate for the early start time by going to bed earlier, studies have shown that workers tend not to go to bed early enough to balance the early wake-up time (19) and often have social obligations that prevent them from more fully adapting their sleep schedules to their work times (7,19).

The increase in sleep time for the evening shift reported by rotating shift workers in comparison to permanent evening shift workers is an interesting finding. It could be a rebound effect in that the workers could be trying to compensate for the decreased amount of sleep that they experience on both day and night shifts (3). Thus, the workers seem to take advantage of a working schedule that allows them to "sleep in" during the morning hours.

The substantial decrease in sleep times following nights in rotating shift schedules when compared to permanent night shifts indicates that permanent night shift workers adjust, at least to some extent, to working at night and sleeping during the day (3). This limited adjustment may be due to the workers having to compensate for the accumulated sleep loss resulting from working several night shifts in a row. Their physiological need for sleep would be increased, thus impelling the workers to sleep more during their off-duty time.

B. Speed of Shift Rotation

In addition to the actual work times of the shifts, rotating shift schedules raise other issues that can impact sleep. One concern is the speed of shift rotation. Most rotating shift systems are classified as either a rapid or a slow rotation. Rapid rotating shifts typically result in 2–3 days in a row on a particular shift and then require the workers to either work on a different shift or have a couple of days off. Slow rotating shifts usually have 5–7 days in a row on a shift and then rotate to days off before working on another shift. The relative benefits of rapid as opposed to slow rotating shifts have been a much debated topic in the sleep and shift work literature (20–26). However, few studies have directly compared the two (27).

Our meta-analysis (3), by quantitatively summarizing across studies in the shift work literature, contributed to this issue. We found that rapidly rotating shifts resulted in generally less sleep (6.52 hr) than slowly rotating shifts (6.93 hr). As seen in the bottom left portion of Figure 2, rapidly rotating shifts resulted in less sleep on morning shifts and night shifts and more sleep on evening shifts than slowly rotating shifts. These results support the conclusion that increased sleep on evening shifts in rotating shift systems may be a rebound effect due to the decreased amount of sleep experienced on other work days. This seems to be especially true in rapidly rotating shifts that result in the most disturbed sleep times for morning and night shifts.

C. Direction of Shift Rotation

Another issue in rotating shifts is the direction of shift rotation. A clockwise rotating shift system has shifts that move first from morning shift then to evening shift and then to night shift. This direction of rotation is also called a phase delay or forward rotation in that the days between shifts are prolonged, similar to flying westward over several time zones. A counterclockwise rotating shift system has shifts that move from nights to evenings to days. This direction of rotation is also called a phase advance or backward rotation because it results in shortened days between shifts, similar to flying eastward over several time zones. Studies on the effects of jet lag and laboratory-based phase shifts suggest that a clockwise rotation results in fewer problems for the endogenous circadian system and thus fewer problems with sleep than a counterclockwise rotation (28,29). Unfortunately, not many studies on shift work have focused directly on the direction of rotation. One study concluded that, as expected, the circadian system would more rapidly adapt to a clockwise rotating system than a counterclockwise system (30). In a short review of the topic, Turek (31) concluded that circadian rhythms are disturbed in both clockwise and counterclockwise rotation, but that clockwise rotation seems to minimize the effect.

Our meta-analysis could not directly address the issue of direction of shift rotation due to a lack of usable data in the literature (3). However, some of the studies used in our meta-analysis reported data on the direction of shift rotation. When we examine the average sleep times reported by the workers in these studies, we see that more sleep was reported under counterclockwise rotation than clockwise rotation (bottom right portion of Figure 2). These results can likely be explained by more closely examining the studies that reported clockwise and counterclockwise rotation for the speed of rotation. When we do that we find that of the 10 studies providing information on counterclockwise rotating shifts, 7 combined it with a slow rotation system. Furthermore, of the 15 studies that provided data on clockwise rotating shifts, 13 used a rapid rotation system. Thus, the sleep times seen in clockwise and counterclockwise rotating shifts may have been due to the speed of shift rotation rather than the actual direction of shift rotation. More studies are needed that address the effects of the direction of shift rotation that control for the speed of rotation to help resolve this issue.

V. Shift Length

An additional matter that may have an impact on both permanent and rotating shifts is the length of the shift. The two most common shift lengths are 8 hr and 12 hr. Although 8-hr shifts may be considered the standard, a variety of work environments are adopting 12-hr shifts, especially healthcare facilities and nuclear plants. The 12-hr shifts result in a "compressed" work week that gives fewer actual days of work and more days off each week. The compressed work

week is often implemented because of the extra time off and the expected benefits in production and morale (32–34).

However, increasing the number of consecutive work hours may have a
detrimental effect on sleep and fatigue. Some studies have reported sleep disturbances (35) and less alertness (36) in 12-hr shift work schedules. Fatigue and
alertness can also be a concern toward the end of a 12-hr shift, especially in jobs
that require monotonous work or heavy physical labor (37). Most studies and previous reviews of the literature, however, have concluded that 12-hr schedules
have no clear detrimental effects on sleep (36,38–40).

When considering 12-hr shifts, it is also important to take into account the
number of consecutive work days and how days off will be interspersed between
work days (41). In a review of the literature, Smith and colleagues (36) concluded
that five or more consecutive 12-hr shifts could result in substantial decrements
in productivity and alertness. As such, they concluded that no more than three or
four consecutive 12-hr shifts should be used in compressed schedules.

VI.   Conclusions

The current review of the effect of shift work on sleep allows us to draw several
conclusions. First, night shifts typically allow for less sleep than either day or
evening shifts, whereas evening shifts permit more sleep than either day or night
shifts. Second, day shifts that are part of a rotating schedule result in less sleep than
permanent day shifts. Third, in rotating shift systems, slowly rotating shifts result
in less disruption to sleep length than rapidly rotating shifts. Lastly, 12-hr shifts for
three to four consecutive days have no clear detrimental effect on sleep in comparison to 8-hr shifts. The major question that we wished to address in this chapter,
however, concerns the best overall shift work compromise. *Given that shift work is
inevitable in our modern society, what is the best way to schedule workers?*

In his classic book, *Sleep and Wakefulness* (42), Kleitman was one of the first
to support the idea of adopting permanent shifts in operational settings. In both edi-
tions, he suggested that permanent shifts, including night shifts, were preferable to
rotating shifts. Of course, when he drew these conclusions he did not have the benefit of many years of shift work studies or the meta-analytical technique. Our meta-
analysis (3) indicated that permanent nights could be a useful addition to a shift
work schedule, especially in those areas where many workers are needed at night.
However, the overall best compromise in shift work scheduling in terms of sleep
length is a slowly rotating shift system. On average, slowly rotating shifts resulted
in more sleep than any of the other shift work schedules that included night shifts.

References

1.   National Sleep Foundation. Omnibus Sleep in America Poll, Washington, DC, 1998.
2.   Åkerstedt T. Psychological and psychophysiological effects of shift work. Scand J
     Work Environ Health 1990; 16:67–73.

3. Pilcher JJ, Lambert BJ, Huffcutt AI. Differential effects of permanent and rotating shifts on self-report sleep length: a meta-analytic review. Sleep 2000; 23:155–163.

4. Härmä M. Individual differences in tolerance to shift-work: a review. Ergonomics 1993; 36:101–109.

5. Penn PE, Bootzin RR. Behavioral techniques for enhancing alertness and performance in shift work. Work Stress 1990; 4:213–226.

6. Wilkinson TT. How fast should the night shift rotate? Ergonomics 1992; 35:1425–1446.

7. Åkerstedt T. Work schedules and sleep. Experientia 1984; 40:417–422.

8. Minors DS, Scott AR. Circadian arrhythmia: shift-work, travel and health. Occup Med 1986; 36:39–44.

9. Rutenfranz J. Occupational health measures for night- and shift workers. J Hum Ergol 1982; 11:67–86.

10. Rutenfranz J, Colquhoun W, Knauth P, Ghata J. Biomedical and psycho-social aspects of shift work. Scand J Work Environ Health 1977; 3:165–182.

11. Åkerstedt T, Gillberg M. Sleep disturbances and shiftwork. In: Reinberg A, Vieux N, Andlauer P, eds. Night and Shift Work: Biological and Social Aspects. Oxford: Pergamon Press, 1981:127–137.

12. Czeisler CA, Weitzmann ED, Moore-Ede MC, Zimmerman CJ. Human sleep: its duration and organization depend on its circadian phase. Science 1980; 210:1254–1267.

13. Gillberg M, Åkerstedt T. Body temperature and sleep at different times of day. Sleep 1982; 5:378–388.

14. Mahan RP, Carvalhis AB, Queen SE. Sleep reduction in night-shift workers: is it sleep deprivation or a sleep disturbance disorder? Percept Mot Skills 1990; 70:723–730.

15. Knauth P. Changing schedules: shiftwork. Chronobiol Int 1997; 14:159–171.

16. Van Loon JH. Diurnal body temperature curves in shiftworkers. Ergonomics 1963; 6:267–273.

17. Tepas DI, Carvalhais AB. Sleep patterns of shiftworkers. Occup Med 1990; 5:199–208.

18. Knauth P. The design of shift systems. Ergonomics 1993; 36:15–28.

19. Folkard S, Barton J. Does the "forbidden zone" for sleep onset influence morning shift sleep duration? Ergonomics 1993; 36:85–91.

20. Dahlgren K. Adjustment of circadian rhythms and EEG sleep functions to day and night sleep among permanent night workers and rotating shift workers. Psychophysiology 1981; 18:381–391.

21. Folkard S. Is there a "best compromise" shift system? Ergonomics 1992; 35:1453–1463.

22. Knauth P, Landau K, Droge C, Schwitteck M, Widynski M, Rutenfranz J. Duration of sleep depending on the type of shift work. Int Arch Occup Environ Health 1980; 46:167–177.

23. Minors DS, Waterhouse JM. Circadian rhythms in deep body temperature, urinary excretion and alertness in nurses on night work. Ergonomics 1985; 28:1523–1530.

24. Ng-A-Tham JEE, Thierry HK. An experimental change of the speed of rotation of the morning and evening shift. Ergonomics 1993; 36:51–57.

25. Olson CM. Shift work. J Emerg Med 1984; 2:37–43.

26. Vokac Z, Magnus P, Jebens E, Gundersen N. Apparent phase-shifts of circadian rhythms (masking effects) during rapid shift rotations. Int Arch Occup Environ Health 1981; 49:53–65.

27. Scott AJ. Chronobiological considerations in shiftworker sleep and performance and shift-work scheduling. Hum Performance 1994; 7:207–233.

28. Aschoff J, Hoffman K, Pohl H, Wever R. Re-entrainment of circadian rhythms after phase shifts of zeitgebers. Chronobiologia 1975; 2:23–78.

29. Klein KE, Wegmenn HM, Hunt BI. Desynchronization as a function of body temperature and performance circadian rhythm as a result of outgoing and homecoming transmeridian flights. Aerospace Med 1972; 43:119–132.

30. Czeisler CA, Moore-Ede MC, Coleman RM. Rotating shift work schedules that disrupt sleep are improved by applying circadian principles. Science 1982, 217:460–463.

31. Turek FW. Circadian principles and design of rotating shift work schedules. Am J Physiol 1986; 251:R636–638.

32. Poor R, ed. 4-Days, 40-hours. Cambridge: Bursk and Poor, 1970.

33. Steward GV, Larsen JM. A four-day-three-day per week application to a continuous production operation. Management Personnel Quar 1971; 10:13–20.

34. Underwood AB. What a 12-hour shift offers. Am J Nurs 1975; 75:1176–1178.

35. Rosa R, Bonnet MH. Performance and alertness on 8h and 12h rotating shifts at a natural gas facility. Ergonomics 1993; 36:1177–1193.

36. Smith L, Folkard S, Tucker P, Macdonald I. Work shift duration: a review comparing eight hour and 12 hour shift systems. Occup Environ Med 1998; 55:217–229.

37. Tepas DI. Flexitime, compressed workweeks and other alternative work schedules. In: Folkard S, Monk T, eds. Hours of work: temporal factors in work scheduling. Chichester: John Wiley & Sons, 1985:147–164.

38. Peacock B, Glube R, Miller M, Clune P. Police officers' responses to 8 and 12 hour shift schedules. Ergonomics 1983; 26:479–493.

39. Tucker P, Barton J, Folkard S. Comparison of eight and 12 hour shifts: impacts on health, well being, and alertness during the shift. Occup Environ Med 1996; 53:767–772.

40. Williamson AM, Gower CGI, Clarke BC. Changing the hours of shiftwork: a comparison of 8- and 12-hour shift rosters in a group of computer operators. Ergonomics 1994; 37:287–298.

41. Smiley A, Moray NP. Review of 12-hour shifts at nuclear generating stations. Report to Atomic Energy Control Board. Ottawa, 1989.

42. Kleitman N. Sleep and wakefulness. Chicago: University of Chicago Press, 1939, 1963.

9

Medications, Drugs of Abuse, and Alcohol

JONATHAN A.E. FLEMING
University of British Columbia, Vancouver, British Columbia, Canada

CLETE A. KUSHIDA
Stanford University, Stanford California, U.S.A.

I. Introduction

Medications, drugs of abuse, and alcohol can affect sleep performance either directly or indirectly. Direct effects, such as the promotion of wakefulness by stimulants, are usually intended therapeutic effects mediated through the central nervous system (CNS), whereas indirect effects may be inadvertent side effects, such as insomnia caused by stimulating antidepressants (1) or the withdrawal of a centrally acting (2) or a systemically acting medication (3).

Information about the effects of medications on sleep is derived from a variety of sources. Sleep disruption may be noted as an adverse effect in placebo-controlled or comparative drug studies; once the medication is introduced into clinical practice, case reports add to the data on sleep-disruptive side effects. From these sources we know how some medications affect sleep performance, but our knowledge is far from complete.

For example, subjective complaints of insomnia should be confirmed by objective measures, and usually these data are missing or are collected from a small number of patients. In addition, we know little about the effects of using drug dosages outside the usual recommended dose range and substantially less about how medications affect sleep performance in special populations such as the medically ill, the very young, and the very old. Furthermore, we know less about how drug-drug interactions affect sleep and the effects of medications when used in combination with over-the-counter, nonprescription medications, dietary supplements (4), and herbal products (5).

Because of the recognized association between disrupted sleep and disturbed behavior it is not surprising that we know much more about the effects of centrally acting medications—particularly the antidepressants, the antipsychotics, and the hypnosedatives—than we do about other drug classes. Often medications with direct central effects, targeted at specific neurotransmitter systems known to affect sleep, are specifically studied by polysomnography in both normal and target populations so that their effects on sleep architecture and sleep performance can be understood. For other medications, where sleep-disturbing side effects are not anticipated, case reports emphasizing subjective complaints about disrupted sleep may or may not be followed by more detailed study.

In this chapter, sleep loss induced by medications and other substances will be reviewed from two perspectives (see Table 1). First we will consider the effects of medications, such as antidepressants, sedatives, analgesics, or other substances specifically designed to have a direct effect on the brain. Second, we will mention medications designed to affect other systems—such as cardiovascular drugs and bronchodilators—which inadvertently have sleep-disrupting effects.

II. Medications and Other Substances with a Primary Central Effect

A. Central Nervous System Depressants

Alcohol

The effects of alcohol on sleep have been studied since the 1930s. Alcohol has direct effects on sleep and also differential effects on sleep during periods of dependence and withdrawal (6).

Acute Alcohol Intoxication

In nonalcoholics who occasionally use alcohol, low and high doses of alcohol initially improve sleep. The hypnotic effect of alcohol may be directly related to brain ethanol metabolism, since a positive correlation was found between ethanol-derived acetaldehyde accumulation in vitro in the brain and this central effect of alcohol in outbred rats and mice in vivo (7). However, tolerance rapidly develops to the sedative effects of alcohol, and sleep disturbances are reported during the second half of the sleep period with high alcohol doses. Acute administration of alcohol inhibits rapid-eye-movement (REM) sleep in normal individuals by increasing REM latency and reducing REM duration; this effect is dose dependent (8). As the blood alcohol concentration declines, a REM sleep rebound may occur during the same night. The rebound of REM sleep typically found after total or REM sleep deprivation is decreased in a dose-dependent manner following alcohol ingestion (8). Interestingly, alcohol intake in rats was significantly elevated during REM sleep deprivation, and there was a rebound decrease in alcohol intake during the REM rebound phase immediately after the REM sleep dep-

Table 1 Medications, Drugs of Abuse, and Alcohol That Induce Sleep Loss

(A) Medications or Other Substances
   With a Primary Central Effect

DEPRESSANTS
   Alcohol
   Barbiturates

ANTIDEPRESSANTS
   Selective serotonin reuptake inhibitors:
      Fluoxetine, Paroxetine, Fluvoxamine,
      Citalopram, Sertaline Aminoketones:
      Bupropion
   Serotonin-norepinehrine reuptake
      inhibitors: Venlafaxine Monoamine
      oxidase inhibitors (non-selective and
      selective): Tran-ylcypromine,
      Phenelzine, Isocarboxazid,
      Moclobemide, Brofaromine

ANTIPSYCHOTICS
   Haloperidol and other high-potency
   antipsychotics
   Clozapine[a]
   Risperidone[a]
   Olanzapine[a]
   Quetiapine[a]

HYPNOTICS and ANXIOLYTICS
   High-potency, short-acting benzodi-
      azepines (e.g., triazolam and alprazo-
      lam)
   Buspirone

STIMULANTS
   Caffeine

Modafinil
Methylphenidate
Dextroamphetamine
Pseudoephedrine
Phenylpropanolamine
Nicotine
Cocaine

HALLUCINOGENS
   Marijuana
   Lysergic acid diethylamide
   Phencyclidine

OPIOIDS
   Neroin
   Morphine
   Cyclazocine

ANTIPARKINSONIAN AGENTS
   L-Dopa
   Selegiline
   Pergolide
   Bromocriptine
   Amantadine
   Pramipexole
   Ropinirole

APPETITE SUPPRESSANTS
   Fenfluramine
   Dexfenfluramine
   Phentermine
   Sibutramine

(B) Medications or Other Substances
   With a Secondary Central Effect

CARDIOVASCULAR DRUGS
   β-Blockers:
      Propanolol
      Atenolol
      Pindolol
   Antihypertensives:
      Clonidine
      Methyldopa
      Carvedilol
      Labetalol
   Hypolipidemic drugs:
      Lovastatin

Histamine$_2$ antagonists:
   Ranitidine
Hormones
Steroids:
   Anabolic steroids
   Prednisone
   Cortisone
   Dexamethasone
   Thyroid preparations
Bronchodilators:
   Theophylline
   Salbutamol
   Salmeterol

[a] These medications are sedating. Their sleep-disruptive effects only occur when they induce sleep
disorders such as restless legs syndrome (see text).

rivation period. A vicious cycle of REM sleep deprivation increasing alcohol consumption and alcohol intake causing REM sleep deprivation was postulated (9). These investigators hypothesize in a separate study that functional alterations in central noradrenergic neurons during REM sleep deprivation may contribute to the concurrent increase in alcohol intake (10).

Alcohol and sleep deprivation independently produce impairments in cognitive and motor performance (11,12), and have synergistic effects on these variables (13). Examples of performance impairments include increased reaction time for low stimulus quality (14); decreased performance accuracy and increased latency of late cortical evoked potential components (15,16); and impaired simulated automobile driving (17). Obstructive sleep apnea independently results in daytime sleepiness and impaired neurocognitive performance; alcohol worsens sleep apnea, even in otherwise healthy, nonobese elderly adults (18).

Chronic Alcohol Dependence and Withdrawal

Alcoholic patients show a marked loss of slow-wave sleep, and the augmentation of slow-wave sleep and delta power seen in healthy adults following sleep deprivation is compromised in these patients (19). Compared with normal controls, primary alcoholic inpatients abstinent for about 17 days took longer to fall asleep, slept less, had poor sleep efficiency, and the maximal number of withdrawal symptoms a patient had ever experienced was inversely related to the amount of delta sleep (20). In chronic alcoholics with delirium tremens (DT), terminal sleep resulted in the alcoholics fully recovering from DT, prompting the investigators to speculate that the terminal sleep probably consists of recovery sleep from sleep deprivation caused by DT and disturbances of consciousness (21). Alcohol withdrawal studies in rats indicate that the electroencephalograms (EEGs) of rats show an initial sleep loss followed by a return of total sleep and a REM sleep rebound several days later (22). Two lines of mice have been selectively bred for differential sleep time responses to ethanol, long sleep (LS) and short sleep (SS); genetically determined central muscarinic cholinergic mechanisms may have a role in the difference in ethanol sensitivity between these two mice strains (23). Human subjects with low amounts of slow-wave sleep showed a faster rate of tolerance development for changes in slow-wave sleep from baseline (abstinent values) to those on alcohol (24). Treatment effects were assessed in the same study; chlordiazepoxide treatment for alcohol withdrawal produced a marked synergism with alcohol withdrawal suppression of slow-wave sleep.

Interactions with Antidepressants

Alcohol use with any antidepressant is actively discouraged; alcohol use with antidepressants in any patient with a sleep disorder is certainly contraindicated (25).

Barbiturates

Barbiturates reduce sleep latency at night but produce sedation the following day as well (26), and insomnia may persist for up to 2 weeks following abrupt discontinuation. This class of medication also reduces REM sleep but may induce a REM sleep rebound, frequently accompanied by nightmares, following cessation of long-term treatment. Non-REM (NREM) stage 2 sleep is prolonged, and the K complexes and slow eye movements during this stage are decreased both during use and during the withdrawal night after a drug night. Non-Rem (NREM) stages 3 and 4 sleep are decreased with short-term use and increased above baseline levels after withdrawal (27). Similar to alcohol, barbiturates selectively reduce the neural output via the hypoglossal nerve and predispose individuals to upper airway occlusion during sleep (28). Barbiturates are contraindicated as hypnotics; however, they still have specific and important medical indications, such as in the management of epilepsy.

γ-Hydroxybutyrate

γ-hydroxybutyrate (GHB, also known as sodium oxybate) is a known drug of abuse. Adverse CNS effects of this drug include seizures, respiratory depression, and profound decreases in level of consciousness, with instances of coma and death. However, GHB has been shown to be effective in managing the cataplectic attacks and daytime sleepiness of narcoleptic patients (29,30). These findings may be due to its positive effects on nocturnal sleep quality; it increased NREM stage 3 sleep, decreased NREM stage 1 sleep, and reduced stage shifts and awakenings in both narcoleptic and normal subjects (31,32). The sedative, anxiolytic, and euphoric effects of GHB are believed to be due to its potentiation of cerebral GABAergic, dopaminergic, and possible serotonergic activities (33). Sleepwalking and periodic limb movements during sleep were associated with GHB use (34); however, no worsening was observed in sleep-disordered breathing in patients with obstructive sleep apnea (35), and improved subjective and objective sleep quality measures were found in patients with impaired sleep (36) and fibromyalgia (37).

B. Antidepressants

The most consistent sleep effect of antidepressants is the change they cause in REM sleep. Typically antidepressants decrease the percentage of REM sleep throughout the night and prolong the REM latency (the time taken from sleep onset to the onset of the first REM period) (38).

Selective Serotonin Reuptake Inhibitors

Although the older, tricyclic antidepressants are relatively "sleep friendly" due to their antihistaminic effects (39), the newer antidepressants, such as the selective serotonin reuptake inhibitors (SSRIs), are generally viewed as being activating medications that can cause or exacerbate insomnia (40).

Pooled data show that in 1728 depressed patients treated with fluoxetine, insomnia was reported as an adverse event in 16%. The incidence of this adverse event increased in the elderly (18%) and in certain patient populations such as those with obsessive compulsive disorder (28%) and bulimia (33%) (41).

A study in 2000 showed that in depressed patients 20 mg of fluoxetine caused more frequent reports of subjective insomnia, but fluoxetine was no more activating than placebo (42). However, most studies suggest that unlike other common adverse events with the SSRIs, insomnia associated with fluoxetine use may be persistent (43) and require treatment (44) with hypnosedatives.

In addition to impairing sleep performance through its activating effects, fluoxetine has been shown to induce new sleep disorders, which in themselves are associated with sleep disruption and nonrestorative sleep. Using polysomnography, Dorsey and colleagues (45) showed that in nine depressed patients fluoxetine reduced sleep efficiency and caused significantly more eye movements and arousals during NREM sleep than in their control group. Both eye movement and arousal counts were significantly correlated, and an additional cause of sleep disruption—clinically significant periodic limb movement disorder (PLMD) (46)—was observed in 44% of the fluoxetine-treated group versus none of the control group. Dorsey and colleagues concluded that a higher incidence of PLMD and frequent transient arousals associated with eye movements might be responsible for the subjective complaint of poor sleep in patients treated with fluoxetine.

Abnormal eye movements were shown in other patients treated with fluoxetine (47), and a case report of treatment-emergent, persistent REM sleep behavior disorder was reported (48). As a class, the SSRIs were shown to induce bruxism, which, in addition to causing dental damage, may result in nonrestorative sleep. Interestingly, buspirone, which appears to have a stimulant effect and causes insomnia (49), may be useful in the management of SSRI-induced bruxism (50).

Clinical trial data for the SSRI class of antidepressants show placebo-adjusted rates of insomnia ranging from 5% to 19% in depressed patients, and these rates are considered similar for the different drugs in this class (38). However, in patients with posttraumatic stress disorder, fluvoxamine was shown to improve sleep by reducing dreams associated with the traumatic event and promoting more restful sleep (51), and in one single-blind, uncontrolled study, citalopram caused no decrements in objective sleep performance when used for 5 weeks (52).

Withdrawal from SSRIs, particularly paroxetine, can cause a measurable SSRI discontinuation syndrome (53) characterized by the development of two or more of the following symptoms: dizziness, light-headedness, vertigo, or feeling faint; shocklike sensations or paresthesia; anxiety; diarrhea; fatigue; gait instability; headache; insomnia; irritability; nausea or emesis; tremor; and visual disturbances. In addition to this discontinuation syndrome, when antidepressants are withdrawn the suppression of REM ceases and a rebound of REM sleep occurs (54), which may result in nightmares, awakenings, and sleep disruption.

Aminoketones

Bupropion, an antidepressant of the aminoketone class that inhibits the uptake of dopamine and norepinephrine, is used both as an antidepressant and as an aid to smoking cessation. Theoretically, bupropion could cause sleep disruption indirectly through the promotion of bruxism or, more rarely, by causing acute dystonic reactions (55). In one sleep laboratory study of seven depressed males, bupropion treatment did not affect sleep performance (56).

Phenethylamines

Venlafaxine, a member of a novel chemical class phenethylamines, inhibits neuronal uptake of serotonin, norepinephrine, and dopamine (in decreasing order of potency) at doses of 75–375 mg/day. It causes subjective insomnia and subjective sleepiness in treated patients. Objective data from normal subjects show that 75–150 mg of venlafaxine given for 4 days induced wakefulness and increased light stage 1 sleep (57). In addition, venlafaxine caused PLMD in 75% of the eight subjects studied. In a double-blind, placebo-controlled study of depressed inpatients, venlafaxine used in dosages of up to 225 mg/day, compared to placebo, increased electroencephalographically recorded wake after sleep onset by about 30 min (58).

Monoamine Oxidase Inhibitors

The monoamine oxidase inhibitors (MAOIs)—tranylcypromine, phenelzine, and isocarboxazid—are all associated with sleep disruption (59) which, despite an antidepressant response, can be severe enough to require stopping treatment. Although safer, the newer, reversible, and selective inhibitors of monoamine oxidase type A—moclobemide (60) and brofaromine (61)—also cause insomnia, which may necessitate discontinuation or treatment with sleep-promoting medications (62). Interactions between MAOIs and other antidepressants are always a concern; moclobemide administered with paroxetine and fluoxetine induces insomnia and myoclonic jerks (63).

Sleep-Conserving Antidepressants (Nefazodone and Mirtazapine)

Stimulation of serotonin-2 ($5\text{-}HT_2$) receptors by SSRIs or serotonin-norepinephrine reuptake inhibitors (SNRIs) is thought to cause subjective insomnia and change sleep. Thus, antidepressant drugs with $5\text{-}HT_2$ blocking properties, such as mirtazapine (64) or nefazodone (65), may promote sleep and improve sleep architecture in patients requiring treatment with antidepressants. However, subjective drowsiness with nefazodone—not confirmed by Multiple Sleep Latency Tests (MSLTs) in nondepressed subjects (66)—is a major side effect with a placebo-adjusted incidence of 6–24% (38).

C. Antipsychotics

Most of the antipsychotic drugs including the older classical and newer atypical agents usually induce drowsiness or sleepiness (54) with the incidence of sedation varying considerably among the class. Sedation is caused by different affinities for cholinergic and histaminic receptors as well as blockage of α_1-adrenore-ceptors (67).

Rarely, antipsychotics can cause insomnia directly, or indirectly, through inducing or worsening a sleep disorder. For example, haloperidol can cause insomnia directly (41) or through the development of extrapyramidal side effects (68) that disturb sleep.

Although the atypical antipsychotics [clozapine (69), risperidone (70), olanzapine (71), and quetiapine (72)] promote sleep, they can cause sleep loss, indirectly, through the development of a new sleep disorder such as restless legs syndrome (73), PLMD (74), or a respiratory sleep disorder (75).

D. Hypnotics and Anxiolytics

Hypnosedatives are commonly used to induce and maintain sleep in a variety of clinical situations. The preferred medications are the benzodiazepines or benzo-diazepine agonists such as zopiclone, zolpidem, and zaleplon. The barbiturates (76) and nonbenzodiazepine hypnotics such as chloral hydrate (77) are unsafe and should not be used.

Although the benzodiazepines are safe, they can cause sleep difficulties through the phenomenon of tolerance and rebound insomnia. Tolerance to the hypnotic effect of the benzodiazepines occurs so that sleep becomes disrupted and the patient may consume more drug to obtain the same initial hypnotic effect.

Rebound insomnia is a sleep disturbance that occurs on discontinuation of hypnotic drugs (78) and other drugs with sedative properties (79). It has been reported in both patients and healthy normal subjects (80) and is characterized by increased wakefulness compared to that measured in the pretreatment period. Typically, it is a disturbance of one or two night's duration that primarily follows discontinuation of short- to intermediate-acting benzodiazepines. It is more likely to occur with high dosages. However, there seems to be clear individual differ-ences in the experience of rebound insomnia although no prospective studies have established which differences predict the phenomenon. Rebound insomnia may be avoided by initiating treatment with the lowest effective dose and tapering the dose upon discontinuation (78).

Short-acting, high-potency benzodiazepines, such as triazolam, are partic-ularly likely to be associated with the development of tolerance (81) and rebound insomnia (82). Early morning awakening, caused by through-the-night with-drawal from a rapidly eliminated hypnotic such as triazolam, has also been observed (83).

E. Central Nervous System Stimulants

Drugs with stimulant effects come from several classes including the xanthines (e.g., caffeine and theophylline) and the amphetamines. Caffeine is used socially and therapeutically as a stimulant to promote vigilance and alertness and is an additive in foodstuffs, such as cola beverages, and medications, such as analgesics (84). Caffeine affects subjective (85) and objective (86) sleep performance and is associated with a withdrawal syndrome (87).

The medications most frequently utilized to treat excessive sleepiness are— with the exception of modafinil—psychomotor stimulants causing behavioral activation with increased arousal, motor activity, and alertness (88). There are three classes of psychomotor stimulants: (a) direct-acting sympathomimetics (e.g., the α_1-adrenergic stimulant phenylephrine); (b) indirect-acting sympathomimetics (e.g., methylphenidate, amphetamine); and (c) stimulants that are not sympathomimetics and have different mechanisms of action (e.g., caffeine). Until recently, the indirect sympathomimetics—dextroamphetamine, methamphetamine and methylphenidate—have been the medications of choice for the management of narcolepsy (89) with the introduction of modafinil further expanding treatment options (88).

Patients with narcolepsy may experience nocturnal sleep disruption (90) as part of their disorder, and this may be worsened when high daytime dosages or late afternoon and evening dosages of stimulants are used. In addition, periodic limb movements occur in nonmedicated narcoleptics (91), and these may be worsened—further disrupting sleep performance—by the tricyclic antidepressants, SSRIs and the SNRIs, that are used to manage cataplexy. With the exception of sodium oxybate (92), all of the drugs used to manage the sleepiness and cataplexy associated with narcolepsy have insomnia or sleep disruption as a known side effect (88).

The introduction of the novel stimulant modafinil, with a more benign side effect profile and low abuse potential (93), has been an important advance for the management of sleepiness associated with narcolepsy and respiratory sleep disorders (94) as well as treating fatigue states (95) and clinical depression (96). Modafinil can cause initial insomnia and sleep disruption, but this is a less common event than with the older stimulants. In 174 narcoleptics treated with 200 mg of modafinil, 4.1% reported insomnia; for the 300-mg and 400-mg dosages the percentages were was 8.4% and 5.5%, respectively (41).

Methylphenidate and amphetamines are widely used in children and adults with attention deficit hyperactivity disorder (ADHD) and, commonly, symptoms attributed to stimulant medication are actually preexisting characteristics of children with ADHD and improve with stimulant treatment. Nonetheless, both of these drugs cause insomnia with dextroamphetamine causing greater sleep disruption than methylphenidate (97) in children.

Pseudoephedrine and phenylpropanolamine (PPA) are two drugs that share similar pharmacological properties with ephedrine but have less potent CNS-stimulating effects. The Food and Drug Administration (FDA) and other regulatory authorities around the world (98) have taken steps to remove phenylpropanolamine from all drug products because of its potential to increase blood pressure and induce hemorrhagic stroke.

Pseudoephedrine is used extensively in cold and cough remedies and, like PPA, has been reported to cause insomnia. In one study, 27% of patients given

120 mg of extended-release pseudoephedrine for a 3-week treatment of allergic rhinitis complained of subjective sleep disruption (99). Objective data on sleep performance and pseudoephedrine use is very limited, but nighttime use was associated with increased wake time during sleep (38).

Nicotine has complex central effects and in withdrawal it can cause marked behavioral disturbances including, in susceptible smokers, delirium (100). More commonly, insomnia is one of several symptoms associated with nicotine withdrawal (101). Treating nicotine dependence through pharmacological interventions [e.g., bupropion (102) and transdermal nicotine (103)] can cause sleep disruption, which may reflect nocturnal nicotine withdrawal or direct stimulant effects.

Cocaine reduces total sleep time, slow-wave sleep, and sleep latency in humans and animals, and REM sleep is significantly suppressed during the first half of sleep (104). In patients studied during cocaine withdrawal (105), shortened REM latencies and increased REM sleep percentages were observed during the second and third weeks. By the third week of withdrawal, the patients were observed to have a sleep pattern characteristic of that of insomniacs, i.e., prolonged sleep latency, an abnormally increased total time awake after sleep onset, and poor sleep efficiency. Cocaine-exposed infants have an increased incidence of the sudden infant death syndrome (SIDS) and significantly disturbed sleep (106); deficits in arousal mechanisms are hypothesized to be the cause of this increased incidence (107).

F. Hallucinogens

In chronic users, marijuana (Δ-9-tetrahydrocannabinol) significantly reduced eye movement activity during sleep and the duration of REM sleep and increased NREM stage 4 sleep (108). Long-term suppression of slow-wave sleep is found with chronic ingestion of marijuana (109). During withdrawal, rebounds in eye movements and REM sleep, as well as a decrease in NREM stage 4 sleep, were observed (108). Marijuana induced aggressive behavior in REM sleep-deprived rats, and brain catecholamines appeared to have a role in this behavior (110). In humans, partial sleep deprivation increased the dose dependence of marijuana effects on heart rate and subjective impairment (111). Prenatal exposure to marijuana caused increased body movements and decreased total quiet sleep in the neonate (112).

Lysergic acid diethylamide (LSD) increases wakefulness and decreases REM sleep in humans and animals (113). Fourteen percent of infants exposed to phencyclidine (PCP) in utero were reported to have sleep problems (114).

G. Opioids

The opioids are natural, semisynthetic, or synthetic substances with opiate-like activity that have complex central effects. Although they are important therapeutic medications, the opioids are among the most widely abused drugs (115) and sleep disruption is a common symptom among opiate addicts (116).

Therapeutic doses of less potent opioid analgesics, such as codeine, pentazocine, and meptazinol, appear to have limited effects on cognitive and psychomotor performance and sleep. Interestingly, narcoleptic patients treated with codeine report subjective clinical improvement, although objective measures of sleep and daytime sleepiness fail to confirm the subjective findings (117). Single doses of morphine and heroin cause disturbed sleep (115). Methadone induces an insomnia comparable to that after single doses of morphine, resulting in increased wakefulness and decreased sleep efficiency. During long-term administration methadone causes less sleep disruption than morphine (118). The mixed opioid agonist-antagonist cyclazocine has similar effects on human sleep to morphine type analgesics, causing sustained periods of waking with little muscle tension and increased urination (119).

H. Antiparkinsonian Medications

Disturbed nocturnal sleep is a common symptom associated both with Parkinson's disease (120) and with the medications used to manage the disorder (121). Objective studies confirm delays in sleep onset and increased wakefulness throughout the night in untreated patients (122), and patients treated with L-Dopa experience subjective insomnia, which has been confirmed by objective evaluation (123).

Selegiline is metabolized to L-methamphetamine and L-amphetamine and has been reported to cause subjective insomnia in 10–32% of users (124), although lower dosages cause less sleep disruption than higher dosages (125). Subjective insomnia has been reported with pergolide affecting about 8% of treated patients (41), although Jeanty and colleagues (126) reported an incidence of 42% in 26 patients. Bromocriptine (127) and amantadine (128) are also associated with subjective sleep disruption.

Although excessive sleepiness is associated with Parkinson's (119), there have been concerns of sudden "sleep attacks" in patients taking antiparkinsonian drugs, including the newer agents pramipexole and ropinirole which, like other dopamine agonists, can induce insomnia (41). Although controversial (129), up to 30% of patients taking dopamine agonists for Parkinson's disease have sleep attacks, and these events are caused by both the older and newer medications (130). Whether or not sudden sleep attacks are associated with a treatment-emergent nocturnal sleep disruption caused by dopamine agonists or by other complex interactions awaits further research.

I. Appetite Suppressants

Although anorectic side effects are common among the stimulants (41), more specific medications have been developed to suppress appetite as a treatment for obesity (131). Fenfluramine and dexfenfluramine were withdrawn from the market because of a high rate of abnormal echocardiograms among users (132). Both drugs were associated with subjective insomnia in users, and the scant objective data suggest that dexfenfluramine (133) had more objective sleep-disruptive effects than fenfluramine (134). Phentermine—which stimulates norepinephrine and dopamine release—is associated with subjective insomnia (135), and sibutramine caused insomnia in 7.3% of 4350 patients treated (41).

III. Medications and Other Substances with a Secondary Central Effect

A. Cardiovascular Drugs

β-Blockers

β-adrenergic blocking drugs are widely used, well-tolerated, and effective interventions for a variety of cardiovascular and noncardiovascular disorders. However, they are associated with CNS side effects including sleep disturbances, dreams, nightmares, and hallucinations (136). The incidence of these side effects is low, with the incidence of insomnia being reported as 2–4.3% (38).

Side effects vary by age of the user, the dose, and the type of drug used. Both objective and subjective sleep disturbance are more common with the lipophilic drugs such as propranolol than with the more hydrophilic drugs such as atenolol (136), although atenolol use causes some sleep disruption in normal subjects (137). For pindolol, which is less lipophilic than propranolol, there is a relationship between dose and sleep disruption, with 60 mg causing more insomnia and nervousness than lower dosages (138).

Although lipophilicity may be the primary determinant of the CNS effects of the β antagonists, sleep disruption may reflect other central processes including the drug's affinity for β_2 (139) or 5-HT receptors or the degree of melatonin suppression (140).

Antihypertensives

Although subjective sedation is the most common side effect associated with the use of α_2 agonists such as clonidine and methyldopa—affecting between 30% and 75% of users (38)—clonidine can cause insomnia (141), and both drugs can cause sleep disruption mediated through nightmares (142).

β antagonists with α_1-blocking activity such as carvedilol that combine β-adrenoreceptor blockade and vasodilation in a single racemic mixture are more commonly associated with fatigue and somnolence, although rare cases of subjective insomnia have been reported (143). Labetalol has also been associated with insomnia (144), but for both of these drugs objective sleep laboratory evidence for sleep-disruptive or sedative effects is lacking.

Although there are limited objective data, the available evidence suggests that other antihypertensives do not adversely affect sleep. Calcium channel blockers such as verapamil and nifedipine are rarely associated with insomnia (41) or sleepiness, although they may decrease the effectiveness of hypnotics and potentiate the effects of stimulants (38). Angiotensin-converting enzyme (ACE) inhibitors such as captopril and cilazapril (145) have a low incidence of central side effects and are not known to disrupt sleep.

Hypolipidemic Drugs

Inhibitors of 3-hydroxy-3-methylglutaryl coenzyme A (HMG-CoA) reductase have become the most widely used medications in the management of elevated plasma cholesterol levels, or hypercholesterolemia (146). Lovastatin has been associated with subjective reports of insomnia (147), and an early sleep laboratory evaluation of the use of lovastatin and pravastatin in 12 normal volunteers (148) showed that lovastatin did not disturb sleep initially during the first week of use. However, with continued use there was a significant and marked increase in both wake time after sleep onset and NREM stage 1 sleep compared with baseline. Pravastatin was not associated with sleep disturbance at any point during the trial, and neither drug caused any sleep disturbance after withdrawal.

The sleep disturbance associated with lovastatin was attributed to its high degree of lipophilicity in contrast with the hydrophilicity of pravastatin, but subsequent studies have not confirmed any significant sleep-disruptive effect of the statin drugs (149–152).

Antiarrhythmic Drugs

Although there are scant data on objective changes in sleep-wake performance with the antiarrhythmic drugs, fatigue is the most common CNS side effect reported by patients taking these medications. The placebo-adjusted incidence from clinical trials for this class ranges from 0 to 10% (38). As discussed above, sleep-disruptive effects of the β-blockers are more prominent than with other antiarrhythmic drugs.

Histamine₂ Antagonists

Although sedation is a primary side effect of the first-generation H_1 antihistamines such as diphenhydramine, the H_2 antagonists (e.g., cimetidine, ranitidine, nizatidine) do not easily cross the blood-brain barrier and are less likely to cause sleep disruption. Cimetidine is not associated with sleep disruption (153), but through competition for the cytochrome P_{450} isoenzyme system that catalyzes the metabolism of benzodiazepines, it can slow their hepatic metabolism (154). Similarly and through the same mechanism when given with cimetidine, the sleep-disruptive effects of theophylline (see below) and some β-blockers may be potentiated.

Although subjective insomnia has been associated with ranitidine use (41), the incidence is unknown. Data from clinical trials and experience suggest that ranitidine is unlikely to cause clinically significant potentiation of medications that are inactivated by the hepatic cytochrome P_{450} enzyme system.

However, likely due to its elevation of gastrointestinal pH allowing for greater absorption of acid-labile triazolam, ranitidine increases the oral absorption of this hypnotic in both young and older people without affecting its half-life (155).

Hormones

Severe psychiatric reactions, which include a sleep disturbance, occurred in approximately 5% of steroid-treated patients (156). Such disturbances usually occurred early in the course of steroid therapy, and risk factors for the development of a steroid-induced psychiatric syndrome include female gender, systemic lupus erythematosus, and high doses of prednisone.

Subjective sleep disturbance, characterized by increased wakefulness (157), associated with steroids (158) is quite common and occurs in nonmedicinal usage and as a treatment-emergent side effect. Forty-eight percent of gay men using anabolic steroids reported insomnia (159) and insomnia is a common side effect of medical steroid use in both adults and children (160).

Although objective studies of sleep disturbance associated with steroid use have been inconsistent and methodologically flawed, the most consistent effect in normal subjects has been a reduction in REM sleep time (161). Dexamethasone, prednisone and cortisol are known to cause sleep disruption (38) whereas the mineralocorticoid aldosterone does not affect sleep (162).

Sleep disturbance is a common feature of hyperthyroidism (163) and other hormonal disorders. Subjective sleep disturbance can be seen with the inappropriate use of iodine-containing compounds (164), deliberate overdosage with thyroid hormones (165), the use of food supplements (166), and as a side effect of treatment with thyroid hormones (41).

Bronchodilators

Nocturnal awakenings occur in about one-third of children with stable, mild to moderate asthma (167), and the use of steroids and bronchodilators (168) can further disrupt sleep.

Theophylline—chemically related to caffeine and used as a respiratory stimulant and bronchodilator—is commonly associated with subjectively disturbed sleep. In a prospective study, 55% of patients treated with theophylline complained of sleep maintenance difficulties (169), and sleep laboratory studies confirm the sleep-disruptive effect of this medication both in normals (170) and in asthmatics (171).

The selective β_2-adrenergic stimulants such as salbutamol are commonly used as bronchodilators for the management of asthma. CNS stimulation in general and insomnia in particular are known adverse effects of this intervention. Salmeterol is an effective alternative with less subjective sleep disruption (172,173).

IV. Conclusions

Sleep disruption, or insomnia, is a common symptom with multiple causes. Clinicians assessing the impact of sleep loss on daytime functioning must determine the cause or causes of the sleep loss before undertaking a treatment plan. Part of the required detailed assessment includes noting all substances the patient consumes—from prescribed mediations through recreational drugs to food supplements—to ensure that drug effects or drug-drug interactions are not contributing significantly to the disturbance.

References

1. Staab JP, Evans DL. Efficacy of venlafaxine in geriatric depression. Depress Anxiety 2000;12 (suppl 1):63–68.
2. Kales A, Kales JD. Sleep laboratory studies of hypnotic drugs: efficacy and withdrawal effects. J Clin Psychopharmacol 1983;3:140–150.
3. McVeigh C. Withdrawal of synthetic hormones during the perimenopause: a case study. J Psychosom Obstet Gynaecol 2000;21:175–178.
4. Bauer BA, Elkin PL, Erickson D, Klee GG, Brennan MD. Symptomatic hyperthyroidism in a patient taking the dietary supplement tiratricol. Mayo Clin Proc 2002;77:587–590.
5. Al-Windi A, Elmfeldt D, Svardsudd K. The relationship between age, gender, well-being and symptoms, and the use of pharmaceuticals, herbal medicines and self-care products in a Swedish municipality. Eur J Clin Pharmacol 2000;56: 311–317.
6. Friedmann PD, Herman DS, Freedman S, Lemon SC, Ramsey S, Stein MD. Treatment of sleep disturbance in alcohol recovery: a national survey of addiction medicine physicians. J Addict Dis 2003;22:91–103.
7. Zimatckin SM, Liopo AV, Slychenkov VS, Deitrich RA. Relationship of brain ethanol metabolism to the hypnotic effect of ethanol. I: Studies in outbred animals. Alcohol Clin Exp Res 2001;25(7):976–981.
8. Lobo LL, Tufik S. Effects of alcohol on sleep parameters of sleep-deprived healthy volunteers. Sleep 1997;20(1):52–59.
9. Aalto J, Kiianmaa K. Increased voluntary alcohol drinking concurrent with REM-sleep deprivation. Alcohol 1984;1(1):77–79.
10. Aalto J, Kiianmaa K. REM-sleep deprivation-induced increase in ethanol intake: role of brain monoaminergic neurons. Alcohol 1986;3(6):377–381.
11. Williamson AM, Feyer AM. Moderate sleep deprivation produces impairments in cognitive and motor performance equivalent to legally prescribed levels of alcohol intoxication. Occup Environ Med 2000;57(10):649–655.
12. Fairclough SH, Graham R. Impairment of driving performance caused by sleep deprivation or alcohol: a comparative study. Hum Factors 1999;41(1):118–128
13. Roehrs T, Roth T. Sleep, sleepiness, and alcohol use. Alcohol Res Health 2001;25(2):101–109.
14. Krull KR, Smith LT, Kalbfleisch LD, Parsons OA. The influence of alcohol and sleep deprivation on stimulus evaluation. Alcohol 1992;9(5):445–450.

15. Peeke SC, Callaway E, Jones RT, Stone GC, Doyle J. Combined effects of alcohol and sleep deprivation in normal young adults. Psychopharmacology 1980;67(3):279–287.

16. Krull KR, Smith LT, Sinha R, Parsons OA. Simple reaction time event-related potentials: effects of alcohol and sleep deprivation. Alcohol Clin Exp Res 1993;17(4):771–777.

17. Roehrs T, Beare D, Zorick F, Roth T. Sleepiness and ethanol effects on simulated driving. Alcohol Clin Exp Res 1994;18(1):154–158.

18. Guilleminault C, Silvestri R, Mondini S, Coburn S. Aging and sleep apnea: action of benzodiazepine, acetazolamide, alcohol, and sleep deprivation in a healthy elderly group. J Gerontol 1984;39(6):655–661.

19. Irwin M, Gillin JC, Dang J, Weissman J, Phillips E, Ehlers CL. Sleep deprivation as a probe of homeostatic sleep regulation in primary alcoholics. Biol Psychiatry 2002;51(8):632–641.

20. Gillin JC, Smith TL, Irwin M, Kripke DF, Schuckit M. EEG sleep studies in "pure" primary alcoholism during subacute withdrawal: relationships to normal controls, age, and other clinical variables. Biol Psychiatry 1990;27(5):477–488.

21. Nakazawa Y, Yokoyama T, Koga Y, Kotorii T, Ohkawa T, Sakurada H, Nonaka K, Dainoson K. Polysomnographic study of terminal sleep following delirium tremens. Drug Alcohol Depend 1981;8(2):111–117.

22. Mendelson WB, Majchrowicz E, Mirmirani N, Dawson S, Gillin JC, Wyatt RJ. Sleep during chronic ethanol administration and withdrawal in rats. J Stud Alcohol 1978;39(7):1213–1223.

23. Erwin VG, Korte A, Jones BC. Central muscarinic cholinergic influences on ethanol sensitivity in long-sleep and short-sleep mice. J Pharmacol Exp Ther 1988;247(3):857–862.

24. Allen RP, Wagman AM, Funderburk FR. Slow wave sleep changes: alcohol tolerance and treatment implications. Adv Exp Med Biol 1977;85A:629–640.

25. Hawton K, Harriss L, Hall S, Simkin S, Bale E, Bond A. Deliberate self-harm in Oxford, 1990–2000: a time of change in patient characteristics. Psychol Med 2003;33:987–995.

26. Roth T, Zorick F, Sicklesteel J, Stepanski E. Effects of benzodiazepines on sleep and wakefulness. Br J Clin Pharmacol 1981;11:31S–35S.

27. Kales A, Kales JD, Bixler EO, Scharf MB. Effectiveness of hypnotic drugs with prolonged use: flurazepam and pentobarbital. Clin Pharmacol Ther 1975;18(3):356–363.

28. Brouillette RT, Thach BT. A neuromuscular mechanism maintaining extrathoracic airway patency. J Appl Physiol 1979;46:772–779.

29. U.S. Xyrem Multicenter Study Group. A randomized, double blind, placebo-controlled multicenter trial comparing the effects of three doses of orally administered sodium oxybate with placebo for the treatment of narcolepsy. Sleep 2002;25(1):42–49.

30. U.S. Xyrem Multicenter Study Group. A 12–month, open-label, multicenter extension trial of orally administered sodium oxybate for the treatment of narcolepsy. Sleep 2003;26(1):31–35.

31. Scrima L, Hartman PG, Johnson FH Jr, Thomas EE, Hiller FC. The effects of gamma-hydroxybutyrate on the sleep of narcolepsy patients: a double-blind study. Sleep 1990;13(6):479–490.

32. Lapierre O, Montplaisir J, Lamarre M, Bedard MA. The effect of gamma-hydroxy-butyrate on nocturnal and diurnal sleep of normal subjects: further considerations on REM sleep-triggering mechanisms. Sleep 1990;13(1):24–30.

33. Gobaille S, Schleef C, Hechler V, Viry S, Aunis D, Maitre M. Gamma-hydroxybutyrate increases tryptophan availability and potentiates serotonin turnover in rat brain. Life Sci 2002;70(18):2101–2112.

34. Bedard MA, Montplaisir J, Godbout R, Lapierre O. Nocturnal gamma-hydroxybutyrate. Effect on periodic leg movements and sleep organization of narcoleptic patients. Clin Neuropharmacol 1989;12(1):29–36.

35. Series F, Series I, Cormier Y. Effects of enhancing slow-wave sleep by gamma-hydroxybutyrate on obstructive sleep apnea. Am Rev Respir Dis 1992;145(6):1378–1383.

36. Mamelak M, Escriu JM, Stokan O. The effects of gamma-hydroxybutyrate on sleep. Biol Psychiatry 1977;12:273–288.

37. Scharf MB, Baumann M, Berkowitz DV. The effects of sodium oxybate on clinical symptoms and sleep patterns in patients with fibromyalgia. J Rheumatol 2003;30(5):1070–1074.

38. Schweitzer PK. Drugs that disturb sleep and wakefulness. In: Kryger MH, Roth T, Dement WC, eds. Principles and Practice of Sleep Medicine. Toronto. WB Saunders, 2000:441–461.

39. Riemann D, Voderholzer U, Cohrs S, Rodenbeck A, Hajak G, Ruther E, Wiegand MH, Laakmann G, Baghai T, Fischer W, Hoffmann M, Hohagen F, Mayer G, Berger M. Trimipramine in primary insomnia: results of a polysomnographic double-blind controlled study. Pharmacopsychiatry 2002;35:165–174.

40. Oberndorfer S, Saletu-Zyhlarz G, Saletu B. Effects of selective serotonin reuptake inhibitors on objective and subjective sleep quality. Neuropsychobiology 2000; 42:69–81

41. Compendium of Pharmaceuticals and Specialties. 37th ed. Ottawa: Canadian Pharmacists Association, 2002.

42. Beasley CM Jr, Nilsson ME, Koke SC, Gonzales JS. Efficacy, adverse events, and treatment discontinuations in fluoxetine clinical studies of major depression: a meta-analysis of the 20–mg/day dose. J Clin Psychiatry 2000;61:722–728.

43. Cooper GL. The safety of fluoxetine—an update. Br J Psychiatry 1988; (suppl 3): 77–86.

44. Thase ME. Antidepressant treatment of the depressed patient with insomnia. J Clin Psychiatry 1999; 60 (suppl 17):28–31.

45. Dorsey CM, Lukas SE, Cunningham SL. Fluoxetine-induced sleep disturbance in depressed patients. Neuropsychopharmacology 1996;14:437–442.

46. Trenkwalder C, Walters AS, Hening W. Periodic limb movements and restless legs syndrome. Neurol Clin 1996;14:629–650.

47. Armitage R, Trivedi M, Rush AJ. Fluoxetine and oculomotor activity during sleep in depressed patients. Neuropsychopharmacology 1995;12:159–165.

48. Schenck CH, Mahowald MW, Kim SW, O'Connor KA, Hurwitz TD. Prominent eye movements during NREM sleep and REM sleep behavior disorder associated with fluoxetine treatment of depression and obsessive-compulsive disorder. Sleep 1992;15:226–235.

49. Manfredi RL, Kales A, Vgontzas AN, Bixler EO, Isaac MA, Falcone CM. Buspirone: sedative or stimulant effect? Am J Psychiatry 1991;148:1213–1217.

50. Ellison JM, Stanziani P. SSRI-associated nocturnal bruxism in four patients. J Clin Psychiatry 1993; 54:432–434.

51. Neylan TC, Metzler TJ, Schoenfeld FB, Weiss DS, Lenoci M, Best SR, Lipsey TL, Marmar CR. Fluvoxamine and sleep disturbances in posttraumatic stress disorder. Journal of Traumatic Stress 2001; 14: 461–467.

52. van Bemmel AL, van den Hoofdakker RH, Beersma DG, Bouhuys AL. Changes in sleep polygraphic variables and clinical state in depressed patients during treatment with citalopram. Psychopharmacology 1993;113:225–230.

53. Black K. Shea C. Dursun S. Kutcher S. Selective serotonin reuptake inhibitor discontinuation syndrome: proposed diagnostic criteria. J Psychiatry Neurosci 2000; 25:255–261.

54. Vogel GW, Buffenstein A, Minter K, Hennessey A. Drug effects on REM sleep and on endogenous depression. Neurosci Biobehav Rev 1990; 14:49–63.

55. Detweiler MB. Harpold GJ. Bupropion-induced acute dystonia. Ann Pharmacother 2002; 36:251–254.

56. Nofzinger EA, Reynolds CF 3rd, Thase ME, Frank E, Jennings JR, Fasiczka AL, Sullivan LR, Kupfer DJ. REM sleep enhancement by bupropion in depressed men. Am J Psychiatry 1995;152:274–276.

57. Salin-Pascual RJ, Galicia-Polo L, Drucker-Colin R. Sleep changes after 4 consecutive days of venlafaxine administration in normal volunteers. J Clin Psychiatry 1997;58:348–350.

58. Luthringer R, Toussaint M, Schaltenbrand N, Bailey P, Danjou PH, Hackett D, Guichoux JY, Macher JP. A double-blind, placebo-controlled evaluation of the effects of orally administered venlafaxine on sleep in inpatients with major depression. Psychopharmacol Bull 1996;32:637–646.

59. Jain KK. Drug-induced sleep disorders. In: Jain KK. Drug-Induced Neurological Disorders. 2nd ed. Toronto: Hogrefe and Huber, 2001:387–396.

60. Chen DT, Ruch R. Safety of moclobemide in clinical use. Clin Neuropharmacol 1993;16 (suppl 2):S63–68.

61. Hoffmans J, Knegtering R. The selective reversible monoamine oxidase-A inhibitor brofaromine and sleep. J Clin Psychopharmacol 1993;13:291–292.

62. Haffmans PM, Vos MS. The effects of trazodone on sleep disturbances induced by brofaromine. Eur Psychiatry 1999;14:167–171.

63. Hawley CJ, Quick SJ, Ratnam S, Pattinson HA, McPhee S. Safety and tolerability of combined treatment with moclobemide and SSRIs: a systematic study of 50 patients. Int Clin Psychopharmacol 1996;11:187–191.

64. Aslan S, Isik E, Cosar B. The effects of mirtazapine on sleep: a placebo controlled, double-blind study in young healthy volunteers. Sleep 2002; 15: 677–679.

65. Rush AJ, Armitage R, Gillin JC, Yonkers KA, Winokur A, Moldofsky H, Vogel GW, Kaplita SB, Fleming JA, Montplaisir J, Erman MK, Albala BJ, McQuade RD. Comparative effects of nefazodone and fluoxetine on sleep in outpatients with major depressive disorder. Biol Psychiatry 1998;44: 3–14.

66. van Laar MW, van Willigenburg AP, Volkerts ER. Acute and subchronic effects of nefazodone and imipramine on highway driving, cognitive functions, and daytime sleepiness in healthy adult and elderly subjects. J Clin Psychopharmacol 1995;15:30–40.

67. Gerlach J, Peacock L. New antipsychotics: the present status. Int Clin Psychopharmacol 1995;10 (suppl 3):39–48.

68. Costa e Silva JA, Alvarez N, Mazzotti G, Gattaz WF, Ospina J, Larach V, Starkstein S, Oliva D, Cousins L, Tohen M, Taylor CC, Wang J, Tran PV. Olanzapine as alternative therapy for patients with haloperidol-induced extrapyramidal symptoms: results of a multicenter, collaborative trial in Latin America. J Clin Psychopharmacol 2001;21:375–381.

69. Hinze-Selch D, Mullington J, Orth A, Lauer CJ, Pollmacher T. Effects of clozapine on sleep: a longitudinal study. Biol Psychiatry 1997;42:260–266.

70. Yamashita H, Morinobu S, Yamawaki S, Horiguchi J, Nagao M. Effect of risperidone on sleep in schizophrenia: a comparison with haloperidol. Psychiatry Res 2002;109:137–142.

71. Salin-Pascual RJ, Herrera-Estrella M, Galicia-Polo L, Laurrabaquio MR. Olanzapine acute administration in schizophrenic patients increases delta sleep and sleep efficiency. Biol Psychiatry. 1999;46:141–143.

72. Hellewell JS. Quetiapine: a well-tolerated and effective atypical antipsychotic. Hosp Med 2002;63:600–603.

73. Kraus T, Schuld A, Pollmacher T. Periodic leg movements in sleep and restless legs syndrome probably caused by olanzapine. J Clin Psychopharmacol 1999;19:478–479.

74. Wetter TC, Brunner J, Bronisch T. Restless legs syndrome probably induced by risperidone treatment. Pharmacopsychiatry 2002;35:109–111.

75. Wirshing DA, Pierre JM, Wirshing WC. Sleep apnea associated with antipsychotic-induced obesity. J Clin Psychiatry 2002;63:369–370

76. Gillin JC, Byerley WF. Drug therapy: the diagnosis and management of insomnia. N Engl J Med 1990;322:239–248.

77. Frankland A, Robinson MJ. Fatal chloral hydrate overdoses: unnecessary tragedies. Can J Psychiatry 2001;46:763–764.

78. Merlotti L, Roehrs T, Zorick F, Roth T. Rebound insomnia: duration of use and individual differences. J Clin Psychopharmacol 1991;11:368–373.

79. Staedt J, Stoppe G, Hajak G, Ruther E. Rebound insomnia after abrupt clozapine withdrawal. Eur Arch Psychiatry Clin Neurosci 1996;246:79–82.

80. Mamelak M, Csima A, Price V. The effects of a single night's dosing with triazolam on sleep the following night. Journal of Clinical Pharmacology 1990; 30:549–555.

81. Soldatos CR, Dikeos DG, Whitehead A. Tolerance and rebound insomnia with rapidly eliminated hypnotics: a meta-analysis of sleep laboratory studies. Int Clin Psychopharmacol 1999;14:287–303.

82. Kales A, Manfredi RL, Vgontzas AN, Bixler EO, Vela-Bueno A, Fee EC. Rebound insomnia after only brief and intermittent use of rapidly eliminated benzodiazepines. Clin Pharmacol Ther 1991;49:468–476.

83. Tan TL, Bixler EO, Kales A, Cadieux RJ, Goodman AL. Early morning insomnia, daytime anxiety, and organic mental disorder associated with triazolam. J Fam Pract 1985;20:592–594.

84. Zhang WY. A benefit-risk assessment of caffeine as an analgesic adjuvant. Drug Saf 2001;24:1127–1142.

85. Hindmarch I, Rigney U, Stanley N, Quinlan P, Rycroft J, Lane J. A naturalistic investigation of the effects of day-long consumption of tea, coffee and water on alertness, sleep onset and sleep quality. Psychopharmacology (Berl) 2000;149:203–216.

86. Lin AS, Uhde TW, Slate SO, McCann UD. Effects of intravenous caffeine administered to healthy males during sleep. Depress Anxiety 1997;5:21–28.

87. Dews PB, O'Brien CP, Bergman J. Caffeine: behavioral effects of withdrawal and related issues. Food Chem Toxicol 2002;40:1257–1261.

88. Mitler MM, Hayduk R. Benefits and risks of pharmacotherapy for narcolepsy. Drug Saf 2002;25:791–809

89. Mitler MM. Evaluation of treatment with stimulants in narcolepsy. Sleep 1994;17(suppl 8):S103–106.

90. Parkes JD, Chen SY, Clift SJ, Dahlitz MJ, Dunn G. The clinical diagnosis of the narcoleptic syndrome. J Sleep Res 1998;7:41–52.

91. van den Hoed J, Kraemer H, Guilleminault C, Zarcone VP Jr, Miles LE, Dement WC, Mitler MM. Disorders of excessive daytime somnolence: polygraphic and clinical data for 100 patients. Sleep 1981;4: 23–37.

92. Borgen LA, Cook HN, Hornfeldt CS, Fuller DE. Sodium oxybate (GHB) for treatment of cataplexy. Pharmacotherapy 2002;22:798–799

93. Malcolm R, Book SW, Moak D, DeVane L, Czepowicz V. Clinical applications of modafinil in stimulant abusers: low abuse potential. Am J Addict 2002;11:247–249.

94. Pack AI, Black JE, Schwartz JR, Matheson JK. Modafinil as adjunct therapy for daytime sleepiness in obstructive sleep apnea. Am J Respir Crit Care Med 2001; 164:1675–1681.

95. Zifko UA, Rupp M, Schwarz S, Zipko HT, Maida EM. Modafinil in treatment of fatigue in multiple sclerosis: results of an open-label study. J Neurol 2002;249(8):983–987.

96. Menza MA, Kaufman KR, Castellanos A. Modafinil augmentation of antidepressant treatment in depression. J Clin Psychiatry 2000;61:378–381.

97. Efron D, Jarman F, Barker M. Side effects of methylphenidate and dexamphetamine in children with attention deficit hyperactivity disorder: a double-blind, crossover trial. Pediatrics 1997;100:662–666.

98. Figueras A, Laporte JR. Regulatory decisions in a globalised world: the domino effect of phenylpropanolamine withdrawal in Latin America. Drug Saf 2002;25:689–693.

99. Bertrand B, Jamart J, Marchal JL, Arendt C. Cetirizine and pseudoephedrine retard alone and in combination in the treatment of perennial allergic rhinitis: a double-blind multicentre study. Rhinology1996;34:91–96.

100. Mayer SA, Chong JY, Ridgway E, Min KC, Commichau C, Bernardini GL. Delirium from nicotine withdrawal in neuro-ICU patients. Neurology 2001;57:551–553.

101. Hughes JR, Hatsukami D. Signs and symptoms of tobacco withdrawal. Arch Gen Psychiatry 1986;43:289–294.

102. Paul MA, Gray G, Kenny G, Lange M. The impact of bupropion on psychomotor performance. Aviat Space Environ Med 2002;73:1094–1099.

103. Gourlay SG, Forbes A, Marriner T, McNeil JJ. Predictors and timing of adverse experiences during trandsdermal nicotine therapy. Drug Saf 1999;20:545–555.

104. Hill SY, Mendelson WB, Bernstein DA. Cocaine effects on sleep parameters in the rat. Psychopharmacology 1977;51(2):125–127.

105. Kowatch RA, Schnoll SS, Knisely JS, Green D, Elswick RK. Electroencephalographic sleep and mood during cocaine withdrawal. J Addict Dix 1992;11(4):21–45.

106. Gingras JL, Feibel JB, Dalley LB, Muelenaer A, Knight CG. Maternal polydrug use including cocaine and postnatal infant sleep architecture: preliminary observations

and implications for respiratory control and behavior. Early Hum Dev 1995;43(3):197–204.

107. Gingras JL, Weese-Mayer D. Maternal cocaine addiction. II: An animal model for the study of brainstem mechanisms operative in sudden infant death syndrome. Med Hypotheses 1990;33(4):231–234.

108. Feinberg I, Jones R, Walker JM, Cavness C, March J. Effects of high dosage delta-9–tetrahydrocannabinol on sleep patterns in man. Clin Pharmacol Ther 1975;17(4):458–466.

109. Freemon FR. The effect of chronically administered delta-9–tetrahydrocannabinol upon the polygraphically monitored sleep of normal volunteers. Drug Alcohol Depend 1982;10:345–353.

110. Musty RE, Lindsey CJ, Carlini EA. 6–Hydroxydopamine and the aggressive behavior induced by marihuana in REM sleep-deprived rats. Psychopharmacology 1976;48(2):175–179.

111. Liguori A, Gatto CP, Jarrett DB, Vaughn McCall W, Brown TW. Behavioral and subjective effects of marijuana following partial sleep deprivation. Drug Alcohol Depend 2003;70(3):233–240.

112. Scher MS, Richardson GA, Coble PA, Day NL, Stoffer DS. The effects of prenatal alcohol and marijuana exposure: disturbances in neonatal sleep cycling and arousal. Pediatr Res 1988;24(1):101–105.

113. Kay DC, Martin WR. LSD and tryptamine effects on sleep/wakefulness and electrocorticogram patterns in intact cats. Psychopharmacology 1978;58(3):223–228.

114. Wachsman L, Schuetz S, Chan LS, Wingert WA. What happens to babies exposed to phencyclidine (PCP) in utero? Am J Drug Alcohol Abuse 1989;15(1):31–39.

115. Obermeyer WH, Benca RM. Effects of drugs on sleep. Neurol Clin 1996;14:827–840.

116. Oyefeso A, Sedgwick P, Ghodse H. Subjective sleep-wake parameters in treatment-seeking opiate addicts. Drug Alcohol Depend 1997;48:9–16.

117. Fry JM, Pressman MR, DiPhillipo MA, Forst-Paulus M. Treatment of narcolepsy with codeine. Sleep 1986;9(1 Pt 2):269–274.

118. Pickworth WB, Neidert GL, Kay DC. Morphinelike arousal by methadone during sleep. Clin Pharmacol Ther 1981;30:796–804.

119. Pickworth WB, Neidert GL, Kay DC. Cyclazocine-induced sleep disruptions in nondependent addicts. Prog Neuropsychopharmacol Biol Psychiatry 1986;10:77–85.

120. Larsen JP, Tandberg E. Sleep disorders in patients with Parkinson's disease: epidemiology and management. CNS Drugs 2001;15:267–275.

121. Schafer D, Greulich W. Effects of parkinsonian medication on sleep. J Neurol 2000; 247 (suppl 4): 24–27.

122. Kales A, Ansel RD, Markham CH, Scharf MB, Tan TL. Sleep in patients with Parkinson's disease and normal subjects prior to and following levodopa administration. Clin Pharmacol Ther 1971;12:397–406.

123. van Hilten B, Hoff JI, Middelkoop HA, van der Velde EA, Kerkhof GA, Wauquier A, Kamphuisen HA, Roos RA. Sleep disruption in Parkinson's disease. Assessment by continuous activity monitoring. Arch Neurol 1994;51:922–928.

124. Crisp P, Mammen GJ, Sorkin EM. Selegiline: a review of its pharmacology, symptomatic benefits and protective potential in Parkinson's disease. Drugs Aging 1991; 228–248.

125. Lavie P, Wajsbort J, Youdim MB. Deprenyl does not cause insomnia in parkinsonian patients. Commun Psychopharmacol 1980;4:303–307

126. Jeanty P, Van den Kerchove M, Lowenthal A, De Bruyne H. Pergolide therapy in Parkinson's disease. J Neurol. 1984;231:148–52.

127. Vardi J, Glaubman H, Rabey J, Streifler M. EEG sleep patterns in Parkinsonian patients treated with bromocryptine and L-dopa: a comparative study. J Neural Transm 1979;45:307–316.

128. Schwab RS, Poskanzer DC, England AC Jr, Young RR. Amantadine in Parkinson's disease. Review of more than two years' experience. JAMA 1972;222:792–795.

129. Horne J. Misperceptions exist about sleep attacks when driving. BMJ 2002; 325: 657.

130. Homann CN, Wenzel K, Suppan K, Ivanic G, Kriechbaum N, Crevenna R, Ott E. Sleep attacks in patients taking dopamine agonists: review. BMJ 2002;324:1483–1487.

131. Steelman M. Pharmacotherapy for obesity. N Engl J Med 2002;346:2092–2093.

132. Weissman NJ. Appetite suppressants and valvular heart disease. Am J Med Sci 2001;321:285–291.

133. Wiegand M, Bossert S, Kinney R, Pirke KM, Krieg JC. Effect of dexfenfluramine on sleep in healthy subjects. Psychopharmacology 1991;105:213–218.

134. Oswald I, Jones HS, Mannerheim JE. Effects of two slimming drugs on sleep. Br Med J 1968; 1:797–799.

135. Groenewoud G, Schall R, Hundt HK, Muller FO, van Dyk M. Steady-state pharmacokinetics of phentermine extended-release capsules. Int J Clin Pharmacol Ther Toxicol 1993;31:368–372.

136. McAinsh J, Cruickshank JM. Beta-blockers and central nervous system side effects. Pharmacol Ther 1990;46:163–197.

137. Van Den Heuvel CJ, Reid KJ, Dawson D. Effect of atenolol on nocturnal sleep and temperature in young men: reversal by pharmacological doses of melatonin. Physiol Behav 1997;61:795–802.

138. Gonasun LM, Langrall H. Adverse reactions to pindolol administration. Am Heart J 1982;104:482–486.

139. Yamada Y, Shibuya F, Hamada J, Sawada Y, Iga T. Prediction of sleep disorders induced by beta-adrenergic receptor blocking agents based on receptor occupancy. J Pharmacokinet Biopharm 1995;23:131–145.

140. Brismar K, Hylander B, Eliasson K, Rossner S, Wetterberg L. Melatonin secretion related to side-effects of beta-blockers from the central nervous system. Acta Med Scand 1988;223:525–530.

141. Kostis JB, Rosen RC, Holzer BC, Randolph C, Taska LS, Miller MH. CNS side effects of centrally-active antihypertensive agents: a prospective, placebo-controlled study of sleep, mood state, and cognitive and sexual function in hypertensive males. Psychopharmacology 1990;102:163–170.

142. Paykel ES, Fleminger R, Watson JP. Psychiatric side effects of antihypertensive drugs other than reserpine. J Clin Psychopharmacol 1982;2:14–39.

143. Dunn CJ, Lea AP, Wagstaff AJ. Carvedilol. A reappraisal of its pharmacological properties and therapeutic use in cardiovascular disorders. Drugs 1997;54:161–185.

144. Pearce CJ, Wallin JD. Labetalol and other agents that block both alpha- and beta-adrenergic receptors. Cleve Clin J Med 1994;61:59–69.

145. Dietrich B, Herrmann WM. Influence of cilazapril on memory functions and sleep behaviour in comparison with metoprolol and placebo in healthy subjects. Br J Clin Pharmacol 1989;27 (suppl 2):249S-261S.

146. Schaefer EJ, Genest JJ, Ordovas JM, Salem DN, Wilson PWF. Familial lipoprotein disorders and premature coronary artery disease. Atherosclerosis 1994;108:S41–S54.

147. Tobert JA, Shear CL, Chremos AN, Mantell GE. Clinical experience with lovastatin. Am J Cardiol1990;65:23F-26F.

148. Vgontzas AN, Kales A, Bixler EO, Manfredi RL, Tyson KL. Effects of lovastatin and pravastatin on sleep efficiency and sleep stages. Clin Pharmacol Ther 1991;50:730–737.

149. Kostis JB, Rosen RC, Wilson AC. Central nervous system effects of HMG CoA reductase inhibitors: lovastatin and pravastatin on sleep and cognitive performance in patients with hypercholesterolemia. J Clin Pharmacol 1994;34:989–996.

150. Roth T, Richardson GR, Sullivan JP, Lee RM, Merlotti L, Roehrs T. Comparative effects of pravastatin and lovastatin on nighttime sleep and daytime performance. Clin Cardiol 1992;15:426–432.

151. Partinen M, Pihl S, Strandberg T, Vanhanen H, Murtomaki E, Block G, Neafus R, Haigh J, Miettinen T, Reines S. Comparison of effects on sleep of lovastatin and pravastatin in hypercholesterolemia. Am J Cardiol 1994;73:876–880.

152. Ehrenberg BL, Lamon-Fava S, Corbett KE, McNamara JR, Dallal GE, Schaefer EJ. Comparison of the effects of pravastatin and lovastatin on sleep disturbance in hypercholesterolemic subjects. Sleep 1999;22:117–121.

153. Orr WC, Duke JC, Imes NK, Mellow MH. Comparative effects of H2–receptor antagonists on subjective and objective assessments of sleep. Aliment Pharmacol Ther 1994;8:203–207.

154. Tanaka E. Clinically significant pharmacokinetic drug interactions with benzodi-azepines. J Clin Pharm Ther 1999;24:347–355.

155. O'Connor-Semmes RL, Kersey K, Williams DH, Lam R, Koch KM. Effect of ranitidine on the pharmacokinetics of triazolam and alpha-hydroxytriazolam in both young (19–60 years) and older (61–78 years) people. Clin Pharmacol Ther 2001;70:126–131.

156. Lewis DA, Smith RE. Steroid-induced psychiatric syndromes. A report of 14 cases and a review of the literature. J Affect Disord 1983;5:319–332.

157. Buysse DJ. Drugs affecting sleep, sleepiness and performance. In: Monk TH, ed. Sleep, Sleepiness and Performance. Toronto: John Wiley and Sons, 1991: 249–306.

158. Gillin JC, Jacobs LS, Fram DH, Snyder F. Acute effect of a glucocorticoid on normal human sleep. Nature 1972 Jun 16;237(5355):398–399.

159. Bolding G, Sherr L, Elford J. Use of anabolic steroids and associated health risks among gay men attending London gyms. Addiction 2002;97:195–203.

160. Drigan R, Spirito A, Gelber RD. Behavioral effects of corticosteroids in children with acute lymphoblastic leukemia. Med Pediatr Oncol 1992;20:13–21.

161. Fehm HL, Benkowitsch R, Kern W, Fehm-Wolfsdorf G, Pauschinger P, Born J. Influences of corticosteroids, dexamethasone and hydrocortisone on sleep in humans. Neuropsychobiology 1986;16:198–204.

162. Born J, Zwick A, Roth G, Fehm-Wolfsdorf G, Fehm HL. Differential effects of hydrocortisone, fluocortolone, and aldosterone on nocturnal sleep in humans. Acta Endocrinol 1987;116:129–137.

163. Deutsch SF. Recent contributions in psychoendocrinology. Psychosomatics 1968; 9:127–134

164. Pagliaricci S, Lupattelli G, Mannarino E. [Hyperthyroidism due to the improper use of povidone-iodine.] Ann Ital Med Int 1999;14:124–126.

165. Hack JB, Leviss JA, Nelson LS, Hoffman RS. Severe symptoms following a massive intentional L-thyroxine ingestion. Vet Hum Toxicol 1999;41:323–326.
166. Bauer BA, Elkin PL, Erickson D, Klee GG, Brennan MD. Symptomatic hyperthyroidism in a patient taking the dietary supplement tiratricol. Mayo Clin Proc 2002;77:587–590.
167. Strunk RC, Sternberg AL, Bacharier LB, Szefler SJ. Nocturnal awakening caused by asthma in children with mild-to-moderate asthma in the childhood asthma management program. J Allergy Clin Immunol 2002;110:395–403.
168. Bailey WC, Richards JM Jr, Manzella BA, Brooks CM, Windsor RA, Soong SJ. Characteristics and correlates of asthma in a university clinic population. Chest 1990;98:821–828.
169. Janson C, Gislason T, Boman G, Hetta J, Roos BE. Sleep disturbances in patients with asthma. Respir Med 1990;84:37–42.
170. Kaplan J, Fredrickson PA, Renaux SA, O'Brien PC. Theophylline effect on sleep in normal subjects. Chest 1993;103:193–195.
171. Richardt D, Driver HS. An evaluative study of the short-term effects of once-daily, sustained-release theophylline on sleep in nocturnal asthmatics. S Afr Med J. 1996;86:803–804.
172. Wiegand L, Mende CN, Zaidel G, Zwillich CW, Petrocella VJ, Yancey SW, Rickard KA. Salmeterol vs theophylline: sleep and efficacy outcomes in patients with nocturnal asthma. Chest 1999;115:1525–1532.
173. Selby C, Engleman HM, Fitzpatrick MF, Sime PM, Mackay TW, Douglas NJ. Links Inhaled salmeterol or oral theophylline in nocturnal asthma? Am J Respir Crit Care Med 1997;155:104–108.

10

Factors Affecting Test Performance

TRACY F. KUO AND CLETE A. KUSHIDA

Stanford University, Stanford, California, U.S.A.

I. Introduction

The most common objective of testing is to determine the subject's current status with respect to a particular domain of functioning (e.g., cognitive, emotional, physical). The test results often are used to aid in clinical decision making or to quantify change from previous levels of functioning due to a disease process or as a result of experimental manipulation. Therefore, obtaining valid and reliable test results are important for making accurate assessments about the subject's current status and rendering inferences about the effects of a particular condition on the individual. There are many factors that can influence performance. The best way to avoid confounds is by preventing them from the start through proper preparation of the subject for testing, adhering to established standard test administration procedures, and using direct inquiry or observation of factors that can affect performance. This chapter broadly reviews factors that can affect performance, with emphasis on sleep-deprived individuals. Considerations of these factors should be an integral part of interpretation of test scores.

II. Subject Factors

The goal of testing and how the results impact the subjects can influence the test takers' response set. Cooperation of test takers can usually be secured by convincing them that it is in their own interests to obtain a valid score. *Will a negative consequence follow poor performance, such as in the case of a pilot who may lose the privilege to fly because of failing a Maintenance of Wakefulness Test (MWT)? Does the subject stand to gain something in the event the testing supports the presence of impairment, as in the case of obtaining disability benefits or through litigation?* In most experimental situations, subjects' performance generally is of no serious consequence. Nevertheless, subtle contingencies may have a role in shaping the subject's response. For example, if a subject learned that falling asleep will terminate an MWT session sooner, he or she may make less effort to stay awake to escape this boring testing situation. In general, based on operant conditioning theory, a person would be motivated to perform in a way that leads to rewards and avoidance of punishment or negative consequences.

The adequate assessment of an individual's cognitive functioning entails a working knowledge of the demographic variables that have an effect on neuropsychological test performance. On standardized tests, when a subject's demographic characteristics are quite different from those of the normative groups, caution should be taken in the interpretation of the scores because the subject's scores are compared and statistically expressed as relative to those of the normative groups. Regardless of whether an individual does or does not match the demographic characteristics of the normative samples, the interpretation of neuropsychological test scores will ultimately depend on multiple factors, including one's definition of normal and abnormal, the goal and context of the assessment, the relationship of current test performance and daily functioning to prior levels of functioning, together with a consideration of the likely impact of the results on diagnostic and treatment decisions. Whenever available, the use of age- and education-corrected norms is advisable (1). As with all clinical information, judgment is required to weigh the importance of false-positive or false-negative error.

A. Subject Characteristics

General intelligence (IQ) is one of the strongest predictors of performance on cognitive tests. Education, which is often considered a proxy for general intelligence, has been found to be significantly related to performance on the majority of cognitive tests. Research on gender differences in ability has found that men and women tend to be equivalent in general intelligence scores. However, men tend to do better on tests that involve manipulating spatial relationships, quantitative skills, physical strength, and simple motor speed, whereas women show advantages on tests of certain verbal abilities (2). However, these differences have not been consistently observed. Personality traits do not significantly influence testing because they are generally stable throughout the adult years (3).

Aging is associated with anatomical and ischemic changes in the brain, along with loss or degeneration of the neurons. Assessment of cognitive functioning in the elderly is often complicated, due to sensorimotor impairments, systemic illnesses, and greater variability in cognitive abilities even among optimally healthy individuals (4,5). Often older individuals are taking multiple medications, which because of reduced hepatic and renal functioning can pose amplified adverse effects in alertness, psychomotor speed, and cognition. As a result of aging, working memory span appears to be reduced, thus reducing the capacity to multitask. Memory decrements are greater on recall than on recognition tasks (6). Nonverbal recall (7) tends to show more of a decrement with age than verbal recall. Verbal fluency for words also decreases with age. Older individuals also tend to use less effective strategies for memory and in problem solving.

Crystallized intelligence is well preserved with age but fluid intelligence is more vulnerable to decline. Crystallized intelligence is measured by tests of knowledge and skills that are acquired in previous learning experiences. Fluid intelligence is considered most dependent on biological factors such as the normal development and continued integrity of the central nervous system. Fluid intelligence includes cognitive flexibility, information processing and psychomotor speed, and spatial visualization skills. This form of intelligence is measured by tasks requiring learning, conceptual, and problem-solving operations, in the context of novel situations. The effects of culture, ethnicity, or race on neuropsychological tests have been reported as minimal.

Handedness is defined as the preferred hand used for a motor activity (manual preference) or the hand most skillful at performing a task (manual proficiency). Approximately 90–95% of the population are right handed (8). It is important to assess hand preference in any neuropsychological evaluation. The dominant hand is expected to perform better than the nondominant hand, so knowledge of hand preference is essential for interpretation of performance on motor and sensory tasks.

B. Arousal, Fatigue, Mood, Affect, and Motivation

Arousal bears an inverted U-shape relationship to performance (9). The condition for optimal performance is when there is a moderate degree of arousal. Hyperarousal and underarousal can adversely affect performance. Anxiety, which also is a related construct to arousal, adversely influences test performance because it can interfere with attention, concentration, and memory retrieval. Performance on other than extremely simple tasks is generally impaired in a state of low and high arousal and is optimal at a midlevel of arousal. In reference to sleep deprivation studies, fatigability and sleepiness may affect alertness and performance (10,11). Performance on auditory vigilance, reaction time, and memory tasks was shown to be impaired by sleep deprivation (12–14). It has been suggested that impairments noted on vigilance and reaction time tests were due to lapses of approximately 1 sec (15). Herscovitch et al. (16) found greater perseveration on the Wisconsin Card Sorting Task (WCST; an executive function test) with sleep loss.

A potential confound exists as to whether cognitive tests of sleep-deprived humans (and animals) actually identify cognitive deficits or simply identify behavioral deficits. *Does a sleep-deprived human or animal actually "forget" how to do a learned task, or is the human or animal not able to perform the learned task because of fatigue, decreased motivation due to sleepiness, or sensory or motor impairments due to sleep loss?* For these reasons, the perfect experiment to assess the effects of sleep loss on learning and memory has not been devised up to this point. Sleep deprivation confounds the experimental design; these factors may result in the human or animal experiencing a decline in performance that may be independent of the variable (e.g., sleep deprivation effects on executive function) under consideration.

A simple reductionist view is that these factors may not be so important. Sleep deprivation produces a constellation of differential effects on alertness, motivation, and sensorimotor systems that are inevitably and inextricably associated with sleep loss. Whether the observed cognitive deficits are the result of the sleep loss or these associated effects is impossible to determine, so one may argue that they must always be considered together.

III. Testing Environment

It is important to realize the extent to which testing conditions may influence performance. Even apparently minor aspects of the testing situation may appreciably alter performance. The most important requirement for obtaining valid and reliable testing is advance preparation. Standardized procedures apply not only to verbal instructions, timing, materials, and other aspects of the test but also to the testing environment. Some attention should be given to the selection of a suitable testing room. Optimally, the testing environment should be one that is quiet, with no foot traffic or distracting views. In most cases, this environment is an examination room that has sufficient artificial light (without glare and reflection), that is kept at a comfortable temperature, and that has adequate ventilation. It is usually best to seat the subject facing away from windows and doors from which his or her activities can be seen, and also to prevent glare. If the external environment is noisy, it may be necessary to use a white noise generator or to take steps to soundproof walls and doors. The office should appear welcoming and friendly. The seating should be comfortable and ergonomically designed. To minimize distractions, test materials should be kept out of sight until needed. The following elements of the testing environment are also of key importance.

A. Establishing Examiner-Subject Rapport

In order to optimize a subject's performance, the examiner should try to gain the cooperation and trust of that individual. One of the first issues addressed should be an explanation of the purpose of the testing and a discussion about how the session will progress. Issues of confidentiality should be discussed. Subjects should be informed that the tasks they will be doing range from easy to hard, and their job is to do their best. Subjects should be encouraged to attempt all test items and, in some cases, take a chance by guessing while the examiner remains supportive and encouraging. In order to avoid giving information about the correctness or incorrectness of an answer, praise should be given for effort, not for the answer itself. To avoid discouraging the subject early, the examiner should start with simpler tasks and, as the tasks become more difficult, acknowledge that an item may have been difficult and that no one gets all the answers right. Praise often helps the subject avoid becoming discouraged but should be given judiciously rather than after every answer.

B. Structuring the Test Session

The scheduling of a test session depends on the purpose of assessment, the nature of the tests being used, and the focus and stamina of the subject. In general, test sessions are limited by the severity of the subjects' presenting problems, their general health, their age, and other factors (see Table 1). In some instances, shorter test sessions are needed to achieve reliable samples of optimal cognitive ability. However, the testing period should include practice sessions, so as to decrease the possibility that "learning effects" might influence the results. In other words, a subject practices a given task to the point that any decrement in task performance is very unlikely due to the process of learning how to perform the task. Another important factor is the well-documented time-on-task decrement, which refers to a systematically decreasing performance as a function of an increasing duration of a cognitive task.

For subjects whose symptomatology includes distractibility and for subjects whose energy level has been compromised, it may be unwise to attempt testing in only 1 day if the goal is to obtain the subjects' best performance across many tasks. On the other hand, if the goal is to assess cognition and mental stam-

Table 1   Important Behavioral Observations during the Clinical Interview

---

- Level of arousal, alertness, including energy level, motor findings such as hyperactivity and speed
- Appearance, including manner of dress, level of grooming, gait and posture, mannerisms, and physical abnormalities
- Level of cooperation, including motivation and effort
- Discourse abilities, including ability to understand and produce conversational speech
- Sensorimotor functioning, including eyesight, hearing, muscle strength, and the use of aids such as glasses, hearing aids, canes, and so forth
- Appropriateness of social skills and level of anxiety
- Speech, including rate, tone, prosody, articulation, fluency, and word choice
- Emotionality, including affect, mood, and appropriateness
- Thought content and processes, including organization and reality testing
- Memory, including retrieval of recent and remote events

---

ina over the course of a day, then administering the tests in a 1-day session would be more appropriate than dividing up the tasks over several sessions. Subjects who may be unable to work consistently well in one session include older adults, very young children, and subjects who suffer from physical pain that is exacerbated by long periods of sitting. In general, the clinician should try to complete the interview and testing in 1 day. This increases the likelihood that the tests will be given under similar circumstances. When test sessions are given on different days, differences in sleep, illness, anxiety, and other situational factors may confound the results and make their interpretation difficult. When tests are given in a single session, the subject should be offered a reasonable number of breaks and time for lunch. Breaks should be taken only between, not during, tests or subtests. Any signs of fatigue or variations in effort should be noted.

C. Administering the Tests

Special steps should be taken to prevent interruptions during the test. There is also evidence to show that the type of answer sheet employed may affect test scores. Use of a separate answer sheet may significantly lower test scores, especially in children. Even more significant at any age level are the possible differences between paper-and-pencil and computer administration of the same tests. In ability tests, the objective calls for careful concentration on the given tasks and for putting forth one's best effort to perform well. In self-report inventories, the objective calls for frank and honest responses to questions about one's usual behavior; in certain projective tests, it calls for full reporting of associations evoked by the stimuli, without any censoring or editing of content. Examiners should expend effort to arouse test takers' interest in the test and to elicit their cooperation for the test. Examiners endeavor to motivate respondents to follow the instructions as fully and conscientiously as possible.

Many other more subtle testing conditions have been shown to affect performance on ability tests as well as personality tests. Whether the examiner is a stranger or someone familiar to the test taker may make a significant difference in test scores. For a child, a friendly, cheerful, and relaxed manner on the part of the examiner is reassuring. A shy, timid child needs more preliminary time to become familiar with the surroundings.

D. Optimizing Motivation and Alertness

To increase the likelihood of adequate motivation, the examiner should spend some time before beginning formal testing explicitly asking the subject whether he or she understands the reasons for the examination and offering an opportunity to ask questions about the session. Some populations of subjects may not be motivated to perform optimally for the examination (see Table 1). Subjects who are medically ill or physically uncomfortable may find it extremely unpleasant to expend mental effort over long periods of time. In addition, questions regarding the quantity and quality of subjects' sleep are important to assess whether the subjects will be able to remain awake and alert during the testing. Questionnaire rating scales of daytime alertness, such as the Epworth and Stanford Sleepiness Scales, may be useful in determining the level of alertness of subjects prior to testing. Elderly subjects and those with psychiatric illnesses or histories of impaired intellectual abilities often are found to be inadequately motivated or uncooperative with long testing. Finally, subjects who are tested as part of a forensic examination are frequently reported as not expending optimal effort. Poor motivation may be manifested by overt signs of distractibility, excessive slowness or carelessness, direct questioning about the usefulness or meaning of the tests, or even expression of contempt toward the examiner.

IV. Summary and Conclusions

There are many key factors that interact in the test environment and influence performance in the test situation. The proper identification of these factors that can affect performance, especially in sleep-deprived individuals, is thus essential in obtaining valid and reliable data.

Comparison of a subject's scores to those of a normative group is important; the use of age- and education-corrected norms should always be considered. One of the strongest predictors of performance on cognitive tests is general intelligence. Performance is also affected by the subject's age, education, and handedness; less consistently affected by gender, and not appreciably affected by personality traits. Factors such as arousal, fatigue, mood, affect, and motivation may directly affect test performance as well. Sleep deprivation, in particular, produces detrimental behavioral effects that, in turn, yield decrements in test performance that are difficult, if not impossible, to differentiate from those related to sleep loss-associated cognitive deficits.

A quiet, comfortable, and well-designed testing room contributes to valid and reliable testing. It is important for the examiner to establish good rapport with the subject; this frequently involves support, encouragement, and judicious praise. The duration of testing must be carefully considered, to allow time for practice sessions, to account for time-on-task decrements, and to factor in the subject's characteristics (e.g., age, health status). In most cases, the interview and testing of the subject should be completed within a 1-day period, with appropriate breaks to minimize subject fatigue. Factors such as the type of test, paper-and-pencil versus computerized testing, and the mood of the examiner can influence test performance. Lastly, a subject's prior night's sleep and current alertness level should always be evaluated prior to the administration of any test.

The factors described in this chapter are critical yet often neglected during the administration of tests. In the case of sleep-deprived subjects, these factors are paramount, especially because subjects suffering from sleep loss already have problems with alertness, motivation, and sensorimotor ability.

References

1. Heaton RK, Ryan L, Grant I, Matthews CG. Demographic influences on neuropsychological test performance. In: Grant I, Adams KM, eds. Neuropsychological Assessment of Neuropsychiatric Disorders. 2nd ed. New York: Oxford University Press, 1996:141–163.
2. Maccoby EE, Jacklin CN. The Psychology of Sex Differences. Stanford, CA: Stanford University Press, 1974.
3. McCrae RR, Costa PT. Personality in Adulthood. New York: Guilford Press, 1990.
4. Valdois S, Joanette Y, Poissant A, Ska B, Dehaut F. Heterogeneity in the cognitive profile of normal elderly. J Clin Exp Neuropsychol 1990; 12(4):587–596.
5. Williams R, Reeve W, Ivison D, Kavanagh D. Use of environmental manipulation and modified informal reality orientation with institutionalized, confused elderly subjects: a replication. Age Ageing 1987; 16(5):315–318.
6. Albert MS. Cognitive function. In: Albert MS, Moss MB, eds. Geriatric Neuropsychology. New York, NY: Guilford Press, 1988:33–53.
7. Shichita K, Hatano S, Ohashi Y, Shibata H, Matuzaki T. Memory changes in the Benton Visual Retention Test between ages 70 and 75. J Gerontol 1986; 41(3):385–386.
8. Annett M. A classification of hand preference by association analysis. Br J Psychol 1970; 61(3):303–321.
9. Hebb DO. A Textbook of Psychology. Philadelphia: WB Saunders, 1958.
10. Anderson RM Jr., Bremer DA. Sleep duration at home and sleepiness on the job in rotating twelve-hour shift workers. Hum Factors 1987; 29(4):477–481.
11. Borland RG, Rogers AS, Nicholson AN, Pascoe PA, Spencer MB. Performance overnight in shiftworkers operating a day-night schedule. Aviat Space Environ Med 1986; 57(3):241–249.
12. Glenville M, Broughton R, Wing AM, Wilkinson RT. Effects of sleep deprivation on short duration performance measures compared to the Wilkinson auditory vigilance task.Sleep 1978; 1(2):169–176.
13. Wilkinson RT, Houghton D. Portable four-choices reaction-time test with magnetic tape memory. Behav Res Meth Instr Comput 1975; 7:441–446.
14. Williams HL, Gieseking CF, Lubin A. Some effects of sleep loss on memory.Percept Mot Skills 1966; 23(3):1287–1293.
15. Broughton R. Performance and evoked potential measures of various states of daytime sleepiness. Sleep 1982; 5 Suppl 2:S135–146.
16. Herscovitch J, Stuss D, Broughton R. Changes in cognitive processing following shortterm cumulative partial sleep deprivation and recovery oversleeping. J Clin Neuropsychol 1980; 2(4):301–319.

11

Attention and Memory Changes

GENEVIÈVE FOREST

University of Ottawa, Ottawa, Ontario, Canada

ROGER GODBOUT

University of Montréal and Hôpital Rivière-des-Prairies, Montréal, Québec, Canada

I. Introduction

Sleep quality is an essential prerequisite for optimal daytime functioning. Since the discovery of rapid-eye-movement (REM) sleep 50 years ago by Aserinsky and Kleitman (1), persistent research efforts have established some of the basic functions of sleep, first at the physiological level and more recently at the cognitive level. One of the major sets of findings is that sleep involves the spontaneous activation of neurobiological systems that are shared with the waking state (2,3). REM sleep and non-REM (NREM) sleep being two complementary states governed by intimately related neural networks (4), sleep disruption is bound to have a significant impact on daytime cognitive performance. Indeed, sleep deprivation induced either by pure sleep loss or through idiopathic sleep disorders is now known to impair behavioral adjustment and cognitive performance during waking. After briefly reviewing some basic facts on sleep and on memory and attention, this chapter will discuss some of the evidence according to which sleep may contribute to waking performance and sleep loss may impair particular cognitive systems.

II. Brief Review of Sleep Organization

A. Sleep Stages and Electroencephalographic Activity

The standard method of sleep stage scoring (5) uses neurophysiological markers to identify five stages of sleep: stages 1–4 and REM sleep (5). Quantified analysis of the electroencephalogram (EEG) and topographic mapping serve as stage-specific indicators of areas that are more or less activated by frequency-specific activity. During the waking state with eyes opened, the EEG is predominantly composed of low-amplitude, high-frequency beta activity (12–30 Hz). In a relaxed state with eyes closed, this pattern changes to slower alpha activity (8–12 Hz), predominant in the occipital area. As sleepiness increases, slower frequency theta waves (4–7 Hz) take over and alpha occupies less than 50% of epochs; this is considered stage 1 sleep. In fact, stage 1 sleep is not truly a sleeping state as measures of behavioral and evoked electroencephalographic potential measures are concerned. Stage 1 is rather considered as a transitional stage between waking and true sleeping, a part of the process of falling asleep (6).

Recordings of increased EEG theta activity upon waking are indeed known to correlate with somnolence (7,8). Shortly after the onset of stage 1, theta waves will progressively gain amplitude and particular electroencephalographic events, referred to as sleep spindles and K complexes, will appear within 10 min. This is the onset of stage 2, considered by most researchers and clinicians as the true onset of sleep. Sleep spindles are phasic bursts of sinusoidal high-frequency activity (12–15 Hz), lasting 0.5 to 2 sec, with maximal occurrence over the frontal and parietal cortices (9,10). Sleep spindles are considered to represent a sleep-protective mechanism by which access of input to the brain is diminished through a deactivation of the thalamocortical loop (11–13); this has been supported in various papers (see, for example, Refs. 9, 14–16). K complexes are negative biphasic waves prominent over the vertex, with a sharp onset and smoother offset, lasting 0.5–1.5 sec, and an amplitude of at least 75 μV. K complexes can be evoked by sensory stimulation, and some authors suggest that they could reflect the brain's increased reactivity to internal or external stimuli during sleep (17–19), suggesting that an excessive number of K complexes could be related to an instability between waking and sleeping maintenance processes. Whether K complexes reflect an arousal reaction or another sleep-protective mechanism is still debated (20–22).

Twenty to forty minutes after sleep onset, electroencephalographic activity will have slowed considerably, showing bouts of high-amplitude delta waves (0.5–4 Hz, > 75 μV). When delta activity contributes to at least 20% of a scoring epoch, the latter is considered as stage 3 sleep whereas proportions greater than 50% are considered as stage 4 sleep epochs; collectively, stages 3 and 4 are known as slow-wave sleep, (SWS). The amount of delta activity, as quantified by quantitative electroencephalographic (qEEG) spectral analysis, may be used as an index of the "density" or "intensity" of NREM sleep, and sleep deprivation is followed by increased delta activity during recovery sleep (23,24), with a maximal intensity over the frontal cortex (25). When selective SWS deprivation is applied, rebound spindle activity is first replaced by rebound SWS (24,26).

REM sleep appears approximately 90 min following sleep onset, featuring a dramatic change in the electroencephalographic picture where delta waves are replaced by low-voltage fast electroencephalographic activity in the beta range. REM sleep "density" is indexed by the number of rapid eye movements during REM sleep. At the electroencephalographic level, spectral analysis has shown that beta activity better characterizes REM sleep-related subcortical neuronal activity (27).

B. Sleep Cycles

A typical night of sleep comprises 50–60% of the total sleep time in stages 1 and 2, whereas the rest of the night is devoted to SWS and REM sleep in almost equal proportions (i.e., 20–25%). The sequence of sleep stages from stage 1 to REM sleep unfolds itself in cycles of 90–120 min and the internal structure of successive cycles evolves throughout the night: SWS is mainly found in the first third of the night whereas the longest bouts of REM sleep are found in the latter half. Sleep deprivation in the first half of the night thus blocks more severely the expression of SWS (or NREM sleep), whereas sleep deprivation in the latter half prevents a large proportion of REM sleep.

III. Brief Review of Physiological Functions of Sleep

Among the commonly held hypotheses on the functions of sleep is the assumption that it serves somatic homeostasis by compensating, reversing, or restoring "expenditures" that have occurred during prior wakefulness. For example, it is known that SWS plays a critical role in growth hormone secretion (28,29), brain protein synthesis (30,31), body temperature regulation and energy conservation (32,33), and immune function and tissue restoration (34–36). Increased amounts and "intensity" of sleep during recovery from sleep deprivation are also consistent with a restorative function of sleep in most mammals (37,38).

Physiological functions of sleep have also been associated with REM sleep. For example, REM sleep contributes to the maturation of the newborn central nervous system by providing endogenous stimulation leading to the formation of new synaptic connections (39), binocular coordination (40), and so forth. Another hypothesis is that REM sleep has a role in the reactivation of innate behaviors that is essential for adaptation and survival (41). Because high levels of brain activity are achieved in REM sleep together with high rates of dream reports upon awakenings from that state, REM sleep is also considered as the perfect physiological support for dream mentation (42).

IV. Cognitive Functions

Sleep is also thought to serve "restorative" function because it reverses sleepiness, the latter being defined in terms of cognitive efficiency. Sleepiness is often defined as a greater need to sleep, or *"how fast can you fall asleep?"*, and this is tested in the clinical sleep laboratory with the Multiple Sleep Latency Test (MSLT). Another side to sleepiness is not being able to stay awake, i.e., *"how hard can you resist falling asleep?"*, which is tested in the clinical sleep laboratory with the Maintenance of Wakefulness Test (MWT) (44). This second face of sleepiness can also be addressed by behavioral tests such as neuropsychological/performance tasks. Such tasks not only detect lapses in performance (errors of omission) but also inappropriate responding (errors of commission). Before we discuss the relationship between sleep deprivation and cognitive performance it is necessary to define the basic concepts to be covered.

A. Definitions

For a certain number of years, researchers in the field of neuropsychology have schematized cognitive operations into well-delineated steps and categorized performance into modules (Fig. 1). This chapter focuses on two main cognitive func-

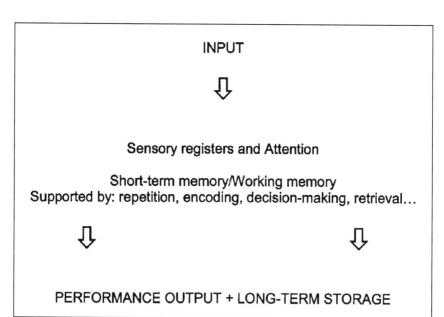

Figure 1 Schematic representation of some of the processing steps in the cognitive treatment of information.

tions have been extensively studied in sleep research: memory and attention processes.

Memory (See Table 1)

Memory allows one to encode, store, and retrieve information for immediate use. It is considered to be a heterogeneous grouping of multiple systems that are constantly interacting with one another. It is important to note that subdivisions of memory can vary among authors. *Short-term memory*, often referred to as *working memory*, is responsible for the active manipulation of information for immediate use (45). Its structure is composed of two subsystems: one for processing language (the phonological loop) and one for visuospatial information (the visuospatial sketch pad). These subsystems are controlled by an executive system, which ensures optimal division of attention resources in order to manipulate two or more pieces of information simultaneously. *Long-term memory* is concerned with the encoding, storing, and retrieval of information, and is composed of *declarative* and *nondeclarative* memories (46). The former involves the representation of semantic information, such as conceptual knowledge about the world, as well as episodic information, such as autobiographical knowledge coded in spatiotemporal terms. Nondeclarative or *procedural memory* is involved with the representation of skills and motor and cognitive programs, each involving different mental processes. Information in long-term memory can be retrieved either explicitly or implicitly. *Explicit recall* corresponds to the voluntary recall of previously learned information, whereas *implicit recall* corresponds to the facilitation in performance of tasks due to prior exposure to the task without explicit reference to the learning episode. Declarative memory is usually associated with explicit recall, whereas procedural memory is usually associated with implicit recall.

Recent studies indicate the presence of a working memory circuit, which connects frontal and parietal cortices (46–50), whereas the executive system is located in the frontal lobe (51). The working memory circuit is independent of the modality used to test it. Research has consistently shown that lesions of the temporal lobe, particularly lesions of the hippocampus and amygdala, are closely related to impairments in explicit/declarative memory (46,52,53). More specifically, regions of the temporal lobe appear to be involved in tasks requiring cued recalls (i.e., contextual clues). However, when the task requires free recall (i.e., without any clues) and relies on strategies to search for information, the frontal lobe (dorsolateral and ventromedian frontal areas) becomes a prominent element (54).

Evidence suggests that an implicit form of memory, known as priming, is associated with the activity of the posterior cortical regions, which are involved in perceptual processing. This implicit memory is also dependent on the basal ganglia and frontal lobes, sharing many connections (55–59). Research has shown that anatomical structures used during implicit memory tasks could be dependent on the type of material presented. For example, an implicit motor task usually requires motor cortical areas (46), whereas a task geared at encoding and retrieving the organization of a time sequence involves the frontal lobes (60–62).

Attention

Attention can be defined as a mobilization and/or orientation of mental resources toward pertinent information in order to accomplish a task. It is also a cognitive function that cannot be considered as a unique concept. In fact, it can be divided into four main components: alertness, sustained attention, selective attention, and divided attention (63,64). *Alertness* can be defined as the capacity to quickly

Table 1   Schematic Organization and Substrates of Memory Systems

Type	Subtype	Capacity	Characteristics	Anatomical correlates
Working memory	Task dependent	Short term	- Immediate memory - Limited storage space - Dependent on attention - Information handling - Allows multitasking	Prefrontal cortex, parietal cortex, posterior areas of the brain (see text for details)
Episodic memory	Declarative/ explicit	Long term	- Autobiographic memory - Large storage space - Spatiotemporal context - Personal data: events, dates, locale, etc.	Temporal lobe (hippocampus, amygdala, etc.), thalamus
Semantic memory	Declarative/ explicit	Long term	- Directory of concepts, meaning of symbols, technical knowledge	Primary and associative cortices, frontal lobes, etc.
Procedural	Nondeclarative/ Implicit	Long term	- "Know-how memory," action, automatisms, cognitive habits, sensorimotor learning	Basal ganglia, frontal lobe, cerebellum. Task dependent

respond (simple reaction time), for a short period of time, to a stimulus that is infrequent and unpredictable. It can also reflect the arousal level of a person. *Sustained attention* requires the mobilization of attention resources for long periods, in relation to unpredictable and infrequent stimuli. It could also involve decision-making processes (65). Many authors use the terms "vigilance" and "sustained attention" interchangeably. *Selective attention* concerns the ability to focus attention resources on one target stimulus despite the presence of other distracting stimuli. It therefore requires the ability to inhibit attention from shifting to nonrelevant stimuli. Finally, *divided attention* is characterized by the ability to deal with two or more types of information simultaneously. It requires the optimal division of attention resources in order to achieve two or more independent goals. This concept is similar to working memory because it also consists of a supervision system that governs the attention resources.

Many anatomical structures are associated with attention processes, most of which are part of a large corticostriatal network. Two main attention systems interacting with one another have been described in the literature (63,66). The first system, called the "posterior attention network," involves the posterior parietal areas, pulvinar and reticular nuclei of the thalamus, as well as different parts of the superior colliculi. This system is responsible for the involuntary and unconscious orientation of attention toward important stimuli. The second system, the "anterior attention network," consists of the cingulate gyrus and parts of the frontal lobe. This system is involved in signal detection and is associated with more voluntary and conscious control mechanisms of attention. These two networks are supervised by a main system located in the frontal lobe (63). A third, less known system has been associated with alertness and arousal, and involves parts of the frontal lobe and locus coeruleus (63).

Despite the fact that cognitive functions are relatively well defined and described as entities, they often interact with one another depending on the task presented. For example, attention processes can be solicited during memory tasks.

B. Protocols for Studying Cognitive Functions During Sleep

With the use of several different approaches, studies have shown that a relationship exists between sleep and cognitive processes in humans. Different types of experimental protocols have been implemented to study such a relationship. One of these methods consists of evaluating the impact of an increased cognitive workload on subsequent sleep parameters (67–70). A second approach is to investigate the effects of sleep deprivation (total, partial, and selective; or sleep fragmentation) on subsequent learning, memory, or cognitive and motor performance (39,71–80). A third method measures nocturnal performance upon awakening during specific stages of sleep (81–84). Finally, the clinical approach determines cognitive and motor deficits associated with sleep disorders or medical conditions affecting sleep (85–87). A brief literature review of these various methods is presented.

Effects of Increased Cognitive Load on Subsequent Sleep

This type of protocol involves imposing a long and/or complex cognitive workload to a participant and measuring its effects on sleep parameters during the following night of sleep, or by performing correlations between performance and subsequent sleep parameters.

In a study evaluating the impact of an increased cognitive workload on subsequent sleep parameters, Mandai et al. (69) found that a complex task requiring new knowledge acquisition (i.e., learning the Morse code) results in an increase in both total REM sleep time and number of REM sleep episodes. Spreux et al. (88) also found that learning a complex task is followed by an increase in oculomotor activity during REM sleep. Similarly, Smith and Lapp (89) noted an increase in REM sleep lasting several days after learning material in a psychology class. Studies have also found that intensive language learning also results in an increase in REM sleep, and this increase is significantly correlated with the efficacy of the learning process (67,68,90). In a study by De Koninck et al. (90), participants were asked to wear lenses that vertically rotated their visual field by 180 degrees for 3 days. This cognitive workload required learning to coordinate body movements in new ways. Results showed an increase in the percentage of REM sleep during subsequent nights. In another study, De Genaro et al. (91) found that prolonged exposure to a visual spatial attention task resulted in an increase in REM sleep duration as well as a decrease in REM sleep latency (increased "REM pressure"). Results from such studies suggest that macroscopic measurements and phasic events of REM sleep are sensitive to previous cognitive experiences.

In addition to changes observed in REM sleep following a cognitive workload, increases in sleep spindles have also been noted (92,93). Indeed, Gais et al. (92) have found that subjects had an increased spindle density in the first part of the night after learning pairs of words (it is noteworthy that 12- to 15-Hz electroencephalographic sigma activity was not associated with learning). Similarly, Meier-Koll et al. (93) found an increase in the amount of sleep spindles and stage 2 sleep after a spatial (maze) memory task. Authors suggested that sleep spindles reflected a level of aptitude for learning certain types of material (94,95). For example, Fogel et al. (94) found that performance on a procedural/implicit task was associated with a 42% increase in the number of sleep spindles in the following night of sleep. Nader et al. (95) found that sleep spindle activity is highly correlated with nonverbal intelligence quotient (IQ), more precisely with tasks that required perceptual and analytical skills. Stage 2 itself may also have a relationship to specific cognitive functions. Indeed, Smith and MacNeil (78) have demonstrated that improvement on a procedural/implicit task (pursuit rotor) is dependent on the amount of stage 2 sleep in sleep following the learning sessions. Walker et al. (96) obtained similar results with another procedural/implicit task (simple finger tapping task), even though the correlation with stage 2 sleep was significant only in the last quarter of nocturnal sleep. In our laboratory, we have studied the possible role of sleep in learning ability and have found a positive correlation between post-sleep performance on an implicit word recall task and the number of sleep spindles during the previous night of sleep (97). In addition, we have found that the sleep spindle index and amount of stage 2 sleep is positively correlated with post-sleep performance on a selective attention task (98).

Effects of Sleep Deprivation on Memory and Attention

The most common manipulation used to study the relationship between sleep and cognition is to measure the effects of sleep deprivation on subsequent cognitive or motor performance as well as on recall of learned material. Several types of sleep deprivation have been used in the literature: short-term or long-term sleep deprivation; total, partial, or selective sleep deprivation; and sleep fragmentation.

Total Sleep Deprivation (See Also Chap. 4)

Most total sleep deprivation studies have shown that a night or more without sleep results in memory deficits. More specifically, research has shown that explicit/declarative memory, procedural/implicit memory and working memory are impaired by a single night of total sleep deprivation. In a study by Aubrey et al. (99), participants were asked to memorize a simple route through the library just before a night of sleep deprivation. An explicit recall task one week later confirmed that sleep had a critical role in spatial memory consolidation. Similarly, Blagrove et al. (100) found that one night of sleep deprivation impairs the immediate and delayed recall for stories. Comparable results were obtained with the learning of nonsense syllables. For example, Idzikowski (101) found that sleep-deprived participants took longer to learn a list of words in comparison with their own baseline. Recognition of paired letters and numbers (102), working memory (serial addition task) (103), implicit sequence learning in a serial reaction task (104), and procedural memory formation, as measured by a visual discrimination task (105), are also affected by one night of total sleep deprivation. Despite two nights of recovery sleep following sleep deprivation, Stickgold et al. (105) could not document any improvements in a visual discrimination task.

Attention processes may also be affected by total sleep deprivation (75,106,107). An impaired performance on simple reaction time tests and vigilance tasks (digit detection, auditory signal detection, Wilkinson Auditory Vigilance Task) has been found after one night of sleep loss (71,72,77). Fisher (106) demonstrated, using dual-task interaction (divided attention), that one night of total sleep deprivation may produce a loss of attention control. Linde and Bergstrom (107) found an impairment in feature selection functions after one night of total sleep deprivation, possibly reflecting selective attention problems. After four consecutive nights of total sleep deprivation, Norton (75) found a significant breakdown in participants' capacity to selectively attend to relevant stimuli presented in a card sorting task. Norton (75) concluded that sleep might be an important factor in maintaining processes involved in selective attention.

Partial Sleep Deprivation (See Also Chap. 5)

In partial sleep deprivation protocols, sleep is partially reduced during one or many consecutive nights. The timing of sleep deprivation during nocturnal sleep is closely related to the type of sleep from which one wants to deprive the participants. Indeed, since SWS is more prominent at the beginning of the night, partial sleep deprivation of the first hours of nocturnal sleep will mostly affect this stage of sleep. On the contrary, since REM sleep is more prominent near the end of nocturnal sleep, partial sleep deprivation of the last few hours of nocturnal sleep will mostly affect REM sleep. Partial sleep deprivation can also be applied by simply delaying sleep onset and advancing wake-up time. Unfortunately, methodological problems arise with this type of protocol, including the confounding factor of a circadian component in performance. Indeed, participants are trained and tested at different circadian times; at the beginning and end of the night for the early night sleep condition, and in the middle and the end of the night for the late night sleep condition. In the late night condition, participants benefit from at least 3 hr of sleep prior to training, which is not the case for participants in the early night condition. Recent findings suggest that prior sleep can in fact influence performance or the ability to learn (108).

Plihal and Born (109) examined the effect of early and late night sleep deprivation on two memory tests: recall of paired-associate lists (declarative memory) and mirror tracing skills (procedural memory). Participants' recall was measured after 3 hr of early or late night sleep. Results indicated that early sleep is sufficient for maintaining a normal performance on the declarative memory test, whereas late sleep is sufficient for maintaining a normal performance in the procedural memory test. The authors suggested that results reflected the specific influence of early night SWS and late night REM sleep. In this study, however, the explicit/declarative task was made of verbal material whereas the procedural/implicit task consisted of nonverbal material, a confounding variability making it difficult to interpret the results. To clarify this issue, the study was replicated using a nonverbal declarative task (recall of spatial location) and a verbal procedural/implicit task (words stem priming task) (110). Results obtained from this study were similar to those of the previous study. Early nocturnal sleep, rich in SWS, was associated with better performance on the nonverbal explicit/declarative task whereas later sleep, rich in REM sleep, was associated with better performance on the verbal procedural/implicit task.

These results are in accordance with those of an older study by Yaroush et al. (111), showing a better consolidation of paired associates after early night sleep. On the other hand, contrary to Plihal and Born (109,110) a 2002 study by Gais et al. (92) showed that late night sleep did not allow improvement on a procedural learning task (visual discrimination skills) whereas early night sleep did. According to the authors, task complexity could explain such contradictory results, whereas "the influence of REM sleep may become increasingly important with more complex tasks," a contention supported by many researchers (3).

Finally, Wagner et al (112) examined the effects of early and late night sleep on the recall of neutral versus emotional texts. Results showed that recall of emotional material is better after late night sleep than early night sleep. These results are in accordance with other reports suggesting that REM sleep may be particularly required when an individual is learning emotionally charged information (113).

Attention processes have also shown sensitivity to partial sleep deprivation. Five nights of early sleep partial sleep deprivation (a loss of 40% of sleep per night) resulted in an impaired performance on the Wilkinson Auditory Vigilance Task as well as on two different reaction time tests (Four-Choice Serial Reaction Time Test, simple reaction time test) (114). Dinges et al. (115) obtained similar results after seven nights of partial sleep deprivation (a loss of 33% of sleep per night, i.e., delayed sleep onset and advanced wake-up time), using a sustained attention task (Psychomotor Vigilance Task). On the other hand, another study failed to demonstrate performance impairment on an auditory vigilance task, after 4 nights of partial sleep deprivation (about 4 hr of sleep per night) and 18 nights of partial sleep deprivation (about 5 hr of sleep per night) (71).

Sleep Fragmentation (See Also Chap. 6)

In sleep fragmentation protocols, participants are awakened several times throughout the night, according to a predetermined schedule. Few studies have used this type of protocol and results have not been systematic. For example, two nights of sleep fragmentation (awakenings every 2 min) did not induce decrements in sustained attention (simulated assembly line task) or divided attention (tracking a moving target and simple reaction time) (76,79). Authors concluded that the task was not sufficiently demanding to induce deficits, since every participant had a 95% success rate. On the other hand, a study by Martin et al. (74) showed that one night of awakenings at 2-min intervals resulted in impairments in sustained attention [placed auditory serial addition task (PASAT) 4-sec test]. Bonnet (116,117) found that two nights of fragmented sleep (every 2 min) impaired alertness (length of task: 10 min) as well as sustained attention (length of task: 30 min), the same way one night of total sleep deprivation did. In contrast, sleep fragmentation every 10 min did not significantly affect the same tasks. In a more recent study, Ficca et al. (118) showed that explicit/declarative memory as measured by an explicit recall of paired words is affected by one night of sleep fragmentation only when NREM-REM sleep cycles are perturbed. Authors conclude that sleep organization, i.e., the regular occurrence of NREM-REM cycles, is more crucial for the retention of verbal material presented before sleep than sleep states per se.

Selective Sleep Deprivation (See Also Chap. 5)

Selective sleep deprivation is a method that allows investigation of the selective relationship between specific sleep stages and cognitive functions. In his review of REM sleep deprivation studies, Smith (70) reported that REM sleep deprivation results in deficits in implicit memory as measured by word priming and the

Tower of Hanoi task, but does not result in deficits in explicit recall of word lists or paired associates. Smith (70) concluded that REM sleep is important for procedural/implicit memory performance, whereas explicit/declarative memory is not related to this stage of sleep. In another study, Smith and MacNeill (78) showed that stage 2 sleep could be important for motor procedural memory, as measured by the pursuit rotor task. More specifically, this study measured the effects of REM sleep deprivation on the consolidation of the pursuit rotor task (procedural/implicit memory). Participants were first trained on the task, then distributed into different sleep deprivation protocols (REM sleep deprivation, NREM sleep deprivation, late night partial sleep deprivation, total sleep deprivation, and no sleep deprivation). Participants were retested 1 week later. Results showed impaired recall when late night sleep was deprived (NREM sleep deprivation, late night partial sleep deprivation, and total sleep deprivation conditions) compared to when the last portion of nocturnal sleep was relatively preserved (REM sleep deprivation and no sleep deprivation conditions). Since REM sleep deprivation in the latter part of the night leaves almost exclusively stage 2 sleep, the authors concluded that stage 2 is responsible for the procedural memory deficits observed in their study. This was replicated in a subsequent study by the same laboratory (119).

For practical reasons, very few data are available on the effects of selective NREM sleep (SWS) deprivation. Indeed, NREM sleep (SWS) deprivation is difficult to achieve because it usually affects the organization of sleep cycles. Studies that have used this type of protocol have not shown any systematic cognitive impairments (76,79,116,117,120). Alertness (task of 10 min) and sustained attention (task of 30 min) were shown to be impaired by SWS deprivation (117,120). However, performance on these tasks was also impaired upon nonselective sleep deprivation of equal duration, suggesting that these cognitive functions may be more sensitive to a general loss of sleep rather than selective SWS deprivation. On the other hand, studies by Stickgold et al. (121) and by Gais et al. (92) showed that performance improvement on a visual discrimination task was positively related to the amount of SWS in the first part of the night and to the amount of REM sleep in the last part of the night while any other sleep parameters were found to be significant.

Results from studies using total sleep deprivation, partial sleep deprivation, sleep fragmentation and selective sleep deprivation protocols thus suggest that sleep in general has a role in explicit/declarative memory; procedural/implicit memory; working memory; alertness; and selective, sustained, and divided attention.

Strengthening of Memory Traces During Sleep

The goal of this technique is to modulate or influence the processing of information that is occurring during sleep. For example, a clue (i.e., auditory stimulus) may be given during a specific stage of sleep following a learning session.

Tilley (122) has shown that it is possible to improve memory consolidation by presenting cued information to participants during stage 2 sleep. In this experiment, participants were exposed to pictures, and researchers then presented words either related or unrelated to these pictures during stage 2 sleep. Results indicated that pictures related to the words presented during stage 2 sleep were better remembered than pictures unrelated to words.

Intensive learning of the Morse code is accompanied by an increase in REM sleep time and number of REM sleep episodes during the following night (see "Effects of Increased Cognitive Load on Subsequent Sleep" in Section IV of this chapter). The same researchers (69,123) injected an auditory stimulation during postlearning REM sleep episodes and found significantly improved Morse code retention despite no increases in REM sleep parameters. Smith and Weeden (124) obtained similar results with a complex logic task. During the learning session, an auditory stimulus (a "click") was administered and repeated during REM sleep episodes the following night. Results showed that participants better recalled the task when auditory stimulation was administered during the night compared to when it was not. It is thought that the auditory stimulation used in such experiments can lead to reactivation of the new neuronal networks formed during the previous learning session. It therefore suggests that such a reactivation produces better consolidation of information during REM sleep.

Using a different experimental protocol, Ikeda and Morotomi (125) applied a simple classical conditioning technique during NREM sleep using heart rate as a response measure. It was found that classical conditioning is possible during SWS, but not during stage 2 sleep. Moreover, it was found that the conditioning effect that took place during sleep could be transferred to wakefulness.

Performance Following Awakenings from Different Stages of Sleep

Another method consists of measuring performance after being awakened from different stages of sleep. This method is based on the hypothesis that the properties of the sleep stage preceding the awakening will carry over and influence the participant's immediate performance. This kind of protocol is different from those previously mentioned because performance is measured after nocturnal awakenings rather than during the day.

Some studies of this type have emerged from the finding that electroencephalographic activity seems to be more intense in the right hemisphere during REM sleep and more intense in the left hemisphere during NREM sleep (126). Results from such studies have indicated that performance on right hemisphere cognitive functions (i.e., spatial memory and form recognition) is facilitated after awakening from REM sleep, whereas performance on tasks involving cognitive functions of the left hemisphere (i.e., verbal memory task and word recognition) is facilitated by awakening from NREM sleep (81–83,127).

With the use of a semantic priming task (implicit memory), Stickgold et al. (84) showed in 1999 that participants awakened from REM sleep demonstrate greater priming effects with weakly associated words (e.g., thief-wrong) than with strongly associated words (e.g., hot-cold). The opposite is found when participants are awakened from NREM sleep. Authors concluded that a shift from NREM to REM sleep takes place in the associative memory system, which may explain the bizarre features incorporated in REM sleep dreaming. Moreover, authors suggested that "brain functioning may be altered during REM sleep to facilitate neurocognitive searches for novel interpretation of pre-existing information and could lead to the strengthening of newly identified associations within memory networks." A study by Wagner et al. (128) showed that implicit face memory is facilitated after awakening from REM sleep. These results constitute further support to the notion that the activity of the brain during the waking state is related to its activity during sleep.

Clinical Approach

The last protocol we will discuss concerns sleep disorders and the cognitive deficits related to them. Three main sleep disorders—insomnia, narcolepsy, and the obstructive sleep apnea syndrome (OSAS)—have been associated with clear and consistent cognitive deficits. Insomnia covers a broad range of complaints, including difficulty in initiating and maintaining sleep. The most common consequences are daytime sleepiness and decreased energy. Memory (explicit/declarative memory, working memory) and attention problems (alertness, sustained attention) have also been associated with insomnia, mainly related to excessive daytime sleepiness (EDS) and/or the sleep disturbance itself (87,129–131).

Narcolepsy is a disease of REM sleep, characterized by chronic sleepiness culminating into REM sleep attacks (the so-called sleep onset REM periods) and by attacks of cataplexy (loss of muscle tone without loss of consciousness). Among other symptoms, persons with narcolepsy report difficulties with concentration/attention (alertness and sustained attention), with memory (working memory and explicit/declarative memory), and, at times, with perception (85,132–135). It was shown, however, that memory impairments reported in narcolepsy are most probably due to nonspecific EDS and not to specific REM sleep processes (136).

Finally, OSAS results in hypoxemic episodes and fragmented sleep, causing EDS. The cognitive impairments most commonly associated with OSAS are lowered general intellectual functioning (IQ); decreased attention (alertness, selective attention, and sustained attention); and difficulties with memory (working memory, explicit/declarative memory), executive functions (planning, mental flexibility, abstract thinking, control of impulsivity), and motor performance (speed and precision) (86,137–143). It was found that attention and memory deficits of patients with OSAS are reversible upon treatment, whereas executive impairments are resistant and related to hypoxemia (144–146), suggesting a lasting effect of anoxia on neural networks involved in executive functions. These clinical observations add to the evidence indicating that sleep has an important role in maintaining cognitive daytime functioning in persons with mental health problems such as schizophrenia (147,148).

V. Conclusions

Many published reports suggest a relationship between sleep, or more particularly between specific stages of sleep, and waking performance. For example, attention processes seem to be influenced by sleep in general, whereas memory processes seem to be related to a particular stage of sleep, depending on the module tested. However, the exact nature of the relationship between the organization of sleep and specific cognitive functions still must be clarified as many unresolved questions remain (149–152). It remains unclear, for example, whether the complexity level of the task or its nature (i.e., emotional or neutral) is the determining factor (113,128). Some studies have shown that explicit/declarative memory tasks may be associated with sleep at times but not all of the time (70,109,110). This could be related to the fact that both slow and fast components are involved in the consolidation mechanisms of these two memory subsystems, which in turn could be related to neurophysiological mechanisms (3,153–155).

Some researchers have recently raised the possibility that it is not the amount of sleep that is important for daytime functioning but rather its quality (105,116,117,156). This is consistent with the study of Pilcher et al. (157) which indicated that the quality rather than the quantity of sleep was associated with a healthier physical and psychological state in young students. According to the *sleep continuity theory* (116,117), for example, periods of continuous sleep must exceed 10 min in order for sleep to have a role in the restoration of functions. Giuditta et al. (156) elaborated this concept and first proposed a *sequential hypothesis of sleep function,* followed by the suggestion that the succession and alternation of NREM and REM sleep through the night are likely crucial elements for daytime cognitive functioning (*dual-process hypothesis*) (92,105,118,156,158). According to this hypothesis, SWS and REM sleep are of equal importance in the processing of information during sleep. As a first step, SWS eliminates irrelevant memory traces and strengthens pertinent memory traces (the so-called discrimination process). During the second step, REM sleep consolidates memory traces in appropriate neuronal networks (the so-called consolidation process). Therefore, any disturbance in one of these two steps, or any disturbance in the natural SWS-REM sleep sequence, could significantly impair daytime cognitive performance.

Stickgold (154) in 2003 proposed a comparable model, suggesting that performance improvement or memory consolidation occurs in a three-step process. The first step occurs while the participant is training. The second and third steps occur during SWS and REM sleep, respectively. Interruption or disruption of one of these three steps results in a significant impairment in cognitive performance. Indeed, using a visual texture discrimination task (procedural memory), Stickgold et al. (105) found that participants' performance is directly related to the amount of SWS in the first part of the night and to the amount of REM sleep in the last part of the night. This suggests that both SWS and REM sleep are required to optimize performance on such tasks. Gais et al. (92) have also shown that SWS is associated with texture skill discrimination (procedural memory task) but that performance is even better after a complete night of sleep. In this case, it is suggested that REM sleep could also be involved in memory formation, but only after a first stage of information processing has occurred. The study by Ficca et al. (118) also supports the notion that sleep cycles or the sequence of sleep stages is important for explicit/declarative memory, rather than just a specific stage of sleep or the amount of sleep. Their results indicate that sleep fragmentation with sleep cycle disruption impairs performance, whereas sleep fragmentation without sleep cycle disruption does not impair performance.

Although the roles of several processes in relation to memory and attention have been examined in this chapter, many other dimensions have escaped a thorough scientific examination. For example, more discussion is needed concerning the role of circadian and homeostatic processes (see Chap. 24). Results from the few studies that have examined this issue tend to show that there is a circadian and homeostatic influence on cognitive performance (92,159–161). Another aspect is that of development: *what is the impact of sleep loss on performance of young vs. older participants? What are the neurophysiological determinants of impaired performance in chronically sleep-deprived adolescent, middle-aged, and elderly individuals?* These questions remain well unexplored and further research will hopefully shed more light for all to share.

References

1. Aserinsky, E., Kleitman, N. (1953). Regularly occurring periods of eye motility, and concomitant phenomena, during sleep. Science 118, 273–274.
2. Kryger MH, Roth T, Dement WC. Principles and Practice of Sleep Medicine. Philadelphia: WB Saunders, 2000.
3. Maquet P, Smith C, Stickgold R. Sleep and Brain Plasticity. New York: Oxford University Press, 2003.
4. Steriade M, McCarley RW. Brainstem Control of Wakefulness and Sleep. New York: Plenum Press, 1990.
5. Rechtschaffen A, Kales A. A Manual of Standardized Terminology, Techniques and Scoring System for Sleep Stages of Human Subjects. Los Angeles: BIS/BRI, University of California at Los Angeles, 1968.
6. Ogilvie RD, Harsh JR, eds. Sleep Onset: Normal and Abnormal Processes. Washington, DC: American Psychological Association, 1994.
7. Cajochen C, Krauchi K, Wirz-Justice A. The acute soporific action of daytime melatonin administration: effects on the EEG during wakefulness and subjective alertness. J Biol Rhythms 1997; 12:636–643.
8. Lafrance C, Dumont M. Diurnal variations in the waking EEG: comparisons with sleep latencies and subjective alertness. J Sleep Res 2000; 9:243–248.
9. Jankel WR, Niedermeyer E. Sleep spindles. J Clin Neurophysiol 1985; 2:1-35.

10. Zeitlhofer J, Gruber G, Anderer P, Asenbaum S, Schimicek P, Saletu B. Topographic distribution of sleep spindles in young healthy subjects. J Sleep Res 1997; 6:149–155.

11. McCormick DA, Bal T. Sleep and arousal: thalamocortical mechanisms. Annu Rev Neurosci 1997; 20:185–215.

12. Steriade M, McCormick DA, Sejnowski TJ. Thalamocortical oscillations in the sleeping and aroused brain. Science 1993; 262:679–685.

13. Steriade M. Brain activation, then (1949) and now: coherent fast rhythms in corticothalamic networks. Arch Ital Biol 1995; 134:5–20.

14. Maquet P, Dive D, Salmon E, Sadzot B, Franco G, Poirrier R, Franck G. Cerebral glucose utilization during stage 2 sleep in man. Brain Res 1992; 571:149–153.

15. Naitoh P, Antony-Baas V, Muset A, Ehrhart J. Dynamic relation of sleep spindles and K-complexes to spontaneous phasic arousals in sleeping human subjects. Sleep 1981; 5:58–62.

16. Bové A, Culebras A, Moore JT, Westlake RE. Relationship between sleep spindles and hypersomnia. Sleep 1994; 17:449–455.

17. Numminen J, Makela JP, Hari R. Distributions and sources of magnetoencephalographic K-complexes. Electroencephalogr Clin Neurophysiol 1996; 99:544–555.

18. Sallinen M, Kaartinen J, Lyytinen H. Precursors of the evoked K-complex in event-related brain potentials in stage 2 sleep. Electroencephalogr Clin Neurophysiol 1997; 102:363–373.

19. Terzano MG, Parrinon L, Mennuni GF. Phasic events and microstructure of sleep. In: Terzano MG, Parrino L, Mennuni GF, eds. Associazione Italiana Di Medicina Del Sonno (AIMS), Lecce (Italia): Martano Editore, 1997:57–106.

20. Bastien CH, Ladouceur C, Campbell KB. EEG characteristics prior to and following the evoked K-complex. Can J Exp Psychol 2000; *54*:255–265.

21. Nicholas CL, Trinder J, Colrain IM. Increased production of evoked and spontaneous K-complexes following a night of fragmented sleep. Sleep 2002; 25:882–887.

22. Peszka J, Harsh J. Effect of sleep deprivation on NREM sleep ERPs and related activity at sleep onset. Int J Psychophysiol 2002; 46:275–286.

23. Aeschbach D, Matthews JR, Postolache TT, Jackson MA, Giesen HA, Wehr TA. Dynamics of the human EEG during prolonged wakefulness: evidence for frequency-specific circadian and homeostatic influences. Neurosci Lett 1997; 19:121-124.

24. Dijk DJ, Hayes B, Czeisler CA. Dynamics of electroencephalographic sleep spindles and slow wave activity in men: effect of sleep deprivation. Brain Res 1993; 29:190–199.

25. Cajochen C, Foy R, Dijk DJ. Frontal predominance of a relative increase in sleep delta and theta EEG activity after sleep loss in humans. Sleep Res Online 1999; 2:65–69.

26. De Gennaro L, Ferrara M, Bertini M. Effect of slow-wave sleep deprivation on topographical distribution of spindles. Behav Brain Res 2000; 116:55–59.

27. Merica H, Blois R. Relationship between the time courses of power in the frequency bands of human sleep EEG. Neurophysiol Clinique/Clin Neurophysiol 1997; 27:116–128.

28. Born J, Muth S, Fehm HL. The significance of sleep onset and slow wave sleep for nocturnal release of growth hormone (GH) and cortisol. Psychoneuroendocrinology 1988; 13:233–243.

29. McGinty DJ, Drucker-Colin RR. Sleep mechanisms: biology and control of REM sleep. Int Rev Neurobiol 1982; 23:391-436.

30. Idzikowski C, Oswald I. Interference with human memory by an antibiotic. Psychopharmacology 1983; 79:108–110.
31. Ramm P, Smith CT. Rates of cerebral protein synthesis are linked to slow wave sleep in the rat. Physiol Beh 1990; 48:749–753.
32. Berger RJ. Slow wave sleep, shallow torpor and hibernation: Homologous states of diminished metabolism and body temperature. Biol Psychol 1984; 10:305–326.
33. Berger RJ, Phillips NH. Energy conservation and sleep. Behav Brain Res 1995; 69:65–73.
34. Irwin M. Effects of sleep and sleep loss on immunity and cytokines. Brain, Behav Immun 2002; 16:503–512.
35. Krueger JM, Obal FJ, Fang J, Kubota T, Taishi P. The role of cytokines in physiological sleep regulation. Ann NY Acad Sci 2001; 933:211-221.
36. Maquet P. Sleep function and cerebral metabolism. Behav Brain Res 1995; 69:75–83.
37. Endo T, Schwierin B, Borbely AA, Tobler I. Selective and total sleep deprivation. Effect on the sleep EEG in the rat. Psychiatry Res 1997; 66:97–110.
38. Horne J. Why We Sleep: The Functions of Sleep in Humans and Other Mammals. Oxford: Oxford University Press, 1988.
39. Roffwarg HP, Muzio JN, Dement WC. Ontogenic development of human sleep-dream cycle. Science 1966; 152:604–619.
40. Berger RJ. Oculomotor control: a possible function of REM sleep. Psychol Rev 1969; 76:144–64.
41. Jouvet M. The function of dreaming: a neurophysiologists point of view. In: Gazzaniga MS, Blackmore C, eds. Handbook of Psychobiology. New York: Academic Press, 1975.
42. Hobson A, McCarley RW. The brain as a dream state generator: an activation-synthesis hypothesis of the dream process. Am J Psychiatry 1977; 134:1335–1348.
43. Carskadon MA, Dement WC, Mitler MM, Roth T, Westbrook PR, Keenan S. Guidelines for the multiple sleep latency test (MSLT): a standard measure of sleepiness. Sleep 1986; 9:519–524.
44. Mitler MM, Gujavarty KS, Browman CP. Maintenance of wakefulness test: a polysomnographic technique for evaluating treatment efficacy in patients with excessive somnolence. Electroencephalogr Clin Neurophysiol 1982; 53:658–661.
45. Baddeley AD, Hitch GJ. Working memory. In: Bower A, ed. The Psychology of Learning and Motivation. Vol. 8. New York: Academic Press, 1974.
46. Squire LR. Memory and Brain. New York: Oxford University Press, 1987.
47. Clark CR, Egan GF, McEarlane AC, Morris P, Weber D, Sonkkilla C, Marcina J, Tochon-Danguy HJ. Updating working memory for words: a PET activation study. Hum Brain Mapping 2000; 9:42–54.
48. Collette F, Salmon E, Van der Linden M, Chicherio C, Belleville S, Degueldre C, Delfiore G, Franck G. Regional brain activity during tasks devoted to the central executive of working memory. Brain research. Cogn Brain Res 1999; 7:411-417.
49. Klingberg T, O'Sullivan BT, Roland PE. Bilateral activation of fronto-parietal networks by incrementing demand in a working memory task. Cerebral Cortex 1997; 7:465–471.
50. Thomas J, Laplante L, Everett J. Schizophrénie et attention sélective. L'Encéphale 1989; 15:7–12.
51. Baddeley A. Working memory: the interface between memory and cognition. In: Schacter, Tulving, eds. Memory Systems. Cambridge MA: MIT Press, 1994.

52. Gabrieli JDE. Cognitive neuroscience of human memory. Annu Rev Psychol 1998; 49:87–115.
53. Squire LR, Zola M. Structure and function of declarative and nondeclarative memory systems. Proc Nat Acad Sci USA 1996; 93:13515–13522.
54. Moscovitch M. Memory and working with memory: evaluation of a component process model and comparisons with other models. In: Schacter, Tulving, eds. Memory Systems. Cambridge, MA: MIT Press, 1994.
55. Butters MA, Kaszniak AW, Glisky EL, Eslinger PJ, Schacter DL. Recency discrimination deficits in frontal lobe patients. Neuropsychology 1994; 8:343–353.
56. Hirosaka O. Role of the basal ganglia in motor learning: a hypothesis. In: Ono T, Squire L.R., eds. Brain Mechanisms of Perception and Memory: From Neuron to Behavior. New York: Oxford University Press, 1993.
57. Moscovitch M. Memory and working-memory: a component process model based on modules and central systems. J Cogn Neurosci 1992; 4:257–267.
58. Saint-Cyr JA, Taylor AE. The mobilization of procedural learning: The "key signature" of the basal ganglia. In: Squire LR, Butters N, eds. Neuropsychology of Memory. New York: Guilford Press, 1992.
59. Saint-Cyr JA, Taylor AE, Lang AE. Procedural learning and neostriatal dysfunction in man. Brain 1988; 111:941-959.
60. Gabrieli JDE, Desmond JE, Demb JB, Wagner AD, et al. Functional magnetic resonance imaging of semantic memory process in the frontal lobes. Psychol Sci 1996; 7:278–283.
61. Janowski JS, Shimura AP, Squire LR. Source memory impairment in patients with frontal lobes lesions. Neuropsychologia 1989; 27:1043–56.
62. Shallice T, Fletcher P, Frith CD, Grasby D, et al. Brain regions associates with acquisition and retrieval of verbal episodic memory. Nature 1994; 368:633–635.
63. Posner MI, Peterson SE. The attention system of the human brain. Annu Rev Neurosci 1990; 13:25–42.
64. Treisman A, Sato S. Conjunction search revisited. J Exp Psychol Hum Percep Perform 1990; 16:459–478.
65. Doran SM, Van Dongen HPA, Dinges DF. Sustained attention performance during sleep deprivation: evidence of state instability. Arch Italiennes Biol Neurosci 2001; 139:253–267.
66. Posner MI, Dehaene S. Attentional networks. Trends Neurosci 1994; 17:75–79.
67. De Koninck J, Lorrain JP, Christ G, Proulx G, Coulombe D. Intensive language learning and increases in REM sleep: evidence for a performance factor. Int J Psychophysiol 1989; 8:33–47.
68. De Konick J, Christ G, Hébert G, Rinfret N. Language learning efficiency, dreams and REM sleep. Psychiatr J Univ Ottawa 1990; 15:91-92.
69. Mandai O, Guerrien A, Sockeel P, Dujardin K, Leconte P. REM sleep modifications following a Morse code learning sessions in humans. Physiol Behav 1989; 46:639–642.
70. Smith C. Sleep states and memory processes. Behav Brain Res 1995; 69:137–145.
71. Blagrove M, Alexander C, Horne JA. The effects of chronic sleep reduction on the performance of cognitive tasks sensitive to sleep deprivation. Appl Cogn Psychol 1995; 9:21-40.
72. Deaton M, Tobias JS, Wilkinson RT. The effect of sleep deprivation on signal detection parameters. Q J Exp Psychol 1971; 23:449–452.

73. Horne JA. Sleep loss and divergent thinking ability. Sleep 1988; 11:528–536.
74. Martin SE, Engleman HM, Deary IJ, Douglas NJ. The effect of sleep fragmentation on daytime function. Am J Respir Cri Care Med 1996; 153:1328–32.
75. Norton R. The effect of acute sleep deprivation on selective attention. Br J Psychol 1970; 61:157–161.
76. Roehrs T, Merlotti L, Petrolucci N, Stepanski E, Roth T. Experimental sleep fragmentation. Sleep 1994; 17:438–443.
77. Smith A, Maben A. Effects of sleep deprivation, lunch, and personality on performance, mood, and cardiovascular function. Physiol Behav 1993; 54:967–972.
78. Smith C, MacNeill C. Impaired motor memory for a pursuit rotor task following stage 2 sleep loss in college students. Sleep Res 1994; 3:206–213.
79. Walsh JK, Hartman PG, Scheitzer PK. Slow-wave sleep deprivation and waking function. J Sleep Res 1994; 3:16–25.
80. Webb WB, Agnew HW. The effects of a chronic limitation of sleep length. Psychophysiology 1974; 11:265–274.
81. Casagrande M, Bertini M, Tests P. Changes in cognitive asymmetries from waking to REM and non-REM sleep. Brain Cogn 1995; 29:180–186.
82. Lavie P, Matanya Y, Yehuda S. Cognitive asymmetries after waking from REM and non-REM sleep in right-handed females. Int J Neurosci 1984; 23:111-116.
83. Reinsel RA, Antrobus JS. Lateralized task performance after awakening from sleep. In: Antrobus JS, Bertini M, eds. The Neuropsychology of Sleep and Dreaming. Hillsdale, NJ: Lawrence Erlbaum, 1992.
84. Stickgold R, Scott L, Rittenhouse C, Hobson JA. Sleep-induced changes in associative memory. J Cogn Neurosci 1999; 11:182–193.
85. Broughton R, Ghanem Q, Hishikawa Y, Sugita Y, Nevsimalova S, Roth B. Life effects of narcolepsy in 180 patients from North America, Asia and Europe compared to matched controls. Can J Neurol Sci 1981; 8:299–304.
86. Décary A, Rouleau I, Montplaisir J. Cognitive deficits associated with sleep apnea syndrome: a proposed neuropsychological test battery. Sleep 2000; 23:369–381.
87. Mendelson WB, Garnett D, Gillin JC, Weingartner H. The experience of insomnia and daytime and nighttime functioning. Psychiatry Res 1984; 12:235–250.
88. Spreux F, Lambert C, Chevalier B, Meriaux H, Freixa I, Baque E, Grubar JC, Lancry A, Leconte P. Modification des caractéristiques du SP consécutif à un apprentissage chez l'homme. Cahier Psychol Cogn 1982; 2:327–334.
89. Smith C, Lapp L. Increases in number of REMs and REM density in humans following an intensive learning period. Sleep 1991; 14:325–330.
90. De Koninck J, Prévost F. Le sommeil paradoxal et le traitement de l'information: Une exploration par l'inversion du champ visuel. Rev Canadienne Psychol 1991; 45:125–139.
91. De Genaro L, Violani C, Ferrara M, Casagrande M, Bertini M. Increase of REM duration and decrease of REM latency after a prolonged test of visual attention. Int J Neurosci 1995; 82:163–168.
92. Gais S, Molle M, Helm K, Born J. Learning-dependent increases in sleep spindle density. J Neurosci 2002; 22:6830–6834.
93. Meier-Koll A, Bussmann B, Schmidt C, Neuschwander D. Walking through a maze alters the architecture of sleep. Percept Mot Skills 1999; 88:1141-1159.
94. Fogel S, Jacob J, Smith C. Increased sleep spindle activity following simple motor procedural learning in humans. Actas Fisiologia 2001; 7:123.

95. Nader RS, Smith C. The relationship between stage 2 sleep spindles and intelligence. Sleep 2001; 24(suppl.):A160.

96. Walker MP, Brakefield T, Morgan A, Hobson JA, Stickgold R. Practice with sleep makes perfect: sleep dependent motor skill learning. Neurons 2002; 35:205–211.

97. Brière ME, Forest G, Lussier I, Godbout R. Implicit verbal recall correlates positively with EEG sleep spindle activity. Sleep 2000; 23 (suppl. 2):A219.

98. Forest G, Godbout R, Riopel L, Lussier I, Stip E. Selective attention correlates with stage 2 and sleep spindle EEG activity in normal young subjects. Soc Neurosci Abs 1997; 23:1848.

99. Aubrey JB, Armstrong B, Arkin A, Smith CT, Rose G. Total sleep deprivation affects memory for a previously learned route. Sleep 1999; 22:401.

100. Blagrove M, Cole-Morgan D, Lambe H. Interrogative suggestibility: the effect of sleep deprivation and relationship with field dependence. App Cogn Psychol 1994; 8:169–179.

101. Idzikowski C. Sleep and memory. Br J Psychol 1984; 75:439–449.

102. Polzella DJ. Effects of sleep deprivation on short-term recognition memory. J Exp Psychol 1975; 104:194–200.

103. Drummond PA, Brown GG, Wong EC, Gillin JC. Sleep deprivation-induced reduction in cortical functional response to serial subtraction. Neuro report 1999; 10:3745–3748.

104. Heuer H, Klein W. One night of total sleep deprivation impairs implicit learning in the serial reaction task, but not the behavioral expression of knowledge. Neuropsychology 2003; 17:507–516.

105. Stickgold R, James LT, Hobson JA. Visual discrimination learning requires sleep after training. Nat Neurosci 2000; 3:1237–1238.

106. Fisher S. The microstructure of dual-task interaction: sleep deprivation and the control of attention. Perception 1980; 9:327–337.

107. Linde L, Bergstrom M. The effect of one night without sleep on problem-solving and immediate recall. Psychol Res 1992; 54:127–136.

108. Beaulieu I, Godbout R. Spatial learning on the Morris water test after a short-term paradoxical sleep deprivation in the rat. Brain Cogn 2000; 40:27–31.

109. Plihal W, Born J. Effect of early and late nocturnal sleep on declarative and procedural memory. J Cogn Neurosci 1997; 9:534–547.

110. Plihal W, Born J. Effects of early and late nocturnal sleep on priming and spatial memory. Psychophysiology 1999; 36:571-582.

111. Yaroush R, Sullivan MJ, Ekstrand BR. Effects of sleep on memory. II. Differential effect of the first second half of the night. J Exp Psychol 1971; 88:361-366.

112. Wagner U, Gais S, Born J. Emotional memory formation is enhanced across sleep intervals with high amount of rapid eye movement sleep. Learning Memory 2001; 8:112–119.

113. Fosse R. REM sleep: a window into altered emotional functioning. Sleep 2001; 24 (suppl.):179.

114. Herscovitch J, Broughton R. Performance deficits following short-term partial sleep deprivation and subsequent recovery oversleeping. Can J Psychol 1981; 35:309–322.

115. Dinges DF, Pack F, Williams K, Gillen KA, Powell JW, Ott GE, Aptowicz C, Pack Al. Cumulative sleepiness, mood disturbance, and psychomotor vigilance performance decrements during a week of sleep restricted to 4–5 hours per night. Sleep 1997; 20:267–277.

116. Bonnet MH. Performance and sleepiness as a function of frequency and placement of sleep disruption. Psychophysiology 1986; 23:263–271.

117. Bonnet MH. Performance and sleepiness following moderate sleep disruption and slow wave sleep deprivation. Physiol Behav 1986; 37:915–918.

118. Ficca G, Lombardo P, Rossi L, Salzarulo P. Morning recall on verbal material depends on prior sleep organisation. Behav Brain Res 2000; 112:159–163.

119. Smith C, Fazekas A. Amounts of REM sleep and stage 2 required for efficient learning. Sleep Res 1997; 26:690.

120. Gillberg M, Akerstedt T. Sleep restriction and SWS-suppression: effects on daytime alertness and night-time recovery. J Sleep Res 1994; 3:144–151.

121. Stickgold R, Whidbee D, Schirmer B, Patel V, Hobson JA. Visual discrimination task improvement: a multi-step process occurring during sleep. J Cogn Neurosci 2000; 12:246–254.

122. Tilley AJ. Sleep learning during stage 2 and REM sleep. Biol Psychol 1979; 9:155–161.

123. Guerrien A, Dujardin K, Madai O, Sockeel P, Leconte P. Enhancement of memory by auditory stimulation during post-learning REM sleep in humans. Physiol Behav 1989; 45:947–950.

124. Smith C, Weeden K. Post training REMs coincident auditory stimulation enhances memory in humans. Psychiatri J Univ Ottawa 1990; 15:85–90.

125. Ikeda K, Morotomi T. Classical conditioning during human NREM sleep and response transfer to wakefulness. Sleep 1996; 19:72–74.

126. Goldstein L, Stoltzfus NM, Gardocki JF. Changes in interhemispheric amplitude relationships in the EEG during sleep. Physiol Behav 1972; 8:811-815.

127. Bertini M, Violani C. Cerebral hemispheres, REM sleep and dream recall. Res Commun Psychol Psychiatry Behav 1984; 9:3–13.

128. Wagner U, Fisher S, Born J. Changes in emotional responses to aversive pictures across periods rich in slow wave sleep vs rapid eye movement sleep. Psychosom Med 2002; 64:627–634.

129. Hauri PJ. Cognitive deficits in insomnia patients. Acta Neurol Belg 1997; 97:113–117.

130. Jennum PJ, Sjol A. Cognitive symptoms in persons with snoring and sleep apnea. An epidemiologic study of 1504 women and men aged 30–60 years. The Dan-MONICA II study. Ugeskrift Laeger 1995; 157:6252–6256.

131. Vignola A, Lamoureux C, Bastien CH, Morin CM. Effects of chronic insomnia and use of benzodiazepines on daytime performance in older adults. J Gerontol B Psychol Sci Soc Sci 2000; 55:P54–P62.

132. Bassetti C, Aldrich MS. Narcolepsy. Neurol Clin 1996; 3:545–571.

133. Broughton R, Ghanem Q. The impact of compound narcolepsy on the life of the patient. In: Guilleminault C, Dement WC, Passouant P, eds. Narcolepsy. New York: Spectrum, 1976.

134. Chaudhary BA, Husain I. Narcolepsy. J Fam Pract 1993; 36:207–213.

135. Rogers AE, Rosenberg RS. Tests of memory in narcoleptics. Sleep 1990; 13:42–52.

136. Aguirre M, Broughton R, Stuss D. Does memory impairment exist in narcolepsy-cataplexy? J Clin Exp Neuropsychol 1985; 7:14–24.

137. Bedard MA, Montplaisir J, Richer F, Rouleau I, Malo J. Obstructive sleep apnea syndrome: pathogenesis of neuropsychological deficits. J Clin Exp Neuropsychol 1991; 1:950–64.

138. Berry DTR, Webb WB, Block AJ, Bauer RM, Switzer DA. Nocturnal hypoxemia and neuropsychological variables. J Clin Exp Neuropsychol 1986; 8:229–238.
139. Bliwise DL. Sleep apnea and cognitive function: where do we stand now? Sleep 1993; 16:S72–S73.
140. Naëgelé B, Thouvard V, Pépin J-L, Lévy P, Bonnet C, Perret JE, Pellat J, Feuerstein C. Deficits of cognitive functions in patients with sleep apnea syndrome. J Am Sleep Dis Assoc Sleep Res Soc 1995; 18:43–52.
141. Rouleau I, Décary A, Chicoine AJ, Montplaisir J. Procedural skill learning in obstructive sleep apnea syndrome. Sleep 2002; 25:401-411.
142. Salorio CF, White DA, Piccirillo J, Duntley SP, Uhles ML. Learning, memory, and executive control in individuals with obstructive sleep apnea syndrome. J Clin Exp Neuropsychol 2002; 24:93–100.
143. Sloan K, Craft S, Walsh JK. Neurospychological function in obstructive sleep apnea with and without hypoxemia. Sleep Res 1989; 18:304.
144. Bédard MA, Montplaisir J, Malo J, Richer F, Rouleau I. Persistent neuropsychological deficits and vigilance impairment in sleep apnea syndrome after treatment with continuous positive airways pressure (CPAP). J Clin Exp Neuropsychol 1993; 15:330–341.
145. Dahlof P, Norlin-Bagge E, Hedner J, Ejnell H, Hetta J, Hallstrom T. Improvement in neuropsychological performance following surgical treatment for obstructive sleep apnea syndrome. Acta Oto-Laryngologica 2002; 122:86–91.
146. Ferini-Strambi L, Baietto C, Di Gioia MR, Castaldi P, Castronovo C, Zucconi M, Cappa SF. Cognitive dysfunction in patients with obstructive sleep apnea (OSA): partial reversibility after continuous positive airway pressure (CPAP). Brain Res Bull 2003; 61:87–92.
147. Poulin J, Daoust AM, Forest G, Stip E, Godbout R. Sleep architecture and its clinical correlates in first episode and neuroleptic-naive patients with schizophrenia. Schizophrenia Res 2003; 62:147–153.
148. Taylor SF, Goldman RS, Tandon R, Shipley JE. Neuropsychological function and REM sleep in schizophrenic patients. Biol Psychiatry 1992; 32:529–538.
149. Blissitt PA. Sleep, memory, and learning. J Neurosci Nursing 2001; 33:208–215.
150. Maquet P. The role of sleep in learning and memory. Science 2001; 294:1048–1052.
151. Siegel JM. The REM sleep-memory consolidation hypothesis. Science 2001; 294:1058–1063.
152. Vertes RP, Eastman KE. The case against memory consolidation in REM sleep. Behav Brain Sci 2000; 23:867–876.
153. Walker MP, Brakefield T, Seidman J, Morgan A, Hobson JA, Stickgold R. Sleep and the time course of motor skill learning. Learning Memory 2003; 10:275–284.
154. Stickgold R. Memory, cognition, and dreams. In: Maquet P, Smith C, Stickgold R, eds. Sleep and Brain Plasticity. New York: Oxford University Press, 2003.
155. Drummond SP, Brown GG, Gillin JC, Stricker JL, Wong EC, Buxton RB. Altered brain response to verbal learning following sleep deprivation. Nature 2000; 403:655–657.
156. Giuditta A, Ambrosi MV, Montagnese P, Mandile P, Cotugno M, Zucconi CG, Vescia S. The sequential hypothesis of the function of sleep. Behav Brain Res 1995; 69:157–166.

157. Pilcher JJ, Ginter DR, Sadowsky B. Sleep quality versus sleep quantity: Relationships between sleep and measure of health, well-being and sleepiness in college student. J Psychol Res 1997; 42:583–586.
158. Peigneux P, Laureys S, Delbeuck X, Maquet P. Sleeping brain, learning brain. The role of sleep and memory systems. Neuroreport 2001; 12:111-124.
159. Carrier J, Monk TH. Circadian rhythms of performance: new trends. Chronobiol Int 2000; 17:719–732.
160. Koulack D. Recognition memory, circadian rhythms and sleep. Percept Mot Skills 1997; 85:99–104.
161. Van Dongen HPA, Dinges DF. Circadian rhythms in fatigue, alertness and performance. In: Kryger MH, Roth T, Dement WC, eds. Principles and Practice of Sleep Medicine. Philadelphia: WB Saunders, 2000:391-399.

12

Cortical and Electroencephalographic Changes

LUCA A. FINELLI

The Salk Institute, La Jolla, California, U.S.A.

I. Introduction

Sleep is a regulated process whose timing, duration, and intensity depend on the prior sleep-wake history (1). Sleep deprivation refers equally to the restriction of sleep or the extension of wakefulness beyond the habitual time span. Sleep propensity, i.e., the need or inclination to initiate and maintain sleep, becomes uncontrollable when sleep deprivation is extensively protracted, even under relaxed conditions. It is accepted that sleep has a restorative function that cannot be substituted simply by resting. Indeed, muscles and most organs can get the same amount of rest in relaxed wakefulness as in sleep [reviewed in (2)]. But for the brain, relaxed wakefulness is not sufficient to substitute for sleep, as revealed by the specific and dramatic effects of sleep deprivation on human neurobehavioral functions (3–7).

What are the neural correlates of these effects? What is altered from normal levels if sleep is restricted? What underlies the emergence of a single perceptual feeling of sleepiness? Is it possible to identify macroscopic continuous correlates to the changes occurring with the progression of waking? One way to approach these questions is to investigate how brain activity changes at different levels of arousal, including sleep. Nowadays several technological innovations have begun to revolutionize our notion of the neural basis of behavior, both in waking and in sleep. These include advances in quantitative methods in electrophysiology and the advent of functional neuroimaging. To this purpose it is convenient to define brain activity by means of spatial and temporal measures of its electrophysiological and metabolic correlates. This chapter provides an overview of neuropsychological, neurophysiological, and neuroimaging studies that focused on these and related questions, and discusses resulting implications as well as additional issues to be addressed.

Sleep and waking are unambiguously defined by typical changes in the pattern of the electroencephalogram (EEG), the most sensitive and widely used state indicator. Yet the sensitivity of the EEG goes beyond the simple distinction of the two vigilance states. Thus, in sleep, the EEG may be used as a physiological indicator (marker) of sleep homeostasis, structure, and intensity. In waking, widespread changes in brain dynamics are reflected in the spectral composition of the spontaneous EEG. If wakefulness is prolonged outside of the habitual boundaries, such changes get significantly intensified. Over the past 15 years, progress has been made in characterizing the electrophysiological correlates of circadian and homeostatic processes involved in the regulation of alertness, sleep propensity, and neurobehavioral performance. Complementary to sleep data, waking data should be carefully considered as they may help to understand the essence of sleepiness and the causes of impaired functioning following sleep deprivation. This chapter reviews changes in brain dynamics as reflected in the EEG during normal and prolonged wakefulness (sleep loss), and then relates them to the changes that characterize sleep and recovery sleep after deprivation. The study of brain rhythms as revealed by the EEG might help elucidate their possible significance for the large-scale organization of brain function.

With the advent of functional neuroimaging, in particular positron emission tomography (PET) and functional magnetic resonance imaging (fMRI), an exceptional portrayal of the spatiotemporal configuration of neuronal activity in the brain can now be reached. These modern and technically challenging approaches display both brain structure and aspects of brain function with millimeter resolution, thereby localizing which areas of the brain are more active or less active during assigned tasks or spontaneous behaviors. The methods do not display neuronal activity but rather changes in glucose metabolism, blood flow, and oxygenation that are thought to be colocalized with fluctuations in neuronal activity. This chapter reviews those imaging studies that used PET or fMRI in combination with sleep deprivation protocols to examine how prolonged wakefulness affects cerebral response across the whole brain during task performance.

II. Basic Electrophysiology of the Waking State

A. Neural Correlates of Wakefulness

Wakefulness is commonly perceived as our default operating state, and we generally appreciate there is something beyond it only when sleepiness emerges or sleep prevails.

The neural correlates of electroencephalographic activation during wakefulness find their primary origin in the brainstem. Some of its nuclei seem to be essential for maintaining normal states of vigilance, as lesions of this deep brain structure may cause coma (8). Pioneering work demonstrated that arousal and its corresponding electroencephalographic patterns can be mimicked by electrically stimulating the mesencephalic reticular formation (MRF) (9,10). These and other observations led to the concept of an ascending reticular activating system that projects via synaptic relays in the thalamus to the cerebral cortex [reviewed in (11)]. Accordingly, neurons in the MRF exert their action on neurons in the thalamus by increasing excitability. This is accomplished by keeping the membrane potential in a state of relative depolarization. As a result, rhythmic burst firing is inhibited, and activated neurons in the thalamus and cortex exhibit tonic single-spike activity typical of the waking state. In addition, the appearance of high-frequency oscillations is promoted, together with a state that is favorable to sensory information processing and eventually cognition (12–16). Thus, in this state the thalamus is the main gateway to the cortex for sensory information (e.g., retinal input through the lateral geniculate nucleus to the visual cortex) (17). In summary, electrophysiology portrays wakefulness as a specific functional state in terms of global modulations of the thalamocortical system.

Although most of the supporting evidence for the activating system mechanisms comes from animal experiments, a human PET study demonstrated that the MRF and intralaminar nuclei are coactivated and tonically engaged in maintaining a state of high vigilance during attentional processing (18).

Furthermore, animal data strengthen the notion that the reticular activating system not only promotes arousal but enhances oscillations in the gamma range (30–40 Hz) (19, 20) and facilitates synchronization of such fast rhythms among spatially separated pools of cortical neurons in response to visual stimuli (21). Synchronization of cortical responses may have an important role in response selection and processing of sensory information (22). As a matter of fact, multiple ascending activating systems have been described in the brainstem, posterior hypothalamus, and basal forebrain. Namely, the posterior hypothalamus and basal forebrain are also innervated by the brainstem reticular formation, and in turn these centers project to and activate the cerebral cortex in a long-lasting and widespread manner [reviewed in (23,24)].

Evidence exists for a descending activating system from the cortex to the thalamus. Synapses from corticothalamic neurons have access to the same K^+ channels that are under ascending control; therefore, they can potentially control the excitability of thalamic neurons. Thus, the control of arousal may not be limited to ascending systems but may also have a cortical component (25).

What are the macroscopic correlates of these neural mechanisms? How do they get modulated by the progression of time awake? The occurrence of local field potential and macroscopic oscillations has been correlated with sensory processing in animals (26–29) along with behavioral and cognitive states in humans (13,30,31). The biophysical and network mechanisms underlying oscillatory activity in neurons have been well characterized [for a review focused on sleep oscillations, see (32)]. Nevertheless, the relationship between the microscopic attributes and global activity of large assemblies of neurons, as revealed by the EEG, remains elusive. A better characterization of the dynamics of EEG oscillations across the sleep-wake cycle might help to establish such a link.

B. Electroencephalographic Activity During Wakefulness

Electroencephalographic data reflect integrated activity from large numbers of cells in distinct regions of the brain. The normal spontaneous human EEG during wakefulness displays a fairly wide frequency spectrum. The range that may be considered important from a psychophysiological point of view lies between 0.1 Hz and 100 Hz. Yet this broad band is not simply a jumble of frequencies. A variety of brain rhythms (identified as oscillatory waveforms of comparable shape and extent recurring regularly) can be detected in the waking EEG, and corresponding frequency bands have been defined and labeled using letters of the Greek alphabet to describe them: *theta* 4–8, *alpha* 8–13, *beta* 13–30, *gamma* >30 Hz.

The boundaries of these bands have been standardized (33), but authors tend to modify them slightly depending on the purpose of their work. As will be discussed throughout this chapter, the frequency content of the waking EEG is not constant, and the changes in brain dynamics accompanying differing levels of arousal and vigilance result in changes in relative intensity of activity in the numerous bands.

Alpha Rhythm

Alpha rhythms surface as transient oscillations in the corresponding frequency range [8–13 Hz (33)]. The classical alpha rhythm is a spontaneous oscillation mainly localized over posterior regions, maximal over occipital areas, and predominant when the eyes are closed in a state of relaxed wakefulness. The EEG exhibits an exquisite sensitivity to changes in mental effort. Thus, the alpha rhythm is attenuated or suppressed by elevated attention and mental activity (e.g., mental arithmetic), as was already observed by Hans Berger (34), the discoverer and pioneer of human electroencephalography. This relationship suggested the interpretation that the alpha rhythm may represent a form of cortical idling [e.g., (35)]. A large number of models and theories for the generation of the alpha rhythm have been proposed [eg., (36–38); see also (39) for interesting open peer annotations]. There is evidence that the generation of cortical alpha rhythms depends on the interaction of thalamocortical and corticocortical components (40).

Mu Rhythm

Frequency-wise indistinguishable from the posterior alpha, the rolandic *mu* (for *mo*tor) rhythm denotes oscillations most prominent on and physiologically related to the sensorimotor cortex (41). Therefore, this oscillation has a different topography over the scalp. In analogy with the suppression of alpha by attention, the mu rhythm is blocked by movement or movement planning (41,42).

Theta Rhythm

The theta range comprises frequencies that seem to be related to many different aspects of brain functioning. In contrast to the alpha rhythm, the theta rhythm cannot be simply elicited by eye closure and generally appears in a less organized fashion than the alpha rhythm. What is more, the theta rhythm is not reduced by mental activity. Rather, rhythmic frontal midline theta activity around 6 and 7 Hz has been associated with performance of a mental task (43). During performance of working memory engaging tasks, the frontal midline theta rhythm increased in magnitude with increased memory load and task difficulty (44) and was sustained during the retention period (45). In addition, a significant enhancement in coherence in the theta range (4–7 Hz) was found between prefrontal and posterior electrodes during 4-sec working memory-retention intervals (46). The increase of frontal theta was interpreted as a reflection of enhanced attention (43,44) or, more precisely, as a consequence of sustained neuronal activity reflecting active maintenance of memory representation (45). Furthermore, subdural recordings from epileptic patients showed task-dependent human theta oscillations lasting several cycles during virtual maze navigation (47). The oscillations were more frequent in more complex mazes, as well as during recall trials than during learning trials.

It is intriguing that slow rhythmic activity encompassing the theta range is associated with states of decreased alertness (48,49). According to standardized criteria, non-REM (NREM) sleep stage 1 (the hypnagogic state) should show "a prominence of activity in the 2–7 cps range", and "the highest voltage 2–7 cps activity (about 50–75 µV) tends to occur in irregularly spaced bursts mostly during the latter portions of the stage" (50).

Increased slow theta activity (3–7 Hz) with slow components was found to be associated with decrements in vigilance during monotonous monitoring tasks, and learned regulation (operant conditioning) of activity in that range affected detection behavior by modulating this inverse relationship (51). Consistent with this finding, 4–6 Hz activity correlated with observed cyclic (15–20 sec) vigilance decrements. This activity was higher before undetected than before detected presentations of brief increases in the level of a continuous background noise in a simulated sonar auditory discrimination task (52). The link between (auditory) detection performance and EEG spectral parameters in drowsiness was shown to be adequately reliable to allow accurate individualized prediction of minute-scale changes in alertness in near-real time by using the combination of spectral analysis, principal component analysis, and neural networks (53). Finally, the time course of activity in the theta range during prolonged wakefulness reflects a homeostatic process possibly involved in the regulation of sleep and wakefulness. This aspect will be reviewed in detail in this chapter.

Fast Oscillations

The frequency range of beta activity during wakefulness is commonly defined as 13–30 Hz (33). The occurrence of spindles during sleep, whose spectral signature may include activity up to 16 Hz (54,55), imposes the use of a higher low boundary for beta during sleep, preferably above 17 Hz (56). Beta and gamma (> 30 Hz) oscillations appear in a sustained manner during highly aroused and attentive states, and large-scale synchrony of these and other oscillations across distant sites seems to play an important role for the emergence of a unified cognitive moment and for the manifestation of coherent behavior and cognition [reviewed in (57)]. The occurrence of spontaneous fast oscillations, coherent over intrathalamic, thalamocortical, and intracortical neuronal networks (19,20,58) might have a significant role in focused attention as well as in the integration of discrete features of an object into a global precept ["binding"; see (22)].

It is common practice to consider electroencephalographic activity during wakefulness as characterized by fast rhythms and irregular fluctuations of usually low amplitude that are believed to reflect desynchronization of neuronal activity. Indeed, the associated electroencephalographic state is commonly referred to as "desynchronized." Such terminology essentially originates from the disruption of high-amplitude and synchronous electroencephalographic waves typical of NREM sleep states. However, the observed coherence and synchronization of theta [e.g., (46)], gamma [e.g., (19,20,22,26,30)], and other oscillations during wakefulness intimates that the use of the term "desynchronized" to designate brain-active states may lead to confusion (59). Therefore, it is advisable to substitute "desynchronized" with the more appropriate term "activated," as originally proposed more than 50 years ago (9).

III. Changes in Alertness and Performance with the Progression of Time Awake

How does the progression of time awake affect brain dynamics and electroencephalographic activity while behaviorally alert? The interest in hour- and day-scale changes in electroencephalographic activity during wakefulness has been intimately linked to the quest for an electrophysiological correlate of alertness, or of its anticorrelated concept: sleepiness.

Across the daily 24-hr light-dark and activity-rest cycle we usually stay awake for about 16 hr and then sleep for the resting 8 hr, typically at night. During the waking period we engage in a multitude of activities and our ability to sustain efficient waking cognition with high levels of performance is not unlimited. However, it has been shown under controlled laboratory conditions that alertness and neurobehavioral function generally remain at a somewhat stable level during the 16 hr that coincide with the normal waking day. Performance and alertness then deteriorate rapidly in correspondence to the late evening secretion of plasma melatonin (60–62) (see Fig. 1). These findings should be interpreted by taking into account the interaction of circadian and homeostatic processes underlying the regulation of neurobehavioral performance, alertness, and sleep propensity [reviewed in (63)]. Circadian and homeostatic factors are thought to apply a continuous, time-dependent influence that becomes extended with the continuous prolongation of wakefulness. The effect of these factors on cortical and electroencephalographic changes during sleep deprivation is the central subject of this review. Other environmental influences (e.g., temperature, bright light, noise), specific behaviors (e.g., physical activity, body posture, stress level), or drugs (e.g., caffeine, nicotine, amphetamine) also exert significant but "discrete" effects on levels of alertness and performance during normal and prolonged wakefulness [see (64) for a review].

A. Circadian and Homeostatic Influences (See Also Chap. 24)

The timing of sleep and wakefulness [1,65 (see below)] as well as fluctuations in many biochemical, physiological, and behavioral variables are regulated by the interaction of circadian and homeostatic processes of variable relative strength. Circadian rhythms epitomize the most widespread instance of cyclic state alternation in biological systems [plants included, as first observed by Jean Jacques d'Ortus De Mairan, 1729; see (66)]. The term "circadian" originates from the Latin expression *circa dies* ("approximately one day") and is used to characterize rhythms showing oscillatory dynamics with a period close to 24 hr. Core body temperature and the secretion of melatonin are well-known examples of physiological variables exhibiting distinct circadian fluctuations. In mammals, circadian rhythmicity is controlled by the biological clock (or pacemaker) in the suprachiasmatic nuclei (SCN) of the hypothalamus, and is regularly entrained to the 24-hr environmental light-dark cycle by external zeitgebers ("time givers," e.g., light).

Homeostasis, a term coined by the physiologist Walter Bradford Cannon in 1929, has been defined as "the coordinated physiological processes which maintain most of the steady states in the organism." The word derives from the two Greek expressions *homeo*, which means "similar," and *stasis*, which means "standing." The concept of sleep homeostasis was introduced in 1980 (67) and refers to the aspect of sleep need that depends on prior sleep and waking (1). Accordingly, in this chapter the term homeostatic will be used as indicative of the processes depending on the prior sleep-wake history, a central theme throughout the present discussion. History-dependent homeostatic components have been found in several variables related to behavior (e.g., alertness and performance; see Chap. 13), physiology (e.g., endocrine function; see Chap. 14), gene expression (see Chap. 18), and electrophysiology (e.g., the waking and sleep EEG). Over the past 20 years circadian and homeostatic influences have been integrated into models of alertness [reviewed in (68)], neurobehavioral performance [reviewed in (69)] and sleep regulation [reviewed in (70)] that offer conceptual frameworks for the development and validation of hypotheses regarding underlying regulating mechanisms. However, in contrast to circadian rhythmicity, the neurobiological substrate of homeostatic changes in sleep propensity and other variables is still unknown and might be diffuse.

B.   Desynchronization of Circadian and Homeostatic Influences

The interaction of circadian and homeostatic regulating components has been studied by adopting sophisticated experimental designs called forced desynchrony (FD) protocols (71,72). Essentially, "desynchronization" (73) of rhythms driven by the endogenous circadian periodicity from the sleep-wake cycle is obtained by living for several weeks in a laboratory environment free of time and other synchronizing cues in which the sleep-wake schedule artificially deviates from the habitual 24-hr day period (e.g., a 20-hr or 28-hr period). Assuming that a 28-hr period is imposed, if the times for sleep and waking are scheduled 4 hr later at each sleep-wake cycle (as if subjects were traveling westward four time zones per day), over the course of the protocol those times will occur at many different circadian phases.

The separate contribution of endogenous homeostatic and circadian influences on the wealth of measurable physiological and neurobehavioral variables is then assessed by phase locking the data over either the imposed sleep-wake cycle, or the measured free-running (i.e., unsynchronized) circadian rhythm (as revealed by, say, core body temperature or plasma melatonin level) (74). Thus, FD protocols allowed estimation of the precisely controlled intrinsic (i.e., free running) period of the human circadian pacemaker, which was shown to be essentially around 24.1–24.2 hr in both young and elderly subjects (74).

C.   Alertness During Wakefulness Is Modulated
by Circadian Phase

Circadian patterns in the level of subjective alertness ratings and performance were reported in early studies (75). Twenty-eight-hour FD experiments confirmed that subjective alertness and cognitive performance are highly sensitive to circadian phase and demonstrated that their circadian rhythm parallels the rhythm of core body temperature (60). Furthermore, it was shown that the phase relationship between circadian and wake-dependent oscillatory processes during entrainment to the 24-hr day (i.e., under normal conditions) "is uniquely timed to facilitate the ability to maintain a consolidated bout of sleep at night and a consolidated bout of wakefulness throughout the day" (76), as predicted by initial simulations (65). In this view, the circadian pacemaker is thought to actively counteract the decrements associated with the monotonic increases of wake time-dependent influences [(77); see below].

Such behavior of adaptive significance enables the organism to anticipate and master temporally changing conditions in the natural environment (73). In a subsequent 20-hr FD protocol, performance in a number of computerized neurobehavioral tests including an addition/calculation task, a digit symbol substitution test, and a psychomotor vigilance task showed significant circadian modulation that exhibited peak levels near the temperature maximum, shortly before melatonin secretion onset (78). Such interval corresponds with what has been referred to as the "wake maintenance zone" (79). Under entrained conditions, this maximal circadian drive for wakefulness would occur near the end of the habitual waking day. Conversely, the circadian nadir of performance appeared at or shortly after the temperature minimum, which, in turn, was shortly after the melatonin maximum (78).

How does the circadian clock influence alertness and performance? Although those variables are in close phase with core body temperature [e.g., (80)], it is not known whether they are directly affected by body temperature or whether body temperature, alertness, and performance simply covary with circadian phase. Data from a 28–hr FD protocol showed that a higher body temperature, associated with but independent of circadian phase, is correlated with higher performance and subjective alertness (81). This result supports the original Kleitman's hypothesis that body temperature is an underlying mechanism modulating performance.

Taken together, the outcomes of FD studies illustrate the exquisite sensitivity of brain dynamics to endogenous circadian phase and homeostatic aspects. *Are there electrophysiological correlates to the observed changes?*

IV. Electrophysiological Changes with the Progression of Time Awake

Investigating the relationship between the EEG, circadian phase, alertness, and performance requires frequent collection of electrophysiological data throughout one full cycle of the circadian rhythm (about 24 hr). Therefore, most studies typically include a sleep deprivation protocol. For that reason, identification and characterization of circadian and homeostatic influences requires careful considerations that are discussed below.

A. Electroencephalographic Activity During Wakefulness Is Correlated with Alertness

Preliminary studies investigated the electroencephalographic changes occurring during sleep deprivation. They mainly tested the ability to generate and sustain eyes closed-alpha, as an index of arousal level [reviewed in (64)]. One of the first reports of electroencephalographic activity in the theta (4–8 Hz) and alpha (8–12 Hz) range as possible correlates of reduced alertness and performance dates back to 1967 (82). A later series of laboratory and field experiments attempted to establish the waking EEG as a practical objective method to quantify hour- and day-scale changes in sleepiness (83). In one such experiment, signals were recorded continuously with a portable device from train drivers engaged in their working routine at day and at night (84). The results showed high intraindividual correlations between electroencephalographic spectral power in the alpha and theta bands and self-rated sleepiness. In a subsequent partial sleep deprivation study, these findings were confirmed, while it was observed that intrusions of slow eye movements and of alpha and theta power during waking, open-eyed activity strongly differentiated between high and low subjective sleepiness (85). These results demonstrated hour- and day-long fine associations between electroencephalographic parameters and subjective alertness, thereby setting the foundation for the use of features extracted from electrophysiological recordings as objective, continuous indicators of the level of vigilance and fatigue. However, the contribution of circadian and homeostatic components could not be analyzed in detail.

B. Constant Routine Protocol

Experimental protocols aimed to investigate associations between the EEG and levels of alertness and performance require careful control and minimization of several external noncircadian factors that may mask the relative contribution of circadian, and to some extent also of sleep-wake-dependent influences to the recorded signals. The spontaneous EEG is very sensitive to body posture (86), physical exercise (87), timing of meals (88), and probably nearly all aspects of behavior. As described previously, sensory stimulation, attention, mental operation, decreased arousal and drowsiness, all affect electroencephalographic rhythms. Therefore, the recording conditions must be carefully standardized.

Especially after prolonged wakefulness, or in particularly boring, monotonous task conditions, microsleep episodes may become frequent. Those episodes should be meticulously prevented by close behavioral and/or polysomnographic control of the subjects to avoid intrusion of electroencephalographic correlates of sleep onset that might sensibly affect the results. These observations equally hold for experiments addressing minute-scale associations between task performance and EEG (see Sect. II in this chapter), PET, or blood oxygenation level dependent (BOLD) signals (see Sect. VI and VII below) at a single circadian phase. In consideration of the circadian modulation of electroencephalographic activity, such experiments should also standardize the circadian phase at which data are acquired.

Protocols such as the constant routine (CR) (89,90), that is, "when rhythmic influences in the environment and sleep-waking pattern have been minimized" (91), are specifically designed to control for the various masking effects. Typically, subjects are kept awake in bed in a propped-up position under constant controlled conditions of physical posture, dim light intensity (< 15 lux), balanced food intake, and attenuated sensory stimulation. They have no access to time information [reviewed in (92)].

C. Electroencephalographic Activity During Wakefulness Is Modulated by Circadian Phase in a Frequency-Specific Manner

Circadian variations in the EEG of sleep-deprived subjects were observed in early studies and were associated with changes in body temperature (93). Although a systematic separation of the mutually interacting circadian and homeostatic processes can be optimally studied by forced desynchrony, quantification of their relative influence on the waking EEG can be estimated by statistical modeling of the time course of spectral power during sleep deprivation. Thus, data from a CR study confirmed that the EEG undergoes a circadian modulation in addition to a wake time-dependent increase (discussed below), showing that the relative contribution of circadian phase and elapsed time awake to the dynamics of the EEG differs across frequency bands (94). Assuming an additive interaction of the two components, a sequential fitting procedure revealed that circadian modulation affected electroencephalographic spectral power (activity) in all bands below 12 Hz. Among those, only in the "high" alpha band (9.25–12.0 Hz) did the homeostatic component vanish, and, interestingly, only in that band did the nadir of the fitted "circadian" cosine function over lapped with the minimum of the endogenous rhythm of core body temperature (94). Thus, only the circadian component of high alpha activity resemble the modulation of body temperature. Conversely, the nadir of the circadian component of activity in the 0.75- to 9.0-Hz range occurred in the evening, about 6 hr before the temperature minimum (94), in coincidence with the wake maintenance zone (79). These results, based on classical frequency bands, motivated further experiments, in which the analysis of spectral components was refined on narrow 1-Hz frequency bins.

Conventionally combined into distinct frequency bands, adjacent 1-Hz bins might display completely different dynamics. Thus, data from a CR study evaluated with analysis of variance (including trend analyses with orthogonal polynomial contrasts) revealed the presence of a sinusoidal time course (quartic trend) with maxima in the afternoon and a minimum during the night that was significant in all bins below 15 Hz. Given the similarity with the pattern of body temperature, this trend was interpreted as the circadian influence (95). Among those bins, the 8.0- to 10.75-Hz range was exclusively affected by circadian changes. Data from a contemporaneous CR study (96) validated and expanded the earlier findings of the same team (94), showing that a circadian component was present up to 9 Hz, plus between 10.25 and 14 Hz, while it vanished at higher frequencies (96). According to this refined analysis (1-Hz bins), the range exclusively affected by circadian changes was composed of only two bins (10.25–12.0 Hz). The circadian components of high-frequency alpha bins (10.25–13.0 Hz) exhibited the nadir close to the temperature minimum. Electroencephalographic spectral power in this frequency band showed positive correlation with the estimated circadian component of subjective alertness and a time course that was closely associated with the circadian rhythms of plasma melatonin and body temperature

(96). Finally, the study illustrated similarities between an observed separate circadian rhythm of theta activity (4.25–8.0 Hz) and the time course of sleep propensity estimated in a previous study, where it was quantified by the amount of sleep in 10-min naps scheduled every half hour around the clock (97). In summary, those data suggested that there may be two circadian rhythms in the waking EEG.

D.   Electroencephalographic Activity, Alertness, Body Temperature and Their Speculative Mutual Connection

The observed positive correlation between the circadian components of alpha power and alertness (96) is in apparent contrast with earlier findings (84,85) discussed above. The discrepancy could be explained by comparing the different definitions of the frequency bands employed in the analyses (10.25–13.0 Hz vs. 8–12 Hz). Nevertheless, even bands defined by clustering fine bins with similar dynamics may vary across studies, depending on the methods used to determine such dynamics. Thus, the absence of a significant wake-dependent component in 1-Hz bins was restricted to different ranges [8.0–10.75 Hz, as in (95), vs. 10.25–12.0 Hz, as in (96)]. A similar analysis based on finer 0.25-Hz bins highlighted the 9.25- to 10.75-Hz range (98). Variations across experimental protocols and interindividual differences (99) may enhance those slight discrepancies. It is interesting to observe that, in contrast to high alpha activity, alertness and performance change rapidly with extended time awake (60). Thus activity in the 9- to 12-Hz range did not correlate with subjective sleepiness and neurobehavioral variables in another CR protocol (61). Yet high alpha activity correlated with the circadian variation of subjective alertness (96), i.e., after removal of the wake-dependent component. Altogether those results suggest that electroencephalographic activity in the high alpha range might represent a valid electrophysiological correlate of the circadian rhythm of alertness and performance. Furthermore, given the close association of high alpha activity with core body temperature (94,96) and recalling Kleitman's hypothesis that body temperature is an underlying mechanism modulating performance (81), one is tempted to speculate further about a possible role for body temperature as the agent modulating electroencephalographic activity in the high alpha range.

E.   Electroencephalographic Activity During Wakefulness Depends on the Amount of Time Spent Awake

With the progression of time awake, substantial changes in brain dynamics are reflected in the spectral composition of the human EEG, and those changes get noticeably intensified when wakefulness is prolonged outside of the habitual boundaries. In addition to a circadian modulation (discussed above), a homeostatic drive is evident in behavioral and electrophysiological variables. When introducing FD protocols it was mentioned that performance and alertness decline rapidly in correspondence of the late evening secretion of plasma melatonin (60–62). If wakefulness is extended past this point, the phase relationship of the homeostatic and the circadian rhythm is such that the two processes do not oppose each other's effects any more (65). Instead, the circadian signal becomes sleep promoting and boosts the homeostatic drive for sleep propensity. Maximal circadian sleep propensity is then observed in correspondence of the minimum of core body temperature (76).

In the past 15 years a number of studies provided convincing evidence for the existence of a homeostatic process in the waking EEG. First, associations between changes in subjective alertness and electroencephalographic parameters (see above) (84,85) showed that power in the theta and alpha range is enhanced after prolonged wakefulness. Further evidence for a dependence of electroencephalographic activity on prior sleep-wake history was collected in consequent studies (100,101). In one of those, the waking EEG was recorded every 2 hr over a period of 40 hr of sleep deprivation. A linear increase of theta and beta power was observed, whereas the variables recovered baseline values after one night of sleep (101). The presence of a putative homeostatic component in the waking EEG could be suggested when a saturating exponential function was reported to fit progressively increasing theta/alpha activity (6.25–9.0 Hz) determined at four time points during 40 hr of sustained wakefulness (102). In fact, in the two-process model of sleep regulation, a saturating exponential function approximates the rising limb of sleep propensity in the course of waking (1,65) (see below).

A more detailed analysis of the changes in different frequency bands, using statistical modeling of electroencephalographic data acquired frequently at shorter time intervals, allowed quantification of a wake time-dependent rise superimposed on the circadian modulation described above (94,96). The rise was more pronounced for frequencies below 9 Hz but could also be identified for frequencies between 12.25 and 25.0 Hz. Similarly, the rise was fitted by saturating exponential functions with different time constants for different bands (96). Robust frequency-specific wake duration-dependent changes were confirmed in three other sleep deprivation studies, but in contrast to the latter findings, a linear function and not a saturating exponential function accounted for the rise in low-frequency activity (2.0–7.75 Hz) (95) and theta power (4.5–8.5 Hz, our reanalysis of data from 61); and 5–8 Hz (98) (Fig. 1).

F. Time Course of Theta Activity During Wakefulness

How does electroencephalographic theta activity change during normal and extended wakefulness? The left panel of Figure 1 illustrates how mean theta power (5.0–8.0 Hz) increases during 40 hrs of wakefulness. This frequency range was selected analyzing the changes in fine 0.25-Hz bins. The EEG was obtained in 14 sessions over successive 3-hr intervals starting at 0700 hr after a normal night of sleep (98). For each session, average spectra were calculated over two 5-min periods with eyes open. Superimposed to a monotonic increase, a circadian modulation is evident. Therefore, the statistical model for the pooled data included a linear function, to account for the homeostatic component, and a superimposed 24-hr sine wave representing circadian variation. The model

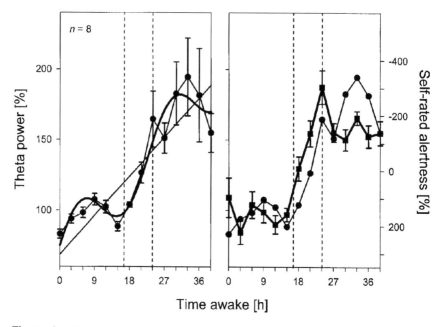

Figure 1   Time course of electroencephalographic power in the theta range (●; 5.0–8.0 Hz; derivation C3A2) and self-rated alertness (■) during 40 hrs of wakefulness. Left: Theta power (mean ± SEM; $n = 8$; for 5 data points $n = 7$) is plotted relative to the mean of the first 24 hr. A linear function with a superimposed 24-hr sine wave was fitted (nonlinear least-squares regression) to theta power (rise rate = 3.08%/h, intercept = 68.7%, amplitude of sine wave = 21.5%). Right: Self-rated alertness (mean ± SEM; $n = 8$; for 3 data points $n = 7$) plotted on a reverse scale (individual z-transformed values expressed as a percent of mean of first 24 hr). For reference, the dashed vertical lines limit the habitual sleep period (23:00–07:00). [Adapted from Ref. 98, Copyright (2000), with permission from Elsevier Science.]

parameters were estimated also for individual records. A significant circadian component was observed for the pooled values and for seven of the eight subjects individually. The rise rates (slopes) of the homeostatic component varied between 1.32 and 3.24%/hr, except for one subject, for whom the rate was 8.69%/hr (see below). Substitution of the linear component with a saturating exponential function did not yield significant results for either individual or pooled data (see also below). Subjective alertness declined with increasing time awake. Self-ratings were plotted on a reversed scale to compare their evolution with theta activity (Fig. 1, right panel). The two patterns were negatively correlated (mean $R = -0.82$; range -0.38 to -0.90). These results support the notion that electroencephalographic activity in the theta range might represent a valid electrophysiological correlate of the homeostatic variation of alertness, discussed above in section III.

Detailed inspection of the time course of theta power reveals the presence of a local maximum at clock time 1600 hr (4 PM) in both the first and second day of the protocol. Closely paralleled by a local minimum in self-rated alertness (occurring earlier on day 1), this feature is reminiscent of the postprandial dip [e.g., (103) (see also Chap. 32)], and can be observed in other reports (61,96,102). Three local minima of theta activity are present: two in the evening of both days at clock time 2200 hr (10 PM), and a third minimum at 1000 hr the second day. The former coincide with the wake maintenance zone (79) (see above), in accordance with prior CR studies (94,96), which used comparable fitting techniques.

G. Electroencephalographic Theta Power Is Maximal at Frontal Derivations During Waking

What is the regional distribution of theta activity on the scalp? Figure 2 illustrates the topographic distribution of absolute electroencephalographic theta power (5.0–8.0 Hz) during prolonged wakefulness derived from 27 recording sites (average reference) (104). Each map relates to one recording session, as in Figure 1, with the corresponding "Time awake [h]" indicated at the top left of each map. The last recording session (lower right corner, "0") took place after the subject had awakened from recovery sleep. In general, the distribution of theta activity exhibits a clear frontal predominance, with a relative pattern that seems fairly invariant to the progression of time awake. However, such invariance arises by plotting each map using the full color range. It becomes equivalent to a normalized map, enhancing within-map regional differences. As shown in Figure 3, the rate of increase of theta power in fact varies from location to location. The maxima of the power maps (located at electrode Fz for maps between 3 and 39 hr of waking) follow a time course with a rise rate similar to that depicted in Figure 1 for theta power at the C3A2 derivation (see Fig. 3). Conversely, power in the alpha range (9.0–12.0 Hz) had the maxima located occipitally in all 14 waking sessions, as expected (data not shown). Note the similarity of the first and last map ("0"), both derived from data recorded shortly after a sleep episode. In those, theta power also shows an occipital component, reminiscent of the occipital distribution of theta power during NREM sleep (55).

H. Electroencephalographic Theta Power Shows the Strongest Increase at Frontal Derivations During Waking

To ascertain whether and how the dynamics of the homeostatic component of the waking EEG differs throughout the scalp, the rise rate of theta activity was estimated systematically for data from each of the 27 electrodes (98). Parametric mapping over the scalp (Fig. 3, top) revealed a rate of increase that was prominent over frontal brain areas in diffused manner. The maximum was located over the frontal cortex (Fz), and the difference with the posterior minimum was significant. This analysis confirmed and extended to full-scalp topography previous reports based

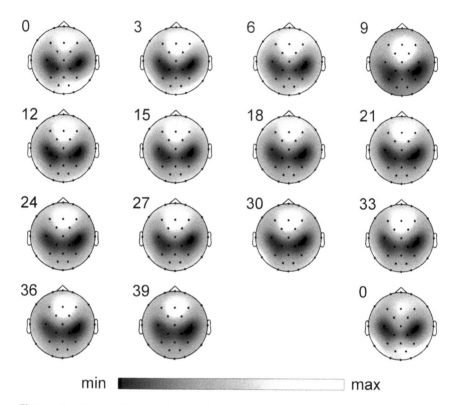

min ▮▮▮▮▮▮▮▮▮▮▮▮▮▮▮▮▮▮▮▮▮▮▮ max

Figure 2 Topographic distribution of absolute electroencephalographic theta power (5.0–8.0 Hz) during prolonged wakefulness. The recording sessions occurred at 3-hr intervals, starting at 07:00 after awakening from baseline sleep. The corresponding "Time awake [h]" is indicated at the top left of each map. The last recording session (lower right corner, "0") took place after awakening from recovery sleep. Maps are based on 27 EEG derivations (average reference; extended 10–20 system). Values are color coded and plotted at the corresponding position on the planar projection of the hemispheric scalp model. Values between electrodes were interpolated (biharmonic spline interpolation). Each map was scaled separately to optimize contrast by using the full color range. Dots indicate the electrode positions of the extended 10–20 system. The maxima of the power maps (max; located at Fz for maps between 3 and 39 hrs of waking) follow a time course qualitatively similar to that depicted in Figure 1 for theta power at the C3A2 derivation. (From Ref. 104.)

on recordings from two bipolar derivations (Fz-Cz and Pz-Oz) (61). The mapping results show that theta power during wakefulness exhibits an evident frontal distribution whose *relative* pattern is less affected by sleep deprivation (Fig. 2). The monotonic (homeostatic) facet of the increase of theta activity associated with prolonged wakefulness has a maximal rate over the same frontal regions (Fig. 3), suggesting that the latter regions may be more sensitive to sleep deprivation.

Rise rate of theta power in waking [% / h]

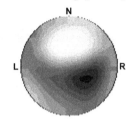

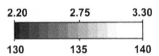

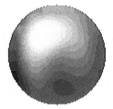

Increase of SWA from baseline to recovery [%]

Figure 3 Topographic distribution of the rise rate of theta power (5.0–8.0 Hz; top panel) during waking and of the increase of SWA (0.75–4.5 Hz; bottom panel) in the first NREM sleep episode from baseline to recovery sleep. Maps as in Figure 2 (N, nasion; L, left; R, right). Values between electrodes were linearly interpolated. The rise rate of theta power was determined by linear regression on pooled data ($n = 8$). The regressions were significant for all derivations ($p < 0.05$). Theta power was standardized as in Figure 1. SWA (% of baseline) was significantly enhanced at all derivations ($p < 0.05$, Wilcoxon signed rank test, $n = 8$). (From Ref. 98, Copyright 2000, with permission from Elsevier Science.)

V. Electroencephalographic Markers of Sleep Propensity for Wakefulness and Sleep

The characterization of a homeostatic component in the waking EEG prompted the question of whether homeostatic markers in the wake and sleep EEG reflect the same process. This new hypothesis had not been previously addressed. The wealth of evidence described in the preceding sections supports the idea that an electroencephalographic correlate of sleep propensity can also be measured during wakefulness, particularly over frontal brain areas. The open question had to be tackled on an individual basis, investigating mutual relationships in the data of single subjects (98).

A. The Two-Process Model and Electroencephalographic Markers of Sleep Homeostasis

The alternation of wakefulness and sleep is a regulated process (1,65) (see Chap. 24). Prolonging the awake state increases the "pressure for sleep" (i.e., sleep propensity), whereas excess sleep triggers the reverse effect. The concept of sleep homeostasis (67) was introduced in Section III, when circadian and homeostatic contributions to alertness and behavioral performance were described. Essentially, alertness and sleepiness are two sides of the same coin, one describing variation in the level of vigilance, the other the need for sleep. Sleep regulation primarily deals with the mechanisms controlling and occurring during sleep rather then wakefulness. In this respect, the homeostatic aspect is particularly interesting because it seems to be deeply interconnected with the still inscrutable function(s) of sleep (see Ref. 105).

The two-process model of sleep regulation posits that sleep propensity rises during waking and declines during sleep (1,65; see 106 for an overview). The time course of this process (process S) was derived from electroencephalographic slow-wave activity (SWA, spectral power in the 0.75- to 4.5-Hz range). The decline in SWA during sleep can be approximated by an exponential decay (107). In an FD protocol it was shown that SWA declines independently of the circadian phase at which sleep occurs, revealing that it is essentially determined by homeostatic factors (108). Hence SWA is traditionally referred to as the electroencephalographic marker of sleep homeostasis. Reflecting the amount of slow waves in the sleep EEG, SWA is also an index of NREM sleep intensity (109–113). In the original formulation of the model (1,65), the rising limb of sleep propensity in the course of waking was approximated by a saturating exponential function. The latter assumption was supported by the changes of SWA during daytime naps scheduled after various waking intervals (114,115); in other words, by sleep electroencephalographic data. Thus, the dynamics of process S in sleep and waking was entirely represented by SWA levels during sleep. The demonstration of a homeostatic component in the human waking EEG might bring together brain dynamics of wakefulness and sleep. Yet those findings raised the question of whether this waking putative physiological indicator of sleep propensity is related to electroencephalographic SWA. The possibility of monitoring the time course, and the intensity of the homeostatic sleep process in the waking EEG would offer interesting practical implications.

B. Electroencephalographic Markers of Sleep Homeostasis During Wakefulness and Sleep Reflect the Same Homeostatic Process

It is well established that sleep deprivation enhances slow-wave sleep and SWA in the recovery night, with the highest rebound in the first NREM sleep episode (e.g., 107). To test the hypothesis of a direct association between electroencephalographic variables during sleep and waking, the increase in SWA in the first NREM sleep episode after 40 hr of sleep deprivation was regressed against the rise rate of theta power during waking (Fig. 4). The data of seven "typical" subjects revealed a remarkable linear relationship between the two measures

Figure 4 Relationship between homeostatic markers in the sleep EEG and waking EEG. The increase (%) of SWA (power in the 0.75- to 4.5-Hz range) in the first NREM sleep episode from baseline to recovery sleep is plotted as a function of the rise rate (%/hr) of theta power (5.0–8.0 Hz) in waking. The linear regression line fitted through seven data points is indicated ($R^2 = 0.724$). The data point of subject 10 was classified as an outlier because of a more than sevenfold increase in theta power in waking and was therefore excluded from the regression. The rise rate of theta power was determined by nonlinear least-squares regression with a linear function and a superimposed 24-hr sine wave (see Fig. 1). (From Ref. 98, Copyright 2000, with permission from Elsevier Science.)

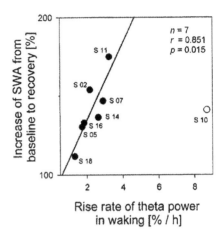

($R = 0.851$, $R^2 = 0.724$, $P = 0.015$). Subjects with a minor increase of SWA in sleep also presented a low-rise theta rate during waking, whereas subjects with stronger SWA responses exhibited higher rates of theta increase. These results show that the intensification of theta activity in the waking EEG is closely associated with sleep homeostasis, mirroring the level of sleep propensity as SWA does. Interestingly, when the SWA data for the first four NREM sleep episodes were used instead of only the first episode, interindividual differences decreased and the correlation with the rise rate of theta power in the waking EEG vanished. These findings of strong intraindividual correspondence demonstrated for the first time that homeostatic EEG markers in sleep (SWA) and in waking (theta activity) are intimately related, both reflecting sleep homeostasis (Fig. 5) (98). This claim was also corroborated by the topographic analysis of the rise rate of theta power in waking and the increase of SWA in sleep, which revealed that the largest values are centered for both over anterior cortical areas (Fig. 3). Thus, it was proposed that those changes are due to a common underlying process (98), a process that may exhibit local features. That is, frontal brain areas may be particularly vulnerable to sleep deprivation (116) (see below), therefore reflecting homeostatic processes more intensely than other cortical regions.

The hypothesis that theta activity in waking may be one of the dual markers of a common homeostatic sleep process was later substantiated in an experimental protocol that included multiple daytime naps. As predicted by this hypothesis, naps attenuated the sleep-wake-dependent increase in frontal electroencephalographic activity in the 1- to 7-Hz range (117).

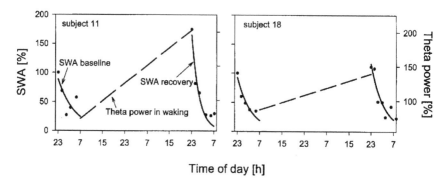

Time of day [h]

Figure 5   Close association between rise of slow-wave activity (SWA) in recovery sleep and theta activity in waking illustrated for two subjects. Mean SWA per NREM sleep episode (•) is plotted at the time corresponding with the beginning of each episode and is expressed relative to the baseline value of the first NREM sleep episode (100%). Exponential functions were fitted through the sleep data points (solid curves). The regression line represents theta power in waking (dashed line). For procedure and standardization, see Figure 1. (From Ref. 98, Copyright 2000, with permission from Elsevier Science.)

C.   Electroencephalographic Theta Activity: Compensatory Mechanisms During Prolonged Wakefulness?

What is the physiological relevance of the homeostatic rise of theta activity during prolonged wakefulness? What mechanisms link it to SWA in sleep? How does it relate to the homeostatic modulation of performance discussed above? The question of whether the homeostatic process during waking rises according to a linear or a saturating exponential function is not only of academic importance but may also be conceptually relevant. The original hypothesis (1,65) of an exponential saturating increase of process S during waking was supported by the changes of SWA during short daytime sleep episodes (114,115). Yet the demonstration of a close relationship between waking and sleep electroencephalographic markers suggests that such a saturating time course might not be an intrinsic property of the process but a consequence of a putative compensatory response taking place during waking. In other words, we proposed that the rise of electroencephalographic theta power during prolonged waking could be not only a sign of a rising sleep propensity but also an indication of an antagonistic mechanism counteracting the rise (98). This would result in a progressive attenuation of the rise rate of process S in waking, shaping a saturating exponential time course of SWA, when tested in daytime sleep episodes.

The gradually increasing occurrence of sleep signs in the waking EEG is well documented in animal studies. In the rat, SWA appears in the waking EEG during enforced wakefulness while the rat is active and behaving (118,119). In the mouse, a waking period as short as 2 hr causes a rise of low-frequency power in the waking EEG (120). The observation that rats subjected to enforced wakefulness for several days lack a prominent slow-wave rebound during recovery sleep (121) may be accounted for by a compensation that may be occurring during wakefulness. Interestingly, when SWA was quantified in mice for sleep episodes following waking periods of variable length, the relationship between the duration of prior wakefulness and subsequent SWA in sleep appeared linear for both spontaneous and enforced periods of wakefulness less than 9 hr (122). However, after 9 hr of sleep deprivation, sleep SWA values were lower as compared with the values after 6 hr of sleep deprivation.

Although the nature of the putative compensatory mechanism acting in wakefulness remains to be determined, joint features at the neuronal level support the idea that the two electroencephalographic markers of sleep homeostasis may be complementary elements of a common restorative network behavior. Thus PET studies have shown that delta (1.5–4.0 Hz) activity in sleep (123) and theta (4.0–7.0 Hz) activity in waking (124) are both correlated with relatively decreased activity in thalamic nuclei. These structures are deeply involved in the control of arousal level (see Section II in this chapter). Once more, the topographic analysis presented in Figure 3 showed that the greatest values of the rise rate of theta power in waking and the increase of SWA in sleep are both distributed over frontal cortical areas (98). Further investigations with brain imaging methods may help to elucidate the nature of a putative waking compensatory process.

D. Local Increase of Electroencephalographic Theta Power: A Manifestation of Use Dependence?

Slow-wave activity in the sleep EEG is a reliable marker of sleep homeostasis and of NREM sleep intensity. Theta activity in the waking EEG is a marker of the level of alertness and of sleep homeostasis. The analysis of the topographic distribution of the increase of SWA in sleep and the rise rate of theta power in waking provided evidence on how the expression of the markers differs across the scalp. This suggested a local manifestation of the underlying neuronal mechanism in the brain (Fig. 3) (98). In particular, the study showed that for both parameters the largest values are distributed over frontal sites.

The predominance of electroencephalographic sleep signs over frontal parts of the brain has been verified repeatedly for baseline sleep (55,125,126), partial sleep deprivation (127,128), and total sleep deprivation (55,98,129,130). When the sleep EEG power spectra were investigated in two or three bipolar derivations along the anteroposterior axis, frequency-specific state-related gradients emerged (125,126). In particular, the frontal predominance of power in the 2-Hz bin during the initial part of sleep suggested that the frontal association areas exhibit higher sleep intensity than other parts of the cortex. In line with this observation, prolonged waking induced the largest rise of SWA at a frontal derivation (129).

Normative data from 27 derivations were obtained to delineate the full-scalp topographic distribution of sleep electroencephalographic power spectra for a baseline night and a recovery night after prolonged waking (55). The study provided the first detailed frequency-specific analysis of electroencephalographic topography of NREM sleep. Exploration of functional changes induced by increased sleep pressure employed the change of electroencephalographic power spectra as a principal indicator. Its topographic distribution was determined by comparing either the baseline night with the recovery night or the first half of the baseline night with the second half. The topographic pattern of the recovery/baseline power ratio was similar to the power ratio between the first and second half of the baseline night. In both cases, higher sleep pressure was associated with an increase in power in the low-frequency range (less than 10.75 Hz), which was largest over frontal brain regions. These findings indicate that frontal brain areas are particularly sensitive to sleep and sleep deprivation (see Sect. VI), possibly owing to a high "recovery need" of frontal heteromodal association areas of the cortex (55). The sleep process is not only a global phenomenon but has local facets. Such interpretations are supported by PET studies, which document a selective deactivation of frontal regions in NREM sleep [(131–135), reviewed in (136)]. A frontal predominance of low-frequency NREM sleep electroencephalographic power could also be demonstrated in animals, both at the beginning of the rest period and after sleep deprivation [rat, (137,138); mouse (139)], which are conditions of high sleep pressure.

Why is there a local high need for (recovery) sleep? Different brain areas are involved in different functions. Hence the local manifestation of the homeostatic markers in sleep and in waking, in conjunction with the PET data, suggest use dependence (see Ref. 140 for a theoretical framework). That is, the markers may result more intensely there, where the underlying brain areas have been particularly "active" during preceding wakefulness. In this view, extended wakefulness could enhance the involvement of frontal cortical areas in brain functioning. However the meaning of the word "active" used here still awaits careful clarification, as the neurobiological substrate of use-dependent "fatigue," i.e., its underlying neuronal mechanisms (see Chap. 15) and/or neurochemical correlates (see Chap. 18), have yet to be determined. For instance, use dependence might include plasticity dependence. Human and animal studies where "activation" was increased locally by augmenting or reducing sensory stimulation to one hemisphere provided evidence for a local, use-dependent character of sleep. Thus, in humans unilateral stimulation by prolonged application of a vibratory stimulus to the dominant hand resulted in a selective increase in SWA over the contralateral somatosensory cortex in the first hour of sleep (141). Similarly in rats, after cutting the vibrissae (whiskers) on one side to reduce waking sensory input, it was found that such unilateral activation of the somatosensory cortex gave rise to a shift of low-frequency power toward the contralateral hemisphere during recovery sleep (142). Overstimulation of cortical regions different from somatosensory areas was performed in humans (143). Six hours of unilateral auditory stimulation (left or right ear) during wakefulness did not generate an asymmetrical pattern in the subsequent sleep EEG. The manipulation resulted in a slow-wave sleep-selective increase of electroencephalographic power within the alpha (8–12 Hz) and sleep spindle (12–15 Hz) range over large scalp areas. The effect could be mainly ascribed to enhanced wave amplitude. The changes in power were accompanied by an increase in coherence between frontotemporal cortical regions within a broad frequency range during slow-wave sleep (143). Taken together, sleep deprivation and asymmetrical stimulation studies support the hypothesis that sleep homeostasis depends not only on the duration of prior wakefulness, but also on use-dependent processes. The finding that the increase of theta power during prolonged wakefulness also has local facets may provide new avenues to explore daytime use dependence of the homeostatic sleep process in awake and behaving individuals.

E.   Electroencephalographic Theta Activity, Attention and Effort

Earlier in this chapter (Sect. II) it was mentioned that during performance of tasks utilizing working memory the frontal midline theta rhythm increases in magnitude with increased task difficulty and memory load (44,45). Such increase was explained as an indication of enhanced attention (43,44) by sustained neuronal activity (45). In children with attention deficits it was shown that quantitative waking EEG abnormalities included increased theta or alpha power, greatest in the frontal regions (144). In addition, evidence from meditation studies supports the hypothesis that frontal theta activity could indicate mental concentration and performance of an attention demanding procedure [see references in (145)]. Careful comparison of the dynamics of the different theta rhythms in those various behavioral circumstances is mandatory before any inference. Nevertheless, in view of these findings it can be alternatively speculated that increased theta activity during prolonged wakefulness may be the manifestation of sustained neuronal activity underlying enhanced mental effort to attend and concentrate on the presented stimuli. See Section VII to compare with the results from fMRI studies of task performance during sleep deprivation. Interestingly, the topographic distribution of theta activity showed a clear frontal predominance throughout a period of 40 hr of extended wakefulness (Fig. 2), with the highest intensification in correspondence of the frontal midline site Fz (Fig. 3) (98). In addition to this, it was reported that during prolonged waking, power in the 5.25- to 9.0-Hz range is higher in natural short sleepers than in long sleepers (146). Whereas the kinetics of the homeostatic process did not differ between the two groups, the sleep-wake-dependent oscillations occurred on a higher level in the short sleepers than in the long sleepers. Assuming that short sleepers tolerate a higher sleep pressure than long sleepers (147), the authors proposed that theta activity may mirror an underlying mechanism "that allows the brain to maintain wakefulness while sleep pressure is high" (146). Such compensation to performance seems conceptually distinct from the compensation to sleep need described above. Further research is necessary to resolve this latent dichotomy.

VI. Neural Correlates of Alertness and Cognitive Performance During Prolonged Wakefulness: PET Studies

At the beginning of this chapter it was argued that the brain is much more susceptible to sleep loss than the body. The explanation is that quiet wakefulness (as in CR protocols) is rest for the body but is not sufficient to prevent the formidable effects of sleep deprivation on higher cognitive functions such as speech (148,149), "divergent" (creative) thinking ability (150), or memory (151,152). It has been proposed that the cerebral cortex, and in particular its prefrontal portion, is the part of the brain particularly vulnerable to sleep deprivation (116). This hypothesis was originally motivated by observing that cognitive deficits after sleep deprivation resemble symptoms characteristic of lesions of the prefrontal cortex (PFC), including reduced word fluency, monotonic voice intonation, apathy, impaired divergent thinking, and elevated exposure to competing distractions (116). As we have discussed, the topographic results presented in the previous sections provide new strong support for this hypothesis in healthy individuals. An interesting association between chronic sleep disruption caused by obstructive sleep apnea and PFC ("executive") dysfunction has also been proposed (153), and the role of the PFC in sleep has been reviewed (154).

What are the neural correlates of the deficits in cognitive performance after sleep loss in healthy individuals? The detrimental effects of sleep deprivation suggest modification in underlying physiology and function. Accordingly, knowledge of the dynamics of metabolic processes in the central nervous system under different conditions of alertness may provide a better understanding of the susceptibility of brain functioning to related alterations. Modern brain imaging techniques offer adequate spatial resolution to identify and study the neuroanatomical substrates possibly affected by sleep deprivation. For instance, PET scanning is a powerful method to acquire images of physiological function under different vigilance states. Thus, PET studies demonstrated that changes in the functional organization of the brain in the course of sleep and waking are reflected by altered patterns of regional cerebral blood flow (rCBF) (135; for an overview, see 136). The PET technique has been comprehensively described elsewhere (155).

A. Brain Metabolic Function During Continuous Performance

When six PET scans (rCBF) and electroencephalographic activity were acquired at 10-min intervals during continuous performance of a 60-min auditory vigilance discrimination task, rCBF decreased as a function of time-on-task in several subcortical (thalamus, substantia innominata, and putamen) and cortical regions (ventrolateral, dorsolateral, and orbital frontal cortex; parietal cortex; and temporal cortex) (124). Blood flow decreases were also found in the temporalis muscles. Simultaneously, rCBF increased in several visual cortical areas. Performance data were analyzed across the six 10-min intervals. The number of hits did not change, but a progressive increase of both the reaction time and theta activity (4.0–7.0 Hz) could be observed across testing. The latter increase was correlated with relatively decreased activity in thalamic nuclei. From these findings it was concluded that the changes in reaction time, electroencephalographic activity, and blood flow in the temporalis muscles and thalamus are related to changes in the level of alertness (124).

B. Brain Metabolic Function During Prolonged Wakefulness

The first quantitative measurement of absolute brain activity changes after extended wakefulness quantified regional cerebral glucose metabolism (rCGM) in young healthy volunteers while performing in a visual vigilance task (156). The method uses PET and [18F]-labeled 2-deoxyglucose (FDG) as a marker, a glucose analog that is taken up like deoxyglucose but is not metabolized (157). After the subject spent 32 hrs awake, absolute glucose metabolic measurements indicated a decrease in thalamus, cerebellum, and basal ganglia. In addition, relative rCGM (i.e., normalized to total brain value) was reduced in the temporal cortex, thalamus, and cerebellum. Sleep deprivation impaired visual vigilance performance. The decrease was correlated with reduced rCGM again in the thalamus, the basal ganglia, and limbic regions. However, no overall decrease in whole-brain metabolism was observed (156).

C. Brain Metabolic Function Across Days of Chronic Total Sleep Deprivation

A notable imaging study investigated the effects of prolonged wakefulness over a much longer period of 85 hr (3 days) from the last awakening (158,159). After a night of normal sleep subjects were scanned either at 9:30, 10:30, 11:30, or 12:30 hr. This procedure was then repeated at the same time after 24, 48, and 72 hr, yielding four scans per subject. Prior to each scan, subjects were injected FDG and underwent a 30-min FDG uptake period, during which they performed an arithmetic serial addition/subtraction task. It is expected that brain systems particularly involved in the task would be more active than others, therefore absorbing a higher amount of radiolabeled FDG. After 24 hr from the baseline scan, decreased performance in the cognitive task was accompanied with decreased global (i.e., averaged across the brain) absolute glucose metabolic rate, and decreased absolute rCGM for many regions throughout most of the brain. Areas of largest decrease included the heteromodal association (prefrontal and posterior parietal) cortices and the thalamus. No brain regions exhibited a significant increase in absolute rCGM (159). In general, these findings persisted at a similar level also after 48 and 72 hr from the first scan, while performance worsened further. In particular, no further decline of global absolute glucose metabolic rate was observed (158). Discrete areas of prefrontal and primary visual cortex and thalamus represented the only exception, showing additional decreases.

D. Comparison to Brain Metabolic Function During Sleep

Comparison of these results with findings from studies of brain metabolic activity during sleep reveals analogous regional changes. Several investigations assessing rCBF by PET using bolus injections of $H_2^{15}O$ reported absolute and relative decreases mostly in prefrontal (and sometimes parietal) cortical activity during NREM stage 1 sleep (160), light sleep (123,133–135), slow-wave sleep (131–135,161), and rapid-eye-movement (REM) sleep (131,135,162). Therefore, it appears that most of the higher order cortical areas differentially affected by prolonged wakefulness are also differentially responsive to the sleep process. Such analogy supports the tenet that these brain regions may be more susceptible to sleep deprivation and consequently have a greater need for the (recuperative) processes underlying sleep.

E. Comparison to Electroencephalographic Data

How do these results relate to EEG data? So far, full scalp electroencephalographic dynamics during cognitive performance over a period of extended wakefulness have not been studied in detail. Thus, it remains to be established whether and how the local changes in the EEG observed during sleep deprivation are related to the circadian and sleep-wake-dependent modulation of performance. Yet the results on dual electroencephalographic markers of sleep homeostasis during wakefulness and sleep exposed in detail in the previous section can be integrated with the findings from the PET studies that showed that the prefrontal cortex was among the brain regions exhibiting the largest reduction of activity during both prolonged wakefulness and sleep. These findings support the argument that a similar topographic distribution of the largest rise of theta power and the largest increase of SWA (Fig. 3) are due to a common underlying homeostatic process, which may be more intense over frontal brain areas.

VII. Neural Correlates of Alertness and Cognitive Performance During Prolonged Wakefulness: fMRI Studies

Magnetic resonance imaging, the tool of choice for the study of functional neuroanatomy of cognitive function, has been used in conjunction with sleep deprivation protocols to investigate the effects of sleep loss on cerebral response during task performance. The fMRI studies described below all defined and measured cerebral activation by using blood oxygenation level dependent (BOLD) fMRI signals, which depend on local changes in deoxyhemoglobin subsequent to variations in neural activity. Namely, altered neuronal activity is accompanied by metabolic and hemodynamic changes in oxygen extraction, blood flow, and blood volume, which in turn affect the local deoxyhemoglobin levels (163; reviewed in 164).

A. Selective Attention

One study investigated the activity changes related to the performance of an attention-demanding task under different levels of arousal: under normal conditions (i.e., after a normal night of sleep), after administration of caffeine, and after 24 hr of sleep deprivation (165). Mean reaction time and total number of mistakes did not vary significantly with arousal level. Different brain regions were active during the attentional task, but in most areas activation did not change as a function of arousal. However, in the ventrolateral thalamus task-induced activity changes were highest after sleep deprivation. The latter finding was interpreted as an indication of the increased effort of maintaining attention during the task after sleep loss. It was concluded that the thalamus is a structure involved in the interaction of attention and arousal in humans (165).

B. Verbal Learning, Arithmetic, and Divided Attention

The aim of a subsequent fMRI study was to compare cerebral activation during performance of a learning task requiring memorization of a list of words (verbal learning), a serial subtraction arithmetic task, also involving working memory, and a divided attention task. In this study subjects underwent functional scanning between 1630 and 1800 hr after both a normal night of sleep (i.e., after about 11 hr of time awake) and after total sleep deprivation (i.e., after about 35 hr of time awake). Sleep deprivation enhanced subjective sleepiness and reduced the self-rated concentration level.

On free recall of the learned words (post-scanning), performance worsened after sleep loss. On the contrary, recognition memory was not affected (166). Surprisingly, despite subjective reports indicated that sleep loss did not enhance effort or task difficulty, activation was higher after sleep deprivation bilaterally in discrete regions of both the PFC and the parietal lobes. In addition, activation in specific areas of those parietal regions was positively correlated with the free-recall performance score. A positive correlation with increased subjective sleepiness was found within the left inferior and right superior/middle frontal gyrus. Relative decreases in activity were found uniquely in the left temporal lobe (166).

The above interesting findings were interpreted as indications that the brain may be able to compensate for the degrading effects of sleep deprivation, trying to keep performance intact, at least during the initial portion of assigned tasks. With increasing time-on-task, performance then declines (6,167). The authors proposed that the active regions may represent the neurophysiological substrate of the initial compensation for sleep deprivation (166). In contrast, the arithmetic task was characterized by relatively decreased activity bilaterally in both the PFC and the parietal lobes. Subjects showed an overall decrease in the proportion of correct responses to the assigned computations (168). These findings are consistent with the hypothesis of high vulnerability of the PFC to sleep deprivation (116) discussed in the previous sections.

Following sleep deprivation, the changes in activation pattern to divided attention was quite similar to the response observed with the verbal learning task (169). Modest behavioral impairment was accompanied by higher activations in brain regions within the right prefrontal cortex, bilateral parietal lobes, and cingulate gyrus. Also with this task, activation in the bilateral parietal lobes was positively correlated with the free recall performance score. Finally, a positive correlation with increased subjective sleepiness was also confirmed within the left inferior frontal gyrus (169).

Taken together these observations were interpreted as an indication that the effects of sleep loss on neurobehavioral performance and the underlying cerebral activation may be task dependent (168).

C. Adaptation and Compensation to Sleep Deprivation Effects

Three of the four reports summarized above support the notion of compensatory mechanisms emerging when wakefulness is extended past the habitual period. This hypothesis was originally advanced 80 years ago when the first systematic studies of sleep deprivation ("experimental insomnia") were performed (170). To explain the finding that subjects could often transiently perform at baseline levels even after more than 60 hr of sleep deprivation, it was proposed that a "new effort" could boost performance but that "the effect of increased effort disappeared when the test became one of endurance" (170). However, except for the study of selective attention (165), subjective assessment of effort level did not change significantly after sleep deprivation in the fMRI studies above. Thus, rather than effort, it was proposed that an adaptive, potentially compensatory cerebral response to cognitive performance was responsible for the increased activity after sleep deprivation (166,169).

How these putative adaptive (compensatory) mechanisms may be expressed in the additional recruitment (coming "on-line") of new brain areas to participate in performance and how this phenomenon may be task-dependent remain to be established. It has been shown that several characteristics of the task employed (e.g., duration and difficulty) strongly influence response performance after sleep loss [reviewed in (64)]. Finally, it must be ascertained whether and how these local effects are related to the circadian- and homeostatic-dependent modulation of performance.

D. Relative Reduction of BOLD Response After
Sleep Deprivation

The review of findings from PET studies opened with the question: What are the neural correlates of the deficits in cognitive performance after sleep deprivation? In concert with impaired performance of arithmetic tasks after prolonged wakefulness, both PET (159) and certain fMRI (168) data supported the tenet of a relative reduction of activity, particularly in frontal areas (116). In addition, areas in the left temporal lobe showed significantly less activity during verbal learning in sleep deprivation as compared to baseline conditions (166).

The apparent contrast with the diffused BOLD increases found in the verbal learning (166) and divided attention tasks (169) was interpreted as an indication that the effects of extended wakefulness on the neural correlates of task performance may depend on the type of cognitive demand (168). It may be worth noting that the fMRI BOLD signal is a sensitive indicator of relative cerebral activation, but for now it is not as a quantifiable, an absolute measure of neural activity (171) as PET. The BOLD signal during the condition of interest is compared to the BOLD signal during a control condition, therefore yielding relative changes in the regional hemodynamic response. Activations and deactivations are not expressed in absolute terms. Yet quantification of absolute brain activity changes during sleep deprivation may be important to characterize and understand the direction and magnitude of regional brain activity alterations.

E. Electroencephalographic Activity During Prolonged Wakefulness and BOLD Response

What are the possible associations between electroencephalographic data during extended wakefulness and the results from fMRI studies? In the last three tasks reported above, a positive correlation with increased subjective sleepiness was found within the left ventral prefrontal cortex. It was shown in Section IV that the time course of theta activity in the waking EEG is positively correlated with the time course of subjective sleepiness. Thus, it can be speculated that increased levels of theta activity after sleep deprivation might be associated with increased BOLD response in discrete frontal areas, reflecting similar underlying mechanisms. Interestingly, full-scalp mapping data showed that the increase of theta activity was most pronounced over the frontal hemisphere (Fig. 3) (98).

Is there a homeostatic component in the BOLD response? The quantitative aspect related to this question still must be clarified. Furthermore, it is experimentally problematical to constantly follow BOLD changes with elapsed time awake. On the other hand, many studies reviewed in this chapter have shown how feasible it is to follow such changes in EEGs. Thus the ideal association of the two techniques, simultaneous electroencephalography and fMRI, may open new avenues to study homeostatic (and circadian) effects on BOLD response during task performance over an extended period of wakefulness.

VIII. Concluding Remarks and Perspectives

Brain dynamics change over time while awake, particularly when wakefulness is extended by means of sleep deprivation. Macroscopic correlates of the variations in brain dynamics occurring with the progression of time awake have been identified in many studies employing several different techniques. However, it is still not clear which are simply correlates and which are in direct causal relationship with the underlying mechanisms. This chapter reviews neuropsychological, neurophysiological, and neuroimaging studies that investigated how brain activity changes with level of arousal, and discusses ensuing implications as well as what should be addressed by future work.

The sleep-wake cycle emerges as a regulated, integrative part of the circadian rest-activity pattern, and is generated by the interaction of a circadian process, which originates from the SCN, and a homeostatic process, which depends on the previous sleep-wake history. The forced desynchrony studies summarized in this review illustrate how subjective alertness, cognitive performance, and, therefore, brain dynamics are sensitive to endogenous circadian phase and wake-dependent aspects.

Electrophysiological correlates to the changes in brain dynamics are reflected in the ongoing EEG during normal and prolonged wakefulness. In reviewing the literature, we distinguish between circadian and homeostatic influences. In general, it is demonstrated that the frequency-specific changes induced in the waking EEG by the circadian pacemaker are distinguishable from the changes induced by the wake-dependent increase of homeostatic sleep pressure. Spectral analysis and statistical modeling of the waking EEG showed that circadian influences are detectable below 15 Hz. In particular, electroencephalographic activity in the (high) alpha range appears to be a valid electrophysiological correlate of the circadian rhythm of alertness and performance.

The homeostatic component of the waking EEG is characterized by a monotonic increase, whose rise rate is more pronounced in the theta range (5–8 Hz). Waking EEG activity in the theta range seems to be not only an electrophysiological correlate of the homeostatic variation of subjective alertness, but also a convincing marker of the homeostatic need for sleep. Furthermore, the strongest increase of theta activity during waking is found over frontal brain areas, suggesting that these may be more sensitive to sleep deprivation in a use-dependent manner.

It is important to note that circadian and homeostatic components are not found at all frequencies. Frequency-selective features are likely to be ascribed to specific neurophysiological mechanisms rather than to nonspecific factors, such as temperature or anatomical characteristics. On the other hand, this chapter summarizes studies that report: (a) a close association of high alpha activity with both core body temperature and alertness, and (b) a direct effect of temperature on alertness and performance, in support of Kleitman's hypothesis. Bearing in mind that it is not known whether the SCN affect thalamic and cortical networks involved in the generation of alpha oscillations actively, through neural connections, or rather passively, through some of their output variables, it is tempting to speculate about a possible role for body temperature as an agent modulating electroencephalographic activity in the alpha range.

The chapter also reviews results indicating how the EEG correlates to the changes in brain dynamics during normal and extended wakefulness are tightly related to the electroencephalographic changes that characterize sleep and recovery sleep after deprivation. In particular, the rise rate of theta activity during waking correlated with the increase in slow-wave activity in the first NREM sleep episode in single individuals. Both parameters were largest in frontal areas. From these results, we suggested that theta activity in waking and slow-wave activity in sleep are markers of a common homeostatic sleep process, a process that may exhibit local features. While discussing a linear versus a saturating exponential time course of theta activity in waking, we proposed that the rise of theta power could also mirror a compensatory response to sleep loss. According to this idea, sleep compensatory mechanisms could already be detected in awake subjects, and the two electroencephalographic markers of sleep homeostasis would represent complementary elements of a common restorative network behavior. The identification of dual electroencephalographic markers of sleep homeostasis in waking and in sleep shed light on the interaction between the arousal system and the sleep system. Additional work is needed to clarify how brain dynamics of wakefulness and sleep are interrelated.

This chapter condenses imaging studies based on PET during normal and extended wakefulness that examined how cerebral response across the whole brain is affected during task performance. After sleep deprivation of variable extent, metabolic parameters revealed by PET during waking are generally found to be reduced in the thalamus, cerebellum, basal ganglia, and several cortical areas, especially heteromodal association cortices (prefrontal and posterior parietal). Comparison of these results with findings from studies of brain metabolic activity during sleep indicates analogous regional changes. Thus, it seems that higher order cortical areas differentially affected by extended wakefulness are also differentially responsive to the sleep process. These findings complement the results from electroencephalographic studies and, taken together, support the hypothesis that higher order (frontal) cortical areas may: (a) be more susceptible to sleep deprivation and (b) have a greater need for the restorative processes occurring during sleep.

Finally, the review summarizes fMRI studies during periods of sleep deprivation. As proposed by J. Christian Gillin, the results indicate that "the brain is dynamic in its efforts to function when deprived of sleep." Accordingly, after sleep loss BOLD activity during a verbal learning and a divided attention task was higher, and not lower, in discrete cortical regions, which may represent the neurophysiological substrate of an initial compensation for sleep deprivation. The data support the alternative view that the brain may be able to compensate for the degrading effects of sleep deprivation in a task-dependent manner.

In this chapter we describe several large-scale measures of brain activity and how they change in time during normal and extended wakefulness. Knowing what type of measurements a given technique permits is of fundamental importance. Only by taking this into consideration can we begin to link hypotheses concerning the nature of the physiological processes occurring across the sleep-wake cycle.

Thus, in view of the interesting but controversial results from imaging studies, it remains to be established to what extent the observed changes in electroencephalographic theta power reflect: (a) a general modification of the organization of brain oscillations with time awake, (b) a compensatory network restorative mechanism, or (c) a neural correlate of an adaptive mechanism to sustain performance, e.g., increased effort or increased use of resources to keep attention focused on a task. These phenomena are not mutually exclusive, and they might all involve (d) local, use-dependent changes.

In this context it is important to note that the electroencephalographic studies summarized in this chapter mostly reported series of mean spectral measures, averaged over 3- to 10-min periods within one frequency band. Such measures provide time-integrated indicators of changes in brain activity, which may correlate with local and global variables such as homeostatic and circadian processes, sleepiness, effort, fatigue, or temperature. Whether and how those electroencephalographic measures reflect all aspects of actual brain dynamics, cortical and subcortical, in the range of milliseconds to seconds still deserve exploration. At the beginning of Section II, we briefly summarized the neuro-physiological mechanisms underlying electroencephalographic activation during wakefulness, discussing the important role of subcortical structures including the brainstem, the thalamus, the posterior hypothalamus, and the basal forebrain. Understanding to what extent circadian and homeostatic processes are represented within those structures, and how their contribution is reflected in the electroencephalographic changes we summarized in this chapter, is an interesting aspect that deserves investigation. Nowadays, multimodal approaches allow scientific exploration of these problems in humans. Studies using combined acquisition modalities (e.g., simultaneous electroencephalography and fMRI) are needed to understand in a unified manner the relevance of electrophysiological parameters and regional changes.

The design of experiments aimed to study how the progression of time awake influences cognitive performance and brain dynamics is challenging. Typically, long and repetitive cognitive tasks are preferred because for short times (less than 10 min) individuals are often able to perform at normal levels. That is, short tasks fail to reflect the effects of sleep loss. However, long tasks might become boring enough to produce light drowsiness and become sleep conducive, rather than sustain alertness. Tasks should not be too long, should be very effective, and the associated brain dynamics (electroencephalographic changes, PET or fMRI activation patterns) should be known in detail for baseline conditions. When pursuing the evolution of features within individuals, sequence-order effects such as adaptation are difficult to control for in sleep deprivation studies. Thus, subjects should be well trained on the tasks before entering the study so to avoid interaction with learning or habituation effects.

In this chapter the numerous rhythms present in the EEG have been discussed. Activity in the different frequency bands is affected by homeostatic and circadian factors, different behaviors, designated tasks, levels of vigilance and, in sleep, by the state and depth of sleep. Therefore, it is important to understand each rhythm in the context of a specific behavioral/vigilance state. For example, the fact that rhythms in the alpha frequency range can be detected in both relaxed wakefulness and sleep does not necessarily imply that the underlying cellular and network mechanisms generating the oscillations are the same. Referring only to the frequency band can be misleading. Also, electroencephalographic rhythms should be placed within the context of interconnected brain networks allowing synchronized activities of neural assemblies. In this respect, electroencephalographic topography helps to distinguish between the underlying generating mechanisms of observed waveforms.

Taken together, the results summarized in this chapter provide strong evidence that specific regions and systems of the brain may be involved in, or highly responsive to, the process of homeostatic sleep regulation, and therefore may be more sensitive to sleep deprivation. The observed signs of locally increased sleep propensity while awake (and sleep intensity while asleep) could reflect the need for a more intense recovery process, a process that may be use dependent.

References

1. Borbély AA. A two process model of sleep regulation. Hum Neurobiol 1982; 1:195–204.
2. Horne JA. Why we sleep. The Functions of Sleep in Humans and Other Mammals. New York: Oxford University Press, 1988.
3. Gulevich G, Dement W, Johnson L. Psychiatric and EEG observations on a case of prolonged (264 hours) wakefulness. Arch Gen Psychiatry 1966; 15:29–35.
4. Horne JA. Mammalian sleep function with particular reference to man. In: Mayes A, ed. Sleep Mechanisms and Functions in Humans and Animals: An Evolutionary Perspective. Workingham, UK: Van Nostrand Reinhold, 1983:262–311.
5. Horne JA. Sleep function, with particular reference to sleep deprivation. Ann Clin Res 1985; 17:199–208.
6. Dinges DF, Kribbs NB. Performing while sleepy: effects of experimentally induced sleepiness. In: Monk TH, ed. Sleep, Sleepiness and Performance. New York: John Wiley and Sons, 1991:97–128.
7. Dinges DF. An overview of sleepiness and accidents. J Sleep Res 1995; 4:4–14.
8. Plum F. Coma and related global disturbances of the human conscious state. In: Peters A, Jones EG, eds. Cerebral Cortex. New York: Plenum Press, 1991:359–425.
9. Moruzzi G, Magoun HW. Brain stem reticular formation and activation of the EEG. Electroencephalogr Clin Neurophysiol 1949; 1:455–473.
10. Bremer F, Stoupel N, van Reeth PC. Nouvelles recherches sur la facilitation et l'inhibition des potentiels évoqués corticaux dans l'éveil réticulaire. Arch Ital Biol 1960; 98:229–247.
11. Steriade M, McCarley RW. Brainstem Control of Wakefulness and Sleep. New York: Plenum Press, 1990.
12. McCormick DA. Neurotransmitter actions in the thalamus and cerebral cortex and their role in neuromodulation of thalamocortical activity. Prog Neurobiol 1992; 39:337–388.
13. Steriade M, McCormick DA, Sejnowski TJ. Thalamocortical oscillations in the sleeping and aroused brain. Science 1993; 262:679–685.

14. McCormick DA, Bal T. Sleep and arousal: thalamocortical mechanisms. Annu Rev Neurosci 1997; 20:185–215.
15. Destexhe A, Contreras D, Steriade M. Spatiotemporal analysis of local field potentials and unit discharges in cat cerebral cortex during natural wake and sleep states. J Neurosci 1999; 19:4595–4608.
16. Steriade M, Timofeev I, Grenier F. Natural waking and sleep states: a view from inside neocortical neurons. J Neurophysiol 2001; 85:1969–1985.
17. Sherman SM, Koch C. The control of retinogeniculate transmission in the mammalian lateral geniculate nucleus. Exp Brain Res 1986; 63:1–20.
18. Kinomura S, Larsson J, Gulyás B, Roland PE. Activation by attention of the human reticular formation and thalamic intralaminar nuclei. Science 1996; 271:512–515.
19. Steriade M, Contreras D, Amzica F, Timofeev I. Synchronization of fast (30–40 Hz) spontaneous oscillations in intrathalamic and thalamocortical networks. J Neurosci 1996; 16:2788–2808.
20. Steriade M, Amzica F, Contreras D. Synchronization of fast (30–40 Hz) spontaneous cortical rhythms during brain activation. J Neurosci 1996; 16:392–417.
21. Munk MH, Roelfsema PR, Konig P, Engel AK, Singer W. Role of reticular activation in the modulation of intracortical synchronization. Science 1996; 272:271–274.
22. Singer W. Synchronization of cortical activity and its putative role in information processing and learning. Annu Rev Physiol 1993; 55:349–374.
23. Jones BE. The neural basis of consciousness across the sleep-waking cycle. Adv Neurol 1998; 77:75–94.
24. Saper CB, Chou TC, Scammell TE. The sleep switch: hypothalamic control of sleep and wakefulness. Trends Neurosci 2001; 24:726–731.
25. von Krosigk M, Monckton JE, Reiner PB, McCormick DA. Dynamic properties of corticothalamic excitatory postsynaptic potentials and thalamic reticular inhibitory postsynaptic potentials in thalamocortical neurons of the guinea-pig dorsal lateral geniculate nucleus. Neuroscience 1999; 91:7–20.
26. Gray CM, Konig P, Engel AK, Singer W. Oscillatory responses in cat visual cortex exhibit inter-columnar synchronization which reflects global stimulus properties. Nature 1989; 338:334–337.
27. Eckhorn R, Bauer R, Jordan W, Brosch M, Kruse W, Munk M, Reitboeck HJ. Coherent oscillations: a mechanism of feature linking in the visual cortex? Multiple electrode and correlation analyses in the cat. Biol Cybern 1988; 60:121–130.
28. Laurent G, Davidowitz H. Encoding olfactory information with oscillating neural assemblies. Science 1994; 265:1872–1875.
29. Patel AD, Balaban E. Temporal patterns of human cortical activity reflect tone sequence structure. Nature 2000; 404:80–84.
30. Rodriguez E, George N, Lachaux JP, Martinerie J, Renault B, Varela FJ. Perception's shadow: long-distance synchronization of human brain activity. Nature 1999; 397:430–433.
31. Miltner WHR, Braun C, Arnold M, Witte H, Taub E. Coherence of gamma-band EEG activity as a basis for associative learning. Nature 1999; 397:434–436.
32. Destexhe A, Sejnowski TJ. Thalamocortical Assemblies. How Ion Channels, Single Neurons, and Large-Scale Networks Organize Sleep Oscillations. Oxford: Oxford University Press, 2001:452.
33. IFSECN. A glossary of terms most commonly used by clinical electroencephalographers. Electroencephalogr Clin Neurophysiol 1974; 37:538–548.

34. Berger H. Über das Elektrenkephalogramm des Menschen. Arch Psychiatr Nervenkr 1929; 87:527–570.
35. Van Winsum W, Sergeant J, Geuze R. The functional significance of event-related desynchronization of alpha rhythm in attentional and activating tasks. Electroencephalogr Clin Neurophysiol 1984; 58:519–524.
36. Lopes da Silva F. Neural mechanisms underlying brain waves: from neural membranes to networks. Electroencephalogr Clin Neurophysiol 1991; 79:81–93.
37. Nunez PL. Neocortical Dynamics and Human EEG Rhythms. New York: Oxford University Press, 1995.
38. Robinson PA, Rennie CJ, Wright JJ, Bahramali H, Gordon E, Rowe DL. Prediction of electroencephalographic spectra from neurophysiology. Phys Rev E Stat Nonlin Soft Matter Phys 2001; 63:021903.
39. Wright JJ, Liley DTJ. Dynamics of the brain at global and microscopic scales: neural networks and the EEG. Behav Brain Sci 1996; 19:285–320.
40. Lopes da Silva FH, Vos JE, Mooibroek J, Van Rotterdam A. Relative contributions of intracortical and thalamo-cortical processes in the generation of alpha rhythms, revealed by partial coherence analysis. Electroencephalogr Clin Neurophysiol 1980; 50:449–456.
41. Gastaut H. Étude électrocorticographique de la reativité des rhythmes rolandiques. Rev Neurol (Paris) 1952; 87:176–182.
42. Pfurtscheller G, Aranibar A. Evaluation of event-related desynchronization (ERD) preceding and following voluntary self-paced movement. Electroencephalogr Clin Neurophysiol 1979; 46:138–146.
43. Mizuki Y, Tanaka M, Isozaki H, Nishijima H, Inanaga K. Periodic appearance of theta rhythm in the frontal midline area during performance of a mental task. Electroencephalogr Clin Neurophysiol 1980; 49:345–351.
44. Gevins A, Smith ME, McEvoy L, Yu D. High-resolution EEG mapping of cortical activation related to working memory: effects of task difficulty, type of processing, and practice. Cereb Cortex 1997; 7:374–385.
45. Jensen O, Tesche CD. Frontal theta activity in humans increases with memory load in a working memory task. Eur J Neurosci 2002; 15:1395–1399.
46. Sarnthein J, Petsche H, Rappelsberger P, Shaw GL, von Stein A. Synchronization between prefrontal and posterior association cortex during human working memory. Proc Natl Acad Sci U S A 1998; 95:7092–7096.
47. Kahana MJ, Sekuler R, Caplan JB, Kirschen M, Madsen JR. Human theta oscillations exhibit task dependence during virtual maze navigation. Nature 1999; 399:781–784.
48. Davis H, Davis PA, Loomis AL, Harvey EN, Hobart G. Changes in human brain potentials during the onset of sleep. Science 1937; 86:448–450.
49. Davis H, Davis PA, Loomis AL, Harvey EN, Hobart G. Human brain potentials during the onset of sleep. J Neurophysiol 1938; 1:24–38.
50. Rechtschaffen A, Kales A. A manual of standardized terminology, techniques and scoring system for sleep stages of human subjects. Bethesda: National Institutes of Health, 1968.
51. Beatty J, Greenberg A, Deibler WP, O'Hanlon JF. Operant control of occipital theta rhythm affects performance in a radar monitoring task. Science 1974; 183:871–873.
52. Makeig S, Jung TP. Tonic, phasic, and transient EEG correlates of auditory awareness in drowsiness. Brain Res Cogn Brain Res 1996; 4:15–25.
53. Jung TP, Makeig S, Stensmo M, Sejnowski TJ. Estimating alertness from the EEG power spectrum. IEEE Trans Biomed Eng 1997; 44:60–69.

54. Uchida S, Maloney T, Feinberg I. Sigma (12–16 Hz) and beta (20–28 Hz) EEG discriminate NREM and REM sleep. Brain Res 1994; 659:243–248.

55. Finelli LA, Borbely AA, Achermann P. Functional topography of the human nonREM sleep electroencephalogram. Eur J Neurosci 2001; 13:2282–2290.

56. Uchida S, Maloney T, Feinberg I. Beta (20–28 Hz) and delta (0.3–3 Hz) EEGs oscillate reciprocally across NREM and REM sleep. Sleep 1992; 15:352–358.

57. Varela F, Lachaux JP, Rodriguez E, Martinerie J. The brainweb: phase synchronization and large-scale integration. Nat Rev Neurosci 2001; 2:229–39.

58. Ribary U, Ioannides AA, Singh KD, Hasson R, Bolton JPR, Lado F, Mogilner A, Llinas R. Magnetic field tomography of coherent thalamocortical 40–Hz oscillations in humans. Proc Natl Acad Sci U S A 1991; 88:11037–11041.

59. Steriade M. Arousal: revisiting the reticular activating system. Science 1996; 272:225–6.

60. Dijk DJ, Duffy JF, Czeisler CA. Circadian and sleep/wake dependent aspects of subjective alertness and cognitive performance. J Sleep Res 1992; 1:112–117.

61. Cajochen C, Khalsa SBS, Wyatt JK, Czeisler CA, Dijk D-J. EEG and ocular correlates of circadian melatonin phase and human performance decrements during sleep loss. Am J Physiol 1999; 277:R640–R649.

62. Doran SM, Van Dongen HP, Dinges DF. Sustained attention performance during sleep deprivation: evidence of state instability. Arch Ital Biol 2001; 139:253–267.

63. Dijk DJ, Lockley SW. Integration of human sleep-wake regulation and circadian rhythmicity. J Appl Physiol 2002; 92:852–862.

64. Bonnet MH. Acute sleep deprivation. In: Kryger MH, Roth T, Dement WC, eds. Principles and Practice of Sleep Medicine. Philadelphia: WB Saunders, 2004. In press.

65. Daan S, Beersma DGM, Borbély AA. Timing of human sleep: recovery process gated by a circadian pacemaker. Am J Physiol 1984; 246:R161–R178.

66. Bünning E. The Physiological Clock: Endogenous Diurnal Rhythms and Biological Chronometry. Berlin: Springer-Verlag, 1964.

67. Borbély AA. Sleep: circadian rhythm versus recovery process. In: Koukkou M, Lehmann D, Angst J, eds. Functional States of the Brain: Their Determinants. Amsterdam: Elsevier, 1980:151–161.

68. Folkard S, Akerstedt T, Macdonald I, Tucker P, Spencer MB. Beyond the three-process model of alertness: estimating phase, time on shift, and successive night effects. J Biol Rhythms 1999; 14:577–587.

69. Jewett ME, Kronauer RE. Interactive mathematical models of subjective alertness and cognitive throughput in humans. J Biol Rhythms 1999; 14:588–597.

70. Borbély AA, Achermann P. Sleep homeostasis and models of sleep regulation. J Biol Rhythms 1999; 14:557–568.

71. Kleitman N. Sleep and Wakefulness. Chicago: University of Chicago Press, 1939.

72. Kleitman N, Kleitman E. Effect of non-twenty-four-hour routines of living on oral temperature and hearth rate. J Appl Physiol 1953; 6:283–291.

73. Aschoff J. Circadian rhythms in man. Science 1965; 148:1427–1432.

74. Czeisler CA, Duffy JF, Shanahan TL, Brown EN, Mitchell JF, Rimmer DW, Ronda JM, Silva EJ, Allan JS, Emens JS, Dijk DJ, Kronauer RE. Stability, precision, and near-24–hour period of the human circadian pacemaker. Science 1999; 284:2177–2181.

75. Akerstedt T, Froberg JE. Interindividual differences in circadian patterns of catecholamine excretion, body temperature, performance, and subjective arousal. Biol Psychol 1976; 4:277–292.

76. Dijk DJ, Czeisler CA. Paradoxical timing of the circadian rhythm of sleep propensity serves to consolidate sleep and wakefulness in humans. Neurosci Lett 1994; 166:63–68.

77. Edgar DM, Dement WC, Fuller CA. Effect of SCN lesions on sleep in squirrel monkeys: evidence for opponent processes in sleep-wake regulation. J Neurosci 1993; 13:1065–1079.

78. Wyatt JK, Ritz-De Cecco A, Czeisler CA, Dijk DJ. Circadian temperature and melatonin rhythms, sleep, and neurobehavioral function in humans living on a 20–h day. Am J Physiol 1999; 277:R1152–R1163.

79. Strogatz SH, Kronauer RE, Czeisler CA. Circadian pacemaker interferes with sleep onset at specific times each day: role in insomnia. Am J Physiol 1987; 253:R172–R178.

80. Johnson MP, Duffy JF, Dijk DJ, Ronda JM, Dyal CM, Czeisler CA. Short-term memory, alertness and performance: a reappraisal of their relationship to body temperature. J Sleep Res 1992; 1:24–29.

81. Wright KP, Jr., Hull JT, Czeisler CA. Relationship between alertness, performance, and body temperature in humans. Am J Physiol Regul Integr Comp Physiol 2002; 283:R1370–R1377.

82. Daniel RS. Alpha and theta EEG in vigilance. Percept Mot Skills 1967; 25:697–703.

83. Åkerstedt T, Torsvall L, Gillberg M. Sleepiness in laboratory and field experiments. In: Koella WP, Rüther E, Schulz H, eds. Sleep '84. Stuttgart: Gustav Fischer Verlag, 1985:125–126.

84. Torsvall L, Åkerstedt T. Sleepiness on the job: continuously measured EEG changes in train drivers. Electroencephalogr Clin Neurophysiol 1987; 66:502–511.

85. Åkerstedt T, Gillberg M. Subjective and objective sleepiness in the active individual. Int J Neurosci 1990; 52:29–37.

86. Caldwell JA, Prazinko BF, Hall KK. The effects of body posture on resting electroencephalographic activity in sleep-deprived subjects. Clin Neurophysiol 2000; 111:464–470.

87. Lardon MT, Polich J. EEG changes from long-term physical exercise. Biol Psychol 1996; 44:19–30.

88. Wells AS, Read NW, Idzikowski C, Jones J. Effects of meals on objective and subjective measures of daytime sleepiness. J Appl Physiol 1998; 84:507–515.

89. Mills JN, Minors DS, Waterhouse JM. Adaptation to abrupt time shifts of the oscillator(s) controlling human circadian rhythms. J Physiol 1978; 285:455–470.

90. Minors DS, Waterhouse JM. The use of constant routines in unmasking the endogenous component of human circadian rhythms. Chronobiol Int 1984; 1:205–216.

91. Minors DS, Waterhouse JM. Does "anchor sleep" entrain circadian rhythms? Evidence from constant routine studies. J Physiol 1983; 345:451–467.

92. Duffy JF, Dijk DJ. Getting through to circadian oscillators: why use constant routines? J Biol Rhythms 2002; 17:4–13.

93. Gundel A, Witthöft H. Circadian rhythm in the EEG of man. Int J Neurosci 1983; 19:287–292.

94. Aeschbach D, Matthews JR, Postolache TT, Jackson MA, Giesen HA, Wehr TA. Dynamics of the human EEG during prolonged wakefulness: evidence for frequency-specific circadian and homeostatic influences. Neurosci Lett 1997; 239:121–124.

95. Dumont M, Macchi MM, Carrier J, Lafrance C, Hebert M. Time course of narrow frequency bands in the waking EEG during sleep deprivation. Neuroreport 1999; 10:403–407.

96. Aeschbach D, Matthews JR, Postolache TT, Jackson MA, Giesen HA, Wehr TA. Two circadian rhythms in the human electroencephalogram during wakefulness. Am J Physiol 1999; 277:R1771–R1779.

97. Wehr TA. A "clock for all seasons" in the human brain. Prog Brain Res 1996; 111:321–42.

98. Finelli LA, Baumann H, Borbély AA, Achermann P. Dual electroencephalogram markers of human sleep homeostasis: correlation between theta activity in waking and slow-wave activity in sleep. Neuroscience 2000; 101:523–529.

99. Finelli LA, Acherman P, Borbely AA. Individual 'fingerprints' in human sleep EEG topography. Neuropsychopharmacology 2001; 25:S57–S62.

100. Corsi-Cabrera M, Ramos J, Arce C, Guevara MA, Ponce-de Leon M, Lorenzo I. Changes in the waking EEG as a consequence of sleep and sleep deprivation. Sleep 1992; 15:550–555.

101. Lorenzo I, Ramos J, Arce C, Guevara MA, Corsi-Cabrera M. Effect of total sleep deprivation on reaction time and waking EEG activity in man. Sleep 1995; 18:346–54.

102. Cajochen C, Brunner DP, Kräuchi K, Graw P, Wirz-Justice A. Power density in theta/alpha frequencies of the waking EEG progressively increases during sustained wakefulness. Sleep 1995; 18:890–894.

103. Monk TH, Buysse DJ, Reynolds CF, Kupfer DJ. Circadian determinants of the postlunch dip in performance. Chronobiol Int 1996; 13:123–133.

104. Finelli LA. Functional mapping of the human brain during sleep and sleep deprivation. Zürich: Swiss Federal Institute of Technology, 2001:218. http://e-collection.ethbib.ethz.ch/show?type=diss&nr=14251

105. Borbély AA, Tononi G. The quest for the essence of sleep. Daedalus 1998; 127:167–196.

106. Borbély AA, Achermann P. Sleep homeostasis and models of sleep regulation. In: Kryger MH, Roth T, Dement WC, eds. Principles and Practice of Sleep Medicine. Philadelphia: WB Saunders, 2000:377–390.

107. Borbély AA, Baumann F, Brandeis D, Strauch I, Lehmann D. Sleep deprivation: effect on sleep stages and EEG power density in man. Electroencephalogr Clin Neurophysiol 1981; 51:483–493.

108. Dijk D-J, Czeisler CA. Contribution of the circadian pacemaker and the sleep homeostat to sleep propensity, sleep structure, electroencephalographic slow waves, and sleep spindle activity in humans. J Neurosci 1995; 15:3526–3538.

109. Blake H. Brain potentials and depth of sleep. Am J Physiol 1937; 119:273–274.

110. Blake H, Gerard RW. Brain potentials during sleep. Am J Physiol 1937; 119:692–703.

111. Feinberg I. Changes in sleep cycle patterns with age. J Psychiatr Res 1974; 10:283–306.

112. Borbély AA, Neuhaus HU. Sleep deprivation: effects on sleep and EEG in the rat. J Comp Physiol [A] 1979; 133:71–87.

113. Neckelmann D, Ursin R. Sleep stages and EEG power spectrum in relation to acoustical stimulus arousal threshold in the rat. Sleep 1993; 16:467–477.

114. Beersma DGM, Daan S, Dijk DJ. Sleep intensity and timing: a model for their circadian control. In: Carpenter GA, ed. Some Mathematical Questions in Biology— Circadian Rhythms. Vol. 19. Providence, RI: American Mathematical Society, 1987:39–62.

115. Dijk DJ, Beersma DGM, Daan S. EEG power density during nap sleep: reflection of an hourglass measuring the duration of prior wakefulness. J Biol Rhythms 1987; 2:207–219.

116. Horne JA. Human sleep, sleep loss and behaviour. Implications for the prefrontal cortex and psychiatric disorder. Br J Psychiatry 1993; 162:413–419.

117. Cajochen C, Knoblauch V, Krauchi K, Renz C, Wirz-Justice A. Dynamics of frontal EEG activity, sleepiness and body temperature under high and low sleep pressure. Neuroreport 2001; 12:2277–2281.

118. Borbély AA, Tobler I, Hanagasioglu M. Effect of sleep deprivation on sleep and EEG power spectra in the rat. Behav Brain Res 1984; 14:171–182.

119. Franken P, Dijk DJ, Tobler I, Borbély AA. Sleep deprivation in rats: effects on EEG power spectra, vigilance states, and cortical temperature. Am J Physiol 1991; 261:R198–R208.

120. Huber R, Deboer T, Tobler I. Effects of sleep deprivation on sleep and sleep EEG in three mouse strains: empirical data and simulations. Brain Res 2000; 857:8–19.

121. Rechtschaffen A, Bergmann BM, Gilliland MA, Bauer K. Effects of method, duration, and sleep stage on rebounds from sleep deprivation in the rat. Sleep 1999; 22:11–31.

122. Franken P, Chollet D, Tafti M. The homeostatic regulation of sleep need is under genetic control. J Neurosci 2001; 21:2610–2621.

123. Hofle N, Paus T, Reutens D, Fiset P, Gotman J, Evans AC, Jones BE. Regional cerebral blood flow changes as a function of delta and spindle activity during slow wave sleep in humans. J Neurosci 1997; 17:4800–4808.

124. Paus T, Zatorre RJ, Hofle N, Caramanos Z, Gotman J, Petrides M, Evans AC. Time-related changes in neural systems underlying attention and arousal during the performance of an auditory vigilance task. J Cogn Neurosci 1997; 9:392–408.

125. Werth E, Achermann P, Borbély AA. Brain topography of the human sleep EEG: antero-posterior shifts of spectral power. Neuroreport 1996; 8:123–127.

126. Werth E, Achermann P, Borbély AA. Fronto-occipital EEG power gradients in human sleep. J Sleep Res 1997; 6:102–112.

127. Werth E, Achermann P, Borbély AA. Regional differences in the sleep EEG. Sleep 1998; 21:207.

128. Ferrara M, De Gennaro L, Curcio G, Cristiani R, Corvasce C, Bertini M. Regional differences of the human sleep electroencephalogram in response to selective slow-wave sleep deprivation. Cereb Cortex 2002; 12:737–748.

129. Cajochen C, Foy R, Dijk DJ. Frontal predominance of a relative increase in sleep delta and theta EEG activity after sleep loss in humans. Sleep Res Online 1999; 2:65–69.

130. Achermann P, Finelli LA, Borbely AA. Unihemispheric enhancement of delta power in human frontal sleep EEG by prolonged wakefulness. Brain Res 2001; 913:220–223.

131. Braun AR, Balkin TJ, Wesensten NJ, Carson RE, Varga M, Baldwin P, Selbie S, Belenky G, Herscovitch P. Regional cerebral blood flow throughout the sleep-wake cycle. An $H_2^{15}O$ PET study. Brain 1997; 120:1173–1197.

132. Maquet P, Degueldre C, Delfiore G, Aerts J, Péters JM, Luxen A, Franck G. Functional neuroanatomy of human slow wave sleep. J Neurosci 1997; 17:2807–2812.

133. Andersson JLR, Onoe H, Hetta J, Lidström K, Valind S, Lilja A, Sundin A, Fasth K-J, Westerberg G, Broman J-E, Watanabe Y, Långström B. Brain networks affected

by synchronized sleep visualized by positron emission tomography. J Cereb Blood Flow Metab 1998; 18:701–715.

134. Kajimura N, Uchiyama M, Takayama Y, Uchida S, Uema T, Kato M, Sekimoto M, Watanabe T, Nakajima T, Horikoshi S, Ogawa K, Nishikawa M, Hiroki M, Kudo Y, Matsuda H, Okawa M, Takahashi K. Activity of midbrain reticular formation and neocortex during the progression of human non-rapid eye movement sleep. J Neurosci 1999; 19:10065–10073.

135. Finelli LA, Landolt HP, Buck A, Roth C, Berthold T, Borbely AA, Achermann P. Functional neuroanatomy of human sleep states after zolpidem and placebo: a $H_2^{15}O$-PET study. J Sleep Res 2000; 9:161–173.

136. Maquet P. Functional neuroimaging of normal human sleep by positron emission tomography. J Sleep Res 2000; 9:207–231.

137. Schwierin B, Achermann P, Deboer T, Oleksenko A, Borbély AA, Tobler I. Regional differences in the dynamics of the cortical EEG in the rat after sleep deprivation. Clin Neurophysiol 1999; 110:869–875.

138. Vyazovskiy VV, Borbely AA, Tobler I. Interhemispheric sleep EEG asymmetry in the rat is enhanced by sleep deprivation. J Neurophysiol 2002; 88:2280–2286.

139. Huber R, Deboer T, Tobler I. Topography of EEG dynamics after sleep deprivation in mice. J Neurophysiol 2000; 84:1888–1893.

140. Krueger JM, Obál F, Jr. A neuronal group theory of sleep function. J Sleep Res 1993; 2:63–69.

141. Kattler H, Dijk D-J, Borbély AA. Effect of unilateral somatosensory stimulation prior to sleep on the sleep EEG in humans. J Sleep Res 1994; 3:159–164.

142. Vyazovskiy V, Borbély AA, Tobler I. Unilateral vibrissae stimulation during waking induces interhemispheric EEG asymmetry during subsequent sleep in the rat. J Sleep Res 2000; 9:367–371.

143. Cantero JL, Atienza M, Salas RM, Dominguez-Marin E. Effects of prolonged waking-auditory stimulation on electroencephalogram synchronization and cortical coherence during subsequent slow-wave sleep. J Neurosci 2002; 22:4702–4708.

144. Chabot RJ, Orgill AA, Crawford G, Harris MJ, Serfontein G. Behavioral and electrophysiologic predictors of treatment response to stimulants in children with attention disorders. J Child Neurol 1999; 14:343–351.

145. Kubota Y, Sato W, Toichi M, Murai T, Okada T, Hayashi A, Sengoku A. Frontal midline theta rhythm is correlated with cardiac autonomic activities during the performance of an attention demanding meditation procedure. Brain Res Cogn Brain Res 2001; 11:281–287.

146. Aeschbach D, Postolache TT, Sher L, Matthews JR, Jackson MA, Wehr TA. Evidence from the waking electroencephalogram that short sleepers live under higher homeostatic sleep pressure than long sleepers. Neuroscience 2001; 102:493–502.

147. Aeschbach D, Cajochen C, Landolt HP, Borbély AA. Homeostatic sleep regulation in habitual short sleepers and long sleepers. Am J Physiol 1996; 270:R41–R53.

148. Harrison Y, Horne JA. Sleep deprivation affects speech. Sleep 1997; 20:871–877.

149. Harrison Y, Horne JA. Sleep loss impairs short and novel language tasks having a prefrontal focus. J Sleep Res 1998; 7:95–100.

150. Horne JA. Sleep loss and "divergent" thinking ability. Sleep 1988; 11:528–536.

151. Williams HL, Gieseking CF, Lubin A. Some effects of sleep loss on memory. Percept Mot Skills 1966; 23:1287–1293.

152. Harrison Y, Horne JA. Sleep loss and temporal memory. Q J Exp Psychol A 2000; 53:271–279.

153. Beebe DW, Gozal D. Obstructive sleep apnea and the prefrontal cortex: towards a comprehensive model linking nocturnal upper airway obstruction to daytime cognitive and behavioral deficits. J Sleep Res 2002; 11:1–16.

154. Muzur A, Pace-Schott EF, Hobson JA. The prefrontal cortex in sleep. Trends Cogn Sci 2002; 6:475–481.

155. Cherry SR, Phelps ME. Imaging brain function with positron emission tomography. In: Toga AW, Mazziotta JC, eds. Brain Mapping: The Methods. San Diego: Academic Press, 1996:191–221.

156. Wu JC, Gillin JC, Buchsbaum MS, Hershey T, Hazlett E, Sicotte N, Bunney WE. The effect of sleep deprivation on cerebral glucose metabolic rate in normal humans assessed with positron emission tomography. Sleep 1991; 14:155–162.

157. Sokoloff L, Reivich M, Kennedy C, Des Rosiers MH, Patlak CS, Pettigrew KD, Sakurada O, Shinohara M. The [14C]deoxyglucose method for the measurement of local cerebral glucose utilization: theory, procedure, and normal values in the conscious and anesthetized albino rat. J Neurochem 1977; 28:897–916.

158. Thomas M, Balkin T, Sing H, Wesensten N, Belenky G. PET imaging studies of sleep deprivation and sleep: implications for behavior and sleep function. J Sleep Res 1998; 7(suppl 2):274.

159. Thomas M, Sing H, Belenky G, Holcomb H, Mayberg H, Dannals R, Wagner H, Thorne D, Popp K, Rowland L, Welsh A, Balwinski S, Redmond D. Neural basis of alertness and cognitive performance impairments during sleepiness. I. Effects of 24 h of sleep deprivation on waking human regional brain activity. J Sleep Res 2000; 9:335–352.

160. Kjaer TW, Law I, Wiltschiotz G, Paulson OB, Madsen PL. Regional cerebral blood flow during light sleep—a $H_2^{15}O$-PET study. J Sleep Res 2002; 11:201–207.

161. Buchsbaum MS, Gillin JC, Wu J, Hazlett E, Sicotte N, Dupont RM, Bunney WE Jr. Regional cerebral glucose metabolic rate in human sleep assessed by positron emission tomography. Life Sci 1989; 45:1349–1356.

162. Maquet P, Péters JM, Aerts J, Delfiore G, Degueldre C, Luxen A, Franck G. Functional neuroanatomy of human rapid-eye-movement sleep and dreaming. Nature 1996; 383:163–166.

163. Ogawa S, Lee TM, Kay AR, Tank DW. Brain magnetic resonance imaging with contrast dependent on blood oxygenation. Proc Natl Acad Sci U S A 1990; 87:9868–9872.

164. Ugurbil K, Adriany G, Andersen P, Chen W, Gruetter R, Hu X, Merkle H, Kim DS, Kim SG, Strupp J, Zhu XH, Ogawa S. Magnetic resonance studies of brain function and neurochemistry. Annu Rev Biomed Eng 2000; 2:633–660.

165. Portas CM, Rees G, Howseman AM, Josephs O, Turner R, Frith CD. A specific role for the thalamus in mediating the interaction of attention and arousal in humans. J Neurosci 1998; 18:8979–8989.

166. Drummond SP, Brown GG, Gillin JC, Stricker JL, Wong EC, Buxton RB. Altered brain response to verbal learning following sleep deprivation. Nature 2000; 403:655–657.

167. Donnell JM. Performance decrement as a function of total sleep loss and task duration. Percept Mot Skills 1969; 29:711–714.
168. Drummond SP, Brown GG, Stricker JL, Buxton RB, Wong EC, Gillin JC. Sleep deprivation-induced reduction in cortical functional response to serial subtraction. Neuroreport 1999; 10:3745–3748.
169. Drummond SP, Gillin JC, Brown GG. Increased cerebral response during a divided attention task following sleep deprivation. J Sleep Res 2001; 10:85–92.
170. Lee MAM, Kleitman N. Studies on the physiology of sleep: II. Attempts to demonstrate functional changes in the nervous system during experimental insomnia. Am J Physiol 1923; 67:114–152.
171. Ogawa S, Menon RS, Kim SG, Ugurbil K. On the characteristics of functional magnetic resonance imaging of the brain. Annu Rev Biophys Biomol Struct 1998; 27:447–474.

13

Physiological and Neurophysiological Changes

MAHESH M. THAKKAR AND ROBERT W. MCCARLEY

Harvard Medical School, Boston VA Healthcare System, Brockton, Massachusetts, U.S.A.

I. Introduction

Humans spend one-third of their lives sleeping. Thus, it is not surprising that the topic of sleep has seized the intellectual curiosity of philosophers, scientists and physicians since ancient times (the Upanishads, Hindu religious texts; written around sixth century BC). No other behavior has generated so much interest, yet few behaviors are as mysterious.

Sleep is a state of behavior with a characteristic immobile posture and diminished, but readily reversible, sensitivity to external stimuli. During a normal sleep cycle, the brain's electrical activity, represented by the electroencephalogram (EEG), undergoes regular transformations. Synchronized or slow-wave or non-REM (NREM) sleep consists of brain waves with low frequency and high voltage, whereas desynchronized or paradoxical or rapid-eye-movement (REM) sleep consists of brain waves with high frequency and low voltage. The NREM sleep in higher mammals is further subdivided into four stages, with stage 1 being a brief transitional phase between wakefulness and "true" sleep and stage 4 being the "true" sleep stage characterized by the presence of high-voltage, slow-wave activity. REM sleep is identified by the simultaneous presence of EEG desynchronization, loss of activity in the antigravity muscles (muscle atonia), and periodic bursts of REM and muscle twitches. The constancy of the temporal elements of the sleep cycle, for any species or individual, suggests a strict central control

265

while its ubiquitous presence in mammals and a compulsion to recover lost sleep suggests that sleep has an important function.

To understand the function of an organ, early physiologists removed the organ in question and observed the ensuing deficiency symptoms. Using the same logic, "monitoring the resultant deficiency following sleep deprivation" would be appropriate to understand the function of sleep. Thus, evaluating the effects of sleep deprivation on physiology and neurophysiology was one way to understand the role of sleep. The central theme of this chapter is to review the effects of sleep deprivation on human and animal physiology and neurophysiology.

II. Physiological Effects of Sleep Deprivation

The physiological effects of total and REM sleep deprivation are discussed in this section. The following physiological systems will be discussed: cardiovascular, respiratory, gastrointestinal, renal, integumentary, and neurological. The effects of sleep deprivation on other physiological systems are discussed elsewhere in this book [immunologic effects (Chap. 17) and metabolic/endocrine effects (Chap. 14)]

A. Cardiovascular Effects

Short self-reported durations are reported to be independently associated with a modestly increased risk of coronary events (1). In hypertensive patients, sleep deprivation resulted in increases in sympathetic nervous system activity (i.e., blood pressure, heart rate, and urine norepinephrine) in the morning after a night of inadequate sleep (2). This raised the hypothesis that activation of the sympathetic nervous system by sleep deprivation may be implicated in triggering cardiovascular events in the early morning hours (2–4). However, the cardiovascular system appears to be variably affected by sleep deprivation.

Resting and maximal heart rate were decreased after 30 hr of sleep deprivation (5). A similar finding led another group of investigators to conclude that downregulation of cardiac autonomic activity during both extended wakefulness and subsequent sleep may provide protection and recovery, respectively, from the temporal extension of cardiac demand (6). However, heart rate was progressively increased in rats deprived of total sleep (7) and REM sleep (8) using the disk-over-water method. In addition, following 114 hr of REM sleep deprivation, normotensive rats showed an increase in waking heart rate and systolic blood pressure (9). Interestingly, REM sleep deprivation induced sustained hypertension only in rats with a partial, rather than total, genetic predisposition to developing hypertension (10).

Lower urinary norepinephrine and heart variability at rest were found for workers with longer working hours compared to those with shorter working hours in a field survey of engineers, prompting the investigators to conclude that the long working hours might lower sympathetic nervous system activity due to chronic sleep deprivation (11). Sleep deprivation appears to markedly disturb or even obliterate the circadian rhythms of cardiovascular variables and urinary norepinephrine excretion (12,13). However, not all studies report a change in heart rate or catecholamine levels with sleep deprivation (14–16). The fact that sleep deprivation results in increased resting blood pressure, decreased muscle sympathetic nerve activity, but no change in heart rate in some studies suggests that the pressor response to sleep deprivation may not be mediated by muscle sympathetic vasoconstriction or tachycardia (16).

B. Respiratory Effects

Several independent studies showed that sleep deprivation results in a significant deterioration in ventilatory performance, as measured by indices such as forced vital capacity, maximal voluntary ventilation, maximal static inspiratory/expiratory pressures, peak CO_2 production, and peak O_2 consumption, and time to exhaustion with exercise (17–20). Sleep deprivation may have a role in progressive respiratory insufficiency in acutely ill patients, who are frequently sleep deprived. This hypothesis is supported by the majority of studies demonstrating that sleep deprivation is associated with a reduction of ventilatory drive (17,21–23); however, one study (76) found dissimilar results.

Sleep deprivation can similarly induce or worsen nocturnal respiratory disturbances. The pathogenesis of this disturbance may be due to inadequate activation of the genioglossus muscle, since sleep deprivation selectively decreases genioglossal electromyographic activity during CO_2 rebreathing in awake older subjects (25). A 24-hr period of prior sleep deprivation also significantly worsened the minimal arterial hemoglobin desaturation and increased the duration of obstruction, the rate at which obstruction could be induced, and the peak negative inspiratory effort at arousal in chronically instrumented tracheostomized dogs in response to repetitive airway obstruction during sleep (26). Sleep deprivation also resulted in significant periodic decrements in ventilation during recovery REM sleep; studies on the effects of acute sleep deprivation on control of diaphragm activity during recovery REM sleep suggested that respiratory control mechanisms in REM sleep are sensitive to the effects of prior sleep deprivation (27).

Fragmentation of sleep also leads to upper airway collapsibility, to a degree that may be more frequent than that observed with sleep deprivation (28). Arousal responses to respiratory stimuli are decreased by sleep fragmentation, as shown by studies on the effects of sleep fragmentation by acoustic stimuli on arousal and ventilatory responses to hyperoxic hypercapnia, isocapnic hypoxia, and chemical stimulation of the larynx during sleep in dogs (29). The arousal response may be dependent on sleep state, irrespective of prior sleep deprivation, since the pattern of a brisker arousal response during REM than NREM sleep to external inspiratory resistive loading reported in normal subjects was also found in healthy subjects who had undergone short-term sleep fragmentation (30).

Studies of sleep-deprived infants and young animals provide some clues to sudden infant death syndrome. In 3-month old healthy infants, investigators found that peripheral chemoresponsiveness increased in magnitude, and respiratory control and the timing of baseline breathing were altered, without any detectable alteration in arousal propensity during short-term sleep deprivation (31). The investigators theorized that this state might be associated with an increased vulnerability to obstructive respiratory events. Another study showed that short-term sleep deprivation in healthy full-term infants resulted in an increased number and timing of respiratory events, particularly obstructive events in active, or REM, sleep (32). A study of the effects of 24-hr sleep deprivation in newborn lambs revealed increased apneas (33), suggesting that the consequences of sleep deprivation upon respiration occur early after birth.

Investigators have studied the effects of sleep deprivation on other respiratory conditions. Ventilatory responses to bronchoconstriction were not impaired by sleep deprivation, except in increasing the subsequent arousal threshold (34). Although sleep loss was also associated with significant decrements in some spirometric performance measures in patients with severe chronic obstructive pulmonary disease, the investigators felt that a single night's loss of sleep in the patient with stable chronic airflow obstruction does not have major clinical consequences (35). Using a rat model of asthma, investigators found that REM sleep contributed to nocturnal asthma, possibly due to an alteration of sympathetic nervous function (36).

C. Gastrointestinal Effects

A significant increase in food intake coupled with a paradoxical decrease in body weight was observed in rats deprived of either total sleep or REM sleep by the disk-over-water method (37). Further investigation revealed that although diet composition affected the time course and development of pathology associated with total or REM sleep deprivation, it exerted negligible effects on body weight regulation (38).

Studies on the proliferative and functional units of the jejunum of Syrian hamsters revealed that peak values in kinetic parameters were significantly reduced with sleep loss (39). In addition, sleep deprivation resulted in lowering the gastric mucosal barrier and stimulated the expression of inducible heat shock protein 70 in the gastric mucosa of rats (40). These studies may provide an explanation for the gastric lesions noted in several studies of sleep-deprived rats (7,8,41). Although similar lesions have not been reported in sleep deprivation studies in humans, poor sleep was reported to result in increased gastrointestinal symptoms the following day among women with irritable bowel syndrome (42).

D. Renal Effects

Charloux and colleagues (43) found the following during a 24-hr period of sleep deprivation compared to normal sleep in human subjects: (a) lower plasma levels and pulse amplitude in the 23:00– to 07:00-hr period; (b) reduced levels and lower pulse frequency and amplitude of plasma renin activity; and (c) slightly enhanced plasma cortisol levels. Diuresis, kaliuresis, and plasma potassium and sodium levels were not affected, but natriuresis significantly increased during sleep deprivation. The investigators concluded that sleep deprivation modifies the 24-hr aldosterone profile by preventing the nocturnal increase in aldosterone release; this leads to altered overnight hydromineral balance.

E. Integumentary Effects

A debilitated appearance coupled with severe ulcerative and keratotic skin lesions on the tails and plantar surface of the paws were observed in rats deprived of total and REM sleep (44). The cause of these pathologic changes could not be explained. Impairment of the cellular or biomechanical mechanisms of tissue repair did not contribute to these changes; a study by Landis and Whitney (45) found no evidence for this hypothesis in rats sleep deprived for 72 hr. Interestingly, in a study on healthy women, sleep deprivation decreased skin barrier function recovery and increased plasma interleukin-1β tumor necrosis factor-α and natural killer cell activity (46).

III. Neurophysiological or Psychological Effects of Sleep Deprivation

Many parameters have been measured following sleep deprivation; however, few are considered "neurophysiological." There is a significant amount of human and animal literature describing the effect of sleep deprivation on psychological and performance measures, including learning and memory; however, these measures are not neurophysiological and therefore are not described in this chapter. (They are discussed in Chaps. 11 and 12.)

Among the neurophysiological measures, the electroencephalogram and thermoregulation are the two most extensively studied neurophysiological measures during and following total and selective sleep deprivation both in humans and animals. Both parameters are appropriate measures of brain function and are sensitive to changes in the cerebral performance. In addition, these measures have shown consistent changes within and across species following sleep deprivation. In fact, it is the EEG that defines sleep, and sleep is necessary for appropriate thermoregulation (47). However, it is important to note that the EEG is a reflection of various underlying neurophysiological processes of which many are still unknown. Likewise, we do not know all the neural mechanisms controlling thermoregulation.

Other neurophysiological parameters measured following sleep deprivation include, in animals, the discharge activities of single unit in vivo and long-term potentiation (LTP) in vitro and, in humans, cerebral functioning by positron emission tomography (PET) and functional magnetic resonance imaging (fMRI).

IV. Total Sleep Deprivation

A. Human Studies

In a typical total sleep deprivation experiment, the subject is kept continuously awake throughout the duration of the experiment. However, it is very difficult to conduct sleep deprivation in inactive subjects, as they tend to fall asleep. Therefore, the subjects have to be kept continuously active and this brings in the issue of stress, one of the most debated and controversial topics in sleep deprivation research. The detailed discussion of stress and sleep deprivation is beyond the scope of this chapter; however, the interested reader is referred to excellent reviews by Horne (47,49,50) and Rechtschaffen (51–53) (see also Chap. 5).

Effects of Total Sleep Deprivation on the Electroencephalogram

Human sleep deprivation research has a history of more than 100 years. Thus, it is not surprising that human sleep deprivation has been the topic of many reviews. After perusing some of the reviews (47,54–57) one can easily conclude that the brain is the most affected organ during and after sleep deprivation, and that the EEG is among the most extensively used neurophysiological measure to understand the effects of sleep deprivation in the functioning of the brain in human subjects.

It is common knowledge that sleep deprivation causes increased sleepiness (increased propensity to sleep). The increased sleepiness or the "sleep pressure" is manifested in the waking EEG during sleep deprivation and, if the human subject is allowed to go to sleep, he or she has a tendency to recover lost sleep (otherwise known as recovery or rebound sleep). Thus, sleep deprivation is a simple approach to evoke the neurophysiological processes involved in sleep regulation, and the analysis of the EEG during and following sleep deprivation may lead us to understand the function as well as the regulation of sleep.

An early study (58) reported that total sleep deprivation caused a progressive reduction in alpha activity (8–12 Hz), a known correlate of relaxed wakefulness. Since then, many investigators have confirmed this finding [reviewed in (47)]. In fact, Johnson et al. (59) reported a complete loss of alpha activity following 240 hr of sleep deprivation and the authors ascribed the reduction in alpha activity as an indicator of increased sleepiness/drowsiness. Electroencephalographic spectral analysis [fast Fourier transformation (FFT) of the EEG, which converts the electroencephalographic data from the time domain to the frequency domain] also confirmed this effect. Naitoh et al. (60,61) reported a substantial reduction in the absolute and relative (percent of total EEG) alpha activity during 204 hr of sleep deprivation. Although there was no change in absolute delta and theta activity, increases in relative delta and theta were observed (62). In another study, Lorenzo et al. (63) also reported a decrease in alpha power with 40 hr of total sleep deprivation.

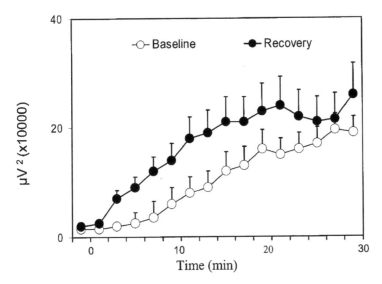

Figure 1   Increase in slow-wave activity during first 30 min of recovery sleep following total sleep deprivation. (Modified from Ref. 16.)

In recent years, the effect of sleep deprivation on the EEG has mainly focused on delta activity. Moderate sleep deprivation of 40 hr or less enhances delta activity during recovery sleep (62,64–66) (Fig. 1).

It has been suggested that a direct correlation exists between the amount of time spent in prior wakefulness and the increase in the delta activity, along with the reduction in spindle activity that occurs during postdeprivation sleep (66). Deep insights into our understanding of the homeostatic regulation of sleep were obtained by studying the effects of total sleep deprivation on the EEG both in humans and in animals (67) (see also Chap. 24).

With regard to EEG evoked responses, Miszczak and Zuzewicz (68) evaluated the effects of 24-hr sleep deprivation on visual evoked potentials in normal healthy adults and reported a rise in the P3–N4 amplitude, whereas 18 hours of sleep deprivation caused a decrease in P3 amplitude and an increase in P3 latency (69). Furthermore, sleep deprivation is also known to decrease the amplitude of the contingent negative variation (CNV) (70,71). The CNV is the brain wave associated with stimulus expectancy (72).

Total sleep deprivation is also known to enhance paroxysmal activity in subjects with a predisposition to epilepsy. Although this effect is rarely observed in normal healthy humans, grand mal seizures have been reported in healthy subjects following total sleep deprivation extending beyond 48–72 hr (73,74).

In summary:

1. One of the most prominent effects of total sleep deprivation in humans is the buildup of sleep pressure or increased propensity to sleep. This increased sleepiness is manifested in the EEG as a buildup of delta activity. If the subject is allowed to sleep after deprivation, there is a rebound of NREM sleep accompanied by increased delta power.
2. Total sleep deprivation in humans decreases alpha activity; however, the underlying mechanism for this increase is unknown.

Effects of Total Sleep Deprivation on Thermoregulation (See Also Chap. 15)

Thermoregulation is an important mechanism by which endotherms, with high metabolic rate, minimize heat loss and conserve energy, and it has been suggested that the primordial function of sleep is energy conservation (48). Resting body temperature is one of the measures by which the thermoregulation of the subject can be evaluated, especially in a thermoneutral environment (defined as the range of ambient temperature within which the metabolic rate is at a minimum and within which temperature regulation, i.e., a stable core temperature, is achieved by nonevaporative physical processes alone). Thus, monitoring the effect of sleep deprivation on body temperature is one of the mechanisms by which we can understand the role of sleep in thermoregulation.

Patrick and Gilbert (75) were the first to report a gradual decrease in the oral temperature during 60 hr of sleep deprivation in humans. Since this initial total sleep deprivation study, several groups have replicated and confirmed the effect of total sleep deprivation on oral temperature [reviewed in (47,57)].

In most cases, sleep deprivation is accompanied by a decrease in body temperature (75–80). However, there are some studies that suggest either an increase or no change in body temperature (63,81). In fact, Naitoh et al. (61) found an initial reduction in oral temperature but a subsequent increase after 70 hr of total sleep deprivation. Whereas Johnson et al. (59) found a reduction in skin temperature, Kreider (82) and Kolka (83,84) found no change in skin temperature. In the case of rectal temperature, Kreider (82) reported a decrease, whereas Savourey and Bittel (85) found no change. Although there is a change in the temperature, the circadian temperature rhythm does not show any change following total sleep deprivation in humans [reviewed in [47,57]].

Temperature is one measure of thermoregulation that has been extensively studied in human sleep deprivation. However, other parameters of thermoregulation, including measurement of sweating during exercise following total sleep deprivation, have also been studied. Kolka and Stevenson (83) reported no change in esophageal temperature at which the onset of sweating occurred; however, the esophageal temperature threshold for sweating tended to be lower. In contrast, Dewasmes et al. (86) observed an increase in the esophageal temperature threshold for the onset of both chest and thigh sweating after 27 hr of sleep deprivation. In addition, Swaka et al. (87) reported a significant loss of dry and evaporative heat during exercise in sleep-deprived subjects along with a drop in resting core temperature. Fiorica et al. (88) did not find any change in the body temperature during sleep deprivation accompanied with cold exposure, whereas Savourey and Bittel (85) reported an increase in mean skin temperature along with an increase in metabolic heat production during sleep deprivation in a cold environment.

In summary, based on the studies described above, it is safe to assume that sleep deprivation impairs thermoregulation with a significant decrease in the body temperature.

Total Sleep Deprivation in Humans: Neuroimaging Studies

In recent years, the effects of sleep deprivation on brain functioning have been examined by neuroimaging techniques. These techniques provide a direct noninvasive method to study the effect of sleep deprivation on cerebral functioning during various tasks including attention and learning. These studies have utilized PET (89,90) and fMRI techniques (91,92). While Portas et al. (91) reported increased activation of the thalamus after a short-term attention task that followed sleep deprivation, both PET studies (91,92) reported a decrease in the global levels of glucose metabolism and a decreased activation in attention and arousal-related brain regions following sleep deprivation. Furthermore, Drummond et al. (92) reported a compensatory activation of the prefrontal cortex and the parietal lobes during verbal learning following 35 hr of total sleep deprivation.

These are only a few studies and it is difficult to draw firm conclusions. However, imaging techniques have tremendous potential and will be very helpful in our quest to understand the regulation and the function of sleep.

B. Animal Studies (See Also Chap. 3)

Like the human sleep deprivation research, sleep deprivation research in animals has a long history and began around the same time as human sleep deprivation research, in the late nineteenth century. During the last 100 years or so, various animal models have been used to study the effects of sleep deprivation with the rat being the animal of choice.

Animal research has contributed tremendously to our understanding of sleep and the sleep processes. In fact, it is from the animal studies that we know that sleep is essential for life and that long-term deprivation leads to the death of the animal (51). Animal studies offer the advantage of using invasive techniques, which is not possible in human subjects. For example, the effect of sleep deprivation on a particular region of the brain can be measured by monitoring the discharge activity of the neurons in vivo before, during, and after sleep deprivation. However, only a few studies have used invasive techniques in animals and monitored neuronal activity in vivo or in vitro following sleep deprivation. Therefore, the EEG has remained the most used parameter for measuring the neurophysiological effects of sleep deprivation.

Effects of Total Sleep Deprivation on the Electroencephalogram

The major changes seen in the EEG following total sleep deprivation are similar among various animal species, including humans. However, there is one major difference observed between humans and animals following total sleep deprivation. Humans show a preferential NREM sleep rebound following total sleep deprivation (discussed in detail above) whereas more that 12 hr of sleep deprivation in animals results first in a large REM sleep rebound although increases in NREM are also observed (93) (Fig. 2). This phenomenon has been observed in various animals, including mice, rats, cats, rabbits, and pigs, and has been confirmed by many investigators (94–112). However, fewer than 12 hr of sleep deprivation does not result in a significant REM sleep rebound in rats (103).

Total sleep deprivation in animals causes a buildup of delta or slow-wave activity similar to what is observed in humans. It has been suggested that the buildup of "sleep pressure" during sleep deprivation is the manifestation of the buildup of delta activity during sleep deprivation. Borbely and his group have elegantly shown this phenomenon in various mammalian species, including humans (113). In fact, animal sleep deprivation studies have provided a great insight into our understanding of the homeostatic regulation of sleep (108). In terms of devel-

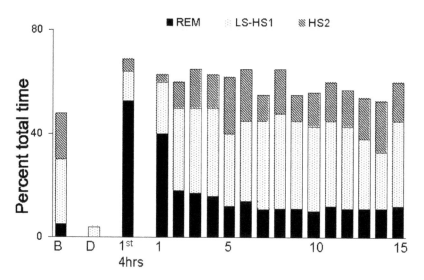

Figure 2 Total sleep deprivation (19 days) causes a large REM rebound during recovery sleep. Sleep stages values as percentage of total time for the mean of baseline days (B), mean of deprivation days (D), first 4 hr of recovery, and each of the first 15 days of recovery sleep are shown. NREM sleep is subdivided into NREM sleep with high EEG amplitude (HS2) and NREM sleep with low and moderate EEG amplitude (LS-HS1). (Modified from Ref. 47.)

opment, neonatal rats (12–14 days old) do not show an increase in slow-wave activity following 3 hr of total sleep deprivation (114), whereas aged rats show a reduced increase in slow-wave activity following 12 hr of sleep deprivation (115). Other data suggest that the homeostatic regulation of sleep is under genetic control (116).

In addition to an increase in delta activity, increase in the amplitude of theta activity is also observed during REM sleep following total sleep deprivation. In fact, Kiyono et al. (94) reported a shift in the theta frequency in the hippocamapal EEG. Lancel et al. (117) obtained EEGs from various subcortical structures including the hippocampus, amygdala and the hypothalamus, and reported increases in the electroencephalographic power density in the delta and theta frequencies during recovery sleep following 12 hr of total sleep deprivation in cats.

The availability of knockout mice has made it possible to study the effects of sleep deprivation on mice lacking a gene. Kopp et al. (118) investigated the effects of 6 hr of total sleep deprivation in mice lacking mPer1 or mPer2 genes. The mPer1 and mPer2 gene products are thought to contribute to the resetting of the circadian clock by light. Sleep deprivation caused an increase in slow-wave activity in NREM sleep for both the mPer1 and the mPer2 knockout mice, suggesting that the homeostatic regulation of sleep was independent of circadian regulation (118).

Antisense technology is another technique used in sleep research to selectively and transiently "knockout" a single gene. The antisense technology is highly specific for receptor subtype, providing a localized, reversible receptor "knock-down," and had been successfully used in many fields including sleep-wakefulness (119). To test the hypothesis of adenosine A1 receptor control of the homeostatic regulation of sleep, the authors employed microdialysis perfusion of antisense oligonucleotides against the mRNA of the A1 receptor in the magnocellular region of the basal forebrain of freely behaving rats. Local perfusion of A1 receptor antisense in the basal forebrain caused a significant decrease in NREM sleep both during spontaneous bouts of sleep-wakefulness and during recovery sleep following 6 hr of sleep deprivation. These data support the hypothesis that adenosine, acting via the A1 receptor, is a key component in the homeostatic regulation of sleep (120) (Fig. 3).

In summary, total sleep deprivation of more than 24 hr causes an initial increase in REM rebound in animals. In contrast, total sleep deprivation in humans shows an initial NREM sleep rebound. The buildup of delta activity during total sleep deprivation is a common phenomenon observed in almost all mammalian species including humans.

Effects of Total Sleep Deprivation on Thermoregulation (See Also Chap. 15)

The first animal sleep deprivation was carried out by Manacéine (121) who found that puppies showed marked hypothermia and died after 92–143 hr of total sleep deprivation. Subsequently, Tarrozi (122) found similar results with total sleep

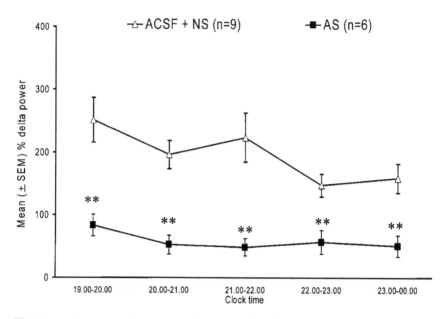

Figure 3 Electroencephalographic delta power (1–4 Hz, Mean ± SEM) following sleep deprivation, expressed as a percentage of each animal's delta power during the same time period on a nondeprivation day (previous day). There was a significant decrease in the delta activity in antisense (antisense oligonucleotides against the mRNA of the adenosine A1 receptor) treated animals (solid squares) during all 5 hr of recovery sleep as compared to the pooled [ACSF (artificial cerebrospinal fluid) and nonsense] controls (open triangles). (Modified from Ref. 74.)

deprivation in dogs. Sleep deprivation studies in rabbits showed a decrease in body temperature (123). However, Legendre (124) and Kleitman (78) did not find any significant change in the body temperature following total sleep deprivation in puppies.

Using the disk-over-water method of sleep deprivation, Rechtschaffen and his colleagues carried out the longest and the most elaborate sleep deprivation studies in animals (reviewed in 51,53,125) (see also Chaps. 4 and 5). The sleep deprivation apparatus consisted of an experimental rat and a yoked control rat, housed on the opposite sides of a divided disk suspended over water. A computer controlled the rotation of the disk, and whenever the experimental rat entered a "forbidden" sleep stage, the disk was automatically rotated, forcing the experimental rat to walk to avoid being carried into the water. The yoked control rat received the same physical stimulation but was allowed to sleep (126). Using this technique, total and selective sleep deprivation was carried out for several weeks or until the animals died (51,97). No other sleep deprivation study in rats has been continued for so long and/or provided such detailed information, especially about the effect of sleep deprivation on thermoregulation and energy metabolism (53). One of the major findings of these studies was that sleep deprivation (total or selective) causes an initial rise in the body temperature followed by a subsequent decline in the body temperature (97,127). This led the authors to suggest that hypothermia may be the primary cause of death in these animals (51,53). The initial increase in the body temperature during total sleep deprivation appeared to be caused by an increase in the temperature set point (128) and large increases in the energy expenditure, leading the authors to suggest that excessive heat loss might be the primary cause for the late decline in the body temperature (51,53). In addition, as the deprivation progressed, the sleep-deprived rats chose higher ambient temperatures. The authors used various strategies including blockade of prostaglandin synthesis (129), opioid antagonism (130), thyroxine administration (131), and lesions of the preoptic hypothalamus (132) to identify the underlying causes of sleep deprivation-induced impairment in thermoregulation. However, none of the strategies provided a clear picture. If the animals were allowed to recover sleep, the body temperature quickly normalized. The data obtained from these studies led the authors to suggest that the increases in temperature during early periods of total sleep deprivation were due to the loss of NREM sleep, whereas the heat loss and decline in the body temperature in the later stages were due to the loss of REM sleep.

Several investigators have studied the effects of short-term (less than 24 hr) sleep deprivation on temperature and thermoregulation. Increases in the cortical temperature during 24 hr of total sleep deprivation and decreases during recovery sleep have also been reported (105,106). In addition, the same authors observed a negative correlation between cortical temperature and NREM sleep; however, there was no correlation between slow wave activity and cortical temperature (106). Tobler et al. (133) carried out 3 hr of total sleep deprivation in rats at two different temperatures and found that the rise in brain temperature was higher in animals that were sleep deprived at a higher ambient temperature. Hansen and Kruger (134) did not find any effect of vagotomy on the increases in the brain temperature during 6 hr of total sleep deprivation.

The effect of total sleep deprivation on thermoregulation is clear. Short-term sleep deprivation causes an increase in the body temperature whereas long-term sleep deprivation eventually causes hypothermia, supporting the hypothesis that one of the functions of sleep is to control and regulate thermoregulation.

Effects of Total Sleep Deprivation on In Vivo and In Vitro Studies of Neuronal Activity

One study (135) monitored the effects of 24-hr sleep deprivation on the discharge activity of dorsal raphe neurons in vivo in freely behaving cats, and found an overall increase in the discharge activity of dorsal raphe neurons during the sleep deprivation period with the maximal effect observed after 15 hr of sleep deprivation. Campbell et al. (136) investigated the effect of total sleep deprivation (12 hr) on neuronal plasticity and found a significant decrease in hippocampal LTP in sleep-deprived rats, suggesting that sleep deprivation impairs neuronal plasticity. Unfortunately, these are the only studies where neuronal discharge activity has been measured following sleep deprivation. Clearly, more in vitro and in vivo studies are needed to fully understand the effects of sleep deprivation at the cellular level.

C. Total Sleep Deprivation: Summary

Based on the review of the literature, we can summarize the effects of total sleep deprivation:

1. Total sleep deprivation builds up sleep pressure (increases sleepiness), and this buildup is reflected in a buildup of delta activity in the EEG.
2. The buildup of delta activity during sleep deprivation is a manifestation of the homeostatic regulation of sleep. Adenosine and its A1 receptor may have a key role in the homeostatic control of sleep.
3. Total sleep deprivation impairs the thermoregulatory process in both humans and animals. However, this effect has not been so prominent in human studies, due to the absence of long-term sleep deprivation.

V. REM Sleep Deprivation (See Also Chap. 5)

Since the discovery of REM sleep and its links to dreaming, REM sleep and the effects of REM sleep deprivation have been extensively studied. There is a large literature base, both human and animal, describing the effects of REM sleep deprivation on various psychological, behavioral, biochemical, and performance measures, including the effects on learning and memory. However, compared to total sleep deprivation, only a handful of studies have monitored the effects of REM sleep deprivation on the neurophysiology of the nervous system (49,51,137–139).

To conduct selective REM sleep deprivation in humans is simple. The EEG of the human subject is closely monitored, and as soon as the subject appears to enter into REM sleep, he or she is awakened. This is known as the arousal technique, and it has been sparingly used in animals because the number of arousals required to conduct long-term REM sleep deprivation becomes very large (137).

The inverted flower pot technique is commonly used to conduct REM sleep deprivation in animals (140–143). The animal is placed on a small platform surrounded by water. Selective REM sleep deprivation occurs because the animal is unable to maintain the posture during REM sleep (due to the muscle atonia) and is awakened by falling into the water (137). Thus, the inverted flower pot technique is a simple, efficient, and easy method for REM sleep deprivation in animals. However, it has been suggested that this technique is confounded by various "stresses." We will not go into details about the pros and cons of the inverted flower pot technique, but rather point the interested reader to various reviews (50,51,53,137,144) (see also Chap 5).

A. Neurophysiological Effects of REM Sleep Deprivation in Humans

In humans, selective REM sleep deprivation is achieved by awakening the subject as soon as he or she enters into REM sleep, and the most significant effect observed with selective REM sleep deprivation is that, as REM sleep deprivation progresses, there is an increase in the frequency of interruption required to awaken the subject from REM sleep (145–149) (Fig. 4). During three nights of selective REM sleep deprivation, the number of interruptions required to awaken the subject from REM sleep on the third night were significantly greater than the number of interruptions required during the first night of selective REM sleep deprivation (149). It appears that selective REM sleep deprivation causes a buildup of REM sleep pressure. However, if the subject is allowed to go for recovery sleep following selective REM sleep deprivation, the REM rebound that follows is limited [reviewed in (50); see also Chap. 5]. In fact, Endo et al. (149) observed REM rebound only during the first night of recovery sleep, though selective REM sleep deprivation was carried out for three nights.

With regard to spectral analysis of the EEG, studies have found a selective decrease in alpha power during REM rebound (149,150). One study reported an increase in cortical excitability in humans following REM sleep deprivation (151).

Based on the studies described above, we can conclude that REM sleep deprivation causes a buildup of REM sleep pressure, and, following REM sleep deprivation, there is a limited REM rebound. Thus, REM sleep may also be under homeostatic control.

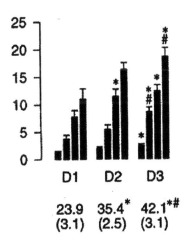

Figure 4 Increase in the number of interruptions required to prevent the subject from entering into REM sleep during REM sleep deprivation, suggesting that the REM sleep is under homeostatic control. Each bar represents mean values of consecutive 2–hr intervals. Numerical values at bottom of figure indicate the average number of sleep interruptions per night (standard error in parentheses; $n = 8$) (D = REM deprivation day; * significant difference from corresponding D1 value; # significant difference from corresponding D2 value). (Modified from Ref. 103.)

B. Neurophysiological Effects of REM Sleep Deprivation in Animals

Early studies done by Dement and co-workers (152–155) suggested that REM sleep deprivation decreased the electrical threshold for waking seizures. A subsequent study confirmed these effects of REM sleep deprivation (156). Dewson et al. (157) reported that REM sleep deprivation facilitated recovery of cortical potentials evoked by auditory stimuli, whereas van Huzlen (158) reported a decrement in the P3–N3 amplitude of the photically evoked response in the visual cortex after 72 hr of REM sleep deprivation in rats. Increases in paleocortical excitability and decreases in the primary sensory afferent pathway, as measured by evoked potentials, were also observed after REM sleep deprivation in cats (159). Thus, along with an increase in cortical excitability, REM sleep deprivation also caused an inhibition of the peripheral stimuli (159) and a reduction in auditory-evoked inhibition (160). In addition, REM sleep deprivation caused increases in the discharge activity of REM-on neurons (neurons with highest discharge during REM sleep), while the discharge activity of presumed noradrenergic REM-off neurons (neurons that are silent during REM sleep) decreases (161). In this study, single units were recorded from the pontine reticular formation in freely behaving animals (161).

There is only one in vitro study following REM sleep deprivation. Shaffery et al. (162) tested the effects of REM suppression on synaptic plasticity in the visual system. The authors used a developmentally regulated type of LTP to measure synaptic plasticity and reported that developmentally regulated LTP could be induced in REM sleep-deprived rats but not in control animals, implicating the importance of REM sleep in brain maturation (162). With regards to the effect of REM sleep deprivation on the EEG, there is an increase in the absolute and relative power in the theta band (7–9 Hz), and a decrease in the delta band relative power during REM sleep deprivation in rats (163).

Most of the studies described above utilized the flower pot technique (or a modified version) to perform REM sleep deprivation. There are few reports, described below, in which REM sleep deprivation was carried out with different techniques.

Using the arousal technique, increases in REM sleep pressure, as reflected by increases in the number of arousals required to prevent REM sleep during REM sleep deprivation and REM sleep rebound indicative of REM sleep homeostasis, have been reported in rats (109,164,165). In addition, REM sleep deprivation suppresses slow-wave activity in NREM sleep, suggesting that increased propensity to REM sleep inhibits slow-wave activity in NREM sleep (109).

Using the disk-over-water technique, Kushida et al. (138) performed selective REM sleep deprivation in rats and found that long-term REM sleep deprivation (16–54 days) led to death, indicating that REM sleep is vital for life. If the animals were allowed to recover, a huge and immediate REM sleep rebound was observed. Selective REM sleep deprivation caused a significant decrease in the body temperature during the course of REM sleep deprivation. However, the decline in intraperitoneal temperature during NREM sleep diminished as REM deprivation progressed and eventually began to rise above the wakefulness values during the final stages of REM sleep deprivation (166). The authors attributed excess heat loss caused by selective REM sleep deprivation as a probable cause for the decline in the body temperature during REM sleep deprivation (51).

To conclude, REM sleep deprivation studies in animals suggest that REM sleep is essential to life and long-term REM sleep deprivation leads to death. Furthermore, REM sleep deprivation increases cortical excitability, increases theta power, and decreases body temperature. In addition, a buildup of REM pressure and REM rebound following REM sleep deprivation suggest that REM sleep may be homeostatically regulated.

C. REM Sleep Deprivation: Summary

1. REM sleep deprivation does not cause any major impairment in humans. However, long-term REM sleep deprivation results in the death of the animals.
2. Both human and animal literature suggests that REM sleep may be homeostatically regulated. This is manifested by an increase in the number of interruptions required to awaken the subject from REM sleep during REM sleep deprivation.
3. Long-term REM sleep deprivation impairs thermoregulatory processes.

VI. Selective NREM Sleep Deprivation

Selective NREM sleep deprivation has been conducted in humans and animals (one single study), and its effects on the functioning of the central nervous system has been investigated. Although there are only a handful of studies, the results are interesting.

A. Neurophysiological Effects of NREM Sleep Deprivation in Humans

In almost all human studies, selective NREM sleep deprivation was carried out using delta activity of the EEG as a marker and an auditory stimulus to arouse the subjects. Thus, in these studies, subjects are not deprived of NREM sleep in entirety; instead, a component of NREM sleep was targeted. Thus, we have used the term selective slow-wave sleep (SWS) delta deprivation.

Lentz et al. (167) conducted selective SWS deprivation and reported decreased pain threshold, whereas Arima et al. (168) did not find any effect on nocturnal jaw-muscle activity and pain-pressure threshold following selective SWS deprivation.

Ferara et al. (169) measured auditory arousal threshold during recovery sleep following selective SWS deprivation and observed an increase in auditory arousal threshold during recovery sleep. The authors concluded that auditory arousal threshold is a reliable index of sleep depth. De Gannaro et al. (170) measured spindle activity in ten subjects during recovery sleep following selective SWS deprivation and reported a reduction of NREM stage 2 in recovery sleep.

Based on these few studies, it is difficult to clearly understand the effects of selective SWS deprivation. However, selective SWS sleep deprivation studies are important and may provide us with insights into the functions of individual stages of NREM sleep.

B. Neurophysiological Effects of NREM Sleep Deprivation in Animals

We found only one animal study in which selective NREM sleep deprivation was performed. Gilliand et al. (171) conducted long-term (23–66 days) selective high-amplitude NREM sleep deprivation in rats by using the disk-over-water method and found that selective NREM sleep deprivation led to death. However, the animals deprived of high-amplitude NREM sleep did not show large decreases in body temperature except at the end (51).

Based on this one study, we can conclude that selective deprivation of high-amplitude NREM sleep also leads to death, further supporting the idea that sleep is necessary for normal life. There is a clear need for more research with selective sleep deprivation to understand the effects of each individual sleep state on the neurophysiology of the brain.

VII.   Conclusions

1. Both NREM and REM sleep are necessary for life.
2. Sleep deprivation, be it total or selective, affects the normal functioning of the brain. The neurophysiological effects of sleep deprivation are most pronounced on thermoregulatory mechanisms.
3. Finally, sleep deprivation studies have provided tremendous insight into our understanding of sleep and sleep processes; however, more research focused on the neurophysiological measures, especially with new and innovative techniques, is necessary and critical to fully understand the functions of sleep.

References

1. Ayas NT, White DP, Manson JE, Stampfer MJ, Speizer FE, Malhotra A, Hu FB. A prospective study of sleep duration and coronary heart disease in women. Arch Intern Med 2003; 163(2):205–209.

2. Lusardi P, Zoppi A, Preti P, Pesce RM, Piazza E, Forari R. Effects of insufficient sleep on blood pressure in hypertensive patients. Am J Hypertens 1999; 12:63–68.

3. Tochikubo O, Ikeda A., Miyajima E, Ishii M. Effects of insufficient sleep on blood pressure monitored by a new multibiomedical recorder. Hypertension 1996;27:1318–1324.

4. Lusardi P, Mugellini A, Preti P, Zoppi A, Derosa G, Fogari R. Effects of a restricted sleep regimen on ambulatory blood pressure monitoring in normotensive subjects. Am J Hypertens 1996; 9:503–505.

5. Chen HI. Effects of 30-h sleep loss on cardiorespiratory functions at rest and in exercise. Med Sci Sports Exerc 1991; 23(2):193–198.

6. Holmes AL, Burgess HJ, Dawson D. Effects of sleep pressure on endogenous cardiac autonomic activity and body temperature. J Appl Physiol 2002; 92(6):2578–2584.

7. Kushida CA, Bergmann BM, Rechtschaffen A. Sleep deprivation in the rat: IV. Paradoxical sleep deprivation. Sleep 1989; 12(1):22–30.

8. Everson CA, Bergmann BM, Rechtschaffen A. Sleep deprivation in the rat: III. Total sleep deprivation. Sleep 1989; 12(1):13–21.

9. DeMesquita S, Hale GA. Cardiopulmonary regulation after rapid-eye-movement sleep deprivation. J Appl Physiol 1992; 72(3):970–976.

10. Neves FA, Marson O, Baumgratz RP, Bossolan D, Ginosa M, Ribeiro AB, Kohlmann O Jr, Ramos OL. Rapid eye movement sleep deprivation and hypertension. Genetic influence. Hypertension 1992; 19(2 suppl):II202–206.

11. Sasaki T, Iwasaki K, Oka T, Hisanaga N, Ueda T, Takada Y, Fujiki Y. Effect of working hours on cardiovascular-autonomic nervous functions in engineers in an electronics manufacturing company. Ind Health 1999; 37(1):55–61.

12. Viola AU, Simon C, Ehrhart J, Geny B, Piquard F, Muzet A, Brandenberger G. Sleep processes exert a predominant influence on the 24-h profile of heart rate variability. J Biol Rhythms 2002; 17(6):539–547.

13. Ahnve S, Theorell T, Akerstedt T, Froberg JE, Halberg F. Circadian variations in cardiovascular parameters during sleep deprivation. A noninvasive study of young healthy men. Eur J Appl Physiol Occup Physiol 1981; 46(1):9–19.

14. Martin BJ, Chen H. Sleep loss and the sympathoadrenal rexponse to exercise. Med Sci Sports Exerc 1984; 16:56–59.

15. Fiorica V, Higgins EA, Iamplietro PF, Lategola MT, Davis AW. Physiological responses of men during sleep deprivation. J Appl Physiol 1968; 24:167–176.

16. Kato M, Phillips BG, Sigurdsson F, Narkiewicz K, Pesek CA, Somers VK. Effects of sleep deprivation on neural circulatory control. Hypertension 2000; 35:1173–1175.

17. Cooper KR, Phillips BA. Effect of short-term sleep loss on breathing. J Appl Physiol 1982; 53(4):855–858.

18. Chen HI. Effects of 30-h sleep loss on cardiorespiratory functions at rest and in exercise. Med Sci Sports Exerc 1991; 23(2):193–198.

19. Keeling WF, Martin BJ. Supine position and sleep loss each reduce prolonged maximal voluntary ventilation. Respiration 1988; 54(2):119–126.

20. Chen HI, Tang YR. Sleep loss impairs inspiratory muscle endurance. Am Rev Respir Dis 1989; 140(4):907–909.

21. Schiffman PL, Trontell MC, Mazar MF, Edelman NH. Sleep deprivation decreases ventilatory response to CO_2 but not load compensation. Chest 1983; 84(6):695–698.

22. White DP, Douglas NJ, Pickett CK, Zwillich CW, Weil JV. Sleep deprivation and the control of ventilation. Am Rev Respir Dis 1983; 128(6):984–986.

23. Phillips B, Cooper KR, Newsome HH, Dewey WL. Effect of sleep loss on beta-endorphin activity, epinephrine levels, and ventilatory responsiveness. South Med J 1987; 80(1):16–20.

24. Spengler CM, Shea SA. Sleep deprivation per se does not decrease the hypercapnic ventilatory response in humans. Am J Respir Crit Care Med 2000; 161(4 Pt 1):1124–1128.

25. Leiter JC, Knuth SL, Bartlett D Jr. The effect of sleep deprivation on activity of the genioglossus muscle. Am Rev Respir Dis 1985; 132(6):1242–1245.

26. O'Donnell CP, King ED, Schwartz AR, Smith PL, Robotham JL. Effect of sleep deprivation on responses to airway obstruction in the sleeping dog. J Appl Physiol 1994; 77(4):1811–1818.

27. Veasey SC, Hendricks JC, Kline LR, Pack AI. Effects of acute sleep deprivation on control of the diaphragm during REM sleep in cats. J Appl Physiol 1993; 74(5):2253–2260.

28. Series F, Roy N, Marc I. Effects of sleep deprivation and sleep fragmentation on upper airway collapsibility in normal subjects. Am J Respir Crit Care Med 1994; 150(2):481–485.

29. Bowes G, Woolf GM, Sullivan CE, Phillipson EA. Effect of sleep fragmentation on ventilatory and arousal responses of sleeping dogs to respiratory stimuli. Am Rev Respir Dis 1980; 122(6):899–908.

30. Gugger M, Keller U, Mathis J. Arousal responses to inspiratory resistive loading during REM and non-REM sleep in normal men after short-term fragmentation/deprivation. Schweiz Med Wochenschr 1998; 128(18):696–702.

31. Thomas DA, Poole K, McArdle EK, Goodenough PC, Thompson J, Beardsmore CS, Simpson H. The effect of sleep deprivation on sleep states, breathing events, peripheral chemoresponsiveness and arousal propensity in healthy 3 month old infants. Eur Respir J 1996; 9(5):932–938.

32. Canet E, Gaultier C, D'Allest AM, Dehan M. Effects of sleep deprivation on respiratory events during sleep in healthy infants. J Appl Physiol 1989; 66(3):1158–1163.

33. Letourneau P, Niyonsenga T, Carrier E, Praud E, Praud JP. Influence of 24–hour sleep deprivation on respiration in lambs. Pediatr Res 2002; 52(5):697–705.

34. Ballard RD, Tan WC, Kelly PL, Pak J, Pandey R, Martin RJ. Effect of sleep and sleep deprivation on ventilatory response to bronchoconstriction. J Appl Physiol 1990; 69(2):490–497.

35. Phillips BA, Cooper KR, Burke TV. The effect of sleep loss on breathing in chronic obstructive pulmonary disease. Chest 1987; 91(1):29–32.

36. Irie M, Nagata S, Endo Y, Kobayashi F. Effect of rapid eye movement sleep deprivation on allergen-induced airway responses in a rat model of asthma. Int Arch Allergy Immunol 2003; 130(4):300–306.

37. Bergmann BM, Everson CA, Kushida CA, Fang VS, Leitch C, Schoeller D, Refetoff S, Rechtschaffen A. Sleep deprivation in the rat: V. Energy use and mediation. Sleep 1989; 12(1):31–41.

38. Everson CA, Wehr TA. Nutritional and metabolic adaptations to prolonged sleep deprivation in the rat. Am J Physiol 1993; 264(2 Pt 2):R376–387.

39. Jazwinska EC. Sleep deprivation alters the cell population kinetics in the jejunum of the male Syrian hamster (*Mesocricetus auratus*). Cell Tissue Kinet 1986; 19(3):335–350.

40. Shen XZ, Koo MW, Cho CH. Sleep deprivation increase the expression of inducible heat shock protein 70 in rat gastric mucosa. World J Gastroenterol 2001; 7(4):496–499.

41. Murison R, Ursin R, Coover GD, Lien W, Ursin H. Sleep deprivation procedure produces stomach lesions in rats. Physiol Behav 1982; 29(4):693–694.

42. Jarrett M, Heitkemper M, Cain KC, Burr RL, Hertig V. Sleep disturbance influences gastrointestinal symptoms in women with irritable bowel syndrome. Dig Dis Sci 2000; 45(5):952–959.

43. Charloux A, Gronfier C, Chapotot F, Ehrhart J, Piquard F, Brandenberger G. Sleep deprivation blunts the night time increase in aldosterone release in humans. J Sleep Res 2001; 10(1):27–33.

44. Kushida CA, Everson CA, Suthipinittharm P, Sloan J, Soltani K, Bartnicke B, Bergmann BM, Rechtschaffen A. Sleep deprivation in the rat: VI. Skin changes. Sleep 1989; 12(1):42–46.

45. Landis CA, Whitney JD. Effects of 72 hours sleep deprivation on wound healing in the rat. Res Nurs Health 1997; 20(3):259–267.

46. Altemus M, Rao B, Dhabhar FS, Ding W, Granstein RD. Stress-induced changes in skin barrier function in healthy women. J Invest Dermatol 2001; 117(2):309–317.

47. Horne JA. A review of the biological effects of total sleep deprivation in man. Biol Psychol 1978; 7(1–2):55–102.

48. Berger RJ, Phillips NH. Energy conservation and sleep. Behav Brain Res 1995; 69(1–2):65–73.

49. Horne JA, McGrath MJ. The consolidation hypothesis for REM sleep function: stress and other confounding factors—a review. Biol Psychol 1984; 18(3):165–184.

50. Horne JA. REM sleep—by default? Neurosci Biobehav Rev 2000; 24(8):777–797.

51. Rechtschaffen A, Bergmann BM, Everson CA, Kushida CA, Gilliland MA. Sleep deprivation in the rat: X. Integration and discussion of the findings. Sleep 1989; 12(1):68–87.

52. Rechtschaffen A, Bergmann BM, Gilliland MA, Bauer K. Effects of method, duration, and sleep stage on rebounds from sleep deprivation in the rat. Sleep 1999; 22(1):11–31.

53. Rechtschaffen A, Bergmann BM. Sleep deprivation in the rat: an update of the 1989 paper. Sleep 2002; 25(1):18–24.

54. Kleitman N. Sleep and Wakefulness. Chicago: University of Chicago Press, 1963.

55. Tucker RP. A review of the effects of sleep deprivation. Univ Mich Med Cent J 1968; 34(3):161–164.

56. Wilkinson RT. Loss of sleep. Proc R Soc Med 1969; 62(9):903–904.

57. Horne JA. Sleep function, with particular reference to sleep deprivation. Ann Clin Res 1985; 17(5):199–208.

58. Blake H, Gerard RW. Brain potentials during sleep. Am J Physiol 1937; 119:692–703.

59. Johnson LC, Slye ES, Dement W. Electroencephalographic and autonomic activity during and after prolonged sleep deprivation. Psychosom Med 1965; 27(5):415–423.

60. Naitoh P, Kales A, Kollar EJ, Smith JC, Jacobson A. Electroencephalographic activity after prolonged sleep loss. Electroencephalogr Clin Neurophysiol 1969; 27(1):2–11.

61. Naitoh P, Kollar EJ, Kales A. The EEG changes after a prolonged sleep loss. Electroencephalogr Clin Neurophysiol 1969; 26(2):238.

62. Dijk DJ, Brunner DP, Borbely AA. Time course of EEG power density during long sleep in humans. Am J Physiol 1990; 258(3 Pt 2):R650–R661.

63. Lorenzo I, Ramos J, Arce C, Guevara MA, Corsi-Cabrera M. Effect of total sleep deprivation on reaction time and waking EEG activity in man. Sleep 1995; 18(5):346–354.

64. Borbely AA, Baumann F, Brandeis D, Strauch I, Lehmann D. Sleep deprivation: effect on sleep stages and EEG power density in man. Electroencephalogr Clin Neurophysiol 1981; 51(5):483–495.

65. Akerstedt T, Gillberg M. Sleep duration and the power spectral density of the EEG. Electroencephalogr Clin Neurophysiol 1986; 64(2):119–122.

66. Dijk DJ. EEG slow waves and sleep spindles: windows on the sleeping brain. Behav Brain Res 1995; 69(1–2):109–116.

67. Borbely AA. A two process model of sleep regulation. Hum Neurobiol 1982; 1(3):195–204.

68. Miszczak J, Zuzewicz W. Variability of the averaged evoked potentials in healthy subjects after 24–hour sleep deprivation. Acta Physiol Pol 1977; 28(1):61–69.

69. Morris AM, So Y, Lee KA, Lash AA, Becker CE. The P300 event-related potential. The effects of sleep deprivation. J Occup Med 1992; 34(12):1143–1152.

70. Gauthier P, Gottesmann C. Influence of total sleep deprivation on event-related potentials in man. Psychophysiology 1983; 20(3):351–355.

71. Naitoh P, Muzet A, Johnson LC, Moses J. Body movements during sleep after sleep loss. Psychophysiology 1973; 10(4):363–368.

72. Horne J. Human slow wave sleep: a review and appraisal of recent findings, with implications for sleep functions, and psychiatric illness. Experientia 1992; 48(10):941–954.

73. Rodin E. Sleep deprivation and epileptological implications. Epilepsy Res Suppl 1991; 2:265–273.

74. Bennett DR, Ziter FA, Liske EA. Electroencephalographic study of sleep deprivation in flying personnel. Neurology 1969; 19(4):375–377.

75. Patrick G, Gilbert J, . On effects of loss of sleep. Psychol Rev 1896; 3:469.

76. Horne JA, Anderson NR, Wilkinson RT. Effects of sleep deprivation on signal detection measures of vigilance: implications for sleep function. Sleep 1983; 6(4):347–358.

77. Kamphuisen HA, Kemp B, Kramer CG, Duijvestijn J, Ras L, Steens J. Long-term sleep deprivation as a game. The wear and tear of wakefulness. Clin Neurol Neurosurg 1992; 94 Suppl:S96–S99.

78. Kleitman N. Studies on the physiology of sleep V. Some experiments on puppies. Am J Physiol 1927; 84:386–395.

79. Scrimshaw NS, Habicht JP, Pellet P, Piche ML, Cholakos B. Effects of sleep deprivation and reversal of diurnal activity on protein metabolism of young men. Am J Clin Nutr 1966; 19(5):313–319.

80. Leproult R, Van Reeth O, Byrne MM, Sturis J, Van Cauter E. Sleepiness, performance, and neuroendocrine function during sleep deprivation: effects of exposure to bright light or exercise. J Biol Rhythms 1997; 12(3):245–258.

81. Corsi-Cabrera M, Arce C, Ramos J, Lorenzo I, Guevara MA. Time course of reaction time and EEG while performing a vigilance task during total sleep deprivation. Sleep 1996; 19(7):563–569.

82. Krieder M. Effect of sleep deprivation on body temperature. Fed Proc 1961; 20:214.

83. Kolka MA, Stephenson LA. Exercise thermoregulation after prolonged wakefulness. J Appl Physiol 1988; 64(4):1575–1579.

84. Kolka MA, Martin BJ, Elizondo RS. Exercise in a cold environment after sleep deprivation. Eur J Appl Physiol Occup Physiol 1984; 53(3):282–285.

85. Savourey G, Bittel J. Cold thermoregulatory changes induced by sleep deprivation in men. Eur J Appl Physiol Occup Physiol 1994; 69(3):216–220.

86. Dewasmes G, Bothorel B, Nicolas A, Candas V, Libert JP, Ehrhart J, et al. Local sweating responses during recovery sleep after sleep deprivation in humans. Eur J Appl Physiol Occup Physiol 1994; 68(2):116–121.

87. Sawka MN, Gonzalez RR, Pandolf KB. Effects of sleep deprivation on thermoregulation during exercise. Am J Physiol 1984; 246(1 Pt 2):R72–R77.

88. Fiorica V, Higgins EA, Iampietro PF, Lategola MT, Davis AW. Physiological responses of men during sleep deprivation. J Appl Physiol 1968; 24(2):167–176.

89. Thomas M, Sing H, Belenky G, Holcomb H, Mayberg H, Dannals R, et al. Neural basis of alertness and cognitive performance impairments during sleepiness. I. Effects of 24 h of sleep deprivation on waking human regional brain activity. J Sleep Res 2000; 9(4):335–352.

90. Wu JC, Gillin JC, Buchsbaum MS, Hershey T, Hazlett E, Sicotte N, et al. The effect of sleep deprivation on cerebral glucose metabolic rate in normal humans assessed with positron emission tomography. Sleep 1991; 14(2):155–162.

91. Portas CM, Goldstein JM, Shenton ME, Hokama HH, Wible CG, Fischer I et al. Volumetric evaluation of the thalamus in schizophrenic male patients using magnetic resonance imaging. Biol Psychiatry 1998; 43(9):649–659.

92. Drummond SP, Brown GG, Gillin JC, Stricker JL, Wong EC, Buxton RB. Altered brain response to verbal learning following sleep deprivation. Nature 2000; 403(6770):655–657.

93. Everson CA, Gilliland MA, Kushida CA, Pilcher JJ, Fang VS, Refetoff S et al. Sleep deprivation in the rat: IX. Recovery. Sleep 1989; 12(1):60–67.

94. Kiyono S, Kawamoto T, Sakakura H, Iwama K. Effect of sleep deprivation upon the paradoxical phase of sleep in cats. Electroencephalogr Clin Neurophysiol 1965; 19:34–40.

95. Borbely AA, Tobler I, Hanagasioglu M. Effect of sleep deprivation on sleep and EEG power spectra in the rat. Behav Brain Res 1984; 14(3):171–182.

96. Trachsel L, Tobler I, Borbely AA. Sleep regulation in rats: effects of sleep deprivation, light, and circadian phase. Am J Physiol 1986; 251(6 Pt 2):R1037–R1044.

97. Everson CA, Bergmann BM, Rechtschaffen A. Sleep deprivation in the rat: III. Total sleep deprivation. Sleep 1989; 12(1):13–21.

98. Mistlberger RE, Landry GJ, Marchant EG. Sleep deprivation can attenuate light-induced phase shifts of circadian rhythms in hamsters. Neurosci Lett 1997; 238(1–2):5–8.

99. Tobler I, Sigg H. Long-term motor activity recording of dogs and the effect of sleep deprivation. Experientia 1986; 42(9):987–991.

100. Tobler I, Borbely AA. Sleep EEG in the rat as a function of prior waking. Electroencephalogr Clin Neurophysiol 1986; 64(1):74–76.

101. Tobler I, Franken P, Scherschlicht R. Sleep and EEG spectra in the rabbit under baseline conditions and following sleep deprivation. Physiol Behav 1990; 48(1):121–129.

102. Tobler I, Scherschlicht R. Sleep and EEG slow-wave activity in the domestic cat: effect of sleep deprivation. Behav Brain Res 1990; 37(2):109–118.

103. Tobler I, Borbely AA. The effect of 3–h and 6–h sleep deprivation on sleep and EEG spectra of the rat. Behav Brain Res 1990; 36(1–2):73–78.

104. Franken P, Tobler I, Borbely AA. Sleep homeostasis in the rat: simulation of the time course of EEG slow-wave activity. Neurosci Lett 1991; 130(2):141–144.

105. Franken P, Dijk DJ, Tobler I, Borbely AA. Sleep deprivation in rats: effects on EEG power spectra, vigilance states, and cortical temperature. Am J Physiol 1991; 261(1 Pt 2):R198–R208.

106. Franken P, Tobler I, Borbely AA. Cortical temperature and EEG slow-wave activity in the rat: analysis of vigilance state related changes. Pflugers Arch 1992; 420(5–6):500–507.

107. Deboer T, Franken P, Tobler I. Sleep and cortical temperature in the Djungarian hamster under baseline conditions and after sleep deprivation. J Comp Physiol [A] 1994; 174(2):145–155.

108. Tobler I. Is sleep fundamentally different between mammalian species? Behav Brain Res 1995; 69(1–2):35–41.

109. Endo T, Schwierin B, Borbely AA, Tobler I. Selective and total sleep deprivation: effect on the sleep EEG in the rat. Psychiatry Res 1997; 66(2–3):97–110.

110. Huber R, Deboer T, Tobler I. Effects of sleep deprivation on sleep and sleep EEG in three mouse strains: empirical data and simulations. Brain Res 2000; 857(1–2):8–19.

111. Huber R, Deboer T, Tobler I. Topography of EEG dynamics after sleep deprivation in mice. J Neurophysiol 2000; 84(4):1888–1893.

112. Schwierin B, Borbely AA, Tobler I. Prolonged effects of 24–h total sleep deprivation on sleep and sleep EEG in the rat. Neurosci Lett 1999; 261(1–2):61–64.

113. Borbely AA. From slow waves to sleep homeostasis: new perspectives. Arch Ital Biol 2001; 139(1–2):53–61.

114. Frank MG, Morrissette R, Heller HC. Effects of sleep deprivation in neonatal rats. Am J Physiol 1998; 275(1 Pt 2):R148–R157.

115. Shiromani PJ, Basheer R, Thakkar J, Wagner D, Greco MA, Charness ME. Sleep and wakefulness in c-fos and fos B gene knockout mice. Brain Res Mol Brain Res 2000; 80(1):75–87.

116. Franken P, Chollet D, Tafti M. The homeostatic regulation of sleep need is under genetic control. J Neurosci 2001; 21(8):2610–2621.

117. Lancel M, van Riezen H, Glatt A. Enhanced slow-wave activity within NREM sleep in the cortical and subcortical EEG of the cat after sleep deprivation. Sleep 1992; 15(2):102–118.

118. Kopp C, Albrecht U, Zheng B, Tobler I. Homeostatic sleep regulation is preserved in mPer1 and mPer2 mutant mice. Eur J Neurosci 2002; 16(6):1099–1106.

119. Thakkar MM, Ramesh V, Cape EG, Winston S, Strecker RE, McCarley RW. REM sleep enhancement and behavioral cataplexy following orexin (hypocretin)-II receptor antisense perfusion in the pontine reticular formation. Sleep Res Online 1999; 2(4):112–120.

120. Thakkar MM, Winston S, McCarley RW. A1 receptor and adenosinergic homeostatic regulation of sleep-wakefulness: effects of antisense to the A1 receptor in the cholinergic basal forebrain. J Neurosci 2003. In press.

121. Manaceine M. de Quelques observations experimentales sur l'influence de l'insomnie absolute. Arch Ital Biol 1894; 21:322–325.

122. Tarrozi G. Sull-influenza dell-insonnio sperimentale sul ricambio materiale. Riv Pat Nerv Ment 1899; 4:1–23.

123. Leake C, Grab JA, Senn M. Studies in exhaustion due to lack of sleep. II Symptomatology in rabbits. Am J Physiol 1927; 92:127–130.

124. Legendre R. The physiology of sleep. Rep Smithsonian Inst 1907; 12:587–602.

125. Rechtschaffen A, Bergmann BM. Sleep deprivation in the rat by the disk-over-water method. Behav Brain Res 1995; 69(1–2):55–63.

126. Bergmann BM, Kushida CA, Everson CA, Gilliland MA, Obermeyer W, Rechtschaffen A. Sleep deprivation in the rat: II. Methodology. Sleep 1989; 12(1):5–12.

127. Bergmann BM, Everson CA, Kushida CA, Fang VS, Leitch CA, Schoeller DA, et al. Sleep deprivation in the rat: V. Energy use and mediation. Sleep 1989; 12(1):31–41.

128. Obermeyer W, Bergmann BM, Rechtschaffen A. Sleep deprivation in the rat: XIV. Comparison of waking hypothalamic and peritoneal temperatures. Sleep 1991; 14(4):285–293.

129. Bergmann BM, Landis CA, Zenko CE, Rechtschaffen A. Sleep deprivation in the rat: XVII. Effect of aspirin on elevated body temperature. Sleep 1993; 16(3):221–225.

130. Zenko CE, Bergmann BM, Rechtschaffen A. Vascular resistance in the rat during baseline, chronic total sleep deprivation, and recovery from total sleep deprivation. Sleep 2000; 23(3):341–346.

131. Bergmann BM, Gilliland MA, Balzano S, Refetoff S, Rechtschaffen A. Sleep deprivation in the rat: XIX. Effects of thyroxine administration. Sleep 1995; 18(5):317–324.

132. Feng PF, Bergmann BM, Rechtschaffen A. Sleep deprivation in rats with preoptic/anterior hypothalamic lesions. Brain Res 1995; 703(1–2):93–99.

133. Tobler I, Franken P, Gao B, Jaggi K, Borbely AA. Sleep deprivation in the rat at different ambient temperatures: effect on sleep, EEG spectra and brain temperature. Arch Ital Biol 1994; 132(1):39–52.

134. Hansen MK, Krueger JM. Subdiaphragmatic vagotomy does not block sleep deprivation-induced sleep in rats. Physiol Behav 1998; 64(3):361–365.

135. Gardner JP, Fornal CA, Jacobs BL. Effects of sleep deprivation on serotonergic neuronal activity in the dorsal raphe nucleus of the freely moving cat. Neuropsychopharmacology 1997; 17(2):72–81.

136. Campbell IG, Guinan MJ, Horowitz JM. Sleep deprivation impairs long-term potentiation in rat hippocampal slices. J Neurophysiol 2002; 88(2):1073–1076.

137. Vogel GW. A review of REM sleep deprivation. Arch Gen Psychiatry 1975; 32(6):749–761.

138. Kushida CA, Bergmann BM, Rechtschaffen A. Sleep deprivation in the rat: IV. Paradoxical sleep deprivation. Sleep 1989; 12(1):22–30.

139. Rechtschaffen A, Bergmann BM, Everson CA, Kushida CA, Gilliland MA. Sleep deprivation in the rat: X. Integration and discussion of the findings, 1989. Sleep 2002; 25(1):68–87.

140. Mallick BN, Thakkar M. Short-term REM sleep deprivation increases acetylcholinesterase activity in the medulla of rats. Neurosci Lett 1991; 130(2):221–224.

141. Thakkar M, Mallick BN. Effect of REM sleep deprivation on rat brain acetyl-cholinesterase. Pharmacol Biochem Behav 1991; 39(1):211–214.

142. Mallick BN, Thakkar M. Effect of REM sleep deprivation on molecular forms of acetylcholinesterase in rats. Neuroreport 1992; 3(8):676–678.

143. Thakkar M, Mallick BN. Rapid eye movement sleep-deprivation-induced changes in glucose metabolic enzymes in rat brain. Sleep 1993; 16(8):691–694.

144. Coenen AM, van Hulzen ZJ. Paradoxical sleep deprivation in animal studies: some methodological considerations. Prog Brain Res 1980; 53:325–330.

145. Sampson H. Psychological effects of deprivation of dreaming sleep. J Nerv Ment Dis 1966; 143(4):305–317.

146. Agnew HW Jr, Webb WB, Williams RL. Comparison of stage four and 1–REM sleep deprivation. Percept Mot Skills 1967; 24(3):851–858.

147. Cartwright RD, Monroe LJ, Palmer C. Individual differences in response to REM deprivation. Arch Gen Psychiatry 1967; 16(3):297–303.

148. Glovinsky PB, Spielman AJ, Carroll P, Weinstein L, Ellman SJ. Sleepiness and REM sleep recurrence: the effects of stage 2 and REM sleep awakenings. Psychophysiology 1990; 27(5):552–559.

149. Endo T, Roth C, Landolt HP, Werth E, Aeschbach D, Achermann P, et al. Selective REM sleep deprivation in humans: effects on sleep and sleep EEG. Am J Physiol 1998; 274(4 Pt 2):R1186–R1194.

150. Roth C, Achermann P, Borbely AA. Alpha activity in the human REM sleep EEG: topography and effect of REM sleep deprivation. Clin Neurophysiol 1999; 110(4):632–635.

151. Kopell BS, Zarcone V, De la PA, Dement WC. Changes in selective attention as measured by the visual averaged evoked potential following REM deprivation in man. Electroencephalogr Clin Neurophysiol 1972; 32(3):322–325.

152. Cohen HB, Dement WC. Sleep: changes in threshold to electroconvulsive shock in rats after deprivation of "paradoxical" phase. Science 1965; 150(701):1318–1319.

153. Dement W, Henry P, Cohen H, Ferguson J. Studies on the effect of REM deprivation in humans and in animals. Res Publ Assoc Res Nerv Ment Dis 1967; 45:456–468.

154. Cohen HB, Duncan RF, Dement WC. Sleep: the effect of electroconvulsive shock in cats deprived of REM sleep. Science 1967; 156(3782):1646–1648.

155. Morden B, Mitchell G, Dement W. Selective REM sleep deprivation and compensation phenomena in the rat. Brain Res 1967; 5(3):339–349.

156. Owen M, Bliss EL. Sleep loss and cerebral excitability. Am J Physiol 1970; 218(1):171–173.

157. Dewson JH, III, Dement WC, Wagener TE, Nobel K. Rapid eye movement sleep deprivation: a central-neural change during wakefulness. Science 1967; 156(773):403–406.

158. van Hulzen ZJ, Coenen AM. Photically evoked potentials in the visual cortex following paradoxical sleep deprivation in rats. Physiol Behav 1984; 32(4):557–563.

159. Satinoff E, Drucker-Colin RR, Hernandez-Peon R. Paleocortical excitability and sensory filtering during REM sleep deprivation. Physiol Behav 1971; 7(1):103–106.

160. Mallick BN, Fahringer HM, Wu MF, Siegel JM. REM sleep deprivation reduces auditory evoked inhibition of dorsolateral pontine neurons. Brain Res 1991; 552(2):333–337.

161. Mallick BN, Siegel JM, Fahringer H. Changes in pontine unit activity with REM sleep deprivation. Brain Res 1990; 515(1–2):94–98.
162. Shaffery JP, Sinton CM, Bissette G, Roffwarg HP, Marks GA. Rapid eye movement sleep deprivation modifies expression of long-term potentiation in visual cortex of immature rats. Neuroscience 2002; 110(3):431–443.
163. Corsi-Cabrera M, Ponce-De-Leon M, Juarez J, Ramos J. Effects of paradoxical sleep deprivation and stress on the waking EEG of the rat. Physiol Behav 1994; 55(6):1021–1027.
164. Benington JH, Woudenberg MC, Heller HC. REM-sleep propensity accumulates during 2–h REM-sleep deprivation in the rest period in rats. Neurosci Lett 1994; 180(1):76–80.
165. Ocampo-Garces A, Molina E, Rodriguez A, Vivaldi EA. Homeostasis of REM sleep after total and selective sleep deprivation in the rat. J Neurophysiol 2000; 84(5):2699–2702.
166. Shaw PJ, Bergmann BM, Rechtschaffen A. Effects of paradoxical sleep deprivation on thermoregulation in the rat. Sleep 1998; 21(1):7–17.
167. Lentz MJ, Landis CA, Rothermel J, Shaver JL. Effects of selective slow wave sleep disruption on musculoskeletal pain and fatigue in middle aged women. J Rheumatol 1999; 26(7):1586–1592.
168. Arima T, Svensson P, Rasmussen C, Nielsen KD, Drewes AM, Arendt-Nielsen L. The relationship between selective sleep deprivation, nocturnal jaw-muscle activity and pain in healthy men. J Oral Rehabil 2001; 28(2):140–148.
169. Ferrara M, De Gennaro L, Casagrande M, Bertini M. Auditory arousal thresholds after selective slow-wave sleep deprivation. Clin Neurophysiol 1999; 110(12):2148–2152.
170. De Gennaro L, Ferrara M, Bertini M. Effect of slow-wave sleep deprivation on topographical distribution of spindles. Behav Brain Res 2000; 116(1):55–59.
171. Gilliland MA, Bergmann BM, Rechtschaffen A. Sleep deprivation in the rat: VIII. High EEG amplitude sleep deprivation. Sleep 1989; 12(1):53–59.

14

Metabolic and Endocrine Changes

KARINE SPIEGEL

Université Libre de Bruxelles, Campus Hôpital Erasme, Brussels, Belgium

RACHEL LEPROULT AND EVE VAN CAUTER

University of Chicago, Chicago, Illinois, U.S.A.

I. Introduction

In humans, endocrine secretions and metabolic function display clear 24-hour rhythms that are mainly controlled by sleep-wake homeostasis and by oscillatory signals generated by the suprachiasmatic nucleus (SCN) of the hypothalamus. The circadian pacemaker in the SCN is primarily entrained by the light-dark cycle. In diurnal species, such as the human, neuronal activity in the SCN is maximal during light exposure and sleep occurs during the dark phase, when SCN neuronal activity is low.

During the last century, the discovery of electricity has profoundly disturbed the 24-hour biological rhythms of humans. The artificial extension of the light phase has resulted for many in the curtailment of the sleep period to the minimum tolerable in order to maximize the time available for work and/or leisure (1,2). In addition, the advent of the 24-hour society has forced millions of individuals to work during the night and sleep during the day, and such schedules almost invariably result in substantial sleep loss (3). Sleep loss due to voluntary bedtime curtailment has thus become a hallmark of modern society (4). Over the past 40 years, Americans have decreased their sleep duration by approximately 2 hours (4–6). Today many individuals are in bed 5 to 6 hours per night on a chronic basis (6). However, several research studies involving extension of the bedtime period for prolonged periods of time have provided strong evidence that an 8-

hour night does not meet the sleep needs of healthy young adults, who may carry a substantial sleep debt even in the absence of obvious efforts at sleep curtailment (7-9). Not surprisingly, contemporary men are more likely to report fatigue and tiredness than men from the 1930s (3). As behavior-related sleep loss affects millions of individuals, it has become crucial to delineate its putative adverse impact on health.

This chapter describes the impact of sleep restriction on endocrine and metabolic functions and provides extensive evidence that supports the importance of the deleterious effects of sleep loss on health. First we review the influence of sleep-wake homeostasis and circadian rhythmicity on hormones and glucose regulation. The following section compares the effects of acute total sleep deprivation with those of chronic partial sleep loss on sleep regulation and suggests that the chronic condition involves adaptive mechanisms with probable long-term adverse health consequences. The third section describes the impact of sleep deprivation, either acute or chronic, on hormones of the hypothalamopituitary axis. The fourth section summarizes the evidence indicating that sleep deprivation affects appetite regulation, suggesting that sleep loss might be a risk factor for weight gain. The fifth section presents the impact of sleep deprivation on glucose metabolism. Finally, the sixth section proposes possible mechanisms mediating adverse effects of sleep deprivation on endocrine and metabolic functions.

II. Influences of Sleep-Wake Cycle and Circadian Rhythmicity on Endocrine and Metabolic Functions

In humans as well as in all mammalian species, the temporal organization of physiological function, including the sleep-wake state, ultimately results from the activity of two interacting time-keeping mechanisms in the central nervous system: endogenous circadian rhythmicity and sleep-wake homeostasis (see also Chap. 24). In mammals, endogenous circadian rhythmicity is generated by a pacemaker located in the paired SCNs of the hypothalamus. Overt rhythms driven by the endogenous circadian pacemaker may be observed for virtually every physiological and behavioral variable, including cognitive function, mood, hormonal secretion, metabolic and cardiovascular functions. The endogenous circadian signal is entrained to the environmental light-dark and social-activity cycles by daily adjustments in the phase of the rhythm (10). This occurs through the presentation of photic and nonphotic stimuli that signal the time of day or state of activity. Sleep-wake homeostasis refers to the increase in propensity to fall asleep, and increased sleep duration and intensity that occur following extended waking. The sleep "homeostat," also referred to as process S, is often represented as an hourglass mechanism relating the amount and intensity of sleep to the duration of prior wakefulness (11). In both humans and rodents, slow-wave activity (SWA or "delta power"; electroencephalographic power density in the low-frequency range < 4 Hz), an index which quantifies the depth of non-REM (NREM)

sleep or "sleep intensity," is the primary marker of sleep-wake homeostasis (11). Figure 1 shows a schematic representation of the interaction of these two time-keeping mechanisms on the control of the sleep-wake state and the generation of 24-hr profiles of hypothalamopituitary hormones. Modulation of pituitary-dependent hormonal release is thought to be mediated by the modulation of the pulsatile activity of hypothalamic releasing and/or inhibiting factors controlling pituitary function. In addition to the input of circadian rhythmicity and the sleep homeostat, other rhythmic and nonrhythmic events during the day, such as postural changes, stress, food intake, and exercise, modulate the overall waveform of the temporal patterns of pituitary hormone release.

In order to delineate the respective contributions of sleep and circadian rhythmicity on endocrine and other physiological functions, protocols involving sleep deprivation during the night and sleep recovery during the day have been used. Such experimental designs allow for the effects of time of day to be observed in the absence of sleep and the effects of sleep to be observed at an abnormal circadian time. Figure 2 shows, from top to bottom, the profiles of plasma growth

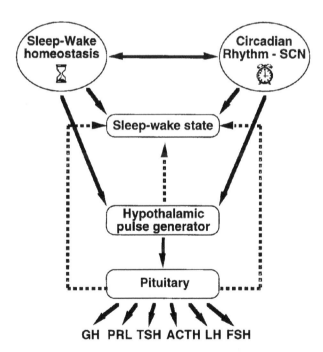

Figure 1 Schematic representation for the control of sleep-wake state and the modulation of pituitary secretions by sleep-wake homeostasis and circadian rhythmicity. SCN, suprachiasmatic nucleus, GH, growth hormone, PRL, prolactin, TSH, thyrotropin, ACTH, adrenocorticotrophic hormone, LH, luteinizing hormone, FSH, follicle stimulating hormone. (Adapted from Ref. 107.)

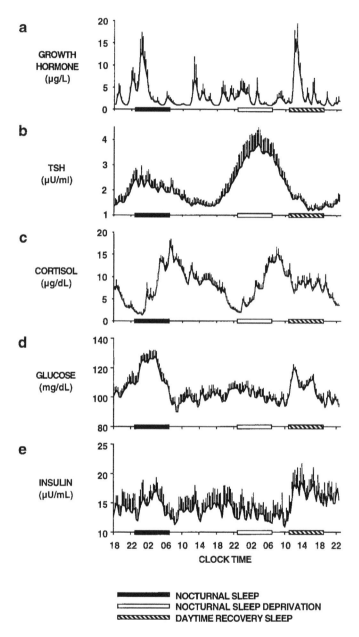

Figure 2 (From top to bottom) Mean (+ SEM) profiles of (a) growth hormone (GH), (b) thyrotropin (TSH), (c) cortisol, (d) glucose, and (e) insulin in a group of eight normal young men (aged 20–27 years) studied during a 53-hr period including 8 hr of nocturnal sleep (black bars), followed by 28 hr of sleep deprivation including a period of nocturnal sleep deprivation (open bars), and 8 hr of daytime recovery sleep (dashed bars). Data were obtained at 20-min intervals under continuous glucose infusion. (Adapted from Refs. 19, 108, 109.)

hormone (GH), thyrotropin (TSH), cortisol, glucose, and insulin in a group of eight normal young men studied during a 53-hr period including 8 hr of nocturnal sleep followed by 28 hr of continuous wakefulness and 8 hr of daytime recovery sleep. For many years, GH has been recognized as a "sleep-dependent" hormone for which the 24-hr profile was primarily determined by the presence or absence of sleep. In contrast, the 24-hr rhythms of TSH and cortisol have long been considered as primarily driven by circadian rhythmicity, with sleep homeostasis exerting little or no effect on the overall profiles. More detailed analyses revealed that all pituitary hormones are under the influence of both systems, some being more strongly affected by sleep and others more by circadian rhythmicity.

Panel a of Figure 2 shows that the secretion of GH is increased during sleep independently of the circadian time at which sleep occurs and that sleep deprivation results in greatly diminished release of this hormone. However, a slight increase may be observed during nocturnal sleep deprivation indicating the existence of a weak circadian component in the control of its secretion. The waveform of the 24-hr cortisol profile consists of an early morning rise, diminishing levels during the daytime, and a quiescent period centered around midnight. As shown in panel c of Figure 2, this profile is only modestly affected by the presence or absence of sleep. Jet lag studies have shown that the cortisol profile takes several days to synchronize to the new schedule (12). Thus, the 24-hr periodicity of corticotropic activity appears primarily controlled by circadian rhythmicity. Nevertheless, the transition from wakefulness to sleep is associated with an inhibition of corticotropic activity whereas the transition from sleep to wakefulness involves a short-term increase in cortisol levels. Thus, during extended wakefulness, including nocturnal sleep deprivation, the excursion of cortisol levels over the 24-hr cycle appears slightly dampened because of the absence of the effects associated with wake-sleep and sleep-wake transitions. Furthermore, evening cortisol levels are elevated following a night of total or partial sleep deprivation.

The activity of the thyrotropic axis is under the control of the two central time-keeping mechanisms in a more balanced manner. Under normal conditions, daytime TSH levels are stable and low, but they increase rapidly in the evening to reach their maximum around the beginning of the sleep period (Fig. 2b). The evening rise of TSH levels is driven by the circadian clock. When sleep is initiated, TSH concentrations decline, suggesting an inhibiting effect of sleep on TSH secretion. This sleep-dependent inhibition of TSH levels is clearly evident under conditions of total sleep deprivation when a large increase in nocturnal TSH levels is apparent, as shown in Figure 2b.

The combined effects of circadian rhythmicity and sleep-wake homeostasis are not limited to hormones of the hypothalamopituitary axes but extend to other aspects of endocrine and metabolic regulation, particularly glucose metabolism. In normal man, glucose tolerance varies with the time of day (13). Plasma glucose responses to oral glucose, intravenous glucose, or meals are markedly higher in the evening than in the morning (13). Diminished insulin sensitivity and decreased insulin secretion in relation to elevated glucose levels are both involved in causing reduced glucose tolerance later in the day (14–16). Using experimental protocols involving intravenous glucose infusion at a constant rate for 24–30 hr, it has been shown that glucose tolerance further deteriorates as the evening progresses, reaching a minimum around the middle of the night (17,18). Since glucose concentrations begin to increase in the late afternoon or early evening, well before bedtime, and continue to rise until approximately the middle of the night, both sleep-independent effects, reflecting circadian rhythmicity, and sleep-dependent effects are involved in producing this overall 24-hr pattern.

Panels d and e of Figure 2 show the mean profiles of plasma glucose and insulin when effects of time of day were dissociated from effects of sleep (19). Caloric intake was exclusively under the form of a glucose infusion at a constant rate. During nocturnal sleep, levels of glucose and insulin secretion increased by approximately 30% and 60%, respectively, and returned to baseline in the morning. During sleep deprivation, glucose levels and insulin secretion rose again to reach a maximum at a time corresponding to the beginning of the habitual sleep period, indicating the existence of an intrinsic circadian modulation of glucose regulation. The magnitude of the rise above morning levels was less than that observed during nocturnal sleep. Daytime sleep was associated with marked elevations of glucose levels and insulin secretion (19), indicating that sleep per se, irrespective of the time of day when sleep occurs, exerts modulatory influences on glucose regulation. Examination of correlations with the temporal variations of the counterregulatory hormones cortisol and GH indicated that the diurnal variation in insulin secretion was inversely related to the cortisol rhythm, with a significant correlation of the magnitudes of their morning to evening excursions. Sleep-associated rises in glucose correlated with the amount of concomitant GH secreted. These studies show that glucose regulation is markedly influenced by circadian rhythmicity and sleep, and suggest that these effects could be partially mediated by cortisol and GH.

III.   Sleep Following Acute Sleep Deprivation and During Chronic Partial Sleep Restriction

While recovery sleep following various durations of total sleep deprivation has been studied extensively, the much more common condition of partial chronic sleep restriction has not received nearly as much attention. A few studies have provided evidence indicating that sleep architecture during chronic sleep restriction cannot be directly inferred from the patterns of sleep recovery following total sleep deprivation because adaptive mechanisms—probably more aptly referred to as maladaptive mechanisms—intervene as the "sleep debt" builds (20,21).

The interaction between the sleep homeostat and circadian signals determines the distribution of the different sleep stages within a sleep period. Rapid-eye-movement (REM) sleep is primarily under the control of the circadian component whereas slow-wave sleep (SWS) mainly reflects the homeostatic process and is therefore influenced by the duration of prior wakefulness. Thus, the beginning of the night is associated with maximal amounts of SWS and SWA that progressively decrease throughout the night. Following acute total sleep deprivation, SWS and SWA are enhanced during recovery sleep (22). Conversely, a decrease in SWS is observed after extended sleep (23,24) or daytime naps (25). It has been proposed that the total amount of SWS is influenced by the duration of prior wakefulness but that the time course of SWS during sleep, i.e., an exponential decline across the sleep period, remains the same irrespective of the duration of prior waking (26). These concepts are well illustrated by the data shown in the upper panels of Figure 3, where recovery sleep was initiated at 11 a.m. following 28 hr of continuous wakefulness. When sleep was recovered during the daytime, accumulation of process S resulted in higher SWA at the beginning of the night with a preserved exponential decline throughout the night. However, when sleep is restricted night after night, rather than acutely eliminated, another pattern of SWA emerges. The lower panels of Figure 3 show the impact of different sleep durations maintained for at least 1 week (12-hr, 8-hr, and 4-hr bedtimes) on the temporal evolution of SWA during sleep. The temporal evolution of SWA during 12-hr and 8-hr nights (lower left and middle panels) conformed to the expected exponential decline of SWA. Unexpectedly, the distribution of SWA after 6 nights of 4 hr in bed (lower right panel) did not conform to the predictions from current theories of SWS homeostasis, which predict: (a) increased SWA during the first cycle when the waking period is extended, and (b) a progressive decrease of SWA with successive sleep cycles. Indeed, as illustrated in the lower right panel of Figure 3, the first SWA cycle was not of higher amplitude during sleep restriction than during sleep extension. Moreover, during sleep restriction, the second SWA cycle was not of lower amplitude than the first SWA cycle. In fact, the major difference in distribution of SWA between the study with chronic sleep restriction and the study with 12-hr bedtimes concerned the amplitude and the amount of delta activity of the second cycle, which were markedly larger during sleep restriction than during sleep extension. These results indicate that adaptive mechanisms are operative during chronic partial sleep loss and that chronic partial sleep deprivation is likely to have a very different impact on human physiology than acute total sleep deprivation.

Figure 4 describes the alterations in sleep architecture when bedtimes are reduced from the recommended 8 hr to 4 hr for 6 days and then extended to 12 hr for 7 days. The data were generated in a study where 11 healthy young men slept during 16 consecutive nights in a sleep laboratory (27). Following 5 days of 8-hr bedtimes at home, the first three study nights involved bedtimes from 23:00 to 07:00 (baseline; B1–B3), the six subsequent nights' bedtimes from 01:00 to 05:00 (debt; D1–D6) and the seven last nights' bedtimes from 21:00 to 09:00 (recovery; R1–R7) (Fig. 4a). Sleep was polygraphically recorded during the last two baseline nights, the last two nights of sleep restriction, the first night of sleep recovery, and the fifth and sixth nights of sleep recovery.

The amount of intrasleep awakenings decreased markedly from the 8-hr bedtime condition to the end of sleep restriction when the total amount of wake was less than 5 min (Fig. 4b). The end of the extension period was associated with

SLOW WAVE ACTIVITY (µV²)

ACUTE SLEEP DEPRIVATION

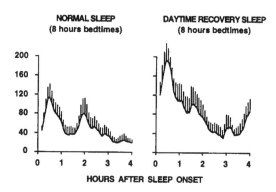

CHRONIC SLEEP RESTRICTION

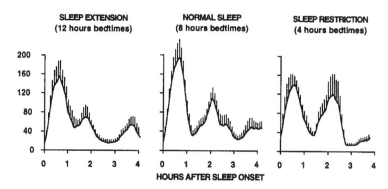

Figure 3 Smoothed mean (+ SEM) SWA profiles during the first 4 hr of sleep. Upper panels, acute sleep deprivation: Profiles obtained in 7 young men (24 ± 0.4 years) during nocturnal sleep with 8-hr bedtimes (left) and during 8 hr of daytime recovery sleep after a night of total sleep deprivation (right). (Unpublished data). Lower panels, chronic sleep restriction: Profiles obtained in 9 young men (22 ± 1 years) after 1 week of 12-hr bedtimes (left), after 1 week of 8-hr bedtimes (middle), and after 1 week of 4-hr bedtimes (right). (Adapted from Ref. 20 and unpublished data.)

increasing amounts of wake, indicating that subjects had partly recovered from the sleep debt. Note that in these healthy young subjects, the amount of sleep obtained during nights 5 and 6 of sleep extension averaged 9 hr 48 min ± 16 min, i.e., 108 min more than the recommended daily amount of sleep and at least 1 more hr than the average sleep duration observed after prolonged sleep extension in previous studies in similar subject populations (7–9). Quantitatively, the major adaptation to

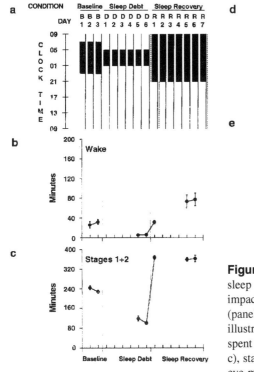

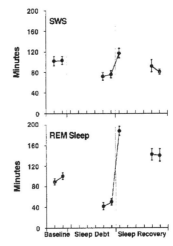

Figure 4 Schematic representation of sleep restriction protocol (panel a) and impact of sleep duration on sleep stages (panels b to e). The sleep stages data are illustrated as the mean ± SEM of minutes spent in wake (panel b), stages 1 + 2 (panel c), stages 3 + 4 (SWS; panel d) and rapid-eye-movement (REM) sleep (panel e) during the last two baseline nights (8-hr bedtimes), the last two nights of sleep restriction (4-hr bedtimes), the first night of sleep recovery (12-hr bedtimes), and the fifth and sixth nights of sleep recovery (12-hr bedtimes). (Adapted from Refs. 20 and 27.)

sleep restriction and extension was achieved by proportional compression or extension of the lighter stages of NREM sleep (stages 1 + 2; Fig. 4c) and of rapid-eye-movement (REM) sleep (Fig. 4e). In contrast, the percentage of deep NREM sleep relative to the other sleep stages (stages 3 + 4, i.e., SWS; Fig. 4d) was highest during sleep restriction, revealing an increased pressure for SWS. SWS appeared better preserved than REM sleep during sleep restriction. Indeed, the increase in REM sleep during the first recovery night averaged 137 ± 7 min (Fig. 4e) over the previous night whereas the rebound in SWS was only 41 ± 8 min (Fig. 4d and e).

IV. Impact of Acute and Chronic Partial Sleep Deprivation on Hypothalamo-Pituitary Hormones

The response to chronic partial sleep restriction is also different from that occurring during acute total sleep deprivation for hormones of the hypothalamo-pituitary axis. Figure 5 compares the profiles of plasma GH, TSH, and cortisol in subjects who had the normal recommended 8 hr of sleep (left panels), in subjects

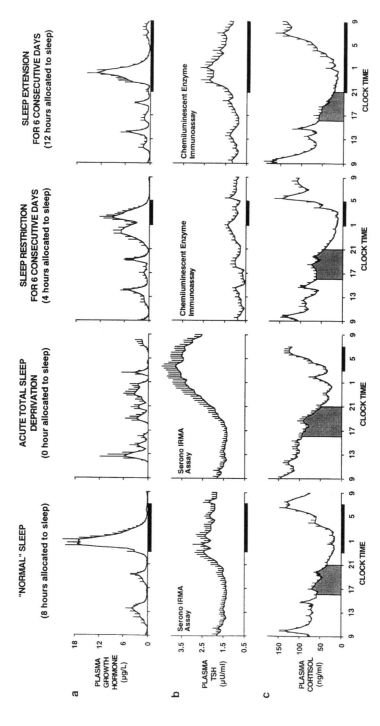

Figure 5 (From top to bottom) 24-hr (+ SEM) profiles of (a) growth hormone (GH), (b) thyrotropin (TSH), and (c) cortisol in subjects who had the normal recommended 8 hr of sleep (left), in subjects who were acutely sleep deprived (second from left), in subjects submitted to partial sleep restriction for 6 days (4-hr bedtimes; third from left), and in subjects who had 12-hr bedtimes for 6 nights (right). The black bars represent the sleep periods. (From Refs. 20 and 27, adapted from Refs. 109 and 110, and unpublished data.)

who were totally sleep deprived for one night (second panels from the left), in subjects submitted to partial sleep restriction (4-hr bedtimes for 6 days; third panels from the left), and in fully rested subjects (12-hr bedtimes for 6 nights; right panels).

A. Somatotropic Axis

Growth hormone (GH) is secreted as a series of pulses throughout the 24-hr cycle. As shown in the left panel of Figure 5a, the most reproducible and generally the largest GH pulse in normal adult men occurs during early sleep, in temporal association with the first phase of SWS (28–31). The amount of GH secreted during the first SWS episode is quantitatively correlated with the duration of SWS (32,33) as well as with the intensity of SWS, as estimated by SWA (34). Pharmacological stimulation of SWS is associated with increased GH secretion with a significant dose-dependent relationship (34,35), indicating that common mechanisms underlie SWS and GH release.

The second panel from the left in Figure 5a shows that acute sleep deprivation results in drastically diminished nocturnal GH secretion. When modest amounts of GH are secreted during nocturnal sleep deprivation (33,36), they are thought to be due to a circadian rhythm in somatostatin tone, with lower activity and thus decreased inhibition of pituitary GH release in the evening and early part of the night (37). Following a night of total sleep deprivation, GH release is increased during the daytime such that the total 24-hr secretion is not significantly affected (38). Recovery from total sleep deprivation, at any time of day, is invariably associated with a robust increase in GH secretion. The rebound in GH secretion following acute sleep deprivation parallels the rebound in SWA that reflects the homeostasis regulation of the sleep-wake cycle. The two right panels in Figure 5a show the 24-hr plasma GH profiles after 6 days of sleep curtailment to 4 hr/night and after 6 days of sleep extension to 12 hr/night in a group of young healthy men. The well-known sleep onset associated GH pulse was observed in all individual profiles for both conditions. However, after chronic partial sleep restriction, all subjects exhibited a GH pulse prior to sleep onset. This pattern contrasts with the mean profiles during sleep extension (right panel of Fig. 5a), which present the usual single nocturnal GH pulse in early sleep as observed during a normal 8-hr sleep period (left panel of Fig. 5a).

After chronic partial sleep restriction, post-sleep-onset GH secretion was negatively related to pre-sleep-onset secretion and tended to be positively correlated with the amount of concomitant SWA, suggesting that pre-sleep-onset GH secretion may have limited SWA in the first cycle, possibly via an inhibition of central GHRH activity.

From studies of acute total sleep deprivation, one would have predicted that chronic sleep loss would have been associated with minimal GH secretion during prolonged wakefulness and with a large secretory pulse associated with high levels of SWA following the initiation of recovery sleep (39). Neither the pattern of

GH secretion (third panel from left of Fig. 5a) nor the distribution of SWA (right lower panel of Fig. 3) conformed to these expectations, indicating that adaptation mechanisms that are not apparent during acute sleep deprivation are operative during chronic partial sleep loss.

B. Thyrotropic Axis

The mean 24-hr TSH profile observed in young healthy subjects under conditions of normal nocturnal sleep with 8-hr bedtimes are represented on the left panel of Fig. 5b. Low and relatively stable daytime levels are followed by a rapid evening elevation culminating around the beginning of the sleep period (40,41). TSH levels then gradually decline during sleep. The nocturnal rise of TSH is controlled by the circadian pacemaker (41–43). The inhibitory influence exerted on TSH during sleep is clearly revealed by the profiles observed in the same subjects during acute total sleep deprivation (Fig. 5b, second panel from left). Indeed, maximal TSH levels are nearly twice as high during nocturnal wakefulness than during nocturnal sleep. Several lines of evidence have indicated that the inhibition of TSH during sleep is associated with SWS (41,44,45). If sleep deprivation is prolonged for a second night, the nocturnal rise of TSH is markedly diminished as compared to that occurring during the first night (46,47). It is likely that, following the first night of sleep deprivation, the elevated thyroid hormone levels, which persist during the daytime period because of the prolonged half-life of these hormones, limit the subsequent TSH rise at the beginning of the next nighttime period. When sleep was restricted for six consecutive nights (Fig. 5b, third panel from left), the nocturnal TSH elevation was markedly dampened, most likely as a result of steadily increasing levels of thyroid hormones, since the free thyroxin index was indeed elevated (27). In contrast, the normal circadian variation of TSH levels was restored by extending the sleep period to 12 hr/night for six consecutive nights (Fig. 5b, right panel).

C. Corticotropic Axis

The 24-hr profile of plasma cortisol under regular sleep-wake conditions in young adults is shown in the left panel of Figure 5c (mean profiles obtained in a group of eight healthy men). As shown in the second panel from left of Figure 5c, which presents the 24-hr cortisol profiles obtained in a group of 17 young men after a night of total sleep deprivation and with recovery sleep being allowed at 2 A.M., the major impact of acute sleep deprivation on the cortisol profile is in the late afternoon and evening hours, when plasma concentrations are generally higher than after a normal night of sleep. Moreover, sleep-wake transitions have been shown to exert modest modulation of the cortisol profile.

A number of studies have indicated that sleep onset is reliably associated with decreasing cortisol secretion (19,48–50). This phenomenon might be related to the inhibitory impact of SWS on cortisol secretion (48,51) or to preparatory mechanisms facilitating sleep onset since cortisol secretion has been shown to present an inverse relationship with SWA, with cortisol decreases preceding SWA increases by about 10 min (52). Under normal conditions, since cortisol secretion is already quiescent in the late evening, this sleep onset effect results in a prolongation of the quiescent period. Therefore, under conditions of sleep deprivation, the nadir of cortisol secretion is less pronounced and occurs earlier than under normal conditions of nocturnal sleep. Conversely, awakenings at the end of the sleep period, as well as awakenings interrupting the sleep period, are consistently followed by a pulse of cortisol secretion (19,51,53,54). During sleep deprivation, these immediate effects of sleep onset and sleep offset on corticotropic activity are absent and the nadir of cortisol levels is higher than during nocturnal sleep (because of the absence of the inhibitory effects of sleep onset) and the morning acrophase is generally lower (because of the absence of the stimulating effects of morning awakening) (second panel from left of Fig. 5c). Overall, the amplitude of the rhythm is reduced by approximately 15% during acute total sleep deprivation as compared to normal conditions.

In addition to the immediate effect of sleep deprivation on cortisol levels at the usual time of sleep onset and sleep offset, acute sleep deprivation appears to affect cortisol secretion the following day (55). Evening cortisol levels (during the time interval 16:00–21:00; shaded areas of Fig. 5c) are significantly higher on the day following total sleep deprivation (second panel from left of Fig. 5c) than after a normal night of sleep (left panel of Fig. 5c). The normal day-long decline of cortisol levels partially reflects the recovery of the hypothalamic-pituitary-adrenal (HPA) axis from the early morning circadian stimulation that occurs in response to increased corticotropin-releasing hormone (CRH) drive during the second part of the night. Elevation of evening cortisol levels might thus reflect an alteration of the rate of recovery of the HPA axis from this endogenous challenge, which is likely to involve an impairment of the feedback regulation of the HPA axis mediated by the hippocampus

The 24-hr cortisol profiles obtained after 6 days of sleep restriction and after 6 days of sleep extension are represented on the two lower-right panels of Figure 5c. These profiles were obtained in the same group of eight healthy men who underwent the 8-hr in-bed condition (Fig. 5c, left panel). The overall waveform of the 24-hr cortisol profile was preserved in the sleep restriction and in the sleep extension conditions. However, when compared to the fully rested condition, the state of sleep debt was associated with alterations of the 24-hr profile of plasma cortisol, including a shorter quiescent period largely due to a nearly 90-min delay in its onset, and elevated levels in the afternoon and early evening (Fig. 5c, shaded areas). As stated above, this alteration may reflect decreased efficacy of the negative-feedback regulation of the HPA axis. Based on the analysis of free cortisol levels in saliva, the rate of decrease of free cortisol concentrations between 16:00 and 21:00 was indeed nearly sixfold slower during sleep restriction than after full sleep recovery.

Both animal and human studies have indicated that deleterious central as well as metabolic effects of HPA hyperactivity are much more pronounced at the time of the usual trough of the rhythm (i.e., in the evening in the human) than at the time of the peak (i.e., in the morning in the human). This is due to the fact that, at the trough of the rhythm, both the high-affinity type I (mineralocorticoid) receptors in the hippocampus and the low-affinity type II (glucocorticoid) receptors in the central nervous system and in the periphery are largely unoccupied (56,57). Thus, the modest elevations in evening cortisol levels that occur in individuals exposed to chronic sleep loss could result both in memory deficits associated with impaired hippocampal function and in the development of peripheral insulin resistance (56,57). The cortisol data obtained in young subjects carrying a sleep debt further suggest the existence of a feed-forward cascade of negative effects. Indeed, nocturnal exposure to increased HPA activity has been shown to promote sleep fragmentation (58,59), and could therefore further impair sleep quality and increase the sleep debt.

V. Impact of Sleep Deprivation on Leptin and Ghrelin Levels and Appetite Regulation

Sleep has an important role in energy balance. In rodents, food shortage or starvation results in decreased sleep (60) and, conversely, total sleep deprivation leads to marked hyperphagia (61). Leptin and ghrelin are both products of peripheral tissues that are involved in energy balance regulation and contribute to the central regulation of food intake (62–65). Leptin, a hormone released by the adipocytes, inhibits appetite (64) whereas ghrelin, a peptide produced predominantly by the stomach, stimulates appetite (65). Leptin levels are elevated during sleep, even when sleep occurs during the daytime (66–68). Ghrelin has been shown to modify sleep-wake patterns in rodents (69) and to stimulate SWS in humans (70).

Figure 6a shows the 24-hr leptin profiles after 6 days of sleep restricted to 4 hr/night and after 6 days of sleep extended to 12 hr/night in a group of healthy, nonobese young men. Leptin profiles in both bedtime conditions exhibited the expected diurnal variation that is largely dependent on meal intake (67). Despite identical amounts of caloric intake, similar levels of physical activity, and stable body mass index, mean leptin levels, acrophase, and amplitude of the diurnal variation were markedly reduced under sleep restriction as compared to sleep extension, and showed respectively a −19%, a −26%, and a −20% decrease. The difference in maximal leptin levels between the two sleep conditions averaged 1.7 ng/mL, i.e., a decrease somewhat larger than that reported to occur in young adults after 3 days of dietary restriction of approximately 900 kcal/day (64).

In another study, which used a randomized crossover design to compare the impact of restricted versus extended sleep, we measured daytime levels of leptin, ghrelin, hunger, and appetite after 2 days of sleep restriction (4-hr bedtime) or sleep extension (10-hr bedtime). Figure 6b shows the daytime leptin (top panel) and ghrelin (bottom panel) profiles obtained in the two bedtime conditions. In this

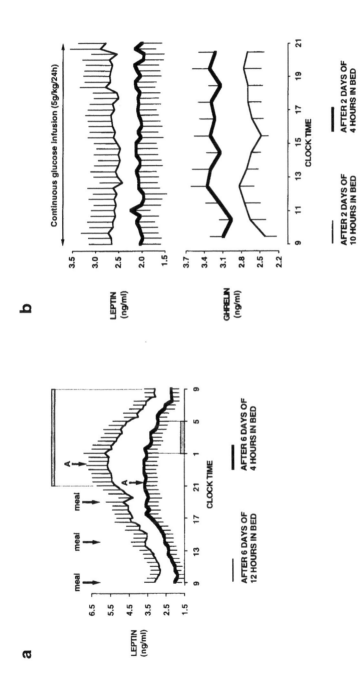

Figure 6 Impact of sleep duration on leptin and ghrelin levels. (a) Mean (± SEM) 24-hr profiles of leptin after 6 days of 4-hr bedtimes and 6 days of 12-hr bedtimes. A, acrophase. Shaded bars represent sleep periods. Mean 24-hr levels and nocturnal acrophase of leptin are markedly decreased after sleep restriction as compared to sleep extension. (b) Mean (± SEM) daytime profiles of leptin and ghrelin after 2 days with 4-hr bedtimes or 2 days with 10-hr bedtimes. Mean daytime leptin levels were 18% lower when sleep was restricted and mean ghrelin levels were 28% higher in the afternoon and early evening when sleep was restricted. (Adapted from Refs. 111 and 112.)

study, leptin levels were stable across the daytime period under both sleep conditions, consistent with the fact that the delivery of calories was exclusively under the form of a constant glucose infusion. Only 2 days with 4-hr bedtimes resulted in a 18% decrease in daytime leptin levels, a nearly 28% increase in afternoon and early evening ghrelin levels, a 24% increase in hunger, and a 23% increase in appetite. The increase in appetite was the largest for foods with high carbohydrate and high fat content, commonly referred to as "junk food" (+33%). There was a robust relationship between the increase in hunger during sleep restriction and the increase in the ratio of ghrelin to leptin concentrations, and analysis of variance revealed that the decrease in leptin was a stronger predictor of changes in hunger than the increase in ghrelin. While these data suggest that the orexigenic effects of sleep restriction are primarily mediated by inhibition of leptin rather than stimulation of ghrelin, further studies monitoring additional factors regulating hunger and appetite, such as cholecystokinin, adiponectin, and peptide YY (PYY), will be needed to elucidate the pathways linking sleep loss and food intake.

In summary, these findings demonstrate that sleep duration has an important role in the regulation of human leptin and ghrelin levels, hunger, and appetite. Since for both studies the experimental protocol was designed to keep energy intake and activity levels (i.e., continuous bed rest) constant for both bedtime conditions, differences in energy balance between the state of sleep loss and the well-rested state were minimal. Sleep loss therefore seems to alter the ability of leptin and ghrelin to accurately signal caloric need and to produce an internal misperception of insufficient energy intake. The findings suggest that sleep loss is likely to increase food intake when food is available ad libitum (unlike in the present studies), consistent with reports of increased food intake in human subjects and in laboratory rodents submitted to total sleep deprivation (61,71).

Taken together with epidemiological data linking body mass index and sleep hours (72,73), these findings suggest that chronic sleep curtailment may contribute to the current epidemic of obesity.

VI. Impact of Sleep Deprivation on Glucose Metabolism

The role of sleep in modulating glucose tolerance across the night has been well documented (13). In subjects who receive an intravenous glucose infusion at a constant rate, plasma glucose levels increase during early sleep and return to presleep levels during late sleep. The increase in plasma glucose appears to be partially related to the predominance of SWS that is associated with a 43% reduction in cerebral glucose metabolism (74). It has been shown that the fall in brain glucose metabolism contributes to about two-thirds of the fall in systemic glucose utilization during sleep (75). The last third would then reflect decreased peripheral utilization. Diminished muscle tone during sleep and rapid anti-insulin-like effects of the sleep-onset GH pulse (76) are likely to both contribute to decreased peripheral glucose uptake. The return of glucose values to presleep values in the later part of the sleep period appears to be partially due to the increase in wake and REM stages (77). Indeed, glucose utilization during REM and wake is higher than during NREM stages (74,75,78,79). In addition, increased insulin sensitivity of peripheral tissues that might result from a delayed effect of low cortisol levels during the evening and early part of the night might participate to the lowering of glucose levels in the later part of the night (80). Under conditions of sleep deprivation, because of the absence of SWS in the first part of the night and related GH secretion, the elevation of glucose levels during early nocturnal sleep is markedly blunted. Thus, sleep has important effects on glucose metabolism, suggesting that sleep disturbances may adversely affect glucose tolerance.

When bedtimes are curtailed to 6 hr/night for 6 days, the glucose response to ingestion of a carbohydrate-rich breakfast is higher than after 6 days of sleep extended to 12 hr/night, despite similar insulin secretory response (27). The magnitude of the difference in peak glucose levels in response to breakfast between the sleep debt and fully rested conditions suggests that, under the sleep restriction condition, the young lean subjects who participated in this study would have responded to a morning standard oral glucose tolerance test in a manner consistent with current diagnostic criteria for impaired glucose tolerance (81,82).

The response to the intravenous glucose tolerance test (IVGTT) following 5 days of sleep restriction confirmed the clinically significant deterioration in glucose tolerance observed after ingestion of a high-carbohydrate breakfast. As apparent in the profiles shown in Figure 7, the rate of disappearance of glucose

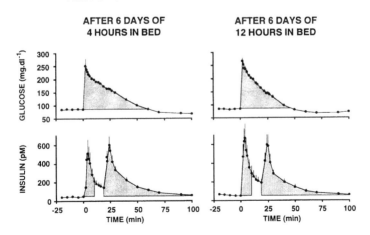

Figure 7 Glucose and insulin profiles obtained in healthy young men during an IVGTT (intravenous glucose administered at 09:00 hr) performed after 6 days of sleep curtailment to 4-hr bedtimes (left) and after 6 days of sleep extension to 12-hr bedtimes (right). (From Ref. 27.)

postinjection (K_G) was 40% slower in the sleep debt condition than after recovery sleep. The difference in K_G between both sleep conditions is similar to that observed in other studies between normal glucose tolerance in young adults and impaired glucose tolerance in older adults (83,84). The acute insulin response to glucose (AIR_G) was also reduced by 30% in the sleep debt condition, compared to postrecovery (lower panels of Fig. 7, left shaded areas). A decrease in AIR_G is an early marker in the development of diabetes and AIR_G decrements of comparable magnitude have been described in aging (85) and gestational diabetes (86). The second phase of insulin secretion tended to be increased (lower panels of Fig. 7, right shaded areas), and insulin sensitivity (S_I) tended to be lower, but the differences did not reach statistical significance.

Abnormalities observed for the counterregulatory hormones cortisol and GH may have contributed to the deterioration in carbohydrate tolerance observed after 1 week of sleep restriction. The biphasic nature of nocturnal GH release after 1 week of sleep restriction resulted in an extended period of elevated GH concentrations as compared to fully rested conditions. By inducing a rapid decrease in muscular glucose uptake (76,87), this extended exposure of peripheral tissues to higher GH levels may have adversely affected glucose regulation. The shortening of the quiescent period of cortisol secretion and the increased evening cortisol concentrations may have been involved in the trend for decreased morning insulin sensitivity. Indeed, even modest elevations of evening glucocorticoid levels result in increased insulin resistance on the following day (88).

VII. Possible Mechanisms Mediating Adverse Effects of Sleep Deprivation on Endocrine and Metabolic Functions

Alterations of autonomic nervous system activity are one of the pathways by which the impact of sleep loss on the central nervous system could be translated to the periphery. Peripheral measures of autonomic nervous system activity that have been used to evaluate the impact of sleep and sleep loss include analyses of cardiac sympathovagal balance, estimations of muscle sympathetic nerve activity (MSNA), and measurements of plasma and/or urinary catecholamine levels.

Analyses of heart rate variability have been widely used to characterize changes in the autonomic nervous system during sleep in healthy humans. The low-frequency (LF) oscillations of heart rate variability, estimated by spectral analysis, are a marker of sympathetic predominance (89) and have been shown to increase during REM sleep (90–93). Conversely, the faster oscillations at the respiratory frequency (high frequency, HF) are a marker of vagal activity and have been shown to predominate during NREM sleep (90–93). Ultradian oscillations in SWA and heart rate variability are inversely coupled during sleep (94–96). Among all electroencephalographic frequency bands, modifications in cardiac vagal activity are predominantly linked to SWA and precede its variations (97).

The autocorrelation of consecutive interbeat intervals (rRR) was introduced as an easy-to-use index of cardiac sympathovagal balance (98-99). Variations in rRR are strongly correlated with variations in LF, HF, and LF/HF, supporting the utility of rRR as an easy-to-monitor, integrative measure of cardiac autonomic activity during sleep.

Sympathetic nerve activity at the level of the muscle (MSNA) is also markedly affected by sleep (100). In comparison with wakefulness, both the amplitude and the frequency of sympathetic bursts are decreased in SWS and increased in REM sleep. As SWA is at its highest during SWS and at its lowest during REM sleep, these results suggest a close temporal link between the evolution of SWA during sleep and sympathetic nerve activity. MSNA is not increased in the morning after a night of total sleep deprivation (101), but this apparently paradoxical observation could be due to the fact that total sleep deprivation prevents REM sleep and the associated increase in sympathetic activity. Here again, findings from studies of acute total sleep deprivation may not generalize to conditions of chronic partial sleep loss.

Studies of acute total or partial sleep deprivation have demonstrated an increase in urinary and plasma catecholamine levels in animals (102) and in humans (103–106) providing further support for the concept that sleep is associated with decreased sympathetic activity and, conversely, that sleep loss is associated with increased sympathetic nervous activity.

Analysis of heart rate variability revealed that 6 days of sleep restriction, as compared to 6 days of sleep extension, is associated with higher values of rRR over the 24-hr period (Fig. 8). Higher rRR values reflect lower levels of heart rate variability due to an elevation of cardiac sympathetic activation and/or a decrease in parasympathetic activation (98). The impact of sleep restriction on sympathovagal balance was particularly important in the morning (27). This relative increase in sympathetic versus parasympathetic tone is the most probable cause

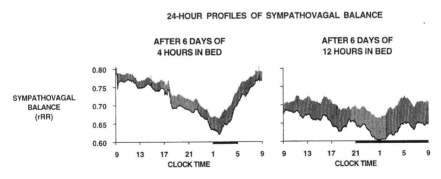

Figure 8 Twenty-four-hour sympathovagal balance (rRR) after 6 days of sleep curtailment to 4-hr bedtimes (left) and after 6 days of sleep extension to 12-hr bedtimes (right). The black bars represent the sleep periods. (From Ref. 112.)

of the decreased leptin levels and β-cell responsiveness during chronic sleep loss. It is also likely to have a deleterious impact on other hormonal systems, cardiac function, blood pressure regulation, and kidney function.

References

1. Bonnet M, Arand D. We are chronically sleep deprived. Sleep 1995; 18:908-911.
2. Broman JE, Lundh LG, Hetta J. Insufficient sleep in the general population. Neurophysiol Clin 1996; 26:30-39.
3. Bliwise DL. Historical change in the report of daytime fatigue. Sleep 1996; 19:462-464.
4. Johnson EO. Sleep in America: 2000. Washington, DC: National Sleep Foundation, 2000:129.
5. Kripke DF, Simons RN, Garfinkel L, Hammond EC. Short and long sleep and sleeping pills. Is increased mortality associated? Arch Gen Psychiatry 1979; 36:103-116.
6. Jean-Louis G, Kripke DF, Ancoli-Israel S. Sleep and quality of well-being. Sleep 2000; 23:1115-1121.
7. Wehr TA, Moul DE, Barbato G, et al. Conservation of photoperiod-responsive mechanisms in humans. Am J Physiol 1993; 265:R846-R857.
8. Roehrs T, Shore E, Papineau K, Rosenthal L, Roth T. A two-week sleep extension in sleepy normals. Sleep 1996; 19:576-582.
9. Harrison Y, Horne JA. Long-term extension to sleep—are we really chronically sleep deprived? Psychophysiology 1996; 33:22-30.
10. Zee P, Turek F. Introduction to sleep and circadian rhythms. In: Zee P, Turek F, eds. Regulation of Sleep and Circadian Rhythms. New York: Marcel Dekker, 1999:1-18.
11. Borbely AA, Achermann P. Sleep homeostasis and models of sleep regulation. J Biol Rhythms 1999; 14:557-568.
12. Van Cauter E, Polonsky KS, Blackman JD, et al. Abnormal temporal patterns of glucose tolerance in obesity: relationship to sleep-related growth hormone and circadian cortisol rhythmicity. J Clin Endocrinol Metab 1994; 79:1797-1805.
13. Scheen AJ, Van Cauter E. The roles of time of day and sleep quality in modulating glucose regulation: clinical implications. Horm Res 1998; 49:191-201.
14. Jarrett RJ. Rhythms in insulin and glucose. In: Krieger D, ed. Endocrine Rhythms. Vol. 1. New York: Raven Press, 1979:247-258.
15. Verrillo A, De Teresa A, Martino C, et al. Differential roles of splanchnic and peripheral tissues in determining diurnal fluctuation of glucose tolerance. Am J Physiol 1989; 257:E459-E465.
16. Lee A, Ader M, Bray GA, Bergman RN. Diurnal variation in glucose tolerance. Cyclic suppression of insulin action and insulin secretion in normal-weight, but not obese, subjects. Diabetes 1992; 41:742-749.
17. Shapiro ET, Polonsky KS, Copinschi G, et al. Nocturnal elevation of glucose levels during fasting in noninsulin-dependent diabetes. J Clin Endocrinol Metab 1991; 72:444-454.
18. Van Cauter E, Desir D, Decoster C, Fery F, Balasse EO. Nocturnal decrease in glucose tolerance during constant glucose infusion. J Clin Endocrinol Metab 1989; 69:604-611.

19. Van Cauter E, Blackman JD, Roland D, Spire JP, Refetoff S, Polonsky KS. Modulation of glucose regulation and insulin secretion by circadian rhythmicity and sleep. J Clin Invest 1991; 88:934-942.

20. Spiegel K, Leproult R, Colecchia EF, et al. Adaptation of the 24-h growth hormone profile to a state of sleep debt. Am J Physiol Regul Integr Comp Physiol 2000; 279:R874-R883.

21. Van Dongen HP, Maislin G, Mullington JM, Dinges DF. The cumulative cost of additional wakefulness: dose-response effects on neurobehavioral functions and sleep physiology from chronic sleep restriction and total sleep deprivation. Sleep 2003; 26:117-26.

22. Borbely AA, Baumann F, Brandeis D, Strauch I, Lehmann D. Sleep deprivation: effect on sleep stages and EEG power density in man. Electroencephalogr Clin Neurophysiol 1981; 51:483-495.

23. Feinberg I, Fein G, Floyd TC. EEG patterns during and following extended sleep in young adults. Electroencephalogr Clin Neurophysiol 1980; 50:467-476.

24. Feinberg I, Fein G, Floyd TC. Computer-detected patterns of electroencephalographic delta activity during and after extended sleep. Science 1982; 215:1131-1133.

25. Feinberg I, March JD, Floyd TC, Jimison R, Bossom-Demitrack L, Katz PH. Homeostatic changes during post-nap sleep maintain baseline levels of delta EEG. Electroencephalogr Clin Neurophysiol 1985; 61:134-138.

26. Borbely AA. A two process model of sleep regulation. Human Neurobiol 1982; 1:195-204.

27. Spiegel K, Leproult R, Van Cauter E. Impact of sleep debt on metabolic and endocrine function. Lancet 1999; 354:1435-1439.

28. Takahashi Y, Kipnis DM, Daughaday WH. Growth hormone secretion during sleep. J Clin Invest 1968; 47:2079-2090.

29. Sassin JF, Parker DC, Mace JW, Gotlin RW, Johnson LC, Rossman LG. Human growth hormone release: relation to slow-wave sleep and sleep-waking cycles. Science 1969; 165:513-515.

30. Honda Y, Takahashi K, Takahashi S, et al. Growth hormone secretion during nocturnal sleep in normal subjects. J Clin Endocrinol Metab 1969; 29:20-29.

31. Van Cauter E, Copinschi G. Interrelations between sleep and the somatotropic axis. Sleep 1998; 21:553-566.

32. Holl RW, Hartmann ML, Veldhuis JD, Taylor WM, Thorner MO. Thirty-second sampling of plasma growth hormone in man: correlation with sleep stages. J Clin Endocrinol Metab 1991; 72:854-861.

33. Van Cauter E, Kerkhofs M, Caufriez A, Van Onderbergen A, Thorner MO, Copinschi G. A quantitative estimation of GH secretion in normal man: reproducibility and relation to sleep and time of day. J Clin Endocrinol Metab 1992; 74:1441-1450.

34. Gronfier C, Luthringer R, Follenius M, et al. A quantitative evaluation of the relationships between growth hormone secretion and delta wave electroencephalographic activity during normal sleep and after enrichment in delta waves. Sleep 1996; 19:817-824.

35. Van Cauter E, Plat L, Scharf MB, et al. Simultaneous stimulation of slow-wave sleep and growth hormone secretion by gamma-hydroxybutyrate. J Clin Invest 1997; 100:745-753.

36. Weibel L, Follenius M, Spiegel K, Gronfier C, Brandenberger G. Growth hormone secretion in night workers. Chronobiol Int 1997; 14:49-60.
37. Jaffe C, Turgeon D, DeMott Friberg R, Watkins P, Barkan A. Nocturnal augmentation of growth hormone (GH) secretion is preserved during repetitive bolus administration of GH-releasing hormone: potential involvement of endogenous somatostatin—a clinical research center study. J Clin Endocrinol Metab 1995; 80:3321-3326.
38. Brandenberger G, Gronfier C, Chapotot F, Simon C, Piquard F. Effect of sleep deprivation on overall 24 h growth-hormone secretion [letter] [In Process Citation]. Lancet 2000; 356:1408.
39. Borbely AA. Processes underlying sleep regulation. Horm Res 1998; 49:114-117.
40. Veldhuis JD, Iranmanesh A, Johnson ML, Lizarralde G. Twenty-four-hour rhythms in plasma concentrations of adenohypophyseal hormones are generated by distinct amplitude and/or frequency modulation of underlying pituitary secretory bursts. J Clin Endocrinol Metab 1990; 71:1616-1623.
41. Brabant G, Prank K, Ranft U, et al. Physiological regulation of circadian and pulsatile thyrotropin secretion in normal man and woman. J Clin Endocrinol Metab 1990; 70:403-409.
42. Parker DC, Rossman LG, Pekary AE, Hershman JM. Effect of 64-hour sleep deprivation on the circadian waveform of thyrotropin (TSH): further evidence of sleep-related inhibition of TSH release. J Clin Endocrinol Metab 1987; 64:157-161.
43. Van Cauter E, Sturis J, Byrne MM, et al. Demonstration of rapid light-induced advances and delays of the human circadian clock using hormonal phase markers. Am J Physiol 1994; 266:E953-E963.
44. Goichot B, Brandenberger G, Saini J, Wittersheim G, Follenius M. Nocturnal plasma thyrotropin variations are related to slow-wave sleep. J Sleep Res 1992; 1:186-190.
45. Gronfier C, Luthringer R, Follenius M, et al. Temporal link between plasma thyrotropin levels and electroencephalographic activity in man. Neurosci Lett 1995; 200:97-100.
46. Van Cauter E, Sturis J, Byrne MM, et al. Demonstration of rapid light-induced advances and delays of the human circadian clock using hormonal phase markers. Am J Physiol 1994; 266:E953-E963.
47. Allan JS, Czeisler CA. Persistence of the circadian thyrotropin rhythm under constant conditions and after light-induced shifts of circadian phase. J Clin Endocrinol Metab 1994; 79:508-512.
48. Weitzman ED, Zimmerman JC, Czeisler CA, Ronda JM. Cortisol secretion is inhibited during sleep in normal man. J Clin Endocrinol Metab 1983; 56:352-358.
49. Born J, Muth S, Fehm HL. The significance of sleep onset and slow wave sleep for nocturnal release of growth hormone (GH) and cortisol. Psychoneuroendocrinology 1988; 13:233-243.
50. Weibel L, Follenius M, Spiegel K, Ehrhart J, Brandenberger G. Comparative effect of night and daytime sleep on the 24-hour cortisol secretory profile. Sleep 1995; 18:549-556.
51. Follenius M, Brandenberger G, Bandesapt J, Libert J, Ehrhart J. Nocturnal cortisol release in relation to sleep structure. Sleep 1992; 15:21-27.
52. Gronfier C, Chapotot F, Weibel L, Jouny C, Piquard F, Brandenberger G. Pulsatile cortisol secretion and EEG delta waves are controlled by two independent but synchronized generators. Am J Physiol 1998; 275:E94-E100.

53. Spath-Schwalbe E, Gofferje M, Kern W, Born J, Fehm HL. Sleep disruption alters nocturnal ACTH and cortisol secretory patterns. Biol Psychiatry 1991; 29:575-584.

54. Van Cauter E, van Coevorden A, Blackman JD. Modulation of neuroendocrine release by sleep and circadian rhythmicity. In: Yen S, Vale W, eds. Advances in Neuroendocrine Regulation of Reproduction. Norwell, MA: Serono Symposia USA, 1990:113-122.

55. Leproult R, Copinschi G, Buxton O, Van Cauter E. Sleep loss results in an elevation of cortisol levels the next evening. Sleep 1997; 20:865-870.

56. Dallman MF, Strack AL, Akana SF, et al. Feast and famine: critical role of glucocorticoids with insulin in daily energy flow. Front Neuroendocrinol 1993; 14:303-347.

57. McEwen B. Protective and damaging effects of stress mediators. N Engl J Med 1998; 338:171-179.

58. Buguet A, Cespuglio R, Radomski MW. Sleep and stress in man: an approach through exercise and exposure to extreme environments. Can J Physiol Pharmacol 1998; 76:553-561.

59. Holsboer F, von Bardelein U, Steiger A. Effects of intravenous corticotropin-releasing hormone upon sleep-related growth hormone surge and sleep EEG in man. Neuroendocrinology 1988; 48:32-38.

60. Danguir J, Nicolaidis S. Dependence of sleep on nutrients' availability. Physiol Behav 1979; 22:735-740.

61. Rechtschaffen A, Bergmann BM. Sleep deprivation in the rat by the disk-over-water method. Behav Brain Res 1995; 69:55-63.

62. Ahima RS, Saper CB, Flier JS, Elmquist JK. Leptin regulation of neuroendocrine systems. Front Neuroendocrinol 2000; 21:263-307.

63. Kolaczynski JW, Considine RV, Ohannesian J, et al. Responses of leptin to short-term fasting and refeeding in humans: a link with ketogenesis but not ketones themselves. Diabetes 1996; 45:1511-1515.

64. Chin-Chance C, Polonsky KS, Schoeller DA. Twenty-four-hour leptin levels respond to cumulative short-term energy imbalance and predict subsequent intake. J Clin Endocrinol Metab 2000; 85:2685-2691.

65. Havel PJ. Peripheral signals conveying metabolic information to the brain: short-term and long-term regulation of food intake and energy homeostasis. Exp Biol Med (Maywood) 2001; 226:963-977.

66. Sinha MK, Ohannesian JP, Heiman ML, et al. Nocturnal rise of leptin in lean, obese, and non-insulin-dependent diabetes mellitus subjects. J Clin Invest 1996; 97:1344-1347.

67. Schoeller DA, Cella LK, Sinha MK, Caro JF. Entrainment of the diurnal rhythm of plasma leptin to meal timing. J Clin Invest 1997; 100:1882-1887.

68. Simon C, Gronfier C, Schlienger JL, Brandenberger G. Circadian and ultradian variations of leptin in normal man under continuous enteral nutrition: relationship to sleep and body temperature. J Clin Endocrinol Metab 1998; 83:1893-1899.

69. Tolle V, Bassant MH, Zizzari P, et al. Ultradian rhythmicity of ghrelin secretion in relation with GH, feeding behavior, and sleep-wake patterns in rats. Endocrinology 2002; 143:1353-1361.

70. Weikel JC, Wichniak A, Ising M, et al. Ghrelin promotes slow-wave sleep in humans. Am J Physiol Endocrinol Metab 2003; 284:E407-E415.

71. Dinges DF, Chugh DK. Physiological correlates of sleep deprivation. In: Kinney JM, Tucker HN, eds. Physiology, Stress, and Malnutrition: Functional Correlates, Nutritional Intervention. Philadelphia: Lippincott-Raven Publishers, 1997.

72. Kripke DF, Garfinkel L, Wingard DL, Klauber MR, Marler MR. Mortality associated with sleep duration and insomnia. Arch Gen Psychiatry 2002; 59:131-136.

73. Vioque J, Torres A, Quiles J. Time spent watching television, sleep duration and obesity in adults living in Valencia, Spain. Int J Obes Relat Metab Disord 2000; 24:1683-1688.

74. Maquet P, Dive D, Salmon E, et al. Cerebral glucose utilization during sleep-wake cycle in man determined by positron emission tomography and [18F]2-fluoro-2-deoxy-D-glucose method. Brain Res 1990; 513:136-143.

75. Boyle PJ, Scott JC, Krentz AJ, Nagy RJ, Comstock E, Hoffman C. Diminished brain glucose metabolism is a significant determinant for falling rates of systemic glucose utilization during sleep in normal humans. J Clin Invest 1994; 93:529-535.

76. Møller N, Jorgensen JO, Schmitz O, et al. Effects of a growth hormone pulse on total and forearm substrate fluxes in humans. Am J Physiol 1990; 258:E86-E91.

77. Scheen AJ, Byrne MM, Plat L, Leproult R, Van Cauter E. Relationships between sleep quality and glucose regulation in normal humans. Am J Physiol 1996; 271:E261-E270.

78. Buchsbaum MS, Gillin JC, Wu J, et al. Regional cerebral glucose metabolic rate in human sleep assessed by positron emission tomography. Life Sci 1989; 45:1349-1356.

79. Maquet P, Dive D, Salmon E, et al. Cerebral glucose utilization during stage 2 sleep in man. Brain Res 1992; 571:149-153.

80. Plat L, Byrne MM, Sturis J, et al. Effects of morning cortisol elevation on insulin secretion and glucose regulation in humans. Am J Physiol 1996; 270:E36-E42.

81. Gumbiner B, Polonsky KS, Beltz WF, Wallace P, Brechtel G, Fink RI. Effects of aging on insulin secretion. Diabetes 1989; 38:1549-1556.

82. VanHelder T, Symons JD, Radomski MW. Effects of sleep deprivation and exercise on glucose tolerance. Aviat Space Environ Med 1993; 64:487-492.

83. Garcia G, Freeman R, Supiano M, Smith M, Galecki A, Halter J. Glucose metabolism in older adults: a study including subjects more than 80 years of age. J Am Geriatr Soc 1997; 45:813-817.

84. Prigeon RL, Kahn SE, Porte D, Jr. Changes in insulin sensitivity, glucose effectiveness, and B-cell function in regularly exercising subjects. Metabolism 1995; 44:1259-1263.

85. Kahn SE, Prigeon RL, McCulloch DK, et al. Quantification of the relationship between insulin sensitivity and beta-cell function in human subjects. Evidence for a hyperbolic function. Diabetes 1993; 42:1663-1672.

86. Catalano PM, Tyzbir ED, Wolfe RR, et al. Carbohydrate metabolism during pregnancy in control subjects and women with gestational diabetes. Am J Physiol 1993; 264:E60-E67.

87. Møller N, Butler PC, Antsiferov MA, Alberti KGMM. Effects of growth hormone on insulin sensitivity and forearm metabolism in normal man. Diabetologia 1989; 32:105-110.

88. Plat L, Leproult R, L'Hermite-Baleriaux M, et al. Metabolic effects of short-term elevations of plasma cortisol are more pronounced in the evening than in the morning. J Clin Endocrinol Metab 1999; 84:3082-3092.

89. Pagani M, Lombardi F, Guzzetti S, et al. Power spectral analysis of heart rate and arterial pressure variabilities as a marker of sympatho-vagal interaction in man and conscious dog. Circ Res 1986; 59:178-193.

90. Zemaityte D, Varoneckas G, Plauska K, Kaukenas J. Components of the heart rhythm power spectrum in wakefulness and individual sleep stages. Int J Psychophysiol 1986; 4:129-141.

91. Berlad II, Shlitner A, Ben-Haim S, Lavie P. Power spectrum analysis and heart rate variability in stage 4 and REM sleep: evidence for state-specific changes in autonomic dominance. J Sleep Res 1993; 2:88-90.

92. Vanoli E, Adamson PB, Ba L, Pinna GD, Lazzara R, Orr WC. Heart rate variability during specific sleep stages. A comparison of healthy subjects with patients after myocardial infarction. Circulation 1995; 91:1918-1922.

93. Bonnet MH, Arand DL. Heart rate variability: sleep stage, time of night, and arousal influences. Electroencephalogr Clin Neurophysiol 1997; 102:390-396.

94. Charloux A, Otzenberger H, Gronfier C, Lonsdorfer-Wolf E, Piquard F, Brandenberger G. Oscillations in sympatho-vagal balance oppose variations in delta-wave activity and the associated renin release. J Clin Endocrinol Metab 1998; 83:1523-1528.

95. Otzenberger H, Simon C, Gronfier C, Brandenberger G. Temporal relationship between dynamic heart rate variability and electroencephalographic activity during sleep in man. Neurosci Lett 1997; 229:173-176.

96. Brandenberger G, Ehrhart J, Piquard F, Simon C. Inverse coupling between ultradian oscillations in delta wave activity and heart rate variability during sleep. Clin Neurophysiol 2001; 112:992-996.

97. Jurysta F, van de Borne P, Migeotte P, et al. A study of the dynamic interactions between sleep EEG and heart rate variability in normal young men. Clin Neurophysical 2003; 114:2140–2145.

98. Kamen PW, Krum H, Tonkin AM. Poincaré plots of heart rate variability allows quantitive display of parasympathetic nervous activity in humans. Clin Sci 1996; 91:201-208.

99. Otzenberger H, Gronfier C, Simon C, et al. Dynamic heart rate variability: a tool for exploring sympathovagal balance continuously during sleep in men. Am J Physiol 1998; 275:H946-H950.

100. Somers VK, Dyken ME, Mark AL, Abboud FM. Sympathetic-nerve activity during sleep in normal subjects. N Engl J Med 1993; 328:303-307.

101. Kato M, Phillips BG, Sigurdsson G, Narkiewicz K, Pesek CA, Somers VK. Effects of sleep deprivation on neural circulatory control. Hypertension 2000; 35:1173-1175.

102. Everson CA. Functional consequences of sustained sleep deprivation in the rat. Behav Brain Res 1995; 69:43-54.

103. Muller HU, Riemann D, Berger M, Muller WE. The influence of total sleep deprivation on urinary excretion of catecholamine metabolites in major depression. Acta Psychiatr Scand 1993; 88:16-20.

104. Irwin M, Thompson J, Miller C, Gillin JC, Ziegler M. Effects of sleep and sleep deprivation on catecholamine and interleukin-2 levels in humans: clinical implications. J Clin Endocrinol Metab 1999; 84:1979-1985.

105. Tochikubo O, Ikeda A, Miyajima E, Ishii M. Effects of insufficient sleep on blood pressure monitored by a new multibiomedical recorder. Hypertension 1996; 27:1318-1324.

106. Lusardi P, Zoppi A, Preti P, Pesce RM, Piazza E, Fogari R. Effects of insufficient sleep on blood pressure in hypertensive patients: a 24-h study. Am J Hypertens 1999; 12:63-68.

107. Van Cauter E, Spiegel K. Hormones and metabolism during sleep. In: Schwartz WJ, ed. Sleep Science: Integrating Basic Research and Clinical Practice. Monographs in Clinical Neuroscience. Vol. 15. Basel: Karger, 1997:144-174.
108. Van Cauter E, Spiegel K. Circadian and sleep control of endocrine secretions. In: Turek FW, Zee PC, eds. Regulation of Sleep and Circadian Rhythms. Vol. 133. New York: Marcel Dekker, 1999:397-426.
109. Frank SA, Roland DC, Sturis J, et al. Effects of aging on glucose regulation during wakefulness and sleep. Am J Physiol 1995; 269:E1006-E1016.
110. Leproult R, Van Reeth O, Byrne MM, Sturis J, Van Cauter E. Sleepiness, performance, and neuroendocrine function during sleep deprivation: effects of exposure to bright light or exercise. J Biol Rhythms 1997; 12:245-258.
111. Spiegel K, Tasali E, Penev P, Van Cauter E. Sleep curtailment in healthy young men is associated with decreased leptin levels, elevated ghrelin levels and increased hunger and appetite. Submitted.
112. Spiegel K, Leproult R, L'Hermite-Balériaux M, Copinschi G, Penev P, Van Cauter E. Leptin levels are dependent on sleep duration: relationships with sympatho-vagal balance, carboxydrate regulation, cortisol, and TSH. J Clin Endocrinol Metab. Submitted.

15

Thermoregulatory Changes

PAUL J. SHAW

The Neurosciences Institute, San Diego, California, U.S.A.

I. Introduction

Past experiments investigating the effects of total sleep deprivation (TSD) on the functioning of the central nervous system have been disappointing. Prolonged sleep deprivation has not revealed changes in: (a) brain histology at the light microscopic level, (b) brain histology using electron microscopy, (c) level and/or turnover of brain monoamines, (d) cholinergic receptor density and affinity, (e) adrenergic receptor binding and affinity, (f) incorporation of 2-deoxyglucose, and (g) the expression of the immediate early gene epidermal growth factor-1 (EGR-1) (see 1 and 2 for review). Although recent studies have begun to reveal more clues using molecular-genetic strategies (see Ref. 3 for review), the nature of the underlying pathological process remains a mystery. These results are somewhat surprising when one considers that long-term TSD is invariably fatal (4,5). Nonetheless, the inability to detect major pathological modifications in the brains of sleep-deprived animals suggest that the deficits produced by TSD result not from a general impairment of the CNS but rather from modifications in specific functional systems (6).

Examination of the systemic physiological and behavioral adjustments that are made by animals subjected to chronic TSD implicate thermoregulatory pathways as major functional targets of sleep loss. Thus, sleep deprivation results in: (a) an initial elevation in waking peritoneal temperature followed by a decline to below baseline levels; (b) an elevation in waking brain temperature that persists well into the fourth quarter of survival time; and (c) a progressive increase in energy expenditure (Fig. 1). Rats that are selectively deprived of paradoxical sleep [i.e., rapid-eye-movement (REM) sleep] also exhibit a progressive increase in energy expenditure but exhibit only a decline in body temperature (Fig. 1) (7). These data have been interpreted to indicate that TSD resulted in both an elevated temperature set point and an inability to retain body heat, whereas paradoxical sleep deprivation produced only an inability to retain body heat (8). Interestingly, these thermoregulatory modifications persist during recovery sleep. The effects of sleep deprivation on thermoregulation in human and animal studies will be discussed below.

II. Body Temperature Regulation

Before discussing the effects of sleep deprivation on thermoregulation, it will be useful to briefly review basic concepts pertaining to the regulation of body temperature. The ability to maintain a relatively constant internal temperature in the face of wide variations in ambient temperature is a common feature of mammals and birds. However, extreme conditions are not uncommon, and animals that are seemingly less equipped to deal with these variations have developed adaptations that take advantage of fundamental properties of heat transfer to ensure survival. Although these strategies can be quite elaborate, as is the case in some fish (9), reptiles (10), and invertebrates (11) that can maintain body temperatures substantially above ambient temperature, most are very rudimentary. Whether simple or elaborate, it is important to emphasize that body temperature regulation is a fundamental requirement for most animals regardless of whether they have been classified as euthermic or poikilothermic (see 12 and 13 for reviews).

A. Heat Transfer

In order to maintain a constant body temperature heat gain must equal heat loss. Heat can be transferred from the environment to the animal or from the animal to the environment only through conduction, radiation, and evaporation. Conduction takes place between two objects that are in physical contact with one another. These objects can be solids, liquids, or gases. Conduction of heat is a direct transfer of kinetic energy of molecular motion from a region of high temperature to a region of low temperature. Objects vary in their conductivity coefficients such that some objects transfer heat very well (e.g., metals) whereas others transfer heat poorly (e.g., air). Animal tissues have relatively high conductivity coefficients because they contain a high proportion of water (about 66%–75%) whereas fur, which can trap large amounts of air, has a markedly lower conductivity coefficient. When air temperature is lower than skin temperature, heat is transferred away from the animal toward the environment. Conversely, when air temperature is above skin temperature heat is transferred to the organism. It is important to remember that in addition to heat transfer between organism and environment,

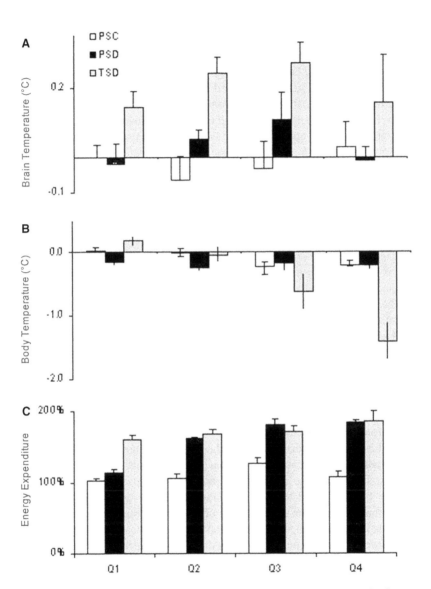

Figure 1 Mean waking brain temperature (A) and peritoneal temperature (B) in paradoxical sleep-deprived (PSD), paradoxical sleep control (PSC), and total sleep-deprived (TSD) rats during each quarter of survival. Data expressed as change in degrees Celsius from their respective baseline means. Mean daily energy expenditure (C) for PSD, PSC, and TSD rats expressed as a percentage of baseline. Error bars indicate standard error.

heat is also transferred within an organism by conduction brought about by local changes in blood flow. Objects that are not in physical contact can transfer heat through radiation. All objects that are above zero Kelvin emit electromagnetic radiation, the intensity and wavelength being dependent on the temperature of the surface of the emitting body. For all intents and purposes, the human skin is able to absorb 100% of all incoming infrared radiation. As with conduction, the direction of heat transfer is always away from the object with the higher temperature. Finally, heat can be transferred through evaporation. To turn 1 g of water at room temperature to water vapor requires 584 calories and as such provides a very efficient way to dissipate heat. Although the transfer of heat to an organism by evaporation is rare, air temperature and humidity will determine the amount of heat that can be lost by evaporation.

B. Autonomic Thermoregulation

Although we speak of body temperature regulation, the temperature of the body is not uniform. Some organs may have higher rates of heat production than others and may differ by as much as 0.5°C or more. These temperature fields can change depending on the heat balance of the organism (14). For example, in the cold, heat transfer to the environment occurs through conduction from the skin to the environment. This heat transfer can be reduced by restricting blood flow (heat) to the periphery; skin and superficial tissues will be several degrees cooler than deeper tissues. However, if heat loss still exceeds metabolic heat production, the organism is placed at risk. Under these conditions, the temperature of vital organs (i.e., heart, liver, brain) may be preserved at the expense of other organs. As blood flow to less vital organs is reduced, the temperature gradient to the environment is also reduced and the amount of insulation between the vital organs and the environment is increased, providing an additional barrier to heat flow; brain temperature may be several degrees higher than that of the peritoneum. In a warm environment, the temperature of organs with elevated metabolic rates can become dangerously high. If the ambient temperature is lower than body temperature, heat can be transferred to the environment, again through conduction. Under these circumstances, the maintenance of internal temperature fields serves to store heat and is maladaptive. Thus, blood flow is increased throughout the animal in order to bring as much heat from deep body tissues to the skin as possible. In contrast to an animal in the cold, then, the temperature of the body is quite uniform. Warmer skin temperature also brings water closer to its vaporization temperature and facilitates evaporative cooling.

The foregoing discussion emphasizes that an organism will respond to specific thermoregulatory challenges by recruiting specific effector mechanisms in order to keep the temperature of one or more regions of the body in a restricted range. It is only by observing the activation of effector mechanisms that we can infer that the temperature of an animal deviates from that range. The temperature range of a body region that does not invoke compensatory thermoregulatory responses is considered to be the temperature set point for that region. As mentioned above, body temperature need not be uniform and, indeed, temperature sensors are located throughout the body, brain, and spinal cord and are able to activate thermoregulatory responses (15,16). What then is the regulated variable? The precise cellular or network mechanisms that generate a temperature set point are not known (17). However, electrophysiological, pharmacological, and lesion studies implicate the preoptic anterior hypothalamus (POAH) as a primary source of thermal feedback for mammals and the center for the coordination of appropriate thermoregulatory responses (18). For example, when the POAH is locally cooled via a thermocouple, the animal responds as if it were cold, increasing the rate of metabolic heat production and reducing its rate of conductive heat loss by decreasing blood flow to the skin (19). Similarly, when the POAH is locally heated, the animal responds as if it were hot by reducing its metabolic heat production and increasing blood flow to the skin to facilitate heat loss (20–22). In this way temperature set point can be defined by describing the range of temperatures that do not result in a thermoregulatory response. It should be noted that the temperature set point of an animal is not constant and is influenced by many variables including heat balance (23), circadian factors (24), and behavioral state (25), to name a few. In that regard it is important to emphasize that monitoring an animal's core temperature does not provide any information about its thermoregulatory status. Not only will a successful thermoregulatory response feed back on the regulated variable, but it may also shift the temperature set point. Thus, although one might assume that a low core temperature indicates that an animal is cold; this need not be the case. For example, the brain temperature of a dog in a hot environment can be substantially below the brain temperature of a dog in a cold environment (26). In the former case, the dog successfully prevented hyperthermia by activating heat loss mechanisms. If one were to evaluate brain temperature alone, one might erroneously conclude that the animal in the cold environment was hyperthermic whereas the animal in the hot environment was hypothermic. In order to asses thermoregulation one must simultaneously monitor core temperature and an appropriate effector such as skin temperature, metabolic rate, or behavior (huddling, shivering, building nests, etc.).

C. Behavioral Thermoregulation

Mammals have evolved both behavioral and autonomic mechanisms to maintain stable body temperatures in response to changing environmental conditions (13,27–29). The recruitment of these mechanisms is under homeostatic control and is believed to be comprised of two primary feedback loops (30). The first feedback loop is for heat gain and/or retention, the second for heat dissipation. When faced with a thermal challenge, behavioral and autonomic mechanisms will be recruited according to their threshold of activation. Although behavioral and autonomic responses are coordinated and are frequently used in combination, several studies suggest that behavioral methods are initially used to increase heat loss whereas autonomic effectors are primarily used to achieve heat gain (31-33). For example, rats given intraperitoneal (IP), intracerebroventricular (ICV), or intrathecal (IT) injections of capsaicin in the absence of an operant showed an immediate fall in core temperature that was mediated by a large increase in tail temperature (i.e., vasodilation) (34). However, when rats were given an operant whereby they could select cool ambient temperatures, both core and tail temperatures decreased, indicating that the rats relied on behavioral responses to a lower core temperature. The preference for behavioral effectors to facilitate heat loss has also been found in squirrel monkeys (35). In that experiment, the medial preoptic area was heated and the animals were allowed to manipulate cage temperature by selecting between air temperatures of 10°C and 50°C. The monkeys were able to maintain stable core and peripheral temperatures by responding on the operant and did not noticeably activate autonomic effectors. The different thresholds of activation seen in response to positive and negative thermal loads are consistent with the observation that behavioral and autonomic responses are functionally and anatomically distinct (13).

D.   Thermoregulation During Sleep

Historically, one of the best predictors of sleep onset has been an increase in the temperature of the distal extremities. This observation, first reported in 1939 by Magnussen, was confirmed by Nathaniel Kleitman in 1948 (36) and again most recently by Krauchi et al. in 1999 (37), thereby emphasizing the interrelationship between these two systems. A thorough review of the relationship between sleep and thermoregulation is beyond the scope of this chapter and will only be discussed briefly. However, several excellent reviews are available and are strongly recommended (38–42).

During the transition from waking to non-REM (NREM) sleep, core temperature normally falls as heat production is reduced and heat loss is enhanced through increased blood flow to the periphery (43). The fall in core temperature during the transition from wake to NREM sleep is ubiquitous, being found in all species studied including armadillo, cat, dog, monkey, opossum, man, mouse, rabbit, and rat (reviewed in 40). The reduction in metabolic heat production which accompanies the fall in core temperature has been found over a range of ambient temperatures indicating that the fall is regulated (44). The drop in core temperature is facilitated not only by decreases in metabolic heat production but also by heat-dissipating mechanisms that appear to be increased during NREM sleep. For example, upon entry into NREM, cats housed at very warm ambient temperature increased vasodilation and tachypnea above waking values to actively regulate core temperature at a lower level (40,45). Using a proportional control model to describe thermoregulation during sleep, Glotzbach and Heller (25) reported that in the kangaroo rat the proportionality coefficients relating changes in POAH temperature to changes in metabolic heat production were lower during NREM sleep than waking; their data also suggested a drop of the lower critical threshold, which is consistent with a regulated fall in temperature set point. These changes in heat production and heat loss appear to be mediated, at least in part, by state-dependent changes in neuronal firing rates of temperature-sensitive neurons in the basal forebrain and medial preoptic area (25,46–50). The proportion of temperature-sensitive neurons decreased during the transition from wake to NREM sleep, consistent with a reduced gain and lowered temperature set point. Thus, the results of many studies from a variety of species measuring many effector systems (i.e., vasomotion, tachypnea, piloerection, metabolic rate) have demonstrated a regulated fall in core temperature during the transition from wake to NREM sleep.

III. Sleep Deprivation

A. Human Studies

The ease with which one can measure body temperature, along with its usefulness in tracking circadian rhythms, has made it one of the most frequently evaluated variables in sleep deprivation experiments. Indeed, body temperature was monitored during the first sleep deprivation experiment ever conducted in humans (51). This pioneering experiment reported that 90 hr of sleep loss resulted in a distinct fall in body temperature. These findings were first confirmed by Nathaniel Kleitman in 1923 (52) and consistently since then (reviewed in Ref. 53). Studies that have monitored body temperature continuously during sleep deprivation have also found that while the circadian variation in core temperature was preserved, both the peak and the nadir of the body temperature rhythm declined over time (54,55). Since then, many other groups have consistently reported a drop in core temperature following even a few hours of sleep deprivation (see 8 and 56 for reviews). Surprisingly, while body temperature is frequently monitored in human sleep deprivation experiments, very few studies have evaluated the effects of sleep loss on thermoregulation per se. Thus, it has not been clear whether the drop in body temperature is due to thermoregulatory adjustments or is a consequence of confounding variables such as circadian time or body posture (8,57).

An additional complication has been the need to impose a relatively discrete thermoregulatory challenge (e.g., cold or heat exposure) to assess the integrity of the system. Under neutral conditions sleep-deprived subjects show signs that suggest thermoregulation may be impaired (i.e., lower body temperature). When challenged, however, sleep-deprived subjects may respond more effectively than controls, indicating that thermoregulation is very much intact (see below). These seemingly contradictory results neglect findings from animal studies that indicate that chronic and acute challenges frequently invoke disparate thermoregulatory strategies and these strategies are in turn influenced by the availability of both internal and external resources. Interestingly, behavioral adjustments, which in many cases are the first line of defense against a thermal challenge, have not been evaluated. Nonetheless, anecdotal reports indicate that sleep-deprived subjects report being cold, eat more without gaining weight, and frequently put on more clothing and turn up the heat when allowed (42). Taken together the data indicate that sleep deprivation impairs heat retention mechanisms in humans.

One of the first studies to specifically evaluate the effects of sleep deprivation on thermoregulation was conducted by Fiorica and colleagues in 1968 (58). Body temperature, skin temperature and metabolic heat production were evaluated following 4 days of sleep deprivation in six male subjects at 27°C and during a brief exposure to ambient temperatures of 10°C. At 27°C, metabolic rate remained unchanged but body temperature declined, indicating increased heat loss. If the reduction in body temperature was the result of a lowered temperature set point and not a deficit in heat retention, one would expect subjects placed into the cold to allow body temperature to fall without invoking compensatory thermoregulatory responses (e.g., increased metabolic rate, decreased skin blood flow). However, sleep-deprived and control subjects responded to cold exposure with similar increases in both rectal temperature and metabolic rate. Skin temperature, on the other hand, was lower in sleep-deprived subjects, indicating that in comparison to controls they mounted a more vigorous defense of core temperature. That is, they responded as if they were colder. Similarly, Savourey and Bittell (59) reported that 2 hr of cold exposure following 27 hr of sleep deprivation resulted in increased sensations of thermal discomfort. Moreover, sleep-deprived subjects began to shiver at warmer body temperatures than controls, indicating that they were less willing to allow their body temperature to drop further. Landis et al. (56) evaluated thermoregulatory adjustments during acute heat and cold exposure in women who had been sleep deprived for 24 hr. As expected, core temperature was reduced following sleep deprivation and the sleep-deprived subjects responded to the negative thermal load with increased vasoconstriction. However, during a second cooling period core temperature fell rapidly, leading the authors to conclude that sleep deprivation weakened thermoregulatory defenses against cooling.

Because metabolic heat production can be increased dramatically during exercise, several investigators have monitored heat gain and heat loss mechanisms in sleep-deprived subjects exercising in cold and hot environments. The increased heat production associated with exercise can be readily stored in cool environments by minimizing heat loss through vasoconstriction. In contrast, exercise in a warm environment frequently induces hyperthermia and thus the need to maximize heat loss through vasodilatation and evaporative cooling. If sleep-deprived subjects are in fact cold, one would expect that they would attempt to minimize heat loss when exercising under both cold and hot conditions. Indeed, Martin and Haney (60) evaluated thermoregulatory responses in sleep-deprived subjects before and after exercise at 0°C. As predicted, 30 hr of sleep deprivation resulted in a lower body temperature than that of controls. However, during exercise in the cold, sleep-deprived and control subjects showed the same increase in metabolic heat production and a similar rise in body temperature. The authors concluded that during exercise in the cold, sleep-deprived subjects lost less heat.

A similar result was obtained during exercise at 0°C following 50 hr of sleep deprivation (61). Interestingly, in the absence of sleep deprivation, physical exertion that is accompanied by repeated exposure to cold, wet environments has been reported to impair vasoconstrictor responses during a subsequent acute cold exposure (62). In any event, heat loss is also minimized when sleep-deprived subjects exercise at mild to warm temperatures. For example, when five subjects were asked to exercise for 40 min at 50% of their peak oxygen uptake following 33 hr of sleep deprivation, both blood flow and sweat rate were reduced compared to controls (63). Similar results have been reported for subjects exercising at warmer ambient temperatures (64,65). Thus, sleep-deprived subjects decrease heat loss when exposed to both positive and negative thermal loads.

While thermoregulatory responses under neutral conditions indicate that sleep deprivation impairs heat retention mechanisms, subjects maintain the ability to mount an appropriate response when sufficiently challenged. A similar result has been found in rats that are exposed to an acute thermoregulatory challenge while being subjected to long-term sleep deprivation (66). However, as the duration of sleep deprivation continues, the animals' ability to respond to the thermal challenge becomes impaired. Thus, one might expect protracted sleep deprivation protocols to produce larger deficits in thermoregulatory responses. Unfortunately, it has not been possible to evaluate thermoregulatory responses following extended TSD in humans. However, the effects of chronic sleep restriction and negative energy balance have recently been evaluated, and results suggest that thermoregulatory deficits may be progressive. Thus, Young et al. (57) evaluated eight men following the completion of the United States Army Ranger School and following 48 hr and 109 days of recovery. During the course of the 9-week training, subjects were exposed to sleep restriction (approximately 4 hr/day) and negative energy balance (4150 kcal expenditure, 3300 kcal intake; average body mass decline of 10%). Thermoregulatory responses were measured while the subjects sat wearing only shorts and socks at 10°C for 4 hr. Results indicated that fatigue coupled with sleep loss and negative energy balance lowered cold tolerance and impaired the individual's ability to maintain a normal body temperature during cold exposure. The loss of body mass presumably facilitated heat loss by decreasing the insulation between the body core and shell. Although the soldiers were able to increase metabolic rate during cold exposure, the rate of metabolic heat production at a given core temperature was reduced in sleep- and nutritionally deprived subjects compared to controls. Furthermore, sleep-deprived soldiers reported more thermal discomfort during cold exposure when they were tired. Interestingly, both the metabolic response to cold and feelings of thermal discomfort were reversed following only 48 hr of sleep and rest.

B. Animal Studies

As with the pioneering human sleep deprivation experiments, body temperature was among the first variables to have been measured in the earliest experiments conducted in animals (reviewed in 53). For example, in 1894 Manacéine deprived puppies of sleep for 4–6 days and observed marked hypothermia. In 1898, Tarozzi kept adult dogs awake for several weeks and reported that body temperature dropped to 25°C. Interestingly, not all of the early experiments reported changes in body temperature. In 1907, Legendre and Pieron found no change in body temperature in dogs deprived of sleep for several weeks. Similarly, Kleitman (67) reported no appreciable changes in body temperature in puppies kept awake for 2–7 days. While these discrepancies are hard to explain, they mirror results seen in a few human studies and may be due to circadian, methodological, or environmental factors. In any event, one might expect larger animals to be less vulnerable to impairments in heat retention mechanisms than smaller animals because the latter have a much larger surface-to-volume ratio that favors heat loss. Surprisingly, while thermoregulatory parameters have been investigated extensively in rodents subjected to short-term sleep deprivation, the focus of these studies has been primarily to elucidate mechanisms involved in sleep regulation, and thus thermoregulatory adjustments have not been characterized as such (68–74). An additional complicating factor has been the use of handling, treadmills, and inverted flower pots to deprive animals of sleep for a few hours. Each of these manipulations would be expected to influence thermoregulation independently of sleep loss [e.g., handling-induced hyperthermia (75)], and the controls used for these procedures have generally been inadequate for use in evaluating thermoregulatory processes. In contrast, long-term sleep deprivation procedures, which necessarily include a period of short-term sleep loss, have been developed to identify the contribution of confounding variables inherent in all sleep deprivation experiments (76). Briefly, both the experimental animal and its control are housed on a single disk suspended over a very shallow pan of water. When sleep is identified in the experimental animal, the disk slowly rotates and both animals walk opposite to the rotation of the disk. In this way both animals are exposed to a stimulus of equal intensity, timing, and duration. Because the disk is stationary when the experimental animal is spontaneously awake, the control animal can sleep (77) (see also Chaps. 4, 5).

Many variables have been investigated since the first rats were subjected to TSD by the disk-over-water method a generation ago. Nonetheless, a core feature of the sleep deprivation pathology continues to focus on the original observation that TSD rats show both a decline in body weight and an increase in food intake. In 1989, this relationship was formalized and used to calculate a measure of total energy expenditure (EE) (78). With the exception of one study (79), in which rats were treated with propylthiouracil to block the synthesis of thyroxine, all rats subjected to total or partial sleep deprivation using the disk-over-water method have shown a progressive increase in EE (reviewed in 80). Consequently, much of the research performed in this laboratory over the last two decades has sought to elucidate the factors that mediate the rise in EE. These studies indicated that EE was elevated in response to an increased calorigenic need rather than by an impaired metabolic mechanism (79,81). When TSD rats were given guanethidine monosulfate, which antagonizes peripheral postganglionic sympathetic activity, EE was not reduced, presumably due to the substitution of epinephrine (EP) for norepinephrine (NE). These data suggested that TSD rats had an increased need for an elevated EE that was obtained by whatever mechanisms were available (81). Similarly, TSD rats that were made hypothyroid and could not increase EE exhibited levels of NE and EP that were greatly enhanced in comparison with normal TSD animals (79). The hypothyroid TSD rats showed severe declines in intraperitoneal temperature (T_{ip}), indicating that the elevation in EE seen in untreated TSD rats was likely a response to an increased calorigenic need. Several lines of evidence suggest that the increased calorigenic need is the result of sleep loss-induced changes in thermoregulation (82).

Based on the observation that the rise in EE was associated with a late decline in T_{ip} (EE was highest when T_{ip} was lowest), Bergmann et al. (80) argued that a primary pathologic process common to both TSD and paradoxical sleep deprived rats was an inability to retain body heat (Fig. 1). Moreover, since TSD rats defended an above baseline T_{ip} in spite of excessive heat loss, it was hypothesized that their pathologic process included an elevated temperature set point (T_{set}). An elevated T_{set} was also indicated for rats selectively deprived of the high-amplitude component of NREM (HS2D) because they also defended an above baseline T_{ip} with an increased EE (83). Taken together, these data were interpreted to indicate that the elevated T_{set} was due to the loss of NREM sleep and that the inability to retain body heat was a consequence of paradoxical sleep loss (8). Although the authors concluded that both an elevated T_{set} and an inability to retain body heat were present early in TSD, they suggested that NREM loss had a larger and more immediate effect on T_{ip} than did paradoxical sleep loss. In addition, the authors proposed that later in the deprivation, the effects of NREM loss on T_{ip} were superseded by accumulated paradoxical sleep deprivation. In other words, the early increase in T_{ip} would predominantly reflect alterations in T_{set} resulting from the loss of NREM sleep; paradoxical sleep loss would exert only a minor counteracting influence. Later in the deprivation, however, the decline in T_{ip} would indicate an inability to retain body heat due to accumulated paradoxical sleep loss, and NREM loss would have a minimal impact on T_{ip}. According to this model, which was first presented by Rechtschaffen et al. in 1989, the evaluation of T_{ip} late in the deprivation would provide an insensitive or inaccurate assessment of T_{set} in both TSD and paradoxical sleep-deprived rats. This ambiguity would necessarily extend to the evaluation of heat loss because it is not possible to determine if heat loss is excessive without knowing the relative position of T_{ip} to T_{set}. Excessive heat loss requires that EE must be above baseline whereas T_{ip} is near or below T_{set}.

Thus, the factors that mediated the rise in EE remained open to alternative interpretations. These interpretations include the following: (a) that the early rise in T_{ip} may have resulted from a nonthermoregulatory increase in resting metabolic rate, which pushed T_{ip} above an unchanged T_{set}; (b) that the later fall in T_{ip} represented appropriate heat loss, and perhaps a lowered T_{set}, in an attempt to dissipate surplus heat created by excess EE; (c) that the fall in T_{ip} may have reflected excessive heat loss *and* a lowered T_{set}; and finally, (d) that paradoxical sleep-deprived rats may have developed an elevated T_{set} that was subsequently masked by excessive heat loss. In isolation, the evaluation of T_{ip} and EE cannot distinguish between alterations in thermoregulation and deficits that would result from a nonthermoregulatory increase in EE. Furthermore, the thermoregulation model of sleep deprivation proposes two counteracting effects on T_{ip} that cannot be separated by examining T_{ip} and EE alone. Therefore, the thermoregulation model of sleep deprivation was reevaluated in both TSD and paradoxical sleep deprived rats by giving them single, short, daily trials in a thermal gradient (84,85). Thermal preference was operationally defined as the temperature at which the animal went to sleep. Immediately after the animal went to sleep, it was placed back into the deprivation apparatus until the following day, when the test was repeated.

As in previous studies, TSD rats showed an initial rise in T_{ip} followed by a decline to below baseline values. The early rise in T_{ip} was associated with an elevated EE and the selection of warmer ambient temperature (T_{amb}) in the thermal gradient. These results favored the hypothesis that TSD resulted in an elevated T_{set} because, if excessive EE had pushed T_{ip} above an unchanged T_{set}, the rats should have selected cooler T_{amb}. In contrast to TSD rats, rats subjected to paradoxical sleep deprivation demonstrated an initial decline in T_{ip}. This decline was associated with an elevated EE and the selection of slightly warmer T_{amb} in the thermal gradient. Again, these results favored the hypothesis that paradoxical sleep deprivation resulted in excessive heat loss early in the experiment becauseif T_{set} were lower one would expect the rats to select cooler T_{amb}. As T_{ip} fell further below baseline, both TSD and paradoxical sleep-deprived rats demonstrated additional increases in EE and selected extremely warm T_{amb} in the gradient, indicating that both groups suffered from excessive heat loss. Nonetheless, T_{set} could not be adequately described late in the deprivation in either of these experiments. That is, although the animals presumably selected high T_{amb} in response to T_{ip} falling below T_{set}, T_{set} could have been higher or lower than baseline. Thus, as predicted by Rechtschaffen et al., T_{ip} did not provide an accurate assessment of T_{set} late in the deprivation.

The ambiguity resulting from the use of T_{ip} to evaluate T_{set} late in the deprivation appeared to be an intractable problem. However, Obermeyer et al. (86) noted that the inability to evaluate T_{set} might be overcome by using a more reliable measure of core temperature in combination with T_{ip}. Specifically, it was hypothesized that in the face of excessive heat loss, the size of the core would be reduced and the peritoneum would be regulated as part of the body shell. Obermeyer argued that, in contrast, brain temperature (T_{br}) would be less affected by heat loss and would provide a more accurate assessment of T_{set}. Consequently, rats were subjected to TSD, and both T_{br} and T_{ip} were evaluated. As in previous studies, T_{ip} showed an initial rise followed by a later decline to below baseline values. T_{br}, on the other hand, rose during the first quarter and remained above baseline until just shortly before the animals' demise (Fig. 1). T_{set} was evaluated using a model that assumed that because T_{br} was the more stable temperature it was held closer to T_{set}. It must be noted that this assumption is not commonly accepted by thermal physiologists (see 12,26,87). Nonetheless, a formal analysis of this model demonstrated an elevated T_{set} for only one-third of the deprivation and excessive heat loss for only the latter three quarters of the experiment. Although this experiment did not prove an elevated T_{set} throughout the entire deprivation, it did provide an important theoretical framework for the future analysis of thermoregulation in sleep-deprived rats. Specifically, this study argued that due to the repartitioning of the body core, an accurate assessment of T_{set} required the evaluation of T_{br} in addition to T_{ip}.

Recently, we have been able to evaluate T_{set} in TSD and paradoxical sleep-deprived rats throughout the entire deprivation by providing the rats with a continuously available operant (88,89). Operant control of T_{amb} provides a more continuous and reliable measure of thermal preference than the short, single, daily trials available with the thermal gradient. TSD rats were given the opportunity to respond for heat over a relatively large range of brain and body temperatures each day. It was assumed that deviations of either T_{br} or T_{ip} from T_{set} would stimulate the rats to produce compensatory changes in T_{amb} (35,90,91). Departures from T_{set} could result from either an inability to retain body heat or failure to achieve an elevated T_{set}. However, evidence for an elevated T_{set} required that on any given day the TSD rats would select warmer T_{amb} not only when T_{ip} or T_{br} were below baseline but also when they were above baseline. In fact, as the deprivation progressed, TSD rats selected warmer T_{amb} at even the highest brain and body temperatures, suggesting that these above baseline temperatures were below an elevated T_{set} (Fig. 2). In contrast to TSD rats, however, paradoxical sleep-deprived rats did not show evidence for an elevated T_{set}. Thus, brain temperature remained near baseline throughout the deprivation. In addition, these rats selected T_{amb} near baseline at all T_{br} and T_{ip} bins indicating that they did not suffer from an elevated T_{set} (Fig. 2). These data provide additional support for the hypothesis that NREM loss results in an elevated T_{set} and that paradoxical sleep loss results in an inability to retain body heat.

Interestingly, several reports indicate that the effects of sleep deprivation persist after the deprivation has stopped and the animals have been allowed to sleep (85,92). Thus, while the fall in body temperature during the transition from waking to NREM sleep is a robust feature of normal sleep, body temperature actually increases above waking values during the transition to NREM during recovery following both short- and long-term TSD (92). Furthermore, this change was temporally associated with high paradoxical sleep pressure, suggesting that it was due to the loss of paradoxical sleep not NREM. In order to evaluate this possibility more thoroughly, brain and body temperatures were evaluated during the transition from wake to NREM in rats selectively deprived of paradoxical sleep (89). These animals are able to obtain approximately 90% of their daily sleep quota such that it was possible to monitor changes in thermoregulation dur-

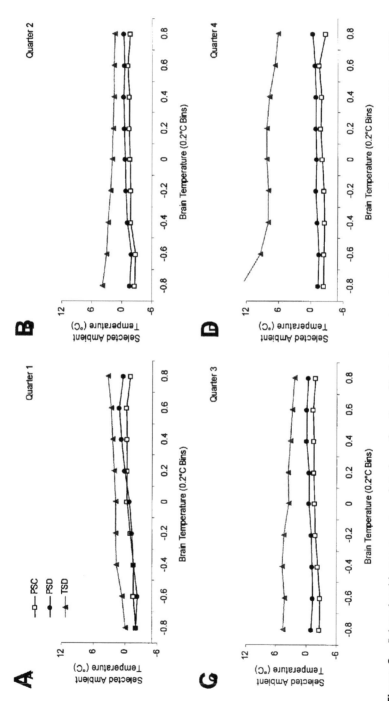

Figure 2 Selected ambient temperature plotted as a function of brain temperature for the four quarters of survival in PSC, PSD, and TSD rats. Epoch values of brain temperature and ambient temperature are expressed as change from baseline. Brain temperature values are divided into 0.2°C bins for each rat. The average ambient temperature for each temperature bin was then calculated (see Ref. 89 for details).

ing sleep while paradoxical sleep pressure accrued (89). Paradoxical sleep loss alone was able to attenuate the normal decline in hypotholauric T_{hy} and to reverse the fall of T_{ip} during the transition from wake to NREM, suggesting that paradoxical sleep loss alters thermoregulation during sleep. An alternative interpretation is that the increase in body temperature over waking values during the transition to NREM represents a redistribution of internal temperature fields in response to an inability to retain body heat. As mentioned above, during the transition from wake to NREM, both T_{br} and T_{ip} are regulated as part of the core and thus fall. Skin temperature, on the other hand, is regulated as part of the shell and increases above waking levels. During chronic sleep deprivation, the peritoneum becomes regulated as part of the body shell and thus behaves like skin temperature; it rises. If the redistribution of internal temperature fields is brought about by an active regulation of blood flow, then this analysis may provide the earliest demonstration of blood flow changes in sleep-deprived rats.

IV. Conclusions

A number of theories on the function of NREM sleep have been presented that postulate the involvement of thermoregulatory mechanisms. One of the most popular is the energy conservation hypothesis. According to this model, the lowered T_{set} during NREM sleep would allow for lower metabolic rates and reduced body temperatures. Under conditions of thermoneutrality, these adjustments should account for only 10% savings in energy expenditure (93). Nonetheless, the data from chronically sleep-deprived rats suggest that the role of NREM sleep in maintaining effective thermoregulation supersedes that of energy savings (8). McGinty and colleagues have made similar arguments (50). These authors noted that one of the costs of endothermy would be the maintenance of brain temperatures that approach damaging levels (50). According to this hypothesis, the function of NREM sleep would be to cool the brain by lowering T_{set}. Although the authors have downplayed the functional aspects of their theory in favor of more mechanistic considerations, they have generated a large body of data implicating thermoregulatory centers in the regulation of NREM sleep. Thus, a subset of warm-sensitive neurons (WSNs) (64%) that are active during NREM sleep displayed both increased firing rates and increased thermosensitivity during NREM compared to waking (47). They also reported that a subset of cold-sensitive neurons (CSNs) discharged more slowly and exhibited decreased thermosensitivity during NREM. The mechanisms by which temperature-sensitive neurons modulate T_{set} changes is controversial. However, most models require an increase in activity of WSNs and a decrease in CSNs to demonstrate a lowered T_{set}. The changes in the activity of temperature-sensitive neurons during NREM are particularly interesting in light of the observation that a lowered T_{set} during NREM is ubiquitous in mammals and birds. The increase in T_{set}, which has been found in TSD rats and attributed to the loss of NREM sleep, lends further support to the hypothesis that NREM sleep is important in regulating some aspects of T_{set}.

It has been suggested that the thermoregulatory function of sleep is only important for small animals with a high thermoregulatory load (42). One of the characteristic features of NREM sleep in mammals and birds of all sizes is a regulated fall in body temperature. Furthermore, several reports indicate that exposure to warm temperatures increases NREM sleep in both small and large animals (74,94). In addition, similar changes in the activity of temperature-sensitive neurons during NREM sleep have been reported in animals with dramatically different thermal loads (24,40,50). Finally, both human and animals studies have found evidence for heat retention deficits following sleep deprivation. Thus, it is unlikely that the thermoregulatory function of NREM sleep is confined to small animals and that the cellular mechanisms for the control of body temperature provide a reasonable avenue for the elucidation of sleep function.

Acknowledgments

Research conducted at The Neurosciences Institute was supported by the Neurosciences Research Foundation.

References

1. Rechtschaffen A, Bergmann BM, Everson CA, Kushida CA, Gilliland MA. Sleep deprivation in the rat: X. Integration and discussion of the findings. 1989. Sleep 2002; 25(1):68-87.
2. Rechtschaffen A, Bergmann BM Sleep deprivation in the rat by the disk over water method. Behav Brain Res 1995; 69: 55 63.
3. Cirelli C. How sleep deprivation affects gene expression in the brain: a review of recent findings. J Appl Physiol 2002; 92(1):394-400.
4. Rechtschaffen A, Gilliland MA, Bergmann BM, Winter JB Physiological correlates of prolonged sleep deprivation in rats. Science 1983 Jul 8;221(4606):182-184.
5. Shaw PJ, Tononi G, Greenspan RJ, Robinson DF. Stress response genes protect against lethal effects of sleep deprivation in Drosophila. Nature 2002; 16; 417(6886):287-291.
6. Landis CA, Collins BJ, Cribbs LL, Sukhatme VP, Bermann BM, Rechtschaffen A, Smalheiser NB, Expression of EGR-1 in the brain of sleep-deprived rats, Mol Brain Res 1993; 17:300-306.
7. Kushida CA, Bergmann BM, Rechtschaffen A. Sleep deprivation in the rat: IV. Paradoxical sleep deprivation. Sleep 1989; 12: 22-30.
8. Rechtschaffen A, Bergmann BM, Everson CA, Kushida CA, Gilliland MA Sleep deprivation in the rat: X. Integration and discussion of the findings. Sleep 1989; 12: 68-87.
9. Block BA. Thermogenesis in muscle. Annu Rev Physiol 1994; 56:535-577.
10. Crawshaw L, Grahn D, Wollmuth L, Simpson L. Central nervous regulation of body temperature in vertebrates: comparative aspects. Pharmacol Ther 1985; 30(1):19-30.

11. Heinrich B. Thermoregulation in endothermic insects. Science 1974; 30;185(153):747-756.

12. Cabanac M. Temperature regulation. Annu Rev Physiol 1975; 37: 415 439.

13. Satinoff E. Neural organization and evolution of thermal regulation in mammals. Science 1978; 201: 16 22.

14. Jessen C Thermal afferents in the control of body temperature. In: Schonbaum E, eds. Thermoregulation: Physiology and Biochemistry. New York: Pergamon Press: 1990;153-183.

15. Simon E, Schmid HA, Pehl U. Spinal neuronal thermosensitivity in vivo and in vitro in relation to hypothalamic neuronal thermosensitivity. Prog Brain Res 1998;115:25-47.

16. Simon E, Pierau F, Taylor DC Central and peripheral thermal control of effectors in homeothermic temperature regulation. Physiol Rev 1986; 2: 235-300.

17. Nagashima K, Nakai S, Tanaka M, Kanosue K. Neuronal circuitries involved in thermoregulation. Auton Neurosci 2000; 85(1-3):18-25.

18. Boulant JA. Role of the preoptic-anterior hypothalamus in thermoregulation and fever. Clin Infect Dis 2000; 31 Suppl 5:S157-S161.

19. Mercer JB, Jessen C. Effects of total body core cooling on heat production of conscious goats. Pflugers Arch 1978; 373(3):259-267

20. Baldwin BA, Ingram DL. Effect of heating and cooling the hypothalamus on behavioral thermoregulation in the pig. J Physiol 1967; 191(2):375-392.

21. Hammel HT, Sharp F. Thermoregulatory salivation in the running dog in response to preoptic heating and cooling. J Physiol (Paris) 1971; 63(3):260-263.

22. Fuller CA, Horwitz BA, Horowitz JM. Shivering and nonshivering thermogenic responses of cold-exposed rats to hypothalamic warming. Am J Physiol 1975; 228(5):1519-1524.

23. Davis JR, Tagliaferro AR, Roberts JS, Hill JO. Effects of early cold adaptation on food efficiency and dietary-induced thermogenesis in the adult rat. Physiol Behav 1982; 29(1):135-140.

24. Van Someren EJ, Raymann RJ, Scherder EJ, Daanen HA, Swaab DF. Circadian and age-related modulation of thermoreception and temperature regulation: mechanisms and functional implications. Ageing Res Rev 2002; 1(4):721-778.

25. Glotzbach SF, Heller HC. Central nervous regulation of body temperature during sleep. Science 1976; 194: 537-539.

26. Hammel HT, Jackson DC, Stolwijk JAJ, Hardy JD, Stromme SB. Temperature regulation by hypothalamic proportional control with an adjustable set point. J Appl Physiol 1963; 18: R1146-R1154.

27. Weiss B, Laties VG. Magnitude of reinforcement as a variable in thermoregulatory behavior. J Comp Physiol Psych 1960; 53: 603-608.

28. Weiss B, Laties VG. Behavioural thermoregulation. Science 1961; 133:1338-1344.

29. Weiss B, Laties VG. Behavioral thermoregulation. In: Verhave T, ed. The experimental analysis of behavior. selected readings. New York: Appleton-Century-Crofts: 1966: 40- 421.

30. Gordon CJ. Temperature Regulation in Laboratory Rodents. New York: Cambridge University Press, 1993.

31. Gordon CJ. 24 hour control of body temperature in rats: I. Integration of behavioral and autonomic effectors. Am J Physiol 1994; 267(1 pt 2): R71-R77.

32. Refinetti R, Carlisle HJ. Complementary nature of heat production and heat intake during behavioral thermoregulation in the rat. Behav Neural Biol 1986; 46: 64-70.

33. Schulze G, Tetzner M, Topolinski H. Operant thermoregulation of rats with anterior hypothalamic lesions. Naunyn Schmiedebergs Arch Pharmacol 1981; 318: 43-48.

34. Dib B. Effects of intrathecal capsaican on autonomic and behavioral heat loss responses in the rat. Pharmacol Biochem Behav 1987; 28(1): 65-70.

35. Adair ER. Evaluation of some controller inputs to behavioral temperature regulation. Int J Biometeorol 1971; 15: 121-125.

36. Kleitman N, Engelman. Variations in skin temperatures of the feet hands and the onset of sleep. Fed Proc 1948; 7:66-73.

37. Krauchi K, Cajochen C, Werth E, Wirz-Justice A. Warm feet promote the rapid onset of sleep. Nature 1999; 401(6748):36-37.

38. Glotzbach SF, Heller HC Thermoregulation. In: Kryger M, Roth T, Dement WC, eds. Principles and Practice of Sleep Medicine. Philadelphia: WB Saunders, 1995; 300-309.

39. McGinty D, Szymusiak R. Keeping cool: a hypothesis about the mechanisms and functions of slow-wave sleep. Trends Neurosci 1990 Dec;13(12):480-487.

40. Parmeggiani PL. Temperature regulation during sleep: a study in homeostasis. In: Physiology in Sleep. New York: Academic Press, 1980: 97-142.

41. Parmeggiani PL. Interaction between sleep and thermoregulation: an aspect of the control of behavioral states. Sleep 1987;10(5):426-435.

42. Horne JA. Why We Sleep: The Functions of Sleep in Humans and Other Mammals. New York: Oxford University Press, 1998.

43. Schmidek WR, Zachariassen KE, Hammel HT. Total calorimetric measurements in the rat: influences of the sleep wakefulness cycle and of the environmental temperature. Brain Res 1983; 288: 261-271.

44. Alfoldi P, Rubicsek G, Cserni G, Obal FJ. Brain and core temperatures and peripheral vasomotion during sleep and wakefulness at various ambient temperatures in the rat. Pflugers Arch 1990; 417: 336-341.

45. Parmeggiani PL, Franzini C. Changes in the activity of hypothalamic units during sleep at different environmental temperatures. Brain Res 1971; 29:347-350.

46. Alam N, McGinty D, Szymusiak R. Neuronal discharge of preoptic/anterior hypothalamic neurons: relation to NREM sleep. Am J Physiol 1995; 269: R1240-R1249.

47. Alam N, McGinty D, Szymusiak R. Preoptic/anterior hypothalamic neurons: thermosensitivity in rapid eye movement sleep. Am J. Physiol 1995; 269: R1250-R1257.

48. Parmeggiani PL, Azzaroni A, Cevolani D, Ferrari G. Polygraphic study of anterior hypothalamic preoptic neuron thermosensitivity during sleep. Electroencephalogr Clin Neurophysiol 1986; 63: 289-295.

49. Glotzbach SF, Heller HC. Changes in the thermal characteristics of hypothalamic neurons during sleep and wakefulness.Brain Res 1984 Aug 20;309(1):17-26.

50. McGinty DJ Szymusiak R. Hypothalamic thermoregulatory control of slow wave sleep. In: Mancia M, Marini G, eds. The Diencephalon and Sleep. New York: Raven Press, 1990: 97-110.

51. Patrick GW, Gillbert JA. On the effects of loss of sleep. Psychol Rev 1896; 3: 469-483.

52. Kleitman N Studies on the physiology of sleep. V. Some experiments on puppies. Am J Physiol 1927; 84:386-395

53. Kleitman N. Sleep and Wakefulness. Chicago: University of Chicago Press, 1963.

54. Murray EJ, Williams HL, Lubin A. Body temperature and psychological ratings during sleep deprivation. J Exp Psychol 1958; 56:271-273.

55. Naitoh P, Kales A, Kollar, EJ, Smith JC, Jacobson A. Electroencephalographic activity after prolonged sleep loss. Electroencephalogr Clin Neurophysiol 1969; 27:2-11.
56. Landis CA, Savage MV, Lentz MJ, Brengelmann GL. Sleep deprivation alters body temperature dynamics to mild cooling and heating not sweating threshold in women. Sleep 1998;21(1):101-108.
57. Young AJ, Castellani JW, O'Brien C, Shippee RL, Tikuisis P, Meyer LG, Blanchard LA, Kain JE, Cadarette BS, Sawka MN. Exertional fatigue, sleep loss, and negative energy balance increase susceptibility to hypothermia. J Appl Physiol 1998;85(4):1210-1217.
58. Fiorica V, Higgins EA, Iampietro PF, Lategola MT, Davis AW. Physiological responses of men during sleep deprivation. J Appl Physiol 1968; 24(2):167-176.
59. Savourey G, Bittel J. Cold thermoregulatory changes induced by sleep deprivation in men. Eur J Appl Physiol Occup Physiol 1994; 69(3):216-220.
60. Martin BJ, Bender PR, Chen H. Stress hormonal response to exercise after sleep loss.Eur J Appl Physiol Occup Physiol 1986;55(2):210-214.
61. Kolka MA, Stephenson LA. Exercise thermoregulation after prolonged wakefulness. J Appl Physiol. 1988; 64(4):1575-1579.
62. Castellani JW, Young AJ, Degroot DW, Stulz DA, Cadarette BS, Rhind SG, Zamecnik J, Shek PN, Sawka MN. Thermoregulation during cold exposure after several days of exhaustive exercise. J Appl Physiol 2001;90(3):939-946.
63. Sawka MN, Gonzalez RR, Pandolf KB. Effects of sleep deprivation on thermoregulation during exercise. Am J Physiol. 1984 Jan;246(1 Pt 2):R72-R77.
64. Dewasmes G, Bothorel B, Hoeft A, Candas V. Regulation of local sweating in sleep-deprived exercising humans. Eur J Appl Physiol Occup Physiol 1993;66(6):542-546.
65. Kolka MA, Martin BJ, Elizondo RS. Exercise in a cold environment after sleep deprivation. Eur J Appl Physiol Occup Physiol 1984;53(3):282-285.
66. Obermeyer W, Bergmann BM, Rechtschaffen A. The effects of sleep deprivation on thermoregulatory responses of rats to phentolamine. Sleep Res 1993;22:340.
67. Kleitman N. Studies on the physiology of sleep. V. Some experiments on puppies. Am J Physiol 1927; 84:386-395.
68. Franken P, Dijk DJ, Tobler I, Borbely AA. Sleep deprivation in rats: effects on EEG power spectra, vigilance states, and cortical temperature. Am J Physiol 1991;261(1 Pt 2):R198-R208.
69. Franken P, Tobler I, Borbely AA. Cortical temperature and EEG slow-wave activity in the rat: analysis of vigilance state related changes. Pflugers Arch 1992;420(5-6):500-507.
70. Franken P, Tobler I, Borbely AA. Effects of 12-h sleep deprivation and of 12-h cold exposure on sleep regulation and cortical temperature in the rat. Physiol Behav 1993;54(5):885-894.
71. Nakao M, McGinty D, Szymusiak R, Yamamoto M. Thermoregulatory model of sleep control: losing the heat memory. J Biol Rhythms 1999;14(6):547-556.
72. Szymusiak R, Steininger T, Alam N, McGinty D. Preoptic area sleep-regulating mechanisms. Arch Ital Biol 2001;139(1-2):77-92.
73. Amici R, Zamboni G, Perez E, Jones CA, Parmeggiani PL. Brain Res 1998;781(1-2):252-258.
74. Moriarty S Szymusiak R, Thompson D, McGinty DJ. Selective increase in non-rapid eye movement sleep following whole body heating in rats. Brain Res 1993; 617:10-16.

75. Briese E, Cabanac M. Stress hyperthermia: physiological arguments that it is a fever. Physiol Behav 1991;49(6):1153-1157.

76. Bergmann BM, Kushida CA, Everson CA, Gilliland MA, Obermeyer W, Rechtschaffen A. Sleep deprivation in the rat: II. Methodology. Sleep 1989;12:5-12.

77. This volume, Chapter 6.

78. Bergmann BM, Everson CA, Kushida CA, Fang VS, Leitch CA, Schoeller DA, Refetoff S, Rechtschaffen A. Sleep deprivation in the rat: V. Energy use and mediation. Sleep 1989; 12:31-41.

79. Pilcher JJ, Bergmann BM, Refetoff S, Fang VS, Rechtschaffen A. Sleep deprivation in the rat: XIII. The effect of hypothyroidism on sleep deprivation symptoms. Sleep 1991; 14: 201-210.

80. Rechtschaffen A, Bergmann BM. Sleep deprivation in the rat: an update of the 1989 paper. Sleep 2002 Feb 1;25(1):18-24.

81. Pilcher JJ, Bergmann BM, Fang VS, Refetoff S, Rechtschaffen A. Sleep deprivation in the rat: XI. The effect of guanethidine induced sympathetic blockade on the sleep deprivation syndrome. Sleep 1990; 13: 218 231.

82. Bergmann BM, Everson CA, Gilliland MA, Kushida CA, Obermeyer W, Pilcher JJ, Prete FR, Rechtschaffen A. Sleep deprivation and thermoregulation. In: Horne J, ed. Sleep '88. New York: Gustav Fischer Verlag, 1989:91-95.

83. Gilliland MA, Bergmann BM, Rechtschaffen A. Sleep deprivation in the rat: VIII. High EEG amplitude sleep deprivation. Sleep 1989;12: 53-59.

84. Prete FR, Bergmann BM, Holtzman P, Obermeyer W, Rechtschaffen A. Sleep deprivation in the rat: XII. Effect on ambient temperature choice. Sleep 1991;14(2): 109-115.

85. Landis CA, Bergmann BM, Ismail MM, Rechtschaffen A. Sleep deprivation in the rat: XV. Ambient temperature choice in paradoxical sleep deprived rats. Sleep 1992;15: 13-20.

86. Obermeyer W, Bergmann BM, Rechtschaffen A. Sleep deprivation in the rat: XIV. Comparison of waking hypothalamic and peritoneal temperatures. Sleep 1991;14: 285-293.

87. Satinoff E. A reevaluation of the concept of the homeostatic organization of temperature regulation. Satinoff E, Teitelbaum P (eds. Handbook of Behavioral Neurobiology. New York: Plenum Press, 1983:443-472.

88. Shaw PJ, Bergmann BM, Rechtschaffen A. Operant control of ambient temperature during sleep deprivation. Am J Physiol 1997 Feb;272(2 Pt 2):R682-R690.

89. Shaw PJ, Bergmann BM, Rechtschaffen A. Effects of paradoxical sleep deprivation on thermoregulation in the rat. Sleep 1998; 21(1):7-17.

90. Laudenslager ML. Proportional hypothalamic control of behavioral thermoregulation in the squirrel monkey. Physiol Behav 1976;17:383-390.

91. Corbit JD. Behavioral regulation of hypothalamic temperature. Science 1969; 166:256-258.

92. Feng P, Shaw PJ, Bergmann BM, Obermeyer W, Tsai LL, Zenko CE, Rechtschaffen A. Sleep deprivation in the rat: XIX. Differences in wake and sleep temperatures during recovery. Sleep 1995; 18(9):797-804.

93. Berger RJ, Phillips N. Energy conservation and sleep. Behav Brain Res 1995;69:65-73.

94. Horne JA, Reid AJ. Night-time sleep EEG changes following body heating in a warm bath. Electroencephalogr Clin Neurophysiol 1985;60:154-157.

16

Biochemical Changes

BIRENDRA N. MALLICK, VIBHA MADAN, AND MOHAMMAD FAISAL
School of Life Sciences, Jawaharlal Nehru University, New Delhi, India

I. Introduction

Sleep and wakefulness are among the basic instinctual behaviors that are expressed in its present form by living species high in the evolutionary ladder. Both sleep and wakefulness are active processes regulated by the brain. However, they may also be modulated by a large number of psychosomatophysiological as well as environmental factors. In spite of unanimity among the experts that sleep is essential, the window for the daily requirement of sleep is fairly wide. Although it is known that loss of sleep adversely affects several physiological, behavioral, and psychological parameters, the detailed function(s) of sleep are as yet unknown (see also Chap. 1).

Although several approaches have been followed to further an understanding of the function(s) of sleep, the deprivation method has been most widely used for this purpose. One of the advantages of the deprivation method is that it may be considered in some respect closer to the normal living condition because most individuals encounter loss of sleep in their lifetime. Nevertheless, a genuine and most common criticism of the deprivation method is assessing the amount of stress experienced by the subject during the course of the experiment. But it may be argued that stress is a complex term. A factor may be stressful to a subject but not to another depending on previous exposure and experience. However, such limitations have been overcome with reasonable success using appropriate and effective control experiments. It has been mentioned earlier in this book that sleep is divided into rapid-eye-movement (REM) sleep and non-REM (NREM) sleep. Studies have been conducted examining the effects of total sleep deprivation (TSD) as well as the selective deprivation of REM sleep. Among the various deprivation methods available, at least for REM sleep deprivation, researchers using animal models have preferred mostly the platform-over-water method (also known as the inverted flower pot method). The effects of total and REM sleep deprivation, primarily with respect to biochemical changes and their significance in understanding sleep and its functions, will be discussed in this chapter.

II. Sleep Deprivation and Biochemical Changes

It is well known that sleep, like any other function in the body, is regulated by neurons in the brain. It follows a circadian rhythm (1) and may be modulated by factor(s) that, in turn, are further modulated by changes in circadian rhythm (2–4). Neurotransmitter agonists or antagonists in specific regions in the brain (5–11) and levels of other chemicals bathing the neurons in the brain may also modulate either or both total sleep and REM sleep. Sleep deprivation is undoubtedly unpleasant as well as distressing. Therefore, behavioral, metabolic, and endocrine responses to lack of sleep have received a great deal of attention. It has been reported in human as well as animal studies that loss of sleep affects several behaviors, leading to anxiety, irritability, aggressiveness (12), fighting (13), hypersexuality (14), and loss of concentration and memory consolidation (15,16). REM sleep-deprived rats become extremely sensitive to tactile stimuli, i.e., flinching, jumping, and squealing, and become very aggressive (17). Thus, gross behaviors are affected after total sleep and REM sleep deprivation (18–20). To understand the underlying mechanism of action it is necessary to study the effects of total and REM sleep deprivation on the behavior of individual neurons and on their activities; however, such studies are very limited. In two such investigations, the effects of REM sleep deprivation were studied on the behavior of single neurons in the brainstem. It was observed that after REM sleep deprivation, the firing rates of REM-off and REM-on neurons (21) as well as the responsiveness of neurons sensitive to auditory stimulation (22) were altered. These observations suggested that sleep deprivation is a generalized phenomenon. Sleep loss or its disturbance is also associated with several disorders including depression and narcolepsy (23,24).

Based on the results mentioned above, it is not difficult to appreciate that there would be changes in the concentration(s) of biomolecules in the body fluid that in turn may influence the neurons in the brain to modulate either or both NREM sleep and REM sleep. Experiments have been conducted after deprivation of either total sleep or REM sleep. These studies may broadly be divided into changes observed in the body fluids, i.e., blood and cerebrospinal fluid (CSF), or in the brain.

A. Changes in Biomolecules in the Blood and CSF After Sleep Deprivation

Initial experiments to investigate the effects of sleep deprivation were performed on animals in 1894 by Marie De Manacéine (25) (see also Chap. 2). She found that puppies died when kept awake for 4–6 days (92–143 hr). At the end of the study there was marked hypothermia, capillary hemorrhages in the cerebral gray matter, and the red blood cell count decreased from 5 million to 2 million. However, the red blood cell count subsequently increased. In another study, three adult dogs were kept awake by being forced to walk when necessary, and the dogs died after 9, 13, and 17 days (26). In yet another study, several dogs were deprived of sleep for periods varying from 30 to 505 hr, but not beyond the point where they showed extreme sleepiness (27). In this study the dogs were not reported to die, possibly because they were not deprived beyond a limit from which they could not recover. In both of the latter studies, histological preparation of the brain showed diffuse chromatolysis and vacuolization in the neurons. The investigators also observed differences in the viscosity and density of the blood before and after sleep deprivation.

Attention was drawn to finding humoral factor(s) that might be responsible for the induction of sleep. That sleep deprivation might affect humoral factor(s) was suspected by studies conducted by Ishimori (28) as early as 1909 in Japan and by Legendre and Pieron (27) at about the same time in France. They deprived dogs of sleep and tried to extract a hypnogenic factor from the tissues of various organs and the body fluid, with the assumption that continued wakefulness or fatigue might bring about the accumulation of such a factor in the body fluids (29). They reported the possible existence of "hypnotoxin" in the blood, CSF, and in the brain of dogs after sleep deprivation for 6–15 days (29). Part of these findings was confirmed in 1939 by Schnedorf and Ivy (30). Other groups later isolated "sleep factors" from the brain and body fluids of sleep-deprived animals. Normal dogs exhibited signs of sleep when injected intravenously or intracerebroventicularly with either the CSF, blood, serum, or emulsion of cerebral tissue taken from sleep-deprived dogs (27). However, normal dogs similarly injected with the blood, serum, or CSF of normally behaving dogs showed no behavioral change.

In the middle of the 1960s, Pappenheimer found that cats infused with fluid from sleep-deprived goats were abnormally sleepy in comparison to cats infused with fluid taken from goats not deprived of sleep. By means of ultrafiltration, two factors, factor S and factor E, were isolated from the CSF of these sleep-deprived goats (31,32). In the late 1960s, Drucker-Colin and his group collected perfusate from the brains of 24-hr sleep-deprived cats and infused it into cats that were made alert by food deprivation. The perfusate increased the duration of NREM sleep and reduced its latency. However, no effect was observed on REM sleep. In a later work, two proteins apparently involved in REM sleep were isolated and partially characterized (33). Prospero-Garcia et al. suggested that the CSF of

REM sleep–deprived donor cats contains a vasoactive intestinal polypeptide (VIP)–like factor (34).

The quest for finding a sleep-promoting factor in the body fluids led to the idea of the presence of endogenous sleep-promoting substances in blood (35), urine (36), CSF (31), and brain tissue (32,37,38). An increasing number of studies in animals demonstrated somnogenic influences of various cytokines such as tumor necrosis factor-α (TNF-α), interferon-γ (IFN-γ), and interleukin-1 (IL-1). Conversely, whether sleep exerts an influence on the production of these cytokines is not clear. A variety of peptides that have been shown to promote sleep in animals also have immunomodulatory effects. These agents include factor-S, muramyl peptides, IL-1, α-interferon, TNF-α (39), VIP (40,41), prostaglandin D_2 (42), and delta sleep–inducing peptide (43). However, only a few substances have been extensively investigated for their involvement in sleep regulation. There is convincing evidence for the involvement of IL-1β, TNF-α, growth hormone–releasing hormone (GHRH), prostaglandin D_2, and adenosine in NREM sleep regulation and prolactin and VIP in REM sleep regulation.

The concentrations of several hormones are altered in the blood with the sleep-waking cycle and with sleep deprivation (2,3). Prolonged sleep deprivation is likely to disrupt numerous complex biochemical rhythms and the interrelationships among metabolic regulators. Thyroid hormone concentration decreases during sleep (44); however, it increases with sleep deprivation (45). There is a decrease in 17-hydrocorticosteroids after sleep deprivation (46–49). The average circulating levels of cortisol are lowest during the initial hours of the night (9 p.m. and midnight) and are highest during the early morning or just before waking (50,51). Sleep deprivation has been reported to affect epinephrine and norepinephrine (NE) in blood (52,53), and NE in urine (54). The pulsatile release of growth hormone (GH) from the anterior pituitary is strongly associated with the sleep/wake rhythm in humans (55) and rats (56). Two hypothalamic peptides, growth hormone–releasing hormone, and somatostatin, control the secretion of GH and have been implicated as sleep factors (57). The serum GH concentration decreases after REM sleep deprivation (57) whereas its intraperitoneal administration in cats and rats induces a significant increase in REM sleep (58). Also it has been observed that a delay in sleep onset induces a delay in GH secretion (59,60), whereas GH release is increased during recovery sleep after sleep deprivation (61). Sleep deprivation has been found to cause loss of body weight and increased food intake associated with hypothermia (52). Sleep deprivation causes increased urea excretion, probably due to the increased protein catabolism required to supply energy needs, and decreased electrolyte excretion (62).

Sleep deprivation also affects the functions of several other systems, including defense against infection (see Chap. 17). Blood polymorphonuclear granulocytes exhibited a decreased ability to phagocytize during sleep deprivation whereas blood lymphocytes showed an increased interferon production after the exposure (63). These findings indicate a diminished host defense during a phase when proper sleep is not achieved, such as a condition associated with irregular work hours (e.g., in the medical and military professions and in conventional industrial shift work). Everson showed that deprivation of sleep impairs whole-organism host defense (64). It was observed that prolonged wakefulness produced a life-threatening systemic infection that was not accompanied by the usual diagnostic symptoms of fever and large-tissue inflammatory reactions. However, a subsequent study supported the notion that short-term sleep deprivation is unlikely to harm the immune system as far as nonspecific acute responses are concerned (65). Other studies have shown that REM sleep deprivation in rats resulted in a reduced primary antibody response to sheep red blood cells (66). Various studies showed that aspects of immune cellular functions are altered with prolonged wakefulness. Pokeweed mitogen (PWM) response and natural killer (NK) cell activity are altered after 40 hr of wakefulness. Although 24-hr mean PWM response showed an overall increase in activity from baseline day 2 to day 4, 24-hr mean NK cell activity decreased over the same time interval in humans (67). Irwin et al. observed similar results, though after partial-night sleep deprivation (68,69). Their data implicates sleep in the homeostatic regulation of natural and cellular aspects of the immune system. Even a modest loss of sleep early in the night can lead to a decrement of NK activity, lymphocyte-activated killer (LAK) cell activity, and lymphocyte production of IL-2 (69). However, contrary to this, Dinges et al. observed that acute loss of sleep to the point of impairment of neurobehavioral function in humans is associated with leukocytosis and increased NK cell counts and activity, and that these outcomes are reversed by recovery sleep (70).

Thus, the studies mentioned above suggest that several molecules change in the blood after total sleep and REM sleep deprivation. However, ascertaining the significance of the changes and their relevance to the normal or abnormal physiological status of the living being requires further investigation.

B. Changes in Biomolecules in the Brain After Sleep Deprivation

It is well known that discrete regions in the brain are involved in the regulation of specific functions including sleep. Since neurotransmitters and other chemical(s) may modulate neuronal functions, the concept of chemical factor(s) regulating sleep was proposed. Although the factor(s) could not be identified for years in the absence of adequate technique and knowledge, Jouvet proposed the aminergic and cholinergic regulation of sleep (5). Injection of an agonist or antagonist of neurotransmitter(s) either locally in the brain or systemically is reported to modulate sleep (9). Hence, it is likely that there would be alterations in the levels of neurotransmitters per se or their respective metabolic enzymes that could change respective neurotransmitter levels in discrete region(s) in the brain during variations, disturbances, or deprivation of sleep.

In the majority of instances, the biochemical changes in the brain have been studied after REM sleep deprivation. It was reported that during REM sleep, noradrenergic neurons in the locus coeruleus cease firing (71,72), whereas (presumably) cholinergic neurons increase firing (73). More recently, the role of (gamma-aminobutyric acid (GABA) in REM sleep regulation has been implicated (74). GABA levels were found to increase in the locus coeruleus during REM sleep (75), and it has been proposed that GABA inhibits the REM-off neurons for the initiation of REM sleep (76). Hence, levels of those neurotransmitters or enzymes that would affect those neurotransmitters in the brain have been estimated after REM sleep deprivation.

Deprivation and Changes in the Aminergic System

An increase in the levels of NE after REM sleep deprivation was initially shown indirectly and later directly using various methods. Increased turnover of NE after REM sleep deprivation was reported by Pujol et al. (77). Subsequently, it was reported that the levels of NE increased after REM sleep deprivation (78). These were supported by the findings that after REM sleep deprivation there were increases in the NE synthesizing enzyme, tyrosine hydroxylase (TH) activity (79), its messenger riabonucleic acid (mRNA) (80,81), and NE transporter mRNA (81). Furthermore, recently it has been confirmed that there is an increase in TH concentration within the neurons in the locus coeruleus after REM sleep deprivation (82). An increased NE may be supported by the finding that after REM sleep deprivation there was a decrease in monoamine oxidase (MAO) (83), the enzyme responsible for the breakdown of NE. MAO-A that is specific for NE degradation was significantly affected; the nonspecific MAO-B was not affected. Interestingly, the medullary MAO-A initially increased even after 1 day of deprivation, which subsequently decreased throughout the brain. An initial increase in MAO-A activity may be to protect the system from excessive NE (due to non-cessation of adrenergic REM-off neurons), possibly a compensatory effect. Subsequently, Perez and Benedito reproduced the effect reported by Thakkar and Mallick of REM sleep deprivation on MAO activity (83,84). Although levels of NE increased after REM sleep deprivation, a cause-and-effect relationship between them could not be confirmed from these studies. Nevertheless, it may be suggested that withdrawal of NE is likely to be a prerequisite for initiation of REM sleep. This is because: (a) REM sleep could not be initiated if levels of NE were increased by reuptake blocker (85) or by injection of adrenoceptor agonist (6); (b) REM sleep could be increased by adrenoceptor blocker (86); and (c) REM sleep was decreased if the locus coeruleus was continuously stimulated (87), which presumably did not allow the REM-off neurons to cease firing, resulting in increased NE in the brain. This increased NE could be responsible for hypothermia (88) during REM sleep deprivation. This is because NE acting on the α_1-adrenoceptor in the medial preoptic area has been reported to cause hypothermia (7), and iontophoretic studies confirmed that the thermosensitive neurons in the medial preoptic area possess α_1-adrenoceptors (89).

A few studies focused on changes in other aminergic neurotransmitters. REM sleep deprivation was found to increase the synthesis and utilization of serotonin in the central nervous system (78,90). Similarly, an increased metabolism of brain serotonin was reported after sleep deprivation in rats (91). Since neurotransmitters act through their respective receptors, it is likely that alteration in the levels of neurotransmitters might alter the receptor concentrations or their sensitivity after sleep or REM sleep deprivation. Aminergic receptor sensitivity was reported to be altered after REM sleep deprivation (92,93). Siegel and Rogawski proposed in their review that REM sleep possibly regulates adrenergic receptor sensitivity (94). This was supported by the finding that following deprivation there was an increase in the adrenergic receptor density in the brain (95). These results suggest an increase in NE in the brain after REM sleep deprivation.

Deprivation and Changes in the Cholinergic System

Cholinergic stimulation induces REM sleep and also wakefulness (96). During REM sleep, adrenergic neurons cease firing and cholinergic neurons increase firing. Pending confirmation, it is proposed that cholinergic induction of REM sleep possibly exerts its effect at the background of NE withdrawal, whereas wakefulness may be induced irrespective of the presence or absence of NE. Acetylcholine (ACh) release is dependent on sleep state and is highest during REM sleep (97). It is expected that levels of ACh would be altered in the brain after sleep deprivation, especially after REM sleep deprivation; however, this must be confirmed. Nevertheless, the following studies support a decrease in the levels of ACh after REM sleep deprivation. Levels of acetylcholinesterase (AChE), an ACh-hydrolyzing enzyme that maintains the levels of ACh, increased after REM sleep deprivation (98). Similar studies were repeated a decade later and confirmed these findings (99). This suggests that effective ACh levels would decrease after REM sleep deprivation, possibly as a compensatory phenomenon. As that of MAO-A, the AChE level also was first affected in the medulla but in an opposite manner (100). The bound form of the enzyme increases more than the decrease in the free form of the enzyme (101). The REM sleep deprivation did not alter the cholinergic receptor concentration in the brain (102). These results suggest a decrease in ACh in the brain after REM sleep deprivation.

Deprivation and Changes in the GABAergic System

In addition to ACh and NE, GABA has been implicated in the regulation of REM sleep (74). The GABA level was found to increase in the locus coeruleus during REM sleep (75). An interaction between NE, ACh, and GABA, at least in the locus coeruleus, for the regulation of REM sleep has been shown (103). Hence, it is expected that GABA levels would be altered during REM sleep deprivation or related disorders. Although GABA levels have not been estimated after REM sleep deprivation, the concentration of glutamic acid decarboxylase (GAD), the enzyme responsible for GABA synthesis, increased within the locus coeruleus neurons only after REM sleep deprivation (82). The increase was not seen in the laterodorsal tegmentum/pedunculopontine tegmentum (LDT/PPT) and the medial preoptic area (mPOA) regions after REM sleep deprivation.

Deprivation and Changes in Other Biomolecules

Based on the studies mentioned earlier it is obvious that sleep and REM sleep deprivation may modulate protein synthetic machinery in the body. Therefore, the effects of deprivation were studied on the expression of immediate early genes (IEGs) in the brain. These genes are expressed rapidly but transiently, primarily in response to disturbance in the cellular membranes. It was noted earlier that some of the neuronal firing rates change during REM sleep and its deprivation. These changes in firing rates would alter neuronal membrane permeability. Also, it has been reported that at least REM sleep deprivation decreases fluidity of the neuronal membrane (104). Hence, there are convincing reasons that NREM sleep and REM sleep deprivation might alter the expression of IEGs in the brain.

Rebound increases in REM sleep after its deprivation or by acoustic stimulation facilitate *c-fos* (an IEG) expression in several nuclei in the brainstem and in the hypothalamus (105,106) (see also Chap. 19). Alternatively, an increase in a REM sleep–like state by microinjection of carbachol, a cholinergic agonist, into the pontine reticular formation also triggered expression of *c-fos* within cells of several brainstem nuclei (107–110). Based on these initial findings, some relationship between REM sleep expressions of IEGs was proposed. However, the subsequent finding that there was induction of *c-fos* in specific brain regions after periods of wakefulness (111), suggests that the expression of IEGs may not be very specific to REM sleep or its deprivation, and may not be functionally correlated to sleep or REM sleep. After sleep deprivation, IL-1 mRNA and TNF-α mRNA increased in the brain (112). In a study in 2000 using a *Drosophila* model, if *Drosophila* organisms were not allowed to rest (in an attempt to simulate sleep deprivation), some genes were upregulated while other genes were downregulated (113). These findings suggest that sleep deprivation affects a large amount of gene expression. As a corollary, these findings also suggest that sleep deprivation is a generalized phenomenon that may directly or indirectly affect a large number of body functions.

It is known that the brain consumes maximal energy to maintain brain excitability status. REM sleep deprivation has been reported to induce hypothermia associated with increased food intake but loss in body weight (52). Although the mechanism of such diverse and sometimes contradictory results is not known, a few studies have looked into the changes in metabolic enzymes after sleep deprivation. In one such study, the activity of glucose-6-phosphatase decreased after REM sleep deprivation whereas the activity of hexokinase increased after sleep deprivation (114). Following REM sleep deprivation, excessive energy is consumed possibly by the increased activity of Na-K ATPase (115) (Fig. 1) and chloride ATPase (116). REM sleep deprivation has also been reported to decrease 5' nucleotidase activity in the brain (117). Galanin is an

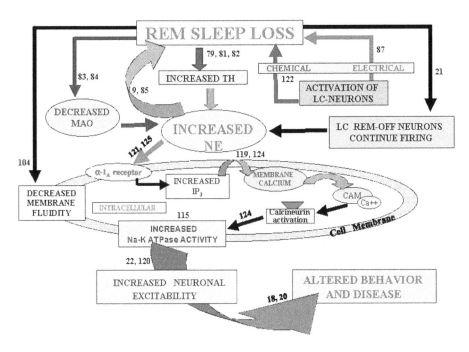

Figure 1 REM sleep deprivation increases Na-K ATPase activity in the brain. This is likely to be the cause of REM sleep loss–induced altered brain excitability and behavior. Numbers represent the cited references.

inhibitory peptide that is found in many brain cell groups that take part in sleep regulation and it is colocalized with other neurotransmitters. REM sleep deprivation has been found to induce galanin gene expression (118). Since the neuronal activities and behaviors are affected after total sleep and REM sleep deprivation, it is likely that there should be alterations in the cellular milieu ionic composition. Although there has not been much study in this direction, some limited studies have estimated different ionic composition in the serum (17). In one such study, calcium concentration in the synaptosome was estimated before and after REM sleep deprivation and also under various control conditions. It was found that the calcium concentration decreased in most of the brain after REM sleep deprivation (119).

III. Sleep Deprivation–Induced Changes in Biomolecules and Physiological Functions

Sleep, including REM sleep, is an instinct behavior and is essential for life process because its absence may lead to several disorders including death in extreme conditions. Several hypotheses have been put forward to explain its function(s). However, there is no definitive answer in this respect and the mechanism of action is far from clear. Some of the reasons for this lacuna in our knowledge are that sleep serves a complex function and its loss affects (directly or indirectly) several physiological parameters simultaneously. Another important lacuna that is evident from the literature is that there have been isolated studies by different groups across the globe. Although the findings of those studies are indicators and form the basis for proposing hypotheses, they do not allow one to draw a definitive conclusion.

Notwithstanding, at least two groups (Rechtschaffen's group and Mallick's group) have used sleep deprivation methods in rats more consistently. Rechtschaffen's group conducted a series of sleep deprivation studies using the disk-over-water method (see Chaps. 4, 5)and measured various biomolecules in the blood as well as in the brain. Although the mechanisms of action of these changes are not clear, it was inferred that sleep may be necessary for effective thermoregulation (88). Based on previous reports and our data it was hypothesized that one of the functions of REM sleep is to maintain brain excitability status, and we carried out a series of REM sleep deprivation studies to investigate the possible mechanism of action (20,120). Although recording of transmembrane potential before and after REM sleep deprivation in freely-behaving conditions would have been the ideal choice, in the absence of such a method due to technical limitations, an alternative method was used to address the issue.

It was proposed that if REM sleep is to maintain brain and neuronal excitability, its deprivation would alter factor(s) affecting the neuronal excitability. One of the primary components involved in maintenance of neuronal excitability is the Na-ion concentration within the neuron and the fact that Na-K ATPase largely maintains its concentration gradient. Hence, Na-K ATPase activity was estimated and was found to increase in the rat brain after REM sleep deprivation (115). Thereafter, the cause of this increase in Na-K ATPase activity was investigated. Since the noradrenergic REM-off neurons do not cease firing after REM sleep deprivation as a result of which there was an increased level of NE, it was hypothesized that NE could cause the increase in Na-K ATPase activity. In fact, it was observed during in vivo as well as in vitro studies that the REM sleep deprivation–induced increase in Na-K ATPase activity in rat brain was due to NE and the effect was mediated through the α_1-adrenoceptor (121). To confirm the results of several isolated studies, a recent in vivo study showed that intermittent (every 6 hr) injection of picrotoxin into the locus coeruleus for 36 hr in an attempt to not allow REM-off neurons to cease firing resulted in decreased REM sleep and increased Na-K ATPase activity (122). Furthermore, it is known that the Ca– ion, inhibitory to Na-K ATPase activity (123), also is affected after REM sleep deprivation (119). Studies were conducted to investigate the relationship between them, and it was observed that increased NE releases membrane-bound calcium and that increased Na-K ATPase activity (124). Further studies to understand the intracellular mechanism of action showed that NE acted on the α_{1A}-adrenoceptor that stimulated the phospholipase C pathway, and activated calcium-calmodulin and dephosphorylated Na-K ATPase to increase its activity (125). Subsequently, prior to undertaking studies to understand the molecular basis of the increase in Na-K ATPase activity a kinetic study was undertaken. It was observed that after REM sleep deprivation there was an increase in both the K_m as well as V_{max} of the enzyme (126). This suggested that REM sleep deprivation increased synthesis posttranslationally as well as allosteric modulation of the enzyme molecules, and both are likely to be increased by NE. The latter may be supported by the fact that NE increased the Na-K ATPase activity in vitro both in the microsome as well as in the synaptosome preparations (127). Subsequently, an increased synthesis of Na-K ATPase molecules has been shown after REM sleep deprivation (128). Furthermore, the molecular mechanisms of action of such increased expression of Na-K ATPase molecules after REM sleep deprivation is under investigation. Thus, these studies show that after REM sleep deprivation there is increased NE in the brain that acts on the α_{1A}-adrenoceptor and increases Na-K ATPase activity. The increased Na-K ATPase activity is likely to be responsible for the REM sleep deprivation–induced altered brain excitability (129). All of these findings have been synthesized in Figure 1, however, whether the change in the enzyme activity is a cause or effect of alteration in excitability has not yet been confirmed.

IV. Could There Be a Biomolecular Marker to Identify Sleep Loss?

We discussed that total sleep and REM sleep deprivation affect several psychobehavioral parameters. They also affect a large number of biomolecules, including neurotransmitters, enzymes, proteins, and so forth in the blood as well as in the brain. It has been argued that since the changes in those factors are due to sleep deprivation, none of these factors could be conclusively taken as a marker for sleep loss. One still has to depend on electrophysiological recordings for the identification of sleep loss. It is now becoming increasingly evident that the body has a capability to compensate for some amount of sleep loss; however, sleep loss has a cumulative effect and thus may be termed as a "slow killer." Therefore, there is a pressing need to identify a marker molecule for sleep deprivation/loss. There is also a need to identify such a molecule in the body fluids for easy identification and for diagnostic purposes. Identification of such an objectively defined marker molecule would also help to maintain the level of deprivation in animals to a uniform level for all studies; this is lacking at the present time.

One of the difficulties in identification of such a molecule is possibly the complex nature of sleep and to try to associate the marker biomolecule, if at all, with NREM sleep– or REM sleep–modulating substance(s). Another factor is that no systematic effort(s) have been made to identify the molecule, especially using modern, more sensitive techniques. One or more (a limited) number of molecules in the blood or CSF is likely to change its concentration with loss of

NREM sleep and/or REM sleep, and that may be termed a marker molecule. Although such a molecule may be correlated with certain sleep loss–associated phenomena, it may not be capable of induction or withdrawal of sleep per se. Such a change is unlikely to be an all-or-none response. We should keep our options open to accept that there may be changes in a molecule with shorter deprivation and that some other molecule might show changes with longer deprivation. This could be due to the fact that with prolonged deprivation some molecules might become degraded and might appear not to alter. In addition, it is also possible that, due to species variation, some molecule(s) might change in one (animal) species while remaining unaffected in another, including humans. There have been some attempts in humans as well as in animals for the identification of a marker molecule after total sleep and/or REM sleep deprivation. Cerebrodiene (a lipid in cats) (130), renin (a protein in humans) (131), and oleamide (a lipid in humans) (132) have been so indicated for this purpose. However, further studies are needed for confirmation. Recently, we have identified a reasonably large monomer molecule in the body fluid that alters its concentration after REM sleep deprivation in a dose-dependent manner (unpublished results). Furthermore, the molecule does not change in controls but recovers after recovery of REM sleep. The biochemical nature and biological properties of the molecule are under current investigation.

V. Summary and Conclusions

The studies reviewed have suggested that total sleep and REM sleep deprivation affect a large number of molecules in the body fluids (blood and CSF) as well as in the brain. The physiological significance of all these changes is not completely known. However, the studies help in understanding the possible mechanism of the action of total sleep or REM sleep deprivation–induced effects. Although there have been isolated studies to identify any molecule as a marker for such deprivation, it has yet to meet with success. One of the limitations is that most of the information has been gathered from studies done independently and in isolation. Nevertheless, based on the results of in-depth follow-up studies, it may at least be suggested that after REM sleep deprivation there is an increase in NE levels in the brain. The increased NE in the brain is at least one of the active components of the REM sleep deprivation–induced increase in Na-K ATPase activity in the brain, which in turn alters brain excitability leading to related disorders.

References

1. Mistlberger RE, Rusak B. Mechanisms and models of the circadian time keeping system. In: Kryger MH, Roth T, Dement WC, eds. Principles and Practice of Sleep Medicine. Philadelphia: WB Saunders, 1989:141–152.

2. Deguchi T, Sinha AK, Dement WC, Barchas JD. Enzyme activity in sleep and sleep deprivation. Pharmacol Biochem Behav 1975; 3(6):957–960.

3. Boyer RM. Sleep related endocrine rhythms. In: Reichlin S, Balsessarini RJ, Martin JB, eds. The Hypothalamus. New York: Raven Press, 1978:373–386.

4. Obal F, Jr., Krueger JM. Hormones and Sleep. In: Mallick BN, Inoue S, eds. Rapid Eye Movement Sleep. New York: Marcel Dekker, 1999:233–247.

5. Jouvet M. The role of monoamines and acetylcholine-containing neurons in the regulation of the sleep-waking cycle. Ergeb Physiol 1972; 64:166–307.

6. Hilakivi I, Leppavuori A. Effects of methoxamine, an alpha-1 adrenoceptor agonist, and prazosin, an alpha-1 antagonist, on the stages of the sleep-waking cycle in the cat. Acta Physiol Scand 1984; 120(3):363–372.

7. Mallick BN, Alam MN. Different types of norepinephrinergic receptors are involved in preoptic area mediated modulation of sleep-wakefulness and body temperature. Brain Res 1992; 591:8–19.

8. Mallick BN, Joseph MM. Role of cholinergic inputs to the medial preoptic area in regulation of sleep-wakefulness and body temperature in freely moving rats. Brain Res 1997; 750:311–317.

9. Depoortere H. Adrenergic agonists and antagonists and sleep-wakefulness stages. In: Wauquier A, Gaillard JM, Monti JM, Radulovacki M, eds. Sleep: Neurotransmitters and Neuromodulators. New York: Raven Press, 1985:79–92.

10. Ali M, Jha SK, Kaur S, Mallick BN. Role of GABA-A receptor in the preoptic area in the regulation of sleep-wakefulness and rapid eye movement sleep. Neurosci Res. 1999 Mar;33(3):245–250.

11. Kaur S, Saxena RN, Mallick BN. GABA in locus coeruleus regulates spontaneous rapid eye movement sleep by acting on GABAA receptors in freely moving rats. Neurosci Lett. 1997 Feb 21;223(2):105–108.

12. Dement W, Fischer C. Experimental intereference with the sleep cycle. J Can Psychiat Assoc 1963; 8:400.

13. Morden B, Conner R, Mitchell G, Dement W, Levine S. Effects of rapid eye movement sleep deprivation on shock induced fighting. Physiol Behav 1968; 3:425–432.

14. Dement W, Henry P, Cohen H, Ferguson J. Studies on the effect of REM deprivation in humans and in animals. Res Publ Assoc Res Nerv Ment Dis 1967; 45:456–468.

15. Fishbein W, Gutwein BM. Paradoxical sleep and memory storage processes. Behav Biol 1977; 19:425–464.

16. Smith CT, Conway JM, Rose GM. Brief paradoxical sleep deprivation impairs reference, but not working, memory in the radial arm maze task. Neurobiol Learn Mem 1998; 69(2):211–217.

17. Kushida CA, Bergmann BM, Rechtschaffen A. Sleep deprivation in the rat: IV. Paradoxical sleep deprivation. Sleep 1989; 12(1):22–30.

18. Vogel GE. A review of REM sleep deprivation. Arch Gen Psychiatry 1975; 82:749–761.

19. Albert IB. REM sleep deprivation. Biol Psychiatry 1975; 10(3):341–351.

20. Gulyani S, Majumdar S, Mallick BN. Rapid eye movement sleep and significance of its deprivation studies: a review. Sleep and Hypnosis 2000; 2:49–68.

21. Mallick BN, Siegel JM, Fahringer H. Changes in pontine unit activity with REM sleep deprivation. Brain Res 1989; 515:94–98.

22. Mallick BN, Fahringer HM, Wu MF, Siegel JM. REM sleep deprivation reduces auditory evoked inhibition of dorsolateral pontine neurons. Brain Res 1991; 552:333–337.

23. Carskadon MA, Dement WC. Normal human sleep: an overview. In: Kryger MH, Roth T, Dement WC, eds. Principles and Practice of Sleep Medicine. Philadelphia: WB Saunders, 1989:3–13.

24. Thorpy MJ. Sleep disorders. Curr Opin Neurol Neurosurg 1991; 4:265–270.

25. Bentivoglio M, Grassi-Zucconi G. The pioneering experimental studies on sleep deprivation. Sleep 1997; 20(7):570–576.

26. Tarozzi G. Sull'influenza dell'insonnio sperimentale sul ricambio materiale. Riv Pat Nerv Ment 1899; 4:1–23.

27. Legendre R, Pieron H. Recherches sur le besoin de sommeil consecutif a une prolongee. Z Allg Physiol 1913; 14:235.

28. Ishimori K. True cause of sleep hypnogenic substance as evidenced in the brain of sleep-deprived animals. Tokyo Igakkai Zasshi 1909; 23:429.

29. Inoue S. Biology of sleep substances. Boca Raton, FL: CRC Press, 1989.

30. Schnedorf JG, Ivy AC. An examination of the hypnotoxin theory of sleep. Am J Psychol 1939; 125:491.

31. Pappenheimer JR, Miller TB, Goodrich CA. Sleep promoting effects of cerebrospinal fluid from sleep-deprived goats. Proc Natl Acad Sci U S A 1967; 58:513–517.

32. Pappenheimer JR, Koski G, Fencl V, Karnovsky ML, Krueger J. Extraction of sleep promoting factor S from cerebrospinal fluid and from brains of sleep deprived animals. J Neurophysiol 1975; 38:1299–1310.

33. Spanis CW, Gutierrez MDC, Drucker-Colin RR. Neurohumoral correlates of sleep: further biochemical and physiological characterization of sleep perfusates. Pharmacol Biochem Behav 1976; 5:165–173.

34. Prospero-Garcia O, Moralis M, Arankowsky-Sandoval G, Drucker-Colin R. Vasoactive intestinal polypeptide (VIP) and cerebrospinal fluid (CSF) of sleep deprived cats restores REM sleep in insomniac recipients. Brain Res 1986; 385:169–173.

35. Monnier M, Hosli L. Humoral transmission of sleep and wakefulness. II. Hemodialysis of sleep inducing humor during stimulation of the thalamic somnogenic area. Pfluegers Arch 1965; 282:60.

36. Krueger JM, Bacsik J, Garcia-Arraras J. Sleep-promoting material from human urine and its relation to factor S from brain. Am J Physiol 1980; 238(2):E116–E123.

37. Drucker-Colin RR. Crossed perfusion of a sleep inducing brain tissue substance in conscious cats. Brain Res 1973; 56:123–134.

38. Nagasaki H, Iriki M, Inoue S, Uchizono K. [Proceedings: Sleep promoting substances in the brain stem of rats]. Nippon Seirigaku Zasshi 1974; 36(8-9):293.

39. Krueger JM, Johannsen L. Bacterial products, cytokines and sleep. J Rheumatol Suppl 1989; 19:52-57.

40. Drucker–Colin R, Bernal–Pedraza J, Fernandez–Cancino F, Oksenberg A. Is vasoactive intestinal polypeptide (VIP) a sleep factor? Peptides 1984; 5(4):837–840.

41. Obal F Jr, Sary G, Alfoldi P, Rubicsek G, Obal F. Vasoactive intestinal polypeptide promotes sleep without effects on brain temperature in rats at night. Neurosci Lett 1986; 64(2):236–240.

42. Ueno R, Honda K, Inoue S, Hayaishi O. Prostaglandin D2, a cerebral sleep-inducing substance in rats. Proc Natl Acad Sci U S A 1983; 80(6):1735–1737.

43. Graf MV, Kastin AJ. Delta-sleep-inducing peptide (DSIP): a review. Neurosci Biobehav Rev 1984; 8(1):83–93.

44. Chan V, Jones A, Liendo-Ch P, McNeilly A, Landon J, Besser GM. The relationship between circadian variations in circulating thyrotrophin, thyroid hormones and prolactin. Clin Endocrinol (Oxf) 1978; 9(4):337–349.

45. Baumgartner A, Haug HJ. Thyroid hormones during sleep deprivation. Biol Psychiatry 1988; 23(5):537–538.

46. Bliss ELCLD, West CD. Studies of sleep deprivation: relationship to schizophrenia. Arch Neurol Psychiatry 1959; 81:348–359.

47. Murawski B, Crabbe J. Effect of sleep deprivation on plasma 17-hydroxycorticosteroids. J Appl Physiol 1960; 15:280–282.

48. Rubin RT, Kollar EJ, Slater GG, Clark BR. Excretion of 17-hydroxycorticosteroids and vanillylmandelic acid during 205 hours of sleep deprivation in man. Psychosom Med 1969; 31:68–79.

49. Akerstedt T, Palmblad J, de la TB, Marana R, Gillberg M. Adrenocortical and gonadal steroids during sleep deprivation. Sleep 1980; 3(1):23–30.

50. Redwine L, Hauger RL, Gillin JC, Irwin M. Effects of sleep and sleep deprivation on interleukin-6, growth hormone, cortisol, and melatonin levels in humans. J Clin Endocrinol Metab 2000; 85(10):3597–3603.

51. Goh VH, Tong TY, Lim CL, Low EC, Lee LK. Effects of one night of sleep deprivation on hormone profiles and performance efficiency. Milit Med 2001; 166(5):427–431.

52. Bergmann BM, Everson CA, Kushida CA, Fang VS, Leitch CA, Schoeller DA, Rechtschaffen A. Sleep deprivation in the rat: V. Energy use and mediation. Sleep 1989; 12(1):31–41.

53. Irwin M, Thompson J, Miller C, Gillin JC, Ziegler M. Effects of sleep and sleep deprivation on catecholamine and interleukin-2 levels in humans: clinical implications. J Clin Endocrinol Metab 1999; 84(6):1979–1985.

54. Netzer NC, Kristo D, Steinle H, Lehmann M, Strohl KP. REM sleep and catecholamine excretion: a study in elite athletes. Eur J Appl Physiol 2001; 84(6):521–526.

55. Goldstein A, Armony-Sivan R, Rozin A, Weller A. Somatostatin levels during infancy, pregnancy, and lactation: a review. Peptides 1995; 16(7):1321–1326.

56. Mitsugi N, Kimura F. Simultaneous determination of blood levels of corticosterone and growth hormone in the male rat: relation to sleep-wakefulness cycle. Neuroendocrinology 1985; 41(2):125–130.

57. Toppila J, Asikainen M, Alanko L, Turek FW, Stenberg D, Porkka-Heiskanen T. The effect of REM sleep deprivation on somatostatin and growth hormone-releasing hormone gene expression in the rat hypothalamus. J Sleep Res 1996; 5(2):115–122.

58. Drucker-Colin RR, Spanis CW, Hunyadi J, Sassin JF, McGaugh JL. Growth hormone effects on sleep and wakefulness in the rat. Neuroendocrinology 1975; 18(1):1–8.

59. Born J, Muth S, Fehm HL. The significance of sleep onset and slow wave sleep for nocturnal release of growth hormone (GH) and cortisol. Psychoneuroendocrinology 1988; 13(3):233–243.

60. Goldstein J, Van Cauter E, Desir D, Noel P, Spire JP, Refetoff S, et al. Effects of "jet lag" on hormonal patterns. IV. Time shifts increase growth hormone release. J Clin Endocrinol Metab 1983; 56(3):433–440.

61. Moldofsky H, Davidson JR, Lue FA. Sleep related patterns of plasma growth hormone and cortisol following 40 hours of wakefulness. Sleep Res 1988; 17:69.

62. Kant GJ, Genser SG, Thorne DR, Pfalser JL, Mougey EH. Effects of 72 hour sleep deprivation on urinary cortisol and indices of metabolism. Sleep 1984; 7(2):142–146.

63. Palmblad J, Cantell K, Strander H, Froberg J, Karlsson CG, Levi L, et al. Stressor exposure and immunological response in man: interferon-producing capacity and phagocytosis. J Psychosom Res 1976; 20(3):193–199.

64. Everson CA. Sustained sleep deprivation impairs host defense. Am J Physiol 1993; 265(5 Pt 2):R1148–R1154.

65. Haack M, Schuld A, Kraus T, Pollmacher T. Effects of sleep on endotoxin-induced host responses in healthy men. Psychosom Med 2001; 63(4):568–578.

66. Solomon GF. Stress and antibody response in rats. Int Arch Allergy Appl Immunol 1969; 35(1):97–104.

67. Moldofsky H, Lue FA, Davidson JR, Gorczynski R. Effects of sleep deprivation on human immune functions. FASEB J 1989; 3(8):1972–1977.

68. Irwin M, Mascovich A, Gillin JC, Willoughby R, Pike J, Smith TL. Partial sleep deprivation reduces natural killer cell activity in humans. Psychosom Med 1994; 56(6):493–498.

69. Irwin M, McClintick J, Costlow C, Fortner M, White J, Gillin JC. Partial night sleep deprivation reduces natural killer and cellular immune responses in humans. FASEB J 1996; 10(5):643–653.

70. Dinges DF, Douglas SD, Zaugg L, Campbell DE, McMann JM, Whitehouse WG, et al. Leukocytosis and natural killer cell function parallel neurobehavioral fatigue induced by 64 hours of sleep deprivation. J Clin Invest 1994; 93(5):1930–1939.

71. Chu NS, Bloom FE. Activity patterns of catecholamine-containing pontine neurons in the dorso-lateral tegmentum of unrestrained cats. J Neurobiol 1974; 5(6):527–544.

72. Aston-Jones G, Bloom FE. Activity of norepinephrine-containing locus coeruleus neurons in behaving rats anticipates fluctuations in the sleep-waking cycle. J Neurosci 1981; 1(8):876–886.

73. McCarley RW, Hobson JA. Single neuron activity in cat gigantocellular tegmental field: selectivity of discharge in desynchronized sleep. Science 1971; 174:1250–1252.

74. Mallick BN, Kaur S, Jha SK, Siegel JM. Possible role of GABA in the regulation of REM sleep with special reference to REM-OFF neurons. In: Mallick BN, Inoue S, eds. Rapid eye movement sleep. New York: Marcel Dekker, 1999:153–166.

75. Nitz D, Siegel JM. GABA release in the locus coeruleus as a function of sleep/wake state. Neuroscience 1997; 78:795–801.

76. Gervasoni D, Darracq L, Fort P, Souliere F, Chouvet G, Luppi PH. Electrophysiological evidence that noradrenergic neurons of the rat locus coeruleus are tonically inhibited by GABA during sleep. Eur J Neurosci 1998; 10:964–970.

77. Pujol JF, Mouret J, Jouvet M, Glowinski J. Increased turnover of cerebral norepinephrine during rebound of paradoxical sleep in the rat. Science 1968; 159:112–114.

78. Stern WC, Miller FP, Cox RH, Maickel RP. Brain norepinephrine and serotonin levels following REM sleep deprivation in the rat. Psychopharmacology 1971; 22:50–55.

79. Sinha AK, Ciaranello RD, Dement WC, Barchas JD. Tyrosine hydroxylase activity in rat brain following "REM" sleep deprivation. J Neurochem 1973; 20:1289–1290.
80. Porkka-Heiskanen T, Smith SE, Taira T, Urban JH, Levine JE, Turek FW et al. Noradrenergic activity in rat brain during rapid eye movement sleep deprivation and rebound sleep. Am J Physiol 1995; 268(6 Pt 2):R1456–R1463.
81. Basheer R, Magner M, McCarley RW, Shiromani PJ. REM sleep deprivation increases the levels of tyrosine hydroxylase and norepinephrine transporter mRNA in the locus coeruleus. Brain Res Mol Brain Res 1998; 57(2):235–240.
82. Majumdar S, Mallick BN. Increased levels of tyrosine hydroxylase and glutamic acid decarboxylase in locus coeruleus neurons after rapid eye movement sleep deprivation in rats. Neurosc Lett 2003; 338(3):193–196.
83. Thakkar M, Mallick BN. Effect of rapid eye movement sleep deprivation on rat brain monoamine oxidases. Neuroscience 1993; 55(3):677–683.
84. Perez NM, Benedito MA. Activities of monoamine oxidase (MAO) A and B in discrete regions of rat brain after rapid eye movement (REM) sleep deprivation. Pharmacol Biochem Behav 1997; 58(2):605–608.
85. Ross RJ, Ball WA, Gresch PJ, Morrison AR. REM sleep suppression by monoamine reuptake blockade: development of tolerance with repeated drug administration. Biol Psychiatry 1990; 28(3):231–239.
86. Makela JP, Hilakivi IT. Effect of alpha-adrenoceptor blockade on sleep and wakefulness in the rat. Pharmacol Biochem Behav 1986; 24(3):613–616.
87. Singh S, Mallick BN. Mild electrical stimulation of pontine tegmentum around locus coeruleus reduces rapid eye movement sleep in rats. Neurosci Res 1996; 24:227–235.
88. Rechtschaffen A, Bergmann BM, Everson CA, Kushida CA, Gilliland MA. Sleep deprivation in the rat: X. Integration and discussion of the findings. Sleep 1989; 12(1):68–87.
89. Mallick BN, Jha SK, Islam F. Presence of alpha-1 adrenoreceptors on thermosensitive neurons in the medial preoptico-anterior hypothalamic area in rats. Neuropharmacology 2002; 42(5):697–705.
90. Hery F, Pujol JF, Lopez M, Macon J, Glowinski J. Increased synthesis and utilization of serotonin in the central nervous system of the rat during paradoxical sleep deprivation. Brain Res 1970; 21(3):391–403.
91. Toru M, Mitsushio H, Mataga N, Takashima M, Arito H. Increased brain serotonin metabolism during rebound sleep in sleep-deprived rats. Pharmacol Biochem Behav 1984; 20(5):757–761.
92. Mogilnicka E. REM sleep deprivation changes behavioral response to catecholaminergic and serotonergic receptor activation in rats. Pharmacol Biochem Behav 1981; 15(1):149–151.
93. Serra G, Melis MR, Argiolas A, Fadda F, Gessa GL. REM sleep deprivation induces subsensitivity of dopamine receptors mediating sedation in rats. Eur J Pharmacol 1981; 72(1):131–135.
94. Siegel JM, Rogawski MA. A function for REM sleep: regulation of noradrenergic receptor sensitivity. Brain Res 1988; 472(3):213–233.
95. Tsai LL, Bergmann BM, Perry BD, Rechtschaffen A. Effects of chronic total sleep deprivation on central noradrenergic receptors in rat brain. Brain Res 1993; 602(2):221–227.
96. Rye DB. Contributions of the pedunculopontine region to normal and altered REM sleep. Sleep 1997; 20(9):757–788.

97. Kodama T, Lai YY, Siegel JM. Enhancement of acetylcholine release during REM sleep in the caudomedial medulla as measured by in vivo microdialysis. Brain Res 1992; 580(1–2):348–350.

98. Thakkar M, Mallick BN. Effects of REM sleep deprivation on rat brain acetylcholinesterase. Pharmacol Biochem Behav 1991; 39(1):211–214.

99. Benedito MA, Camarini R. Rapid eye movement sleep deprivation induces an increase in acetylcholinesterase activity in discrete rat brain regions. Braz J Med Biol Res 2001; 34(1):103–109.

100. Mallick BN, Thakkar M. Short-term REM sleep deprivation increases acetylcholinesterase activity in the medulla of rats. Neurosci Lett 1991; 130(2):221–224.

101. Mallick BN, Thakkar M. Effect of REM sleep deprivation on molecular forms of acetylcholinesterase in rats. Neuroreport 1992; 3:676–678.

102. Tsai LL, Bergmann BM, Perry BD, Rechtschaffen A. Effects of chronic sleep deprivation on central cholinergic receptors in rat brain. Brain Res 1994; 642(1–2):95–103.

103. Mallick BN, Kaur S, Saxena RN. Interactions between cholinergic and GABAergic neurotransmitters in and around the locus coeruleus for the induction and maintenance of rapid eye movement sleep in rats. Neuroscience 2001; 104(2):467–485.

104. Mallick BN, Thakkar M, Gangabhagirathi R. Rapid eye movement sleep deprivation decreases membrane fluidity in the rat brain. Neurosci Res 1995; 22:117–122.

105. Merchant-Nancy H, Vazquez J, Aguilar-Roblero R, Drucker-Colin R. c-fos proto-oncogene changes in relation to REM sleep duration. Brain Res 1992; 579(2):342–346.

106. Merchant-Nancy H, Vazquez J, Garcia F, Drucker-Colin R. Brain distribution of c-fos expression as a result of prolonged rapid eye movement (REM) sleep period duration. Brain Res 1995; 681(1–2):15–22.

107. Shiromani PJ, Malik M, Winston S, McCarley RW. Time course of Fos-like immunoreactivity associated with cholinergically induced REM sleep. J Neurosci 1995; 15(5 Pt 1):3500–3508.

108. Shiromani PJ, Winston S, McCarley RW. Pontine cholinergic neurons show Fos-like immunoreactivity associated with cholinergically induced REM sleep. Brain Res Mol Brain Res 1996; 38(1):77–84.

109. Yamuy J, Mancillas JR, Morales FR, Chase MH. C-fos expression in the pons and medulla of the cat during carbachol-induced active sleep. J Neurosci 1993; 13(6):2703–2718.

110. Yamuy J, Sampogna S, Lopez-Rodriguez F, Luppi PH, Morales FR, Chase MH. Fos and serotonin immunoreactivity in the raphe nuclei of the cat during carbachol-induced active sleep: a double-labeling study. Neuroscience 1995; 67(1):211–223.

111. Cirelli C, Pompeiano M, Tononi G. Sleep deprivation and c-fos expression in the rat brain. J Sleep Res 1995; 4(2):92–106.

112. Taishi P, Chen Z, Obal F Jr, Hansen MK, Zhang J, Fang J, Krueger JM. Sleep-associated changes in interleukin-1beta mRNA in the brain. J Interferon Cytokine Res 1998; 18(9):793–798.

113. Cirelli C, Tononi G. Gene expression in the brain across the sleep-waking cycle. Brain Res 2000; 885(2):303–321.

114. Thakkar M, Mallick BN. Rapid eye movement sleep-deprivation-induced changes in glucose metabolic enzymes in rat brain. Sleep 1993; 16(8):691–694.

115. Gulyani S, Mallick BN. Effect of rapid eye movement sleep deprivation on rat brain Na-K ATPase activity. J Sleep Res 1993; 2(1):45–50.

116. Mallick BN, Gulyani S. Rapid eye movement sleep deprivation increases chloride-sensitive Mg- ATPase activity in the rat brain. Pharmacol Biochem Behav 1993; 45(2):359–362.

117. Thakkar M, Mallick BN. Effect of rapid eye movement sleep deprivation on 5'-nucleotidase activity in the rat brain. Neurosci Lett 1996; 206(2–3):177–180.

118. Toppila J, Stenberg D, Alanko L, Asikainen M, Urban JH, Turek FW, Porkka-Heiskanen T. REM sleep deprivation induces galanin gene expression in the rat brain. Neurosci Lett 1995; 183(3):171–174.

119. Mallick BN, Gulyani S. Alteration in synaptosomal calcium concentrations after rapid eye movement sleep deprivation in rats. Neuroscience 1996; 75:729–736.

120. Mallick BN, Thakkar M, Gulyani S. Rapid Eye Movement sleep deprivation induced alteration in neuronal excitability: possible role of norepinephrine. In: Mallick BN, Singh R, eds. Environment and Physiology. New Delhi: Narosa, 1994:196–203.

121. Gulyani S, Mallick BN. Possible mechanism of rapid eye movement sleep deprivation induced increase in Na-K ATPase activity. Neuroscience 1995; 64(1):255–260.

122. Kaur S, Panchal M, Faisal M, Madan V, Nangia P, Mallick BN. Long term blocking of GABA-A receptor in locus coeruleus by bilateral microinfusion of picrotoxin reduced rapid eye movement sleep and increased brain Na-K ATPase activity in freely moving normally behaving rats. Behav Brain Res 2004; 151:185–190.

123. Davis PW, Vincenzi FF. Ca-ATPase activation and Na-K ATPase inhibition as a function of calcium concentration in human red cell membranes. Life Sci II 1971; 10(7):401–406.

124. Mallick BN, Adya HVA. Norepinephrine induced alpha-adrenoceptor mediated increase in rat brain Na-K ATPase activity is dependent on calcium ion. Neurochem Int 1999; 34:499–507.

125. Mallick BN, Adya HVA, Faisal M. Norepinephrine-stimulated increase in Na-K ATPase activity in the rat brain is mediated through alpha1A-adrenoceptor possibly by dephosphorylation of the enzyme. J Neurochem 2000; 74(4):1574–1578.

126. Adya HV, Mallick BN. Uncompetitive stimulation of rat brain Na-K ATPase activity by rapid eye movement sleep deprivation. Neurochem Int 2000; 36(3):249–253.

127. Adya HVA, Mallick BN. Comparison of Na- K ATPase in the rat brain synaptosome under different conditions. Neurochem Int 1998; 33:283–286.

128. Majumdar S, Faisal M, Madan V, Mallick BN. Increased turnover of Na-K ATPase molecules in the rat brain after rapid eye movement sleep deprivation. J Neurosci Res 2003; 73(6):870–875.

129. Mallick BN, Majumdar S, Faisal M, Yadav V, Madan V, Pal D. Role of norepinephrine in the regulation of rapid eye movement sleep. J Biosci 2002; 27:539–551.

130. Lerner RA, Siuzdak G, Prospero-Garcia O, Henriksen SJ, Boger DL, Cravatt BF. Cerebrodiene: a brain lipid isolated from sleep-deprived cats. Proc Natl Acad Sci U S A 1994; 91(20):9505–9508.

131. Brandenberger G, Charifi C, Muzet A, Saini J, Simon C, Follenius M. Renin as a biological marker of the NREM-REM sleep cycle: effect of REM sleep suppression. J Sleep Res 1994; 3:30–35.

132. Mendelson WB, Basile AS. The hypnotic actions of the fatty acid amide, oleamide. Neuropsychopharmacolohy 2001; 25 (suppl 5):536–539.

17

Immunologic Changes

SAROSH J. MOTIVALA AND MICHAEL IRWIN

University of California–Los Angeles, Los Angeles, California, U.S.A.

I. Introduction

Disordered sleep shows a high prevalence with between 10–50% of the general population reporting difficulty sleeping, depending on the methods used to assess insomnia and the population studied (1,2). In addition, sleep disturbance and loss of sleep occur in association with many psychiatric disorders as well as multiple medical conditions including cardiovascular, infectious, and inflammatory diseases (3–5). Epidemiological data increasingly implicate sleep loss as a predictor of cardiovascular and noncardiovascular disease mortality (3,6), and sleep loss is thought to adversely affect resistance to infectious disease, increase cancer risk, and alter inflammatory disease progression.

In this chapter, we review human and animal studies linking sleep, sleep deprivation, and immunity. In humans, normal sleep is associated with a redistribution of circulating lymphocyte subsets, increases of natural killer (NK) cell activity, increases of interleukin-2 (IL-2) and IL-6 expression, and a relative shift toward Th1 (T helper cell subset) cytokine expression that is independent of circadian processes. Conversely, sleep deprivation suppresses natural killer cell activity and IL-2 production, although prolonged sleep loss has been found to enhance measures of innate immunity and proinflammatory cytokine expression. In clinical populations that show disordered sleep (e.g., depression, bereavement, and alcoholism), alterations of natural and cellular immune function coincide with sleep loss and disturbances of sleep architecture. Decreases of sleep continuity and/or increases of rapid-eye-movement (REM) sleep are associated with increases in the nocturnal and daytime expression of IL-6, possibly with consequences for daytime fatigue.

This chapter will also consider the bidirectional actions of cytokines on sleep. In animals, cytokines have both somnogenic and inhibitory effects on sleep depending on the cytokine, plasma level, and circadian phase. In humans, much less is known about the sleep regulatory effects of cytokines. Expression of the anti-inflammatory cytokine IL-10 prior to sleep predicts amounts of delta sleep during the nocturnal period. In contrast, peripheral administration of the proinflammatory cytokine IL-6 reduces delta sleep. Finally, this chapter will describe the use of sleep deprivation as an experimental probe to examine sleep-immune interactions, and how this strategy might be used to provide insights into the potential role of cytokine abnormalities in predicting disordered sleep in psychiatric and medical populations.

A. Cellular Components of Immune System

The immune system is the body's defense against invading external pathogens such as viruses and bacteria and from abnormal internal cells such as tumors. Innate immunity refers to the body's resistance to pathogens that operates in a nonspecific way without recognition of the different nature of various pathogens, whereas specific immunity is acquired in response to the identification of non-self molecules called antigens. Macrophages and granulocytes are examples of nonspecific immune cells that react to tissue damage by consuming debris and invading organisms. In contrast, each T cell or B cell is genetically programmed to attack a specific target by secreting antibodies (B cell) or by killing cells of the body that harbor a virus (T cell). Both innate and specific immunity are orchestrated by the release of interleukins or cytokines from immune cells, and this cytokine network aids in the differentiation of the immune response and in the coordination of its magnitude and duration as noted below.

Cellular components of the immune system are termed leukocytes and are composed of a number of different cell types including granulocytes, monocytes and lymphocytes. Twenty to forty percent of leukocytes are lymphocytes, which include the T-, B-. and NK-cell populations. T cells are essential for regulation of antigen recognition and response generation. Following stimulation, B cells produce and secrete immunoglobulins, a diverse family of proteins that bind to a particular protein, carbohydrate, lipid, or other macromolecule ligands. Unlike T or B cells, NK cells do not require stimulation to kill their targets—tumor cells and virally infected cells.

Monocytes, representing 2–10% of leukocytes, circulate in vasculature, migrate into tissue, and transform into macrophages. Macrophages perform a number of functions, including phagocytosis, antigen presentation to lymphocytes, and removal of cellular debris. Macrophages also play an important role in launching and regulating an inflammatory response.

Granulocytes (including basophils, eosinophils, neutrophils, and mast cells) account for 60–80% of leukocytes. This population of cells lacks the memory and antigen specificity of T and B lymphocytes, yet they secrete powerful enzymes and are capable of phagocytic activity. For example, mast cells secrete histamine, which is associated with inflammation and allergic reactions.

B. Cytokines in the Regulation of Immunity

As noted above, leukocytes communicate with each other via chemical messengers called cytokines. More than 100 different cytokines have been identified, serving functions that include but are not limited to local and systemic inflammation, wound healing, and hematopoiesis. Cytokines are peptides or glycoproteins produced by immune cells and act in an autocrine, paracrine, or endocrine manner to initiate, maintain, and modulate immune responses. Cytokines can influence the stimulation, differentiation, or activity of target cells. Across cytokines, function can be synergistic, stimulatory, or inhibitory; the cytokine network incorporates a high degree of redundancy. Cytokines can be categorized by their effects on target cells. For example, T cells can be distinguished as Th1 or Th2 based on the kinds of cytokines they release. Th1 cells secrete cytokines such as interferon-γ (IFN-γ), which have important roles in T-cell activation and differentiation. In contrast, Th2 cells secrete IL-4 and IL-10, which regulate B-cell antibody production (7). Th1/Th2 cytokines show an intraservice rivalry in the regulation of cellular and humoral immune response (8). Cytokines can also be conceptualized as inflammatory or anti-inflammatory. Inflammatory cytokines act as stimulators of inflammatory responses by spurring liver production of acute phase proteins, activation and expansion of leukocyte population and promotion of increased vascular perfusion and increased capillary permeability. Lastly, another important cytokine, IL-2, originally termed T-cell growth factor, is a potent stimulator of a number of different cell types, especially T cells and NK cells. However, all of these immunoregulatory processes cannot be fully understood without taking into account the organism and the internal and external milieu in which innate and specific immune responses occur. Hence, studies have been carried out on the role of behavior and sleep in the modulation of immunity.

C. Cytokines: Behavioral Effects

Cytokines released by immune cells are increasingly implicated as messengers in the bidirectional interaction between the peripheral immune system and the brain. For example, the release of IL-1 following activation of macrophages with virus or other stimuli induces alterations of brain activity and changes in the metabolism of central norepinephrine, serotonin, and dopamine in discrete brain areas. Many recent data have focused on how these cytokines signal the brain given their large molecular size and inability to readily cross the blood-brain barrier. It is now known that IL-1 and possibly other inflammatory cytokines communicate with the brain by stimulating peripheral afferent nerves such as the vagus (9). In sum, the immune system acts in many ways like a sensory organ, conveying information to the brain, which ultimately regulates neuroendocrine and autonomic outflow and the course of the immune response.

Numerous behavioral studies have also found that immune activation leads to changes of peripheral physiology and behaviors that are similar to a stress response. With peripheral immune activation, proinflammatory cytokines are expressed in the central nervous system, corticotropin-releasing hormone is released by the hypothalamus, and there is an induction of a pituitary-adrenal response and autonomic activity. Coincident with these physiological changes, animals show reductions in activity, exploration of novel objects, social interactions, willingness to engage in sexual behaviors, and intake of food and water. Taken together, this pattern of behavioral changes (i.e., sickness behaviors) is similar to that found in animals exposed to fear- or anxiety-arousing stimuli, and can be reproduced by the central or peripheral administration of IL-1. In contrast, central administration of an IL-1 antagonist blocks these effects. These cytokine-brain processes are also implicated in increased sensitivity to pain stimuli and the hyperalgesia found following nerve or tissue injury. This chapter will discuss the links between cytokines and sleep processes in humans and in animals.

II. Sleep and Immunity

A. Infectious Agents and Sleep

Early observations suggested an association between infectious processes and sleep. In animals, administration of infectious agents (e.g., lipopolysaccharide, peptidoglycan) has somnogenic effects. For example, Krueger and colleagues have found that injection of bacteria produces initial increases in slow-wave sleep (SWS) time followed by decreases in SWS time in rabbits (10). Likewise, viral infections such as influenza produce increases in SWS in rabbits and mice (10). In humans, administration of low-dose endotoxin has also been found to alter sleep. Following the administration of endotoxin, increases of proinflammatory cytokines such as tumor necrosis factor (TNF) and IL-6 occur with consequent increases of non-REM (NREM) sleep in the first half of the night (11,12).

B. Sleep Processes, Sleep Deprivation, and Infection

Reciprocal interactions have also been identified in which sleep and sleep loss influence infectious processes. For example, prolonged sleep loss, leads to death and this outcome is related in part to insufficient immune responses to infectious challenge.

When loss of sleep is sustained over 3 weeks, a hypercatabolic state develops that ultimately ends in death (13), resembling in many ways the changes found following septic challenge. For example, the hypercatabolic state induced by sustained sleep deprivation is marked by increases of heart rate, plasma nor-epinephrine, and leukocyte counts, along with the development of skin lesions. Evaluation of blood cultures in such sleep-deprived rats shows the presence of lethal bacteria, yet the rats are afebrile. Moreover, in a subsequent study, Everson and Toth (14) found that prolonged sleep deprivation led to progressive increases of indigenous, lethal bacteria in the mesenteric lymph nodes, ileum, cecum, and lungs starting within 5 days of deprivation and continued to be present through days 10, 15, and 20 (Fig. 1). Taken together, these observations of a growing presence of bacteria in lymph nodes suggest impairments of immune-related response mechanisms (14). However, not all investigators have found evidence that sleep deprivation alters immune responses. Benca and colleagues (15) failed to identify immunological differences between healthy rats and severely sleep-deprived rats;

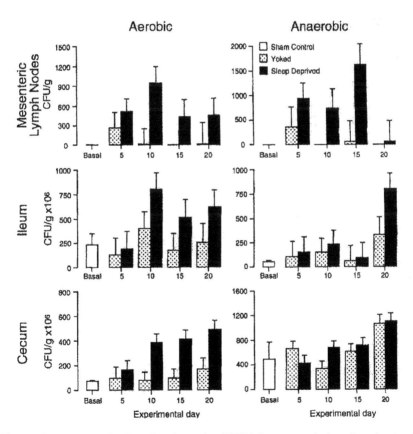

Figure 1　Number of colony-forming units (CFUs) in mesenteric lymph nodes (top), ileum (middle), and cecum (bottom) of sham-control, yoked, and sleep deprived rats, cultured under aerobic (left) and anaerobic (right) conditions. Geometrical means ± SD. (From Ref. 14.)

number of splenic cells, spleen size, or mitogenic response did not differ between sleep-deprived animals and controls.

In addition to the deleterious effects of prolonged sleep deprivation, basic sleep processes can influence survival and immune responsivity following infectious challenge. For example, the amount of SWS and amplitude of electroencephalographic delta waves predicted survival following intravenous injection of an infectious agent in rabbits (16). Other studies have found that sleep deprivation alters the organism's ability to mount an immune response to an infectious challenge. Brown and colleagues (17) inoculated rats with influenza virus and compared the effects of sleep deprivation on viral clearance. Mice that slept following inoculation showed total viral clearance following a subsequent intranasal viral challenge. However, in mice that were sleep deprived for 7 hrs, viral clearance was impaired, indicating that sleep deprivation attenuated the beneficial effects of the prior inoculation or immunization (17).

Translation of these basic observations linking sleep to infectious challenges in humans is limited. One study found that 40 hr of wakefulness followed by administration of low-dose endotoxin produced blunting of the pyrogenic response (18). In contrast, one night of sleep deprivation following administration of low-dose endotoxin was not associated with changes in pyrogenic response (19).

C. Cytokines and Sleep

The immune system's cytokine network may be one mechanism by which an infectious agent influences sleep. Indeed, animal studies have demonstrated that administration of proinflammatory cytokines such as IL-1 and TNF influence sleep quality and depth in ways similar to administration of infectious agents (20–22). In rabbits, central administration of TNF produces increases in NREM sleep and decreases in REM sleep (21). Similarly, central and peripheral administration of IL-1β produces increases in NREM and decreases in REM sleep (Fig. 2) (20). Similar findings are found in human studies. Endotoxin administration induces increases of TNF and IL-6 and is associated with increases in NREM sleep in healthy volunteers (12,23). In contrast to the sleep-promoting effects of proinflammatory cytokines, administration of the anti-inflammatory cytokine IL-10 has the opposite effect. In rats, intracerebroventricular administration of IL-10 20 min before sleep onset produces decreases in NREM sleep and no change in REM sleep (24).

Administration of cytokine antagonists or alteration of cytokine receptor expression extends these pharmacological studies and further indicate that cytokines have a role in the physiological regulation of sleep. The central administration of either TNF or IL-1β receptor fragments, that antagonizes the endogenous action of these cytokines, produces decreases in NREM sleep over a 22-hr period (21,25). Furthermore, administration of a TNF receptor fragment blocks the sleep-related effects of infectious agents such as muramyl peptides (22). Importantly, the effects of cytokine antagonists are dose dependent. Opp and Krueger (25) found that lower doses of anti IL-1β did not produce any effect on

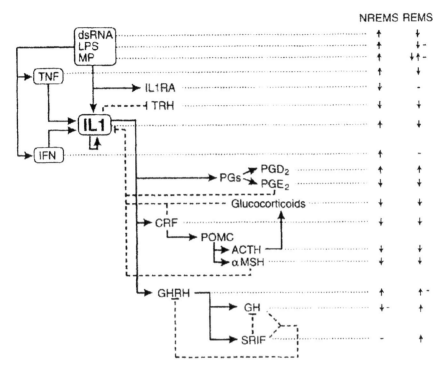

Figure 2 Possible interactions between putative sleep-promoting substances (*left*) and the effects of those substances on sleep (*right*). During infection when supplies of microbial products are enhanced, sleep enhancement is probably mediated via enhanced cytokine production, e.g., interleukin-1 (IL-1). IL-1 enhances production/release of several neuropeptides, some of which enhance and others of which inhibit sleep. The timing and location of these events remain unknown. Abbreviations: dsRNA, double-stranded RNA; LPS, lipopolysaccharide; MP, muramyl peptide; TNF, tumor necrosis factor; IFN, interferon; IL-1, interleukin-1; IL-1RA, interleukin-1 receptor antagonist; TRH, thyroid-releasing hormone; PG, prostaglandin; CRF, corticotropin-releasing factor; POMC, proopiomelanocyte corticotropin; ACTH, adrenocoricotropic hormone; MSH, melanocyte-stimulating hormone; GH, growth hormone; GHRH, growth hormone–releasing hormone; SRIF, somatostatin. On the left side of the figure, solid arrows (→) indicate stimulation and dashed arrows indicate inhibition. On the right side of the figure (under NREMS and REMS columns), the arrows indicate sleep effects; ↑ increase, ↓ decrease and – no effect on sleep. (Reprinted from Ref. 60.)

sleep, but higher doses did have an effect on sleep. Finally, an intriguing study by Fang and colleagues (26) found that TNF receptor knockout mice did not show any changes in sleep parameters following centrally administered TNF. Yet when these knockout mice were administered IL-1β, increases of NREM sleep were found. Together these data indicate an inherent redundancy in the cytokine network in which multiple cytokine pathways alter sleep.

From these studies, it might be concluded that proinflammatory cytokines induce NREM sleep whereas anti-inflammatory cytokines lead to decreases of NREM sleep, and that these actions would be readily translated to humans with similar conclusions. However, in healthy volunteers, peripheral administration of IL-6 4-hr before sleep onset produces a decrease in SWS in the first half of the night and an increase in in SWS the second half (27) of the night. Similarly, peripheral administration of low doses of IFN-α 4-hr before sleep onset also produces decreases in SWS in the first half of the night (28). In contrast, expression of the anti-inflammatory cytokine IL-10 prior to sleep correlates with the amount of delta sleep in the subsequent interval (29). Higher levels of IL-10 predicted greater amounts of delta sleep in the first half of the night (Fig. 3). Further studies in humans have also temporally evaluated the expression of IL-6 and TNF across the night in relation to sleep. Circulating levels of IL-6 in the middle of the night (03:00 hr) predict amounts of REM sleep in the second half of the night. Interestingly, REM sleep was not correlated with circulating levels of IL-6 upon awakening. Together these data in humans supported the

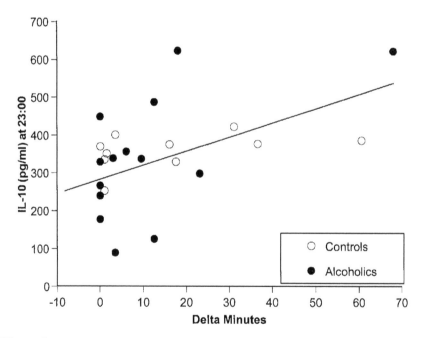

Figure 3   Relation between delta sleep (minutes) and concanavalin A–stimulated production of IL-10 by peripheral blood mononuclear cells at 23:00 hr in control (open circles, ○) and alcoholic (filled circles, ●) African-American subjects. In the total sample, expression of IL-10 at 23:00 hr was positively correlated with delta sleep amounts (Spearman ρ = 0.46, $p < 0.05$). (Reprinted from Ref. 29.)

notion that cytokines influence amounts of delta and REM sleep during the night. However, in humans it also appeared that the effects of proinflammatory and anti-inflammatory cytokines on sleep are divergent from basic studies; proinflammatory cytokine expression temporally predicted amounts of REM sleep, whereas anti-inflammatory cytokine expression predicted increases of delta sleep.

D. Fluctuations in the Immune System During Normal Sleep

Naturalistic studies have found that normal sleep is associated with changes in the distribution of immune cells in the periphery, in cytokine levels, and in the functional activity of immune cells. However, changes of immune parameters across the night are not necessarily driven by sleep, as circadian factors can also influence immunity. Thus, as discussed below, experimental strategies have used a combination of baseline and sleep deprivation nights to determine whether nocturnal changes in immune parameters are due to either sleep or circadian factors.

In regard to cellular trafficking, human studies have shown that the number of neutrophils, monocytes and lymphocytes (including T cells) in the periphery decreases throughout the night (30,31). However, this drop in cellular trafficking is abrogated during one night of total sleep deprivation (TSD), suggesting that changes in the distribution of cells are sleep related.

For NK cells, it is less clear if changes occur during sleep. One study reported no change in NK cell number across the night (30), but other studies have reported a nocturnal decrease in natural killer cells (31,32). For measures of the killing ability of NK cells, Kronfol and colleagues (30) reported a circadian rhythm such that natural killer cell activity peaked at noon and reached its nadir at midnight, staying low during the night. Redwine et al. (29) found increases of NK cell activity across the nocturnal period in normal volunteers but not in alcoholic subjects who had substantial disturbances of sleep with impairments in sleep continuity and loss of delta sleep.

Cytokines also show a diurnal rhythmicity that appears to be related to sleep. In rats, TNF peaks with sleep onset, decreases through the night, and reaches its nadir with sleep offset (33). Likewise in humans, circulating levels of IL-6 peak at night, following sleep onset. When sleep onset is delayed during early evening partial sleep deprivation (PSD), early evening increases of IL-6 are abrogated until the onset of sleep later in the night (34).

Ex vivo production of IL-2 is increased in association with sleep. During one night of TSD, nocturnal increases of IL-2 are abrogated (Fig. 4) (31). Petrovsky and Harrison (35) have also identified nocturnal increases in ex vivo production of IFN-γ and IL-10; as the night progressed, production of IFN-γ remained elevated, whereas IL-10 levels decreased. Similarly, the Th1/Th2 ratio (IFN-γ/IL-10) increased across the nocturnal period in normal volunteers but not in alcoholic subjects who had disordered sleep (Fig. 5) (29). Thus, in contrast with IL-6 and IL-2, which increase early following sleep onset, it appears that the

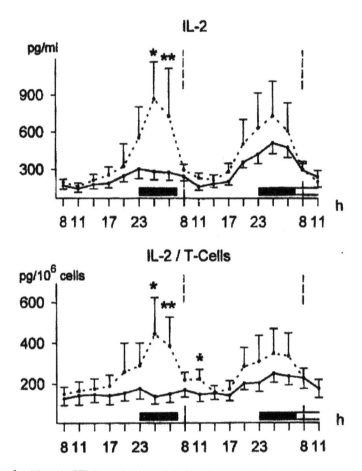

Figure 4 Mean (± SEM) production of IL-2 during two 51–hr sessions. One of the sessions included two regular wake-sleep cycles (dashed lines); the other included a night of sleep deprivation followed by a night of recovery sleep (solid lines). Top: Absolute production of IL-2 in whole-blood samples stimulated with phytohemagglutinin (PHA). Middle: Production of IL-2 per T cells stimulated with mitogen. Horizontal bars indicate time spent in bed between 23:00 and 07:00 hr (first night) and between 23:00 and 11:00 hr (second night); $n = 10$. Statistical analysis was performed on z-transformed values. **, $p < 0.01$; *, $p < 0.05$, for pairwise comparisons of the time courses during both sessions. (Reprinted from Ref. 31.)

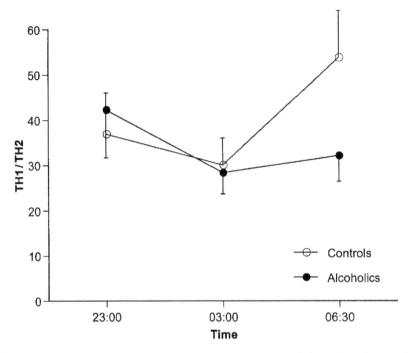

Figure 5 Concanavalin A–stimulated production of Th1 and Th2 cytokines by peripheral blood mononuclear cells in control (open circles, O) and alcoholic (filled circles, ●) African-American subjects. The ratio of the Th1 to Th2 was determined by dividing the Th1 cytokine interferon (IFN) by the Th2 cytokine IL-10. A significant group × time interaction was found ($F(2,42) = 4.1$, $p < 0.02$). The Th1/Th2 ratio increased from 03:00 hr to 06:30 hr ($p < 0.01$) in the controls, whereas the IFN/IL-10 ratio decreased from 23:00 h to 03:00 ($p < 0.05$) and remained low from 03:00 hr to 06:30 hr in the alcoholics. (Reprinted from Ref. 29.)

ratio of IFN-γ/IL-10 or the Th1/Th2 cytokine balance increases toward the latter part of the night, indicating a phasic shift toward more prominent Th1 activity with awakening.

III. Sleep Deprivation and Immunity

A. Total Sleep Deprivation Studies and Altered Immunologic Status

As described earlier, basic studies indicate that prolonged sleep deprivation lasting approximately 3 weeks results in a hypercatabolic state, increases of lethal bacteria in tissue and eventual death (14). Despite progressive increases of harmful bacteria, the immune system appears unable to mount a successful response.

Human TSD studies have followed much shorter time courses for obvious ethical reasons, and typically involved periods of wakefulness lasting greater than 24 hr but generally no longer than 96 hr (4 days) (36).

In terms of cellular trafficking, one of the earliest studies examining TSD and immunity was conducted by Palmblad and colleagues (37), in which eight women underwent 77 hr of TSD in conjunction with simulated battlefield noises. No significant changes in leukocyte counts during or following TSD were found, although this study confounded sleep deprivation with noxious auditory stimulation. In contrast, Dinges and colleagues (38) reported that 64 hr of TSD in 20 men and women produced progressive increases in white blood cells, granulocytes, and monocytes measured nightly, whereas T-helper cell numbers decreased and B cells showed no change. Interestingly, NK cell numbers decreased after 39 hr of sleep deprivation, but then increased as the sleep deprivation was maintained for 53 hr. Decreases of NK cell number using shorter periods of TSD (24 hr) were also found in two other studies (39,40). Finally, Born and colleagues (31) administered TSD to 10 healthy men with blood sampling every 3 hr during the day and night. Sleep deprivation abrogated the typical nocturnal decreases in monocytes, NK cells, lymphocytes, B cells, and T cells. Taken together, it appears that nocturnal decreases of immune numbers during a night of normal sleep are attenuated during one night of sleep deprivation. However, when sleep deprivation is continued beyond one night, increases in cellular trafficking are found.

Natural killer cell activity is also altered by sleep deprivation, and TSD is associated with increases of NK responses as the duration of sleep loss lengthens. For example, Dinges and colleagues have reported that NK cell activity is similar to baseline levels after 15 and 39 hr of sleep deprivation, whereas cytotoxic activity increases with 63 hours of sleep deprivation (Fig. 6) (38). A study by Matsumoto and colleagues (41) also found increased NK cell activity after 28 hr of wakefulness. However, as will be discussed in the subsequent section on partial sleep deprivation, as little as four hours of sleep loss is associated with decreased NK cell activity (Fig. 7) (42,43). Thus it appears that sleep deprivation has an impact on NK cells, the nature of which may depend on the duration of deprivation.

In terms of ex vivo cytokine production, TSD produces varying effects based on the cytokine measured, the duration of TSD, and the type of measurement strategy adopted (i.e., in vivo versus ex vivo). In the study by Palmblad and colleagues (37) involving 77-hr TSD in conjunction with battlefield noise, ex vivo IFN production was increased from baseline at 28 hr and 76 hr into TSD, and 5 days after sleep recovery. Moldofsky and colleagues (44) found that 40 hr of TSD in men produced elevations in IL-1 and IL-2 expression. However, both assays were actually indirect estimates of IL-1 and IL-2 activity, and assays were done on only half of the 10 subjects in the study due to technical problems. Nevertheless, Dinges and colleagues also found a trend for an increase in plasma levels of IL-1β at 39 hr, although IL-1β levels decreased at 15 hr after sleep recovery. In regard to IL-2, production of this cytokine by T cells increases during sleep, and this nocturnal

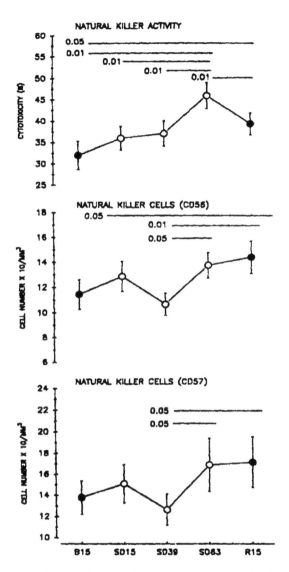

Figure 6 Means and standard errors of the means (SEM) for natural killer cell activity and counts of CD56 and CD57 cells from 20 healthy young adults. Measures were obtained immediately at 22:00 hr on each of five consecutive days: predeprivation baseline day after 15 hr awake (B15), first day of sleep deprivation after 15 hr awake (SD15), second day of sleep deprivation after 39 hr awake (SD39), third day of sleep deprivation after 63 hr awake (SD63) and the first day after recovery sleep after 15 hr awake (R15). Data from days on which sleep was deprived are designated by open circles. Horizontal lines show the results of critical difference comparisons (Newman-Keul tests) carried out among means for those variables in which a statistically significant F ratio was obtained from analyses of variance across days. Means that differ significantly have a horizontal line in common, with the significance level of the difference shown at the left end of the line. (Reprinted from Ref. 38.)

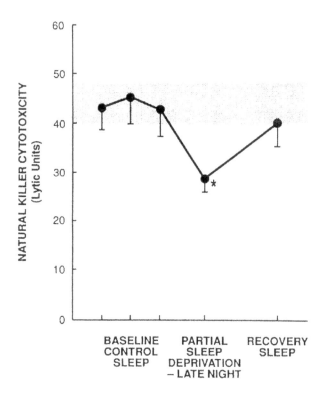

Figure 7 Effects of partial sleep deprivation (from 3 A.M. to 7 A.M.) on natural killer cell activity (mean ± standard error of the mean lytic units) in 23 healthy men. A repeated-measures analysis of variance demonstrated a significant time effect ($F(4, 88) = 3.6$; $p = .01$) in which the values of natural killer cell activity after partial sleep deprivation were significantly ($p < 0.05$) lower than values after control baseline and recovery nights. The stippled area displays the mean ± standard error of the mean of the three control baseline values. (Reprinted from Ref. 42.)

increase fails to occur during a night of sleep deprivation (31). Partial sleep deprivation is also associated with declines of IL-2 production, although partial night sleep loss is not associated with changes in circulating levels of IL-2 (43,45). In summary, these data suggest an initial increase of circulating levels and stimulated expression of IL-1 during sleep deprivation. In contrast, sleep deprivation is associated with decreases of IL-2 production (31), although there are inconsistent findings when the duration of sleep loss is sustained (36,44).

For IL-6, sleep deprivation may influence circulating levels at night with effects that persist into the daytime. For example, Vgontzas and colleagues found that in eight healthy men, a 40-hour TSD protocol produced significant elevations in daytime levels of IL-6 (Fig. 8) (46). This finding was corroborated in an 88-hr TSD study with 19 healthy men and women in which circulating levels of IL-6 were elevated during TSD (47). Findings from partial sleep deprivation studies indicate that during sleep IL-6 levels increase in the hour after sleep onset and that partial sleep deprivation abrogates this increase (Fig. 9) (34). Thus, sleep loss of only a few hours has been shown to block typical nocturnal increases in IL-6; longer lasting sleep loss may produce increases in circulating IL- 6. However, Dinges and colleagues (36) did not find any changes in nocturnal levels of IL-6 during or following TSD.

These contrasting results in regards to sleep deprivation and IL-6 highlight a number of methodological issues related to timing and frequency of blood draws as well as to how the cytokine was assayed (e.g., ex vivo stimulated expression versus in vivo circulating concentrations) that might impact any conclusions. For example, without frequent blood sampling, it may not be possible to accu-

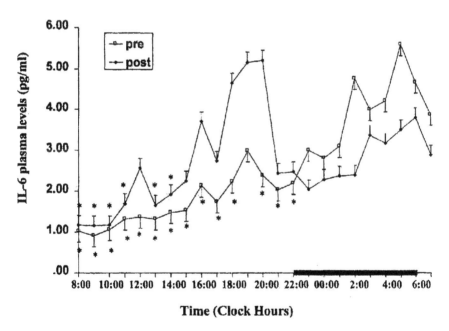

Figure 8 Twenty-four-hour plasma IL-6 concentrations before and after sleep deprivation in eight healthy young men. Each data point represents the mean ± standard error of the mean. *, $P < 0.05$ indicates statistical significance from the peak value within 24 hr for each condition (MANOVA followed by Dunnett post hoc test). The darkened area indicates the sleep recording period. (Reprinted from Ref. 46.)

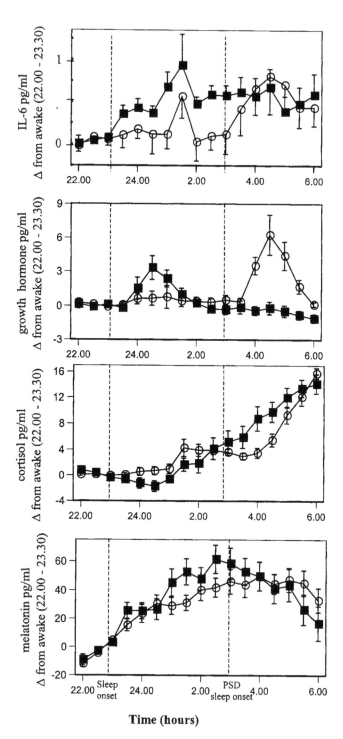

rately discern the effects of sleep deprivation on cytokine expression. Dinges and colleagues (36) obtained single blood samples for the assay of IL-6 at 22:00 hr each night, whereas Vgontzas sampled blood every hour (Fig. 8) (46). Both studies found that nocturnal levels of IL-6 at 22:00 hr were similar during baseline and TSD. However, the conclusions of Vgontzas and colleagues about the effects of TSD on IL-6 differed from those of Dinges and colleagues because the frequent sampling of IL-6 identified daytime increases of IL-6 between 17:00 and 20:00 hr during TSD as compared to baseline. Thus, repeated measures provide a more refined evaluation of the effects of TSD on the cytokine secretory profile.

Another important methodological issue relates to cytokine measurement strategies such as in vivo levels versus ex vivo production. In vivo measurement reflects ambient levels of cytokine in peripheral blood, whereas ex vivo measurement reflects production of cytokine in whole blood or peripheral mononuclear blood cells (PMBCs) when incubated with a particular antigen, such as lipopolysaccharide. As such, the measures provide different information about cytokine expression. In general, it is advantageous to use both measurement strategies; however, for particular cytokines, in vivo measurement is difficult. For example, IL-2 is rapidly degraded so that measurement of in vivo levels is unlikely to be as useful as measurement of ex vivo stimulated production.

In summary, human TSD studies have demonstrated that sleep deprivation has acute effects on cellular trafficking, functional measures, and the cytokine network. Cellular trafficking, which typically decreases during sleep, tends to progressively increase during TSD, as does NK cell activity. For cytokines, the findings are less clear and seem to depend on the measurement strategy adopted and the timing and frequency of blood draws.

B. Partial Sleep Deprivation Studies: Cellular Immunity

Partial sleep deprivation studies provide an opportunity to examine the role of sleep deprivation on immunity in a way that more closely relates to sleep loss in clinical populations such as patients with primary insomnia, clinical depression,

---

Figure 9 Averaged change scores from awake (± SEM) for circulating levels of IL-6, growth hormone, cortisol, and melatonin in subjects during baseline (filled squares, ■) and PSD-E (partial sleep deprivation–experimental) nights (open circles, ○). The vertical dashed line at 23:00 hr indicates the average time that the subjects were asleep on the baseline night; the vertical dashed line at 03:00 hr indicates the time that the subjects were asleep on the PSD-E night. For IL-6, change in the early part of the night was elevated during the baselines—as compared to the PSD-E night ($t = 2.4$, $p < 0.05$). For growth hormone, late-night change scores were elevated in the PSD-E night as compared to baseline ($t = -3.9$, $p < 0.01$). For cortisol, late-night change scores were decreased in the PSD-E as compared to baseline ($t = 6.7$, $p < 0.001$). For melatonin, there were no differences between the PSD-E and baseline nights. (Reprinted from Ref. 34.)

and alcohol dependence (48). These clinical samples report symptoms of early or late insomnia, rather than sleep loss throughout an entire night.

Partial sleep deprivation has been found to produce significant reductions in cellular immunity, as measured by decreased NK cell number or activity, IL-2-stimulated cytotoxic activity, and stimulated production of IL-2 (42,43). The effects of partial sleep loss on NK cell responses appeared to be due to an impairment of NK cell function and not due to changes in the number of NK cells. Even after controlling for the decrease in NK cells, decreases of NK cell activity after partial sleep deprivation remained significant (43). Similarly, partial sleep deprivation alters the responsivity of NK cells to IL-2. In vitro stimulation of peripheral blood lymphocytes with IL-2 ordinarily produces prominent stimulation of NK cells, promoting differentiation, activation, and proliferation when incubated with cultured tumor cells. After partial sleep deprivation, there were prominent decreases in IL-2-stimulated cytotoxicity,—even after controlling for the number of cells expressing the NK cell phenotype and IL-2 receptor. Lastly, partial sleep deprivation led to decreased IL-2 production, which is primarily secreted by T cells and monocytes. This is consistent with the finding that TSD also abrogates the usual nocturnal increases in IL-2 production (31). Together, these findings extend previous investigations in humans on the immunological effects of prolonged or total night sleep deprivation and show that even a modest disruption in sleep produces an acute reduction of NK cell, T cell and monocyte function.

The clinical implications of reduced immune cell function such as NK cell activity are not known. Although NK cells mediate protection against primary herpes virus infections and compromised natural immunity may be a prognostic factor for recurrence in patients with malignant disease (49), it remains unclear whether decreases of NK cell activity and IL-2 production as measured from peripheral blood samples represent declines of host defense mechanisms. In rats, Dhabhar and McEwen (50) reported that acute stress produced decreased NK cell activity in the peripheral blood, but promoted a redistribution of NK cells to other tissue compartments where NK cell activity was increased. Secondly in contrast to partial sleep deprivation, TSD increased NK cell activity as the duration of sleep deprivation lengthened (38). Finally, after administration of partial sleep deprivation, NK cell activity levels returned to normal baseline levels with recovery sleep (42,43), suggesting only a transient change of immune system function with partial sleep loss. Nevertheless, this period of immune decline may identify a period in which vulnerability to infectious challenge is increased.

The mechanisms by which this recovery in NK cell activity occurs is unclear, but it is possibly driven by interactions between SWS, IL-1, and IL-2. Endogenous IL-1 may play a role in driving the recovery of SWS following sleep loss; Opp and Krueger (25) found that administration of antibodies to IL-1 antagonizes rebound increases of SWS in animals following sleep deprivation. SWS also correlates with increased production of IL-2, which may ultimately stimulate activity of NK cells (51). In other words, we speculate that increases of SWS during recovery sleep induce increases of IL-2 production, which promotes greater NK cell activity.

C. Partial Sleep Deprivation Studies: Cytokines

Only a few studies have examined the effects of partial night sleep deprivation on cytokine expression, and these have primarily focused on IL-2 or IL-6. In regard to IL-2, Irwin and colleagues (45) found that circulating concentration of IL-2, measured in half-hour intervals, slightly increases in the first hour after sleep and quickly returns to waking levels as the night progresses. Partial sleep deprivation had no effect on circulating levels of IL-2 levels, and there was no association between sleep activity and change of circulating levels of IL-2 (45). The lack of a sleep deprivation effect on circulating levels of IL-2 is consistent with the effects of 64-hr TSD (38).

These observations with circulating levels of IL-2 contrast with studies that have measured ex vivo production of IL-2. As noted above, sleep is associated with increased production of IL-2 and sleep deprivation abrogates this increase (31,44,51). This disparity between measurements of circulating levels versus stimulated production may be due to the rapid utilization and/or degradation of circulating levels of IL-2 and the fact that circulating IL-2 is rapidly bound to soluble IL-2 receptors for uptake. Thus, circulating levels of IL-2 may not reliably demonstrate sleep-related alterations in the patterns of expression and release of this cytokine.

Circulating levels of IL-6, in contrast to IL-2, are readily detected, and this cytokine is thought to exhibit potent systemic effects (52). IL-6 levels in peripheral blood are related to sleep, circadian rhythms, and daytime fatigue. IL-6 shows a circadian rhythm such that concentrations are low during daytime and increase during the night (53). In patients with sleep disturbance, the diurnal secretory profile of circulating concentrations of TNF and IL-6 are altered (46,54), suggesting that circadian variations of IL-6 are related to sleep.

Indeed in a recent study that addresses the relationship between sleep and IL-6, IL-6 showed a nocturnal maxima only after sleep onset (Fig. 9) (34). In this study, 31 healthy men had nocturnal blood sampling every 30 min. In addition to IL-6, melatonin, cortisol and growth hormone were also measured. Growth hormone is thought to be sleep-dependent (55,56), whereas cortisol and melatonin show a stronger circadian influence (57,58). Change scores were calculated for each time point in relation to awake levels and were used to evaluate the effects of sleep and sleep deprivation on IL-6, growth hormone, cortisol, and melatonin levels. Redwine and colleagues (34) found that IL-6 had a nocturnal profile similar to the sleep-dependent hormone, growth hormone. Following sleep onset, levels of IL-6 increased with peak values occurring 2.5 hr after sleep onset. However, during a partial sleep deprivation condition, the nocturnal increase of IL-6 did not occur until after sleep onset at 03:00 hr. Sleep deprivation did not influence the nocturnal secretion of cortisol or melatonin, which taken together suggest that sleep, rather than a circadian pacemaker, influences nocturnal IL-6 and growth hormone secretion (34). A sleep-induced increase of IL-6 is in contrast to findings by Born and colleagues (31), who found that IL-6 concentrations were flat during sleep and during sleep deprivation. However, blood sampling was limited to 3-hr intervals. Thus, the frequency of blood sampling may not have been adequate to ascertain nocturnal increases in IL-6 during normal sleep or the effects of sleep deprivation on this cytokine.

Redwine and colleagues (34) also compared levels of IL-6 between sleep stages. Circulating concentrations of IL-6 was higher during stages 1–2 sleep and REM sleep as compared to levels during the awake period. Levels of IL-6 were similar between the awake period and stages 3–4 sleep. These findings are consistent with studies that have found a negative correlation between SWS and IL-6 release (46). In sleep deprivation studies, sleep recovery nights are usually associated with increases in SWS; during recovery night, Vgontzas and colleagues found lower levels of IL-6 (46).

Sleep deprivation studies suggest that sleep loss may be a possible pathway by which individuals experiencing psychological stress or psychiatric conditions show signs of immune system dysregulation (27,59). Furthermore, because a number of studies in both basic and human research have found that cytokines have effects on sleep depth (27,46,60), disturbances of sleep architecture may lead to abnormalities in the sleep-related secretion of cytokines, most notably the systemic cytokine IL-6. In clinical conditions such as alcohol dependence and depression where there is a relative increase of REM sleep at the expense of SWS (59), it is possible that abnormal increases of IL-6 occur during sleep with implications for inflammatory and cardiovascular disease risk in these populations (61,62). Sleep deprivation studies have primarily studied healthy subjects. The next step in the study of sleep-immune relationships is to extend these findings to clinical populations.

IV. Sleep Loss and Immunity: Clinical Samples

Extension of findings relating sleep disruption and immunity to clinical populations is limited. Our goal in this next part of the chapter is to discuss sleep deficits and immune function in four distinct populations. In particular, the senior author (Irwin) has conducted a number of partial sleep deprivation studies with alcohol-dependent subjects. We offer this paradigm as a model to study sleep disruption in other populations with immune dysregulation (e.g., depression), immunodeficiency [e.g., human immunodeficiency virus (HIV)], and autoimmune disorders (e.g., rheumatoid arthritis).

A. Disturbed Sleep and Immune Dysregulation in Alcohol-Dependent Subjects

Disturbed sleep in alcohol-dependent subjects is characterized by severe loss of sleep continuity and depth that can last for months and years after abstinence.

These individuals show a marked loss of SWS. In addition, immune function may be impaired as well; alcoholics are at increased risk for a number of infectious illnesses including HIV, tuberculosis, and hepatitis C. The risk is especially increased in African-American alcoholics (63).

In a recent study, African-American ethnicity and alcohol dependence were associated with more profound losses of delta sleep as measured by polysomnographic and spectral sleep analyses than those found in European-American alcoholics (64). African-American alcoholics also had significantly lower levels of NK cell activity and IL-2-stimulated NK cell activity than the other three groups (63). Production of the proinflammatory cytokine IL-6 was significantly lower in the African-American alcoholics than in the other three groups. In contrast, IL-10 was significantly increased in the African-American alcoholics as compared with controls and European-American alcoholics. The increased IL-10 and the decreased IL-6 suggested an alteration in the ratio of Th1 to Th2 cytokines. Dysregulation in these cytokines may have an effect on an individual's susceptibility to infectious conditions such as hepatitis C (65). Chronic infection with this virus is common in alcoholics; furthermore, its chronicity is related to a lack of Th1 cytokine production and/or an increase of Th2 cytokine release. For example, Woitas and colleagues (66) found that hepatitis C–seropositive blood donors without viremia showed increased Th1 cytokine production (IFN, IL-2) in response to hepatitis C core protein, whereas seropositive donors with viremia show increases in IL-10 producing T cells. Thus, alcoholics, and African-American alcoholics in particular, appeared to exhibit profound deficits in SWS in conjunction with a shift to a Th2 cytokine profile. It would be of interest to determine if clinical management of sleep difficulties would influence immunity in this population.

B. Disturbed Sleep and Immune Dysregulation in Clinically Depressed Subjects

As many as 90% of clinically depressed individuals report sleep complaints typically involving difficulty falling asleep, frequent waking during the night, and early morning waking (67). In addition, depressed individuals also show reductions in lymphocyte responses and NK cell activity (68,69) as well as elevated levels of plasma IL-6 and soluble IL-6 receptor (70,71).

In depressed patients, NK cell activity has been found to be negatively correlated with severity of insomnia symptoms ($r = -0.33$, $p < 0.05$) but not with other depressive symptoms. In addition, polysomnographic sleep assessment is also related to NK cell activity. In depressed patients, total sleep time, sleep efficiency, and duration of NREM sleep positively correlate with lytic activity such that individuals with lower amounts of electroencephalographic sleep and sleep continuity also show lower NK cell activity (72). However, whether cytokines or other peptides with sleep-immune effects are altered in depressed patients to produce coincident changes of sleep and NK cell activity remains to be elucidated.

C. Disturbed Sleep in Populations with Immunodeficiency

HIV infection is a progressive condition in which there are marked decrements in cellular immunity, leading to a greatly increased susceptibility to a number of opportunistic infections. In addition, TNF levels as well as ex vivo production of TNF are elevated in HIV-seropositive individuals (73). Fatigue and sleep complaints are common in HIV (74), and HIV patients only sleep an average of 6.5 hr/night (75). Moreover, in patients with advanced HIV infection, there are marked declines in the amount of SWS as compared with control subjects (76). It is of interest that these studies also showed a significant correlation between TNF levels and electroencephalographic delta frequency amplitude in controls, whereas in individuals with advanced HIV infection this relationship between TNF and electroencephalographic delta sleep was not found, leading the authors to suggest that there may be an uncoupling of sleep-cytokine interactions in advanced HIV infection (76).

Recent work using an animal model has indicated that chemokines, a select class of cytokines involved in inflammation and chemotaxis of immune cells, also have somnogenic effects (77). At least 10 different chemokines, such as CCR3, CCR5, and CXCR4, also behave as coreceptors for HIV, and additional studies are needed to determine if HIV-related immunological disruptions, specifically in the cytokine/chemokine network, have effects on sleep disruption and fatigue.

D. Sleep and Autoimmune Disorders

Rheumatoid arthritis (RA) is a chronic autoimmune condition in which proinflammatory cytokines play a major role in disease activity (78). TNF, IL-1, and IL-6 have been suggested as pivotal in the etiologic progression and pathogenesis of rheumatoid arthritis (79). IL-1 and TNF have been associated with destruction of cartilage and bone (80), and plasma levels of IL-6 and TNF predict disease activity (52). Treatment with a TNF receptor antagonist is associated with slower disease progression (81).

More than half of RA patients report abnormal sleep (82) in addition to the traditional symptoms associated with rheumatoid arthritis, such as morning stiffness, pain, functional debility, and fatigue (83). Importantly, disordered sleep in RA patients is not solely due to pain. Although pain has been offered as a causative agent in disrupting sleep in this population, abnormalities of polysomnographic recordings are independent of nocturnal pain (84). The mechanisms that account for disordered sleep in this clinical population are not known. Specifically, it is not known whether disordered sleep in rheumatoid arthritis contributes to overexpression of proinflammatory cytokines. Despite the prevalence of sleep complaints, few studies have examined objective measures of sleep in RA patients (84), and no study has integrated objective measures of sleep with measures of proinflammatory cytokines. Since cytokines are intimately involved in disease pathogenesis in RA and because studies in healthy individuals indicate proinflammatory cytokines influence daytime fatigue, studies examining interactions between sleep disruption and cytokines in this population could help determine the impact of sleep and cytokines on prominent RA symptoms, such as fatigue and morning stiffness.

V. Conclusions

Sleep is vital to healthy functioning and prolonged sleep deprivation is associated with severe morbidity and death (14). The sleep loss and dysregulation are prominent problems in a number of medical conditions, and insomnia is a predictor of cardiovascular and inflammatory disease mortality (5,6). The mechanisms by which disordered sleep impacts overall health are likely multifactorial. It appears that sleep loss affects host defense by impacting susceptibility to viral and bacterial pathogens (14), and these impairments may be mediated via the immune system. Sleep and the immune system appear to have a bidirectional relationship. Cytokines such as IL-1 and TNF can be somnogenic, influencing amounts of NREM sleep (60). In addition, sleep can affect the cytokine network; it produces increased IL-6 secretion (34) and IL-2 production (44,45), and these increases are blunted during sleep deprivation. Sleep deprivation studies provide an experimental manipulation of sleep/wakefulness and thus provide an opportunity to study dynamic fluctuations in the immune system as a function of sleep and/or circadian factors. In addition, extension of the paradigm from healthy subjects to clinical populations may provide valuable information regarding how sleep loss and disruption can impact disease processes.

References

1. Johnson, E.O., Breslau, N., Roth, T., Roehrs, T., and Rosenthal, L., Psychometric evaluation of daytime sleepiness and nocturnal sleep onset scales in a representative community sample. Biol Psychiatry, 1999. 45(6): p. 764–770.
2. Ohayon, M., Epidemiological study on insomnia in the general population Sleep, 1996. 19(3 Suppl): p. S7–S15.
3. Foley, D.J., Monjan, A.A., Brown, S.L., Simonsick, E.M., Wallace, R.B., and Blazer, D.G., Sleep complaints among elderly persons: an epidemiologic study of three communities Sleep, 1995. 18(6): p. 425–432.
4. Benca, R.M., Obermeyer, W.H., Thisted, R.A., and Gillin, J.C., Sleep and psychiatric disorders. A meta-analysis Arch Gen Psychiatry, 1992. 49(8): p. 651–668; discussion 669–670.
5. Bloom, B.J., Owens, J.A., McGuinn, M., Nobile, C., Schaeffer, L., and Alario, A.J., Sleep and its relationship to pain, dysfunction, and disease activity in juvenile rheumatoid arthritis J Rheumatol, 2002. 29(1): p. 169–173.
6. Mallon, L., Broman, J.E., and Hetta, J., Sleep complaints predict coronary artery disease mortality in males: a 12–year follow-up study of a middle-aged Swedish population J Intern Med, 2002. 251(3): p. 207–216.
7. Jordan, S., C. and Fredrich, R., *Cytokines and lymphocytes*, in *Cytokines in Health and Diseae*, J.S.F. Daniel G. Remick, Editor. 1997, Marcel Dekker: New York. p. xx, 678.

8. Mosmann, T.R. and Coffman, R.L., TH1 and TH2 cells: different patterns of lymphokine secretion lead to different functional properties Annu Rev Immunol, 1989. 7: p. 145–173.

9. Watkins, L.R., Maier, S.F., and Goehler, L.E., Cytokine-to-brain communication: a review and analysis of alternative mechanisms Life Sci, 1995. 57(11): p. 1011–1026.

10. Krueger, J.M. and Majde, J.A., Microbial products and cytokines in sleep and fever regulation Crit Rev Immunol, 1994. 14(3–4): p. 355–379.

11. Trachsel, L., Schreiber, W., Holsboer, F., and Pollmacher, T., Endotoxin enhances EEG alpha and beta power in human sleep Sleep, 1994. 17(2): p. 132–139.

12. Pollmacher, T., Schreiber, W., Gudewill, S., Vedder, H., Fassbender, K., Wiedemann, K., Trachsel, L., Galanos, C., and Holsboer, F., Influence of endotoxin on nocturnal sleep in humans Am J Physiol, 1993. 264(6 Pt 2): p. R1077–R1083.

13. Everson, C.A., Sustained sleep deprivation impairs host defense Am J Physiol, 1993. 265(5 Pt 2): p. R1148–R1154.

14. Everson, C.A. and Toth, L.A., Systemic bacterial invasion induced by sleep deprivation Am J Physiol Regul Integr Comp Physiol, 2000. 278(4): p. R905–R916.

15. Benca, R.M., Kushida, C.A., Everson, C.A., Kalski, R., Bergmann, B.M., and Rechtschaffen, A., Sleep deprivation in the rat: VII. Immune function Sleep, 1989. 12(1): p. 47–52.

16. Toth, L.A., Tolley, E.A., and Krueger, J.M., Sleep as a prognostic indicator during infectious disease in rabbits Proc Soc Exp Biol Med, 1993. 203(2): p. 179–192.

17. Brown, R., Pang, G., Husband, A.J., and King, M.G., Suppression of immunity to influenza virus infection in the respiratory tract following sleep disturbance Reg Immunol, 1989. 2(5): p. 321–325.

18. Hermann, D.M., Mullington, J., Hinze-Selch, D., Schreiber, W., Galanos, C., and Pollmacher, T., Endotoxin-induced changes in sleep and sleepiness during the day Psychoneuroendocrinology, 1998. 23(5): p. 427–437.

19. Haack, M., Schuld, A., Kraus, T., and Pollmacher, T., Effects of sleep on endotoxin-induced host responses in healthy men Psychosom Med, 2001. 63(4): p. 568–578.

20. Opp, M.R. and Krueger, J.M., Interleukin 1–receptor antagonist blocks interleukin 1–induced sleep and fever Am J Physiol, 1991. 260(2 Pt 2): p. R453–R457.

21. Takahashi, S., Kapas, L., Fang, J., and Krueger, J.M., Somnogenic relationships between tumor necrosis factor and interleukin-1 Am J Physiol, 1999. 276(4 Pt 2): p. R1132–R1140.

22. Takahashi, S., Kapas, L., and Krueger, J.M., A tumor necrosis factor (TNF) receptor fragment attenuates TNF-alpha- and muramyl dipeptide-induced sleep and fever in rabbits J Sleep Res, 1996. 5(2): p. 106–114.

23. Bauer, J., Hohagen, F., Gimmel, E., Bruns, F., Lis, S., Krieger, S., Ambach, W., Guthmann, A., Grunze, H., Fritsch-Montero, R., and et al., Induction of cytokine synthesis and fever suppresses REM sleep and improves mood in patients with major depression Biol Psychiatry, 1995. 38(9): p. 611–621.

24. Opp, M.R., Smith, E.M., and Hughes, T.K., Jr., Interleukin-10 (cytokine synthesis inhibitory factor) acts in the central nervous system of rats to reduce sleep J Neuroimmunol, 1995. 60(1–2): p. 165–168.

25. Opp, M.R. and Krueger, J.M., Anti-interleukin-1 beta reduces sleep and sleep rebound after sleep deprivation in rats Am J Physiol, 1994. 266(3 Pt 2): p. R688–R695.

26. Fang, J., Wang, Y., and Krueger, J.M., Mice lacking the TNF 55 kDa receptor fail to sleep more after TNFalpha treatment J Neurosci, 1997. 17(15): p. 5949–5955.

27. Spath-Schwalbe, E., Hansen, K., Schmidt, F., Schrezenmeier, H., Marshall, L., Burger, K., Fehm, H.L., and Born, J., Acute effects of recombinant human interleukin-6 on endocrine and central nervous sleep functions in healthy men J Clin Endocrinol Metab, 1998. 83(5): p. 1573–1579.

28. Spath-Schwalbe, E., Lange, T., Perras, B., Fehm, H.L., and Born, J., Interferon-alpha acutely impairs sleep in healthy humans Cytokine, 2000. 12(5): p. 518–521.

29. Redwine, L., Dang, J., Hall, M., and Irwin, M., Disordered sleep, nocturnal cytokines and immunity in alcoholics Psychosom Med, in press.

30. Kronfol, Z., Nair, M., Zhang, Q., Hill, E.E., and Brown, M.B., Circadian immune measures in healthy volunteers: relationship to hypothalamic-pituitary-adrenal axis hormones and sympathetic neurotransmitters Psychosom Med, 1997. 59(1): p. 42–50.

31. Born, J., Lange, T., Hansen, K., Molle, M., and Fehm, H.L., Effects of sleep and circadian rhythm on human circulating immune cells J Immunol, 1997. 158(9): p. 4454–4464.

32. Bourin, P., Mansour, I., Doinel, C., Roue, R., Rouger, P., and Levi, F., Circadian rhythms of circulating NK cells in healthy and human immunodeficiency virus–infected men Chronobiol Int, 1993. 10(4): p. 298–305.

33. Floyd, R.A. and Krueger, J.M., Diurnal variation of TNF alpha in the rat brain Neuroreport, 1997. 8(4): p. 915–918.

34. Redwine, L., Hauger, R.L., Gillin, J.C., and Irwin, M., Effects of sleep and sleep deprivation on interleukin-6, growth hormone, cortisol, and melatonin levels in humans J Clin Endocrinol Metab, 2000. 85(10): p. 3597–3603.

35. Petrovsky, N. and Harrison, L.C., Diurnal rhythmicity of human cytokine production: a dynamic disequilibrium in T helper cell type 1/T helper cell type 2 balance? J Immunol, 1997. 158(11): p. 5163–5168.

36. Dinges, D.F., Douglas, S.D., Hamarman, S., Zaugg, L., and Kapoor, S., Sleep deprivation and human immune function Adv Neuroimmunol, 1995. 5(2): p. 97–110.

37. Palmblad, J., Cantell, K., Strander, H., Froberg, J., Karlsson, C.G., Levi, L., Granstrom, M., and Unger, P., Stressor exposure and immunological response in man: interferon-producing capacity and phagocytosis J Psychosom Res, 1976. 20(3): p. 193–199.

38. Dinges, D.F., Douglas, S.D., Zaugg, L., Campbell, D.E., McMann, J.M., Whitehouse, W.G., Orne, E.C., Kapoor, S.C., Icaza, E., and Orne, M.T., Leukocytosis and natural killer cell function parallel neurobehavioral fatigue induced by 64 hours of sleep deprivation J Clin Invest, 1994. 93(5): p. 1930–1939.

39. Ozturk, L., Pelin, Z., Karadeniz, D., Kaynak, H., Cakar, L., and Gozukirmizi, E., Effects of 48 hours sleep deprivation on human immune profile Sleep Res Online, 1999. 2(4): p. 107–111.

40. Heiser, P., Dickhaus, B., Schreiber, W., Clement, H.W., Hasse, C., Hennig, J., Remschmidt, H., Krieg, J.C., Wesemann, W., and Opper, C., White blood cells and cortisol after sleep deprivation and recovery sleep in humans Eur Arch Psychiatry Clin Neurosci, 2000. 250(1): p. 16–23.

41. Matsumoto, Y., Mishima, K., Satoh, K., Tozawa, T., Mishima, Y., Shimizu, T., and Hishikawa, Y., Total sleep deprivation induces an acute and transient increase in NK cell activity in healthy young volunteers Sleep, 2001. 24(7): p. 804–809.

42. Irwin, M., Mascovich, A., Gillin, J.C., Willoughby, R., Pike, J., and Smith, T.L., Partial sleep deprivation reduces natural killer cell activity in humans Psychosom Med, 1994. 56(6): p. 493–498.

43. Irwin, M., McClintick, J., Costlow, C., Fortner, M., White, J., and Gillin, J.C., Partial night sleep deprivation reduces natural killer and cellular immune responses in humans FASEB J, 1996. 10(5): p. 643–653.

44. Moldofsky, H., Lue, F.A., Davidson, J.R., and Gorczynski, R., Effects of sleep deprivation on human immune functions FASEB J, 1989. 3(8): p. 1972–1977.

45. Irwin, M., Thompson, J., Miller, C., Gillin, J.C., and Ziegler, M., Effects of sleep and sleep deprivation on catecholamine and interleukin-2 levels in humans: clinical implications J Clin Endocrinol Metab, 1999. 84(6): p. 1979–1985.

46. Vgontzas, A.N., Papanicolaou, D.A., Bixler, E.O., Lotsikas, A., Zachman, K., Kales, A., Prolo, P., Wong, M.L., Licinio, J., Gold, P.W., Hermida, R.C., Mastorakos, G., and Chrousos, G.P., Circadian interleukin-6 secretion and quantity and depth of sleep J Clin Endocrinol Metab, 1999. 84(8): p. 2603–2607.

47. Shearer, W.T., Reuben, J.M., Mullington, J.M., Price, N.J., Lee, B.N., Smith, E.O., Szuba, M.P., Van Dongen, H.P., and Dinges, D.F., Soluble TNF-alpha receptor 1 and IL-6 plasma levels in humans subjected to the sleep deprivation model of spaceflight J Allergy Clin Immunol, 2001. 107(1): p. 165–170.

48. Irwin, M., Effects of sleep and sleep loss on immunity and cytokines Brain Behav Immun, 2002. 16(5): p. 503–512.

49. Trinchieri, G., Biology of natural killer cells Adv Immunol, 1989. 47: p. 187–376.

50. Dhabhar, F.S., Miller, A.H., McEwen, B.S., and Spencer, R.L., Stress-induced changes in blood leukocyte distribution. Role of adrenal steroid hormones J Immunol, 1996. 157(4): p. 1638–1644.

51. Moldofsky, H., Lue, F.A., Eisen, J., Keystone, E., and Gorczynski, R.M., The relationship of interleukin-1 and immune functions to sleep in humans Psychosom Med, 1986. 48(5): p. 309–318.

52. Isomaki, P. and Punnonen, J., Pro- and anti-inflammatory cytokines in rheumatoid arthritis Ann Med, 1997. 29(6): p. 499–507.

53. Bauer, J., Hohagen, F., Ebert, T., Timmer, J., Ganter, U., Krieger, S., Lis, S., Postler, E., Voderholzer, U., and Berger, M., Interleukin-6 serum levels in healthy persons correspond to the sleep-wake cycle Clin Invest, 1994. 72(4): p. 315.

54. Vgontzas, A.N., Papanicolaou, D.A., Bixler, E.O., Kales, A., Tyson, K., and Chrousos, G.P., Elevation of plasma cytokines in disorders of excessive daytime sleepiness: role of sleep disturbance and obesity J Clin Endocrinol Metab, 1997. 82(5): p. 1313–1316.

55. Perras, B., Marshall, L., Kohler, G., Born, J., and Fehm, H.L., Sleep and endocrine changes after intranasal administration of growth hormone–releasing hormone in young and aged humans Psychoneuroendocrinology, 1999. 24(7): p. 743–757.

56. Jarrett, D.B., Greenhouse, J.B., Miewald, J.M., Fedorka, I.B., and Kupfer, D.J., A reexamination of the relationship between growth hormone secretion and slow wave sleep using delta wave analysis Biol Psychiatry, 1990. 27(5): p. 497–509.

57. Youngstedt, S.D., Kripke, D.F., and Elliott, J.A., Melatonin excretion is not related to sleep in the elderly J Pineal Res, 1998. 24(3): p. 142–145.

58. Gronfier, C., Chapotot, F., Weibel, L., Jouny, C., Piquard, F., and Brandenberger, G., Pulsatile cortisol secretion and EEG delta waves are controlled by two independent but synchronized generators Am J Physiol, 1998. 275(1 Pt 1): p. E94–E100.

59. Benca, R.M., Obermeyer, W.H., Thisted, R.A., and Gillin, J.C., Sleep and psychiatric disorders: a meta analysis Arch Gen Psychiatry, 1992. 49: p. 651–668.

60. Krueger, J.M. and Toth, L.A., Cytokines as regulators of sleep Ann N Y Acad Sci, 1994. 739: p. 299–310.
61. Musselman, D.L., Evans, D.L., and Nemeroff, C.B., The relationship of depression to cardiovascular disease: epidemiology, biology, and treatment Arch Gen Psychiatry, 1998. 55(7): p. 580–592.
62. Papanicolaou, D.A., Wilder, R.L., Manolagas, S.C., and Chrousos, G.P., The pathophysiologic roles of interleukin-6 in human disease Ann Intern Med, 1998. 128(2): p. 127–137.
63. Irwin, M. and Miller, C., Decreased natural killer cell responses and altered interleukin-6 and interleukin-10 production in alcoholism: an interaction between alcohol dependence and African-American ethnicity Alcohol Clin Exp Res, 2000. 24(4): p. 560–569.
64. Irwin, M., Miller, C., Gillin, J.C., Demodena, A., and Ehlers, C.L., Polysomnographic and spectral sleep EEG in primary alcoholics: an interaction between alcohol dependence and African-American ethnicity Alcohol Clin Exp Res, 2000. 24(9): p. 1376–1384.
65. Mendenhall, C.L., Moritz, T., Rouster, S., Roselle, G., Polito, A., Quan, S., and DiNelle, R.K., Epidemiology of hepatitis C among veterans with alcoholic liver disease. The VA Cooperative Study Group 275 Am J Gastroenterol, 1993. 88(7): p. 1022–1026.
66. Woitas, R.P., Lechmann, M., Jung, G., Kaiser, R., Sauerbruch, T., and Spengler, U., CD30 induction and cytokine profiles in hepatitis C virus core-specific peripheral blood T lymphocytes J Immunol, 1997. 159(2): p. 1012–1018.
67. Riemann, D., Berger, M., and Voderholzer, U., Sleep and depression—results from psychobiological studies: an overview Biol Psychol, 2001. 57(1–3): p. 67–103.
68. Irwin, M., Immune correlates of depression Adv Exp Med Biol, 1999. 461: p. 1–24.
69. Irwin, M., Brown, M., Patterson, T., Hauger, R., Mascovich, A., and Grant, I., Neuropeptide Y and natural killer cell activity: findings in depression and Alzheimer caregiver stress FASEB J, 1991. 5(15): p. 3100–3107.
70. Musselman, D.L., Miller, A.H., Porter, M.R., Manatunga, A., Gao, F., Penna, S., Pearce, B.D., Landry, J., Glover, S., McDaniel, J.S., and Nemeroff, C.B., Higher than normal plasma interleukin-6 concentrations in cancer patients with depression: preliminary findings Am J Psychiatry, 2001. 158(8): p. 1252–1257.
71. Sluzewska, A., Rybakowski, J., Bosmans, E., Sobieska, M., Berghmans, R., Maes, M., and Wiktorowicz, K., Indicators of immune activation in major depression Psychiatry Res, 1996. 64(3): p. 161–167.
72. Irwin, M., Smith, T.L., and Gillin, J.C., Electroencephalographic sleep and natural killer activity in depressed patients and control subjects Psychosom Med, 1992. 54(1): p. 10–21.
73. Lau, A.S. and Livesey, J.F., Endotoxin induction of tumor necrosis factor is enhanced by acid-labile interferon-alpha in acquired immunodeficiency syndrome J Clin Invest, 1989. 84(3): p. 738–743.
74. Darko, D.F., McCutchan, J.A., Kripke, D.F., Gillin, J.C., and Golshan, S., Fatigue, sleep disturbance, disability, and indices of progression of HIV infection Am J Psychiatry, 1992. 149(4): p. 514–520.
75. Lee, K.A., Portillo, C.J., and Miramontes, H., The influence of sleep and activity patterns on fatigue in women with HIV/AIDS J Assoc Nurses AIDS Care, 2001. 12 Suppl: p. 19–27.

76. Darko, D.F., Miller, J.C., Gallen, C., White, J., Koziol, J., Brown, S.J., Hayduk, R., Atkinson, J.H., Assmus, J., Munnell, D.T., and et al., Sleep electroencephalogram delta-frequency amplitude, night plasma levels of tumor necrosis factor alpha, and human immunodeficiency virus infection Proc Natl Acad Sci U S A, 1995. 92(26): p. 12080–12084.

77. Hogan, D., Hutton, L.A., Smith, E.M., and Opp, M.R., Beta (CC)-chemokines as modulators of sleep: implications for HIV-induced alterations in arousal state J Neuroimmunol, 2001. 119(2): p. 317–326.

78. Feldmann, M. and Maini, R.N., The role of cytokines in the pathogenesis of rheumatoid arthritis Rheumatology (Oxford), 1999. 38 Suppl 2: p. 3–7.

79. Feldmann, M. and Maini, R.N., Anti-TNF alpha therapy of rheumatoid arthritis: what have we learned? Annu Rev Immunol, 2001. 19: p. 163–196.

80. Brennan, F.M., Maini, R.N., and Feldmann, M., Role of pro-inflammatory cytokines in rheumatoid arthritis Springer Semin Immunopathol, 1998. 20(1–2): p. 133–147.

81. Charles, P., Elliott, M.J., Davis, D., Potter, A., Kalden, J.R., Antoni, C., Breedveld, F.C., Smolen, J.S., Eberl, G., deWoody, K., Feldmann, M., and Maini, R.N., Regulation of cytokines, cytokine inhibitors, and acute-phase proteins following anti-TNF-alpha therapy in rheumatoid arthritis J Immunol, 1999. 163(3): p. 1521–1528.

82. Drewes, A.M., Pain and sleep disturbances with special reference to fibromyalgia and rheumatoid arthritis Rheumatology (Oxford), 1999. 38(11): p. 1035–1038.

83. Callahan, L.F., The burden of rheumatoid arthritis: facts and figures J Rheumatol Suppl, 1998. 53: p. 8–12.

84. Drewes, A.M., Svendsen, L., Taagholt, S.J., Bjerregard, K., Nielsen, K.D., and Hansen, B., Sleep in rheumatoid arthritis: a comparison with healthy subjects and studies of sleep/wake interactions Br J Rheumatol, 1998. 37(1): p. 71–81.

18

Changes in Gene Expression

CHIARA CIRELLI

University of Wisconsin–Madison, Madison, Wisconsin, U.S.A.

I. Introduction

Knowledge of the molecular consequences of sleep and sleep deprivation is essential to understand the restorative processes occurring during sleep, the cellular mechanisms of sleep regulation, and the functional consequences of sleep loss. This chapter reviews the available data about behavioral state-dependent changes in neural gene expression across sleep, waking, and sleep deprivation, starting with older studies focusing on total ribonucleic acid (RNA) or protein content. Then it discusses the results of more recent studies in which a candidate gene approach was used to analyze the expression of specific genes, particularly transcription factors. Finally, the chapter focuses on a recent whole-genome analysis in which our laboratory used first messenger RNA (mRNA) differential display and nylon membrane microarray, and then GeneChip technology to compare brain gene expression among sleep, spontaneous waking, and different periods of sleep deprivation ranging from a few hours to several days.

II. Global Brain Changes of RNA and Protein Content Related to Sleep and Sleep Deprivation

Early studies examined changes in RNA content (1) or synthesis (2,3), as well as overall changes in protein synthesis (4–7) in relation to sleep and waking or to sleep deprivation. Giuditta et al. (3) injected [^{3}H]orotate intraventricularly and measured its incorporation into newly synthesized RNA during the following hour. In a fraction of neuronal perikarya in the cerebral cortex, the relative content of radioactive RNA was increased in sleep with respect to waking in the nuclear but not in the cytoplasmic compartment. Panov (1) found variations in protein and RNA content in individual neurons and glial cells of some brainstem nuclei after 1–4 days of total or selective rapid-eye-movement (REM) sleep deprivation. Bobillier et al. (4) reported a generalized decrease of [^{3}H]amino acid incorporation into the proteins of telencephalon and brainstem after 3 hr of total sleep deprivation in rats. Conversely, a striking increase of labeled proteins was found in rats that were allowed to sleep for 1.5 hr after 1.5 hr of total sleep deprivation. Ramm and Smith (6) found that in the rat higher rates of cerebral protein synthesis were associated with a higher slow-wave sleep score. In rhesus monkeys Nakanishi et al. (7) found that protein synthesis, as measured by L-[1-^{14}C]leucine incorporation, was positively correlated with deep sleep in most brain regions. Thus, these studies were the first indication that significant changes in gene expression could occur among sleep, wakefulness, and sleep deprivation. However, they did not address the question of how many and which genes were changing in a state-dependent manner.

III. Gene Expression in Sleep and Wakefulness

A. Gene Expression Between Sleep and Wakefulness as Revealed by Candidate Gene Approaches: c-fos and Other Transcription Factors (See Also Chap. 19)

Most initial studies have focused on immediate early genes (IEGs) such as *c-fos, NGFI-A, c-jun*, and *junB*. IEGs are among the first genes to be turned on or off in the cascade of molecular events that leads to changes in the expression of other genes. Their protein products have specific DNA-binding domains by which they act as nuclear transcription factors (8). We and several other laboratories [reviewed in (9)] looked at IEGs expression with targeted approaches such as in situ hybridization and immunocytochemistry, using probes specific for the mRNA and/or the protein product of these genes. It was found that the expression of *c-fos, NGFI-A*, and other IEGs is powerfully modulated by behavioral state. Specifically, our studies (10–12) showed that their expression is low or absent in most brain regions if the animals had spent most of the previous 3–8 hr asleep, whereas it is high if the animals had been either spontaneously awake or sleep deprived for a few hours before sacrifice. One of the most important conclusions derived from these studies was that the strong state-dependent modulation of IEGs expression could indicate widespread transcriptional changes between sleep and wakefulness. Indeed, as mentioned before, many IEGs are transcription factors, and therefore their up- or downregulation in sleep and wakefulness could be an early event heralding and possibly triggering changes in the pattern of expression of many other genes. Thus, it became necessary to take advantage of more systematic approaches to study state-dependent gene expression.

B. Whole-Genome Analysis of Gene Expression in Sleep and Waking

A genome-wide expression analysis has been conducted in several laboratories to isolate genes regulated by the circadian clock. These studies have identified hundreds of transcripts cycling in the brain and in peripheral tissues of mice (13–16) and flies (17–21) as a function of circadian time. Cycling genes are involved in extremely diverse biological functions, from protein synthesis and immune response to metabolism, and may thus play a role in biological processes that change between day and night, including wakefulness and sleep. However, as mentioned above, until recently it was not known to what extent changes in gene expression between day and night depend on circadian time or on behavioral state. Most importantly, it was not known whether there are genes whose expression is increased during sleep and, if so, which they might be.

In order to address these questions, over the last several years we have employed mRNA differential display (mRNA DD), nylon membrane arrays, and, more recently, GeneChip technology, to systematically establish the differences in gene expression that occur across behavioral states (22–25). Brain gene expression was compared among rats that had been asleep for the first 3 or 8 hr of the light period, in rats that had been spontaneously awake for the first 3 or 8 hr of the dark period, and rats that had been sleep deprived during the light period for 3 or 8 hr. This experimental paradigm allowed us to distinguish between changes in gene expression related to sleep and waking per se as opposed to circadian time or to the sleep deprivation procedure. In addition, we also examined gene expression in the brain of rats chronically deprived of sleep for long periods [4–14 days (26)] using the disk-over-water (DOW) (27) method. As discussed in Chapters 4 and 5, the DOW is the method of choice for long-term sleep deprivation. Most of our studies focused on the cerebral cortex because it generates the characteristic electrical rhythms of sleep (28), it responds to prolonged wakefulness with increasing sleep pressure (29), it is responsible for the cognitive defects observed after sleep deprivation (30,31), and it is at the center of most hypotheses concerning the functions of sleep (28,32–35).

The findings summarized in this review are relative to the recent analysis of an estimated 15,000 transcripts using Affymetrix GeneChip technology [GeneChips RGU34A, B, C (25)] as well as to an older analysis of about 10,000 transcripts performed using mRNA DD and nylon membrane arrays (22–24). Since the number of genes expressed in the rat cerebral cortex is likely to range between 15,000 and 30,000 (36,37), this screening represents the most extensive (yet probably still not exhaustive) analysis of state-dependent changes in gene expression performed so far. The main analysis focused on sustained periods of sleep and waking (8 hr) and used all the techniques mentioned before. An older and more limited analysis of short periods (3 hr) of sleep and waking only used mRNA DD and nylon membrane arrays and will be briefly discussed first.

C. Short Periods (3 hr) of Wakefulness Upregulate Transcription Factors and Mitochondrial Genes

Two classes of genes are induced by 3 hr of spontaneous wakefulness or sleep deprivation: IEGs/transcription factors and mitochondrial genes (22). The IEGs group includes *Arc, c-fos, NGFI-A,* the rat homologue of the human Zn-15 related zinc finger (*rlf*) gene, which has been implicated in transcriptional regulation, and AA117313, probably similar to the human global transcription activator SNF2/SWI2. We also found that the transcription factor CREB is differentially phosphorylated depending on the behavioral state of the animals. P-CREB immunolabeling is low in rats sacrificed after a few hours of sleep and high after 3 hr of either spontaneous or forced wakefulness (24). CREB phosphorylation (P-CREB) at Ser^{133} follows increases in the intracellular concentration of Ca^{2+} or cAMP, and the activation of CREB-dependent transcription plays a crucial role in the acquisition of different forms of long-term memory in the hippocampus and the cerebral cortex [see references in (24)].

The rapid regulation in the expression of mitochondrial genes was an unexpected finding. The mitochondrial genes include the subunit I of cytochrome *c* oxidase, the subunit 2 of NADH dehydrogenase, and the 12S ribosonal RNA (rRNA). Cytochrome *c* oxidase is the terminal enzyme of the respiratory chain and plays a crucial role in the regulation of oxidative metabolism (38). The enzyme is made up of several subunits, some of which (e.g., subunit I) are coded by the mitochondrial genome, whereas others (e.g., subunit IV) are coded by the nuclear genome. Interestingly, we found that changes in mRNA levels between sleep and wakefulness involve only the mitochondrial genes coded by the mitochondrial genome and not those coded by the nuclear genome. Mitochondria seem to contain excess amounts of nuclear-encoded cytochrome *c* oxidase subunits. Changes in neuronal activity and energy demand affect the transcription of mitochondrially encoded subunits of cytochrome *c* oxidase more quickly and more significantly than that of the nuclear subunits (38). Thus, it is the synthesis of mitochondrially encoded subunits followed by the holoenzyme assembly, that is governed by dynamic local energy needs. Cerebral glucose is almost exclusively metabolized through mitochondrial oxidative phosphorylation and glucose metabolism is 20–30% higher in wakefulness than in non-REM (NREM) sleep in several species, including the rat (39). The increased expression of mitochondrial genes after 3 hr of wakefulness suggests a previously unsuspected mechanism by which neurons and/or glia can adapt to the increased metabolic demand of wakefulness relative to sleep. The functional role of this mitochondrial upregulation is supported by the finding that the expression of subunit I of cytochrome *c* oxidase increases after periods of wakefulness also in species, such as the fruitfly, that are phylogenetically very distant from the rat. Indeed, in a completely independent gene screening project, we found that subunit I of cytochrome c oxidase mRNA levels are higher after periods of wakefulness and sleep deprivation relative to comparable periods of sleeplike behavior in the brain of *Drosophila melanogaster* (40).

D. Extensive and Divergent Effects of 8 hr of Wakefulness or Sleep on Brain Gene Expression

As mentioned above, the most extensive analysis we have performed so far focused on differences in gene expression after 8 hr of sleep, sleep deprivation, and spontaneous wakefulness (25). The following conclusions were derived from this study:

(1) Up to about 5% of the transcribed sequences tested in the cerebral cortex (about 800 out of 15,000) were found to be up- or downregulated in rats that had slept for 8 hr relative to rats that had been spontaneously awake or sleep deprived for a similar period. These sequences included both known (annotated) transcripts as well as expressed sequence tags (ESTs). In the cerebral cortex of the same animals, a similar number of transcribed sequences was found to change their expression because of time of day rather than because of behavioral state. Thus, daytime/nighttime and sleep/wakefulness appear to influence gene expression in the cerebral cortex to a similar extent. A direct implication of these results is that changes in behavioral state should be taken into account in all gene expression studies.

(2) The number of known transcripts upregulated during wakefulness (wake-related genes) was similar (about 100) to the number of transcripts upregulated during sleep (sleep-related genes). Thus, although sleep is a state of behavioral inactivity, it is associated with the increased expression of many genes in the brain. Moreover, the increased expression in the brain during sleep was found to be specific, since transcripts that were sleep related in the brain were not sleep related in other tissues such as liver and skeletal muscle (25).

(3) Many (about 40%) of the genes wake-related in the cerebral cortex were also wake-related in the cerebellum. Similarly, many (50%) of the cortical sleep-related genes were also sleep related in the cerebellum. The finding that molecular correlates of sleep and wakefulness are found in the cerebellum indicates that cellular processes associated with sleep may occur in brain structures that are not known for generating sleep rhythms. This suggests that, at the cellular level, functions associated with sleep may take place whether or not electrographic signs of sleep can be recorded.

(4) Finally, and most importantly, a functional analysis of transcripts modulated by behavioral state suggests that sleep and wakefulness may favor different cellular processes. Several transcripts involved in energy metabolism (mitochondrial genes, *GLUT1*), excitatory neurotransmission (*Narp, Vesl/Homer*), transcriptional activation (*Per2, NGFI-A, NGFI-B, CHOP*), memory acquisition (*Arc, NGFI-A, BDNF*), and cellular stress (*HSPs, Bip*) were wake-

fulness related. Among sleep-related transcripts was *Dbp*, which in other tissues is regulated by the circadian clock. Sleep-related transcripts also included a two-pore domain potassium channel controlling resting membrane potential (*TREK-1*); key components of the translational machinery (*translation elongation factor 2, initiation factor 4AII*); and genes involved in depotentiation and depression as well as in the consolidation of long-term memory (e.g., *calcineurin, calmodulin-dependent protein kinase IV*). A large number of sleep-related transcripts are involved in membrane trafficking and maintenance, including synaptic vesicle turnover (*Rab genes, NSF; ARF1, ARF3*), glia/myelin function (*MOBP, MAG, plasmolipin, carbonic anhydrase II*) and synthesis and transport of glia-derived cholesterol (e.g., *HMG-CoA synthase, squalene synthase*), the limiting factor for synapse formation and maintenance. Thus, wakefulness-related transcripts may help the brain to face high energy demand, high synaptic excitatory transmission, high transcriptional activity, the need for synaptic potentiation in the acquisition of new information, as well as the cellular stress that may derive from one or more of these processes. An analysis of brain sleep–related transcripts supports an involvement of sleep in protein synthesis and in complementary aspects of neural plasticity such as synaptic depression, and suggests, for the first time, that sleep may play a significant role in membrane trafficking and maintenance. Thus, in line with intracellular recording studies (28), our findings suggest that sleep, far from being a quiescent state of global inactivity, may actively favor specific cellular functions.

IV.   Gene Expression and Neuromodulatory Systems

Many transcripts upregulated during wakefulness are induced diffusely in the cerebral cortex and in many other brain regions. We hypothesized that a key factor responsible for their induction might be the level of activity of neuromodulatory systems such as the noradrenergic and the serotonergic systems. These systems project diffusely to most of the brain and their activity is strictly state dependent.

Noradrenergic neurons of the locus coeruleus fire regularly at very low rates during sleep, whereas during wakefulness they fire at higher rates and emit phasic, short bursts of action potentials in response to salient events (41). Norepinephrine enhances brain information transmission, promotes attentive processes, and can enable various forms of activity-dependent synaptic plasticity by stimulating gene transcription [reviewed in (24)]. To assess the role of the noradrenergic system in the induction of gene expression during wakefulness, we studied behavior, brain electrical activity, and messenger RNA levels of several genes in normal rats and in rats in which the central noradrenergic system had been lesioned either bilaterally or unilaterally (24,42). We found that after the lesion of the locus coeruleus waking behavior associated with a normal low-voltage fast-activity electroencephalogram was not accompanied by the induction of molecular markers of plasticity such as *c-fos, NGFI-A, P-CREB, Arc,* and *BDNF.* These results indicate that: (a) the activation of the EEG can be dissociated from the activation of gene expression; (b) the noradrenergic system plays a major role in the induction of plasticity-related genes during wakefulness (48). Nevertheless, the available findings suggest that the reduced expression of plasticity-related genes due to the reduced firing of locus coeruleus neurons may be a key factor that determines why the ability to learn new material is impaired during sleep.

Like locus coeruleus cells, serotonergic neurons of the dorsal raphe also fire at higher levels during wakefulness and decrease their firing during sleep (43). However, in sharp contrast to noradrenergic neurons, dorsal raphe cells are activated during repetitive motor activity such as locomoting, grooming, or feeding and are inactivated during orientation to salient stimuli (44). Interestingly, lesions of the dorsal raphe nucleus were unable to affect the expression of *c-fos, NGFI-A, P-CREB, Arc,* and *BDNF,* either during wakefulness or during sleep (45). Thus, the noradrenergic, but not the serotonergic, system plays a crucial role in state-dependent brain gene expression.

V. Genes Induced by Long Periods of Sleep Deprivation

Most of the waking-related and sleep-related genes discussed above did not change their expression if sleep loss was prolonged. One important exception is represented by the enzyme arylsulfotransferase (AST), which is induced more markedly after several days than after several hours of sleep deprivation (26). The progressively stronger induction of AST is the first demonstration of a molecular response in the brain that is related to the duration of sleep loss. AST is responsible for the sulfonation of norepinephrine, dopamine, and, to a lesser extent, serotonin. AST induction during sleep deprivation may therefore constitute a homeostatic response to the uninterrupted activity of the central noradrenergic system during wakefulness. This could indicate that at least some of the detrimental effects of sleep loss may be dependent on the continuous activation of the noradrenergic system and that an important function of sleep is that of counteracting the effects of continued monoaminergic discharge. We are currently testing this hypothesis by looking at the molecular, electrophysiological, and behavioral aspects of the long-term sleep deprivation syndrome in normal rats and in rats in which the central noradrenergic system has been pharmacologically lesioned.

VI. Long-Term Sleep Deprivation, Brain Cell Death, and Oxidative Stress

It has been suggested that sustained waking can significantly damage brain cells through excitotoxic or oxidative mechanisms [see references in (46)]. If this were true, massive cell death could explain the fatal consequences of sleep deprivation in rats and other animal species (27). To test the hypothesis that sustained wakefulness can cause brain cell degeneration, we looked for evidence of cell death in the brain of rats sleep deprived for several (4–14) days with the DOW method (46). The presence and extent of DNA fragmentation (a marker of cell death) was analyzed with two techniques (TUNEL and Fluoro-Jade staining), and with both methods the results were invariably negative. In addition, we found that the expression of several apoptosis-related genes did not change between long-term sleep-deprived rats and their yoked controls, nor between these two experimental groups and rats sacrificed after 8 hr of sleep or wakefulness. Thus, molecular studies provided no evidence that prolonged wakefulness could cause brain cell death.

Even if sleep deprivation does not cause brain cell death, it is still possible that prolonged sleep loss represents an oxidative challenge for the brain and that sleep has a protective role against oxidative damage. To test this hypothesis, we have measured in rats the effects of sleep loss on markers of oxidative stress (oxidant production and antioxidant enzyme activities) and on markers of cellular oxidative damage [lipid peroxidation and protein oxidation (47)]. The analyses were performed in the brain and in peripheral tissues (liver and skeletal muscle), after short-term sleep deprivation (8 hr), long-term sleep deprivation (3–14 days), and during recovery sleep after 1 week of sleep loss. Short-term sleep deprivation was performed by gentle handling; long-term sleep deprivation was performed using the DOW method. No evidence of oxidative damage was observed at the lipid and/or at the protein level in long-term sleep-deprived animals relative to their yoked controls, neither in the cerebral cortex nor in peripheral tissues. Also, no consistent change in antioxidant enzymatic activities was found after prolonged sleep deprivation, nor was any evidence of increased oxidant production in the brain or in peripheral tissues found. Thus, the available data do not support the assumption that prolonged wakefulness may cause oxidative damage or that it can represent an oxidative stress for the brain or for peripheral tissue such as liver and skeletal muscle.

VII. Conclusions

In order to determine the molecular changes that occur in the brain during the sleep-waking cycle and after sleep deprivation, we have performed a systematic screening of brain gene expression in rats that have been either sleeping or spontaneously awake for a few hours and in rats that have been sleep deprived for different periods of time ranging from a few hours to several days. The data summarized here refer to the completed analysis of about 15,000 transcripts expressed in the cerebral cortex. The expression of the majority (about 95%) of these genes does not change between sleep and wakefulness or after sleep deprivation, even when forced wakefulness is prolonged for several days. A few hours of wakefulness, either spontaneous or forced by sleep deprivation, increases the expression of several transcripts involved in energy metabolism, excitatory neurotransmission, transcriptional activation, memory acquisition, and cellular stress. The about 100 genes whose expression increases during sleep, on the other hand, provide molecular support for the proposed involvement of sleep in protein synthesis and neural plasticity, and point to a novel role for sleep in membrane trafficking and maintenance. The pattern of changes in gene expression after long periods of sleep deprivation is unique and does not resemble that of short-term sleep deprivation or spontaneous wakefulness. However, a notable exception is represented, by the enzyme arylsulfotransferase, whose induction appears to be related to the duration of previous wakefulness. In rodents, this enzyme plays a major role in the catabolism of catecholamines, suggesting that an important role for sleep may be that of interrupting the continuous activity, during wakefulness, of brain catecholaminergic systems.

References

1. Panov A. RNA and protein content of brain stem cells after sleep deprivation. Riv Biol 1982; 75:95–99.
2. Vitale-Neugebauer A, Giuditta A, Vitale B, Giaquinto S. Pattern of RNA synthesis in rabbit cortex during sleep. J Neurochem 1970; 17:1263–1273.
3. Giuditta A, Rutigliano B, Vitale-Neugebauer A. Influence of synchronized sleep on the biosynthesis of RNA in two nuclear classes isolated from rabbit cerebral cortex. J Neurochem 1980; 35:1259–1266.
4. Bobillier P, Sakai F, Seguin S, Jouvet M. Deprivation of paradoxical sleep and in vitro cerebral protein synthesis in the rat. Life Sci 1971; 10:1349–1357.
5. Brodskii VIa, Gusatinskii VN, Kogan AB, Nechaeva NV. Variations in the intensity of H3-leucine incorporation into proteins during slow-wave and paradoxical phases of natural sleep in the cat associative cortex. Dokl Akad Nauk SSSR 1974; 215:748–750.
6. Ramm P, Smith CT. Rates of cerebral protein synthesis are linked to slow wave sleep in the rat. Physiol Behav 1990; 48:749–753.
7. Nakanishi H, Sun Y, Nakamura RK, Mori K, Ito M, Suda S, Namba H, Storch FI, Dang TP, Mendelson W, Mishkin M, Kennedy C, Gillin JC, Smith CB, Sokoloff L. Positive correlations between cerebral protein synthesis rates and deep sleep in *Macaca mulatta*. Eur J Neurosci 1997; 9:271–279.
8. Sheng M, Greenberg ME. The regulation and function of c-fos and other immediate early genes in the nervous system. Neuron 1990; 4:477–485.
9. Cirelli C, Tononi G. On the functional significance of c-fos induction during the sleep/waking cycle. Sleep 2000; 23:453–469.
10. Pompeiano M, Cirelli C, Tononi G. Immediate-early genes in spontaneous wakefulness and sleep: expression of c-fos and NGFI-A mRNA and protein. Sleep 1994; 3:80–96.
11. Cirelli C, Pompeiano M, Tononi G. Sleep deprivation and c-fos expression in the rat brain. Sleep 1995; 4:92–106.
12. Pompeiano M, Cirelli C, Ronca-Testoni S, Tononi G. NGFI-A expression in the rat brain after sleep deprivation. Mol Brain Res 1997; 46:143–153.
13. Panda S, Antoch MP, Miller BH, Su AI, Schook AB, Straume M, Schultz PG, Kay SK, Takahashi JS, Hogenesch JB, Coordinated transcription of key pathways in the mouse by the circadian clock. Cell 2002; 109:307–320.
14. Ueda HR, Chen W, Adachi A, Wakamatsu H, Hayashi S, Takasugi T, Nagano M, Nakahama K, Suzuki Y, Sugano S, Iino M, Shigeyoshi Y, Hashimoto S. A transcrip-

tion factor response element for gene expression during circadian night. Nature 2002; 418:534–539.

15. Storch KF, Lipan O, Leykin I, Viswanathan N, Davis FC, Wong WH, Weitz CJ. Extensive and divergent circadian gene expression in liver and heart. Nature (2002) 417:78–83.

16. Akhtar RA, Reddy AB, Maywood ES, Clayton JD, King VM, Smith AG, Gant TW, Hastings MH, Kyriacou CP. Circadian cycling of the mouse liver transcriptome, as revealed by cDNA microarray, is driven by the suprachiasmatic nucleus. Curr Biol 2002; 12:540–550.

17. McDonald MJ, Rosbash M. Microarray analysis and organization of circadian gene expression in *Drosophila*. Cell 2001; 107:567–578.

18. Claridge-Chang A, Wijnen H, Naef F, Boothroyd C, Rajewsky N, Young MW. Circadian regulation of gene expression systems in the *Drosophila* head. Neuron 2001; 32:657–671.

19. Ueda HR, Matsumoto A, Kawamura M, Iino M, Tanimura T, Hashimoto S. Genome-wide transcriptional orchestration of circadian rhythms in Drosophila. J Biol Chem 2002; 277:14048–14052.

20. Lin Y, Han M, Shimada B, Wang L, Gibler TM, Amarakone A, Awad TA, Stormo GD, Van Gelder RN, Taghert PH. Influence of the period-dependent circadian clock on diurnal, circadian, and aperiodic gene expression in *Drosophila melanogaster*. Proc Natl Acad Sci USA 2002; 99:9562–9567.

21. Ceriani MF, Hogenesch JB, Yanovsky M, Panda S, Straume M, Kay SA. Genome-wide expression analysis in Drosophila reveals genes controlling circadian behavior. J Neurosci 2002; 22:9305–9319.

22. Cirelli C, Tononi G. Differences in gene expression between sleep and waking as revealed by mRNA differential display. Mol Brain Res 1998; 56:293–305.

23. Cirelli C, Tononi G. Gene expression in the brain across the sleep-waking cycle. Brain Res 2000; 885:303–321.

24. Cirelli C, Tononi G. Differential expression of plasticity-related genes in waking and sleep and their regulation by the noradrenergic system. J Neurosci 2000; 20:9187–9194.

25. Cirelli C, Gutierrez CM, Tononi G. Extensive and divergent effects of sleep and wakefulness on brain gene expression. Neuron 2004; 41:35–43.

26. Cirelli C, Tononi G. Changes in gene expression in the cerebral cortex of rats after short-term and long-term sleep deprivation. Sleep 1999; 22(S1):113.

27. Rechtschaffen A, Bergmann BM. Sleep deprivation in the rat: an update of the 1989 paper. Sleep 2002; 25:18–24.

28. Steriade M., Timofeev I. Neuronal plasticity in thalamocortical networks during sleep and waking oscillations. Neuron 2003; 37: 563–576.

29. Borbély AA, Achermann P. Sleep homeostasis and models of sleep regulation. J Biol Rhythms 1999; 14: 557–568.

30. Horne JA. Why We Sleep. The Functions of Sleep in Humans and Other Mammals. Oxford, Oxford University Press, 1988.

31. Van Dongen HPA, Maislin G, Mullington JM, Dinges DF. The cumulative cost of additional wakefulness: dose-response effects on neurobehavioral functions and sleep physiology from chronic sleep restriction and total sleep deprivation. Sleep 2003; 26: 117–126.

32. Moruzzi G. The sleep-waking cycle. Ergeb Physiol 1972; 64: 1–165.

33. Krueger JM, Obal FJr, Kapas L, Fang J. Brain organization and sleep function. Behav Brain Res 1995; 69: 177–186.
34. Maquet P. Sleep function(s) and cerebral metabolism. Behav Brain Res 1995; 69:75–83.
35. Tononi G, Cirelli C. Sleep and synaptic homeostasis: A hypothesis. Brain Res Bull 2003; 62:143–150.
36. Milner FD, Sutcliffe JG. Gene expression in rat brain. Nucleic Acid Res 1983; 11:5497–5520.
37. Velculescu VE, Madden SL, Zhang L, Lash AE, Yu J, Rago C, Lal A, Wang CJ, Beaudry GA, Ciriello KM, Cook BP, Dufault MR, Ferguson AT, Gao Y, He TC, Hermeking H, Hiraldo SK, Hwang PM, Lopez MA, Luderer HF, Mathews B, Petroziello JM, Polyak K, Zawel L, Kinzler KW, et al. Analysis of human transcriptomes. Nat Genet 1999; 23:387–388.
38. Wong-Riley MTT, Mullen MA, Huang Z, Guyer C. Brain cytochrome oxidase subunit complementary DNAs: isolation, subcloning, sequencing, light and electron microscopic in situ hybridization of transcripts, and regulation by neuronal activity. Neuroscience 1997; 76:1035–1055.
39. Ramm P, Frost BJ Regional metabolic activity in the rat brain during sleep-wake activity. Sleep 1983; 6: 196–216.
40. Shaw PJ, Cirelli C, Greenspan RJ, Tononi G. Correlates of sleep and waking in *Drosophila melanogaster*. Science 2000; 287:1834–1837.
41. Aston-Jones G, Bloom FE. Activity of norepinephrine-containing locus coeruleus neurons in behaving rats anticipates fluctuations in the sleep-waking cycle. J Neurosci 1981; 1:876–886.
42. Cirelli C, Pompeiano M, Tononi G. Neuronal gene expression in the waking state: a role for the locus coeruleus. Science 1996; 274:1211–1215.
43. McGinty DJ, Harper RM. Dorsal raphe neurons: depression of firing during sleep in cats. Brain Res 1976; 101:569–575.
44. Jacobs BL, Fornal CA. Activity of serotonergic neurons in behaving animals. Neuropsychopharmacolopy 1999; 21:9S-15S.
45. Tononi G, Cirelli C, Shaw PJ. The Molecular correlates of sleep, waking, and sleep deprivation. In: Borbély A, Hayaishi O, Sejnowski TJ, Altman JS, eds. Human Frontier Workshop VIII, The Regulation of Sleep. Strasbourg, Human Frontier Scientific Press, 2000:155–167.
46. Cirelli C, Shaw PJ, Rechtschaffen A, Tononi G. No evidence of brain cell degeneration after long-term sleep deprivation in rats. Brain Res 1999; 840:184–193.
47. Gopalakrishnan A, Ji LL, Cirelli C. Oxidative stress and cellular damage after sleep deprivation. Sleep 2004; 27:27–35.
48. Cirelli C, Tononi G. Locus ceruleus control of state-dependent gene expression. J Neurosci 2004; 24:5410–5419.

19

Criteria for Classifying Genes as Sleep or Wake Genes

PRIYATTAM J. SHIROMANI, DMITRY GERASHCHENKO,
CARLO BLANCO-CENTURION, ERIC MURILLO-RODRIGUEZ, AND
FRANK DESARNAUD

West Roxbury Veterans Administration Medical Center, and Harvard Medical School,
West Roxbury, Massachusetts, U.S.A.

I. Introduction

Virtually all organisms manifest regular periods of behavioral quiescence and activity. In mammals and birds these periods have evolved into regular episodes of wakefulness and sleep. The need for sleep begins with the onset of wakefulness. There is a slow time course of buildup of sleep drive with wakefulness and the dissipation of this drive with sleep. Most importantly, cumulative bouts of sleep are necessary to dissipate the sleep drive following sleep loss. The waxing and waning of the sleep process has intrigued investigators because it identifies a need for sleep. What is actually restored or replenished during sleep is not known. Sleep researchers are working to unravel the mysteries of sleep in much the same way as researchers in other areas of neuroscience such as circadian rhythms (reviewed in 1) and feeding (reviewed in 2). Sleep shares many similarities with those behaviors in that it is oscillatory, driven by discrete brain areas, and, like feeding, is associated with a need and satiety. An important goal for sleep researchers is to understand the intracellular and molecular events related to sleep and sleep loss. By understanding these events it will be possible to determine how cells adapt (or fail to adapt) to changing environmental demands (e.g., sleep loss). The long-term goal is to identify and block any destructive cascade that follows extensive periods of sleep loss.

In a previous review (3) we hypothesized that changes at the molecular level would ultimately be responsible for the sleep process. For instance, extracellular factors (cytokines, adenosine, neurotransmitters, etc.) would determine the excitability of sleep-active versus wake-active neurons from the single cell to the network level (Fig. 1). At the single-cell level, receptor and channel openings would influence second messengers [such as cyclic adenosine aronophosphate (cAMP) and calcium] resulting in phosphorylation of specific kinases. This would feed back onto the receptor/channel so that membrane excitability could be modulated rapidly (minutes). Activation of transcription factors would transduce the signal to the nucleus and activate specific genes. These genes could encode receptor, neurotransmitter-synthesizing enzymes, and enzymes subserving critical cell functions. The activation of these genes would dictate the responsivity of the cell over the long term (hours to days).

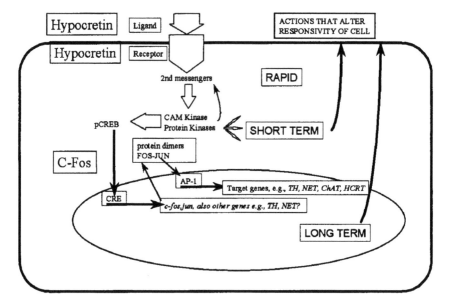

Figure 1 Intracellular cascades involved in sleep-wake regulation. Sleep and wakefulness are regulated in large part by homeostatic factors. Neuronal firing would release specific ligands onto receptors, setting off an intracellular cascade that would dictate excitability levels of the neuron. Rapid and short-term intracellular events initiated by ligand-receptor coupling might regulate the transitions between sleep and wakefulness. However, slow cascades such as those involving transcription factors would be necessary to achieve long-term sleep-wake homeostasis. Deletion of specific genes, such as *hypocretin*, would cause a defect in the cascade. Mutation in the hypocretin receptor, as occurs in canine narcolepsy, would also cause a defect in the cascade. As a defect in both the ligand or the receptor cause narcolepsy, we conclude that hypocretin is a "wake" gene.

An important question is where in the brain to look for changes at the molecular level? We will argue that the molecular changes responsible for regulating sleep or wakefulness are likely to occur in those neurons responsible for generating each of the sleep-wake states. Such has been the case in other areas of neurobiology, most notably in the area of circadian biology where expression of the clock genes is observed in the suprachiasmatic nucleus (SCN) (1). Indeed, it would be odd if expression of the clock genes did not occur in the SCN. However, while the SCN is a clearly defined structure, the neurons responsible for sleep and wakefulness are juxtaposed with neurons subserving other behaviors. Moreover, multiple brain regions have been implicated in generating wakefulness, non-REM (NREM) sleep, and rapid-eye-movement (REM) sleep. Thus, the task faced by sleep neurobiologists is to first identify the neurons responsible for each of the three states of consciousness and to then investigate which genes are expressed in those neurons.

In this chapter we will summarize the recent progress that has been made to identify the neurons responsible for wakefulness, NREM sleep and REM sleep (summarized in Fig. 2). We will also review the current data regarding molecular changes associated with sleep. Because investigators are identifying gene expression in many brain regions, we propose a set of criteria for classifying genes as wake or sleep genes (Table 1). We argue that such criteria are necessary for the molecular changes to have heuristic value.

II. Using Gene Expression to Delineate Sleep-Wake Circuitry

Our current understanding of the neuronal circuitry underlying wakefulness and sleep is based largely on electrophysiological studies wherein investigators monitor the discharge pattern of neurons during individual episodes of wake, NREM sleep, or REM sleep. By definition such studies are correlational, but investigators have ascribed a cause-and-effect relationship to the neuronal activity patterns and current sleep theories are based on such correlational observations (reviewed in 4). From the perspective of molecular biology, gene expression is likely to occur in these neurons. To identify neurons activated during wakefulness compared to sleep, we have used the marker *c-fos*. *C-fos* belongs to a family of immediate-early genes that are rapidly and transiently expressed in cells in response to cell signaling (5). Peak levels of *c-fos* mRNA occur 45 min after stimulation while the peak protein levels are seen 60–90 min after the stimulation. The protein returns to basal levels 3–6 hr after the stimulation. One reason that investigators are interested in immediate-early genes, such as *c-fos*, is that these genes are rapidly activated in response to cellular stimulation, and the resultant proteins modulate the activity of target genes. In this way cells are able to produce a short-term and a long-term response to changes at the membrane level.

The presence of *c-fos* serves two purposes in that it identifies the cell but also indicates gene expression. By using *c-fos* as a marker of both cell activa-

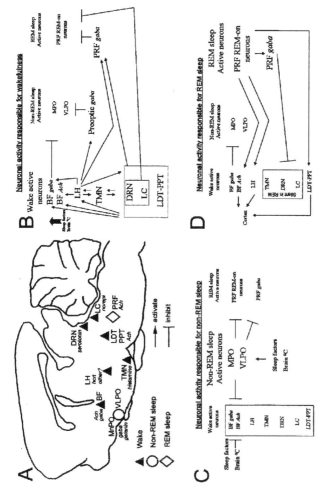

Figure 2 Neuronal circuitry responsible for generating wakefulness, NREM sleep, and REM sleep. Panel A identifies the regions and the neurotransmitters implicated in generating each of the three states of consciousness. Panels B–D identify in more detail the dominant pattern of neuronal activity during each of the behavioral states. Other factors, such as sleep factors and brain temperature would also influence specific neuronal populations. In our model, the lateral hypothalamus (LH) is central to maintaining wakefulness and the balance between sleep and wakefulness. Lesioning the LH and the hypocretin neurons would result in a cascade effect of not activating the arousal neurons located rostral and caudal to it, resulting in hypersomnolence. Insommia would result from lesioning the sleep-active neurons in the median preoptic and ventral lateral preoptic area. Our model also incorporates the influence of sleep factors and brain temperature in the sleep process. Both increase during wakefulness (panel B) and inhibit wake-active neurons. These factors also stimulate sleep-active neurons. It is not clear how the switch to REM sleep occurs. However, the hypocretin neurons play a central role in gating REM sleep also, since their elimination triggers REM during waking behavior (see Ref. 13 for example of REM sleep during waking behavior in rats).

Table 1 Criteria for Classifying Genes as Sleep or Wake Genes[a]

1. Gene and protein expression are associated with a specific behavioral state (i.e., wakefulness, NREM, or REM) independent of circadian time.
2. Gene and its protein product are expressed in cell type(s) implicated in behavioral state control.
3. Feedback loops involving positive and negative elements control transcription/translation of specific genes.
4. These loops are activated by action of putative sleep factors (neurotransmitters, adenosine, prostaglandin D_2, etc.) onto specific receptors.
5. Manipulation of gene (mutation/knockout/knockin/inducible) has a distinct effect on the behavioral state.
6. Evolutionary conservation of gene/protein across species that sleep.

[a]In order for a particular gene to be classified as a sleep or wake gene it should satisfy each of these criteria, from the most general (criterion 1) to the most stringent (criterion 6). A number of genes oscillate with sleep (criterion 1) and deletion of some (such as hypocretin) also affects behavioral state (criterion 5). For each of these genes, it is necessary to satisfy the other criteria so that the function of the gene in the sleep process is fully understood.

tion and gene expression one can proceed to identify the phenotype of the neuron and connectivity to other brain areas. Identification of the chemical signature of the neuron makes it possible to use newer methods such as laser capture microscopy to focus on specific genes that are expressed in that neuron relative to other neurons.

A. Gene Expression in Wake-Active Neuronal Populations

Neurons responsible for wakefulness are located in the forebrain and brainstem regions and include the major neurotransmitters acetylcholine (basal forebrain and pons), norepinephrine (locus coeruleus), histamine (tuberomammillary nucleus), and serotonin (dorsal raphe) (Fig. 2). To this mix a peptidergic system was added. The neuropeptide hypocretin (HCRT), which is also known as orexin (ORX), was discovered by two independent groups using different approaches (6–8). In the central nervous system, HCRT/ORX-containing neurons are located only in the lateral hypothalamus from where they project to the entire brain and spinal cord, providing especially heavy innervation to the arousal populations (7,9). Such innervation suggests that the classical neurotransmitter neuronal populations might be driven by this peptide system and that lesions of the HCRT/ORX neurons could decrease waking behavior and trigger sleep. Indeed, hypocretin was implicated in the human sleep disorder narcolepsy based on the findings that canines with narcolepsy possess a mutation in the hypocretin-2 receptor (10). When the hypocretin neurons are removed either by genetic ablation in mice (11,12) or by use of a saporin-based neurotoxin in rats (13), the animals exhibit symptoms of narcolepsy. In human narcolepsy there is a massive loss of hypocretin neurons (14,15), and consistent with such a neuronal loss, levels of hypocretin-1 are undetectable in the cerebrospinal fluid of human narcoleptic patients (16).

Since the wake-active neuronal populations have been identified, it should be possible to focus on these neurons exclusively and identify whether specific genes are expressed. *C-fos* expression occurs in response to wakefulness in basal forebrain cholinergic neurons (17), histamine neurons of the tuberomammillary nucleus (18), and the HCRT/ORX neurons (19). During sleep, *c-fos* expression is diminished or absent in these neurons. In fact, during sleep *c-fos* is rapidly degraded (20) in all of the wake-active neurons. For instance, with as little as 15 min of sleep, *c-fos* disappears from wake-active neurons (20). The functional significance of such a rapid clearance of a protein is still not known, but we have speculated that it might be one of the functions of sleep, i.e., to prepare the cell/neuron for the next wake-active cycle (3). Increasing *c-fos* in wake-active neurons would place a homeostatic load on the cell, which would force it to slow down so that sleep can occur and the protein can be cleared. One test of this hypothesis would be that animals deficient in *c-fos* should sleep less. Indeed, we have found that *c-fos*-null mice have a selective decrease in NREM sleep, whereas REM sleep is not changed (21). In contrast, mice missing another member of the fos family, *fos B*, have intact NREM sleep but are deficient in REM sleep (21).

Fos is a transcription factor responsible for initiating target genes. From a sleep perspective, the target genes would include genes associated with the key neurotransmitters and their synthesizing enzymes. Of these, we have found that the expression of choline acetyltransferase, the acetylcholine-synthesizing enzyme, is strongly linked to sleep (22). It is low during wakefulness, rises during NREM sleep, and is highest during REM sleep. We find this very intriguing because it suggests a function for sleep, i.e., replenishment of stores depleted during waking behavior.

Hypocretin levels increase with waking behavior (23,24) and its deletion leads to narcolepsy, suggesting that this is a key "wake gene." *C-fos* is present in hypocretin neurons and is induced with wakefulness, suggesting a linkage between immediate-early genes and hypocretin, but this remains to be demonstrated. Of the other neurotransmitters linked with wakefulness, histamine decarboxylase–null mice have decreased wakefulness only at lights-off and fall asleep faster when exposed to a new environment (25). Histamine could be a candidate for a "wake gene" classification. *C-fos* is expressed in histamine neurons in response to wakefulness (26).

Above we have focused on those genes expressed in neurons implicated in generating and maintaining wakefulness. However, virtually all brain neurons are active during wakefulness, even though these specific regions are not responsible for the state. *What would be the purpose of gene expression in these regions and would those genes represent sleep genes?* For instance, subtractive hybridization methods have been used to screen gene expression in the rat cerebral cortex after spontaneous sleep, spontaneous waking, and sleep deprivation (27,28). Out of thousands of genes screened, only a few were found to be expressed at a higher level in awake rats than in rats that were asleep: three were transcription factors, including *c-fos* and *NGFI-A*, three others corresponded to genes of mitochondrial origin encoding key enzymes for energy metabolism, i.e., cytochrome *c* oxidase, NADH dehydrogenase, and 12S rRNA. Five other genes did not correspond to any known sequences. We suggest that expression of these genes in the cortex is not responsible for sleep or wakefulness but their expression in the cortex would meet the demands of the cortical cells for energy during wakefulness. These genes would oscillate with sleep-wakefulness, but since they are not located in neurons implicated in the state, their loss would not adversely affect the sleep-wake state. As such, according to our criteria, these genes would not be classified as sleep genes.

B. Gene Expression in Sleep-Active Regions

Nauta's experiments led him to conclude that there was a sleep center because discrete lesions of the preoptic area (POA) produced insomnia (29). In the succeeding years, a great body of evidence has accumulated to support Nauta's conclusions. In rats, rabbits and cats, bilateral electrical lesions of the POA produce insomnia (30–34). Temporary inactivation of the POA with marcane produces reversible insomnia (35). Electrical stimulation of the POA induces both polygraphic and behavioral indices of sleep (36,37).

The POA is one of only two areas in the brain [the other is in the medulla (38)] where neuronal activity increases during sleep. In virtually every brain region that is examined, sleep is associated with a decline in neuronal discharge. Sleep-active neurons are found in the POA and adjacent basal forebrain in rats, cats, and rabbits (39–42). These neurons begin to fire during drowsiness, and peak activity is seen during NREM sleep.

We have used *c-fos* to identify sleep-active neurons in the POA and found a cluster in the ventral lateral preoptic (VLPO) nucleus (43). Szymusiak's group has now identified another cluster in the median POA (44). The VLPO *fos-ir* cells project to the histaminergic tuberomammillary neurons and to pontine wake-active populations (45). The median preoptic area *c-fos* neurons project to the lateral hypothalamus. Both groups contain inhibitory neurotransmitter gamma aminobutyric acid (GABA) and are galanin positive, and as such their release at target wake-active neuronal populations would shut them off, triggering sleep. The likelihood that the VLPO cells play an important role in sleep is further substantiated by findings that a majority of cells in this region are sleep active (46). We demonstrated that lesions of the VLPO produce long-lasting insomnia (47). Another group investigated the in vitro properties of the VLPO cells (48).

To date only *c-fos* expression has been identified in these neurons (43,44) and *c-fos*-null mice sleep less (21). Expression of other genes should be identified in these cell clusters. Part of the difficulty is that these are fairly small regions and difficult to remove even by micropunch methods.

C. Gene Expression in REM Sleep–Active Regions

Transection, lesion, and pharmacological stimulation studies have demonstrated that REM sleep originates from the pons (summarized in 49). Based largely on electrophysiological studies, it is hypothesized that REM sleep begins in the pons as a result of cessation of activity of REM-off cells in the dorsal raphe and locus coeruleus (LC). The cholinergic neurons located in the lateral dorsal tegmental (LDT) and pedunculopontine tegmental (PPT) nuclei become disinhibited and they begin to have high discharge rates. A subset of these cells innervates the medial pontine reticular formation (PRF) and activates possibly glutaminergic cells, which in turn activate LDT-PPT cholinergic cells. Medial PRF neurons might also activate GABA neurons that hyperpolarize dorsal raphe serotonergic neurons. In the dorsal raphe increased GABA, as measured by microdialysis, is seen during REM sleep relative to waking and NREM sleep (50). In the raphe, serotonin levels are lower during REM sleep compared to waking and NREM sleep. The discovery of hypocretin/orexin and the finding that loss of the ligand, hypocretin/orexin (located in neurons rostral to the pons), can trigger cataplexy and REM sleep onset in mice and rats demonstrates that forebrain mechanisms also control REM sleep.

It is very difficult to identify gene expression during REM sleep because the state lasts for only about 2 min in rats and 5 min in cats. To prolong the state, investigators typically have used one of the following methods: cholinergic stimulation (51), auditory stimulation (52), or REM sleep deprivation (53). These methods have drawbacks since the brain is not being studied under natural REM sleep conditions. Nevertheless, *c-fos* expression has been identified in pontine neurons implicated in REM sleep (52,54–56). Changes in expression of target genes in the pons have not been seen. However, there is expression of *c-fos* in pontine cholinergic (52–55) and GABA neurons (57,58) indicating that target genes might be affected. It will be difficult to assess these genes under natural REM sleep conditions because the REM sleep state lasts for only a short time.

An alternative approach is to examine mice with deletion of specific genes. Of interest are those genes whose deletion leads to increased, rather than decreased, REM sleep. Mice with deletion of the serotonin 5-HT$_{1B}$ receptor have higher amounts of REM sleep and less NREM sleep (59). This is consistent with other evidence that stimulation of the serotonin receptor would be inhibitory to REM sleep and that deletion of this receptor would result in increased REM sleep. Thus, the serotonin 5-HT$_{1B}$ receptor gene could qualify as a "REM sleep gene" because its deletion leads to changes in REM sleep in a predictable manner.

III. Sleep and Genetics in *Drosophila* (See Also Chap. 3)

The need for a simple model to understand sleep has led to the demonstration of a sleeplike state in the fruit fly, *Drosophila melanogaster* (60,61). In the fruit fly, rest shares features with mammalian sleep, including prolonged immobility, decreased sensory responsiveness, increased activity in response to caffeine, and a homeostatic rebound after rest deprivation (61,62).

Screening for changes in sleep in various *Drosophila* mutants has provided important clues about the effects of prolonged periods of activity on gene expression and subsequent rest. During the active period numerous genes are activated (62). Many of these transcripts, such as the mitochondrial gene cytochrome oxidase subunit I, the endoplasmic reticulum chaperone BiP and arylalkylamine *N*-acetyltransferase are also found in greater abundance during wakefulness than sleep in the rat cortex (62). Homozygous *Drosophila* mutants in which the transcription and activity of the enzyme arylalkylamine *N*-acetyltransferase is reduced have a rest rebound that is almost twice the magnitude of wild-type controls (62). This result suggests a link between monoamine catabolism and the rebound response in *Drosophila*. Increased waking is also related to increased activity of the cAMP response element binding (CREB) protein (63). Phosphorylated CREB (pCREB) is one of the transcription factors involved in triggering another transcription factor *c-fos*. Both of these transcription factors are activated in rat cortex and elsewhere in wake-active neurons in response to prolonged waking (64), and they are rapidly degraded from these same neurons after brief periods of sleep (20).

Because there is activation of numerous genes during activity, it is reasonable to theorize that an abnormality in downstream pathways could adversely affect the organisms. Indeed, homozygous *Drosophila* cycle [cyc(01)] mutants rest more after prolonged periods of activity, but more importantly they die after 10 hr of activity (65). If heat-shock genes are activated before the periods of activity then the flies do not die. This reveals an important role for heat-shock genes during periods of activity. Heat-shock proteins are a group of proteins that are present in all cells. They are induced in cells in response to various types of environmental stresses like heat, cold, and oxygen deprivation. As such they are also called stress proteins. These proteins are responsible for transporting other proteins (act as chaperones) and preparing old proteins for disposal. These results suggest that if these proteins are not abundant or mutated then it could compromise the cell's normal functioning, ultimately proving lethal.

IV. Criteria for Classifying Genes as "Sleep Genes"

A number of investigators are identifying gene expression during sleep. We argue that in order for these data to be of heuristic value it is necessary to define a set of criteria for labeling a gene as a wake gene or a sleep gene. In proposing these criteria we are borrowing heavily from the area of circadian biology where investigators have found an intricate intracellular cascade that regulates circadian rhythms (1).

(1) *Gene and protein expression are associated with a specific behavioral state (i.e., wakefulness, NREM, or REM) independent of circadian time.* We propose that if a gene is regulating a behavioral state, it should oscillate with the state

in a predictable manner, independent of circadian time. It is possible that the expression of the gene occurs in one state, such as wakefulness, and the protein product may occur during sleep. Such out-of-phase expression would indicate a time lag between the mRNA and protein and could be useful in determining whether the protein could be made if sleep did not occur. This could be used to determine the function of sleep. Such a lag between mRNA and protein is found in the SCN (1).

(2) *Gene and its protein product are expressed in cell type(s) implicated in behavioral state control.* Having identified that a particular gene is expressed during sleep (or wakefulness), the next step is to determine whether it is expressed in the neurons involved in the behavioral state. We believe this to be the most important criteria. Currently, studies have identified expression of genes in cortex during wakefulness (28), but these genes must be identified in neurons responsible for the wake state.

(3) *Feedback loops involving positive and negative elements control transcription/translation of specific genes.* Such feedback loops have been identified in the regulation of clock genes (1). Because sleep, and REM sleep in particular, is brief, it will be difficult to identify these loops. However, these loops could dictate sleep need versus satiety, just as they have in appetite control (2). *C-fos* expression could be representative of activation of such loops.

(4) *These loops are activated by action of putative sleep factors (neurotransmitters, adenosine, prostaglandin D_2, etc.) onto specific receptors.* There is considerable evidence that alterations in levels of sleep factors regulate sleep homeostasis. The strongest evidence is for adenosine (66) and prostaglandin D_2 (67). Adenosine levels increase with wakefulness and begin to inhibit wake-active neurons. Adenosine levels decline with ensuing sleep. However, the changes at the extracellular level must be communicated to the intracellular level to produce a coordinated action. There is new evidence that adenosine activates the transcription factor nuclear factor kappa β (NF-Kβ) (68). The author's conclusion that such activation might be representative of a "sleep debt" signal is consistent with our hypothesis (3). It is important to determine whether NFKβ activation occurs in adenosine receptor knockout mice, which would denote specificity of activation.

(5) *Manipulation of gene (mutation/knockout/knockin/inducible) has a distinct effect on the behavioral state.* Thus far, sleep investigators have accumulated only correlative evidence regarding the expression of specific genes during wakefulness or sleep. Deleting the gene and then observing changes in wakefulness or sleep will demonstrate cause and effect. If the gene is present in neurons generating the behavioral state then its deletion should bring about change in the behavioral state. Such is the case with hypocretin. It is present in neurons involved in generating the state, i.e., the lateral hypothalamus, and its deletion leads to narcoleptic behavior. As such, we would classify hypocretin as a "wake gene." Similarly, the histamine decarboxylase gene could be classified as a "wake gene" because its deletion leads to a predictable effect, i.e., sleep. The sleep-active neurons in the POA are GABA and galanin positive, but there is no evidence that their genes oscillate with behavioral state.

(6) *Evolutionary conservation of gene/protein across species that sleep.*
Sleep is present in virtually all mammals. It also appears that the same neurotransmitters, peptides, and sleep factors are responsible for each of the three states
of consciousness in mammals that have been tested, i.e., mice, rats, cats, dogs,
and humans. In flies, the mechanism appears to be conserved since they respond
to caffeine in much the same way as mammals (63). Deletion of the hypocretin
gene or its receptor causes narcoleptic behavior in mice, rats, dogs, and humans.
Cholinergic stimulation increases REM sleep in rats, cats, dogs, and humans
(reviewed in 51). This suggests that the genes and their proteins that cause sleep
are conserved across mammals. This has been the case in circadian neurobiology
(1), although a different set of genes could have evolved to undertake the same
function. For instance, the *timeless* gene is present in *Drosophila* but there does
not appear to be a true mammalian homologue of this gene (1). Even in mammals,
different organs could have evolved a different set of genes to accomplish the
same behavior. For instance, in murine liver and heart, a different set of genes
from those present in the brain's SCN regulates circadian behavior of these
organs (69).

V. Conclusions

To determine how sleep is generated and regulated investigators have monitored
neuronal firing along with the resultant ligand-receptor interactions. However,
such events are relatively fast (seconds to minutes) and only partially explain the
generation and regulation of sleep and wakefulness. Neuronal firing can account
for state generation but not the waxing and waning of the sleep process. Sleep factors could account for the rise and fall of the sleep process. However, the finding
that multiple bouts of sleep are necessary to dissipate the sleep drive indicates that
other slower cascades are also involved. Moreover, sleep factors cannot adequately explain the time course of the alternation between waking to SWS to
REM sleep.

We have suggested that an alternation between relatively rapid events, such
as phosphorylation/dephosphorylation, and long-term events such as target gene
expression and protein synthesis, could regulate sleep-wake cycles. Abnormality
at any step could adversely affect sleep. The fly model is a very useful tool in rapidly identifying which of these steps is key. However, ultimately for the gene to
be classified as a wake gene or a sleep gene, the gene would have to be identified
in specific neuronal populations subserving a specific state, and these investigations require mice or rats.

Acknowledgments

Supported by grants from the National Institutes of Health and Veterans
Administration Medical Research Service.

References

1. Shearman, LP., Sriram, S., Weaver, DR., Maywood, ES., Chaves, I., Zheng, B., Kume, K., Le, CC., van de Horst, GTJ., Hastings, MH., Reppert, SM. Interacting molecular loops in the mammalian circadian clock (2000) Science, 288: 1013–1019.
2. Schwartz, MW, Woods, SC., Porte, D., Seeley, RJ., Baskin, DG. Central nervous system control of food intake. (2000) Nature 404:661–671.
3. Shiromani, PJ. Sleep circuitry, regulation and function: Lessons from c-fos, leptin and timeless. In: Progress in Psychobiology and Physiological Psychology, Edited by A. Morrison and C. Fluharty, Academic Press, San Diego, pp. 67–90, 1998.
4. Pace-Shot, E., Hobson, JA., The neurobiology of sleep: Genetics, cellular physiology and subcortical networks (2002) Nat Rev 3: 591–605.
5. Sheng M, Greenberg ME The regulation and function of c-fos and other immediate early genes in the nervous system. Neuron 4:477–485.(1990)
6. De Lecea L, Kilduff TS, Peyron C, Gao X, Foye PE, Danielson PE, Fukuhara C, Battenberg EL, Gautvik VT , Bartlett FS, Frankel WN, Van den Pol AN, Bloom FE, Gautvik KM, Sutcliffe JG (1998) The hypocretins: hypothalamus-specific peptides with neuroexcitatory activity. Proc.Natl.Acad.Sci.U.S.A. 95:322–327.
7. Peyron C, Tighe DK, Van den Pol AN, De Lecea L, Heller HC, Sutcliffe JG, Kilduff TS (1998) Neurons containing hypocretin (orexin) project to multiple neuronal systems. J Neurosci 18:9996–10015.
8. Sakurai T, Amemiya A, Ishii M, Matsuzaki I, Chemelli RM, Tanaka H, Williams SC, Richarson JA, Kozlowski GP, Wilson S, Arch JR, Buckingham RE, Haynes AC, Carr SA, Annan RS, McNulty DE, Liu WS, Terrett JA, Elshourbagy NA, Bergsma DJ, Yanagisawa M (1998) Orexins and orexin receptors: a family of hypothalamic neuropeptides and G protein–coupled receptors that regulate feeding behavior. Cell 92:573–585.
9. Kilduff TS, Peyron C (2000) The hypocretin/orexin ligand-receptor system: implications for sleep and sleep disorders. Trends Neurosci 23: 359–365.
10. Lin L, Faraco J, Li R, Kadotani H, Rogers W, Lin X, Qiu X, deJong PJ, Nishini S, Mignot E (1999) The sleep disorder canine narcolepsy is caused by a mutation in the hypocretin (orexin) receptor 2 gene. Cell 98:365–376.
11. Chemelli RM, Willie JT, Sinton CM, Elmquist JK, Scammell T, Lee C, Richardson JA, Williams SC, Xiong Y, Kisanuki Y, Fitch TE, Nakazato M, Hammer RE, Saper CB, Yanagisawa M (1999) Narcolepsy in orexin knockout mice: molecular genetics of sleep regulation. Cell 98:437–451.
12. Hara J, Beuckmann CT, Nambu T, Willie JT, Chemelli RM, Sinton CM, Sugiyama F, Yagami K, Goto K, Yanagisawa M, Sakurai T (2001) Genetic ablation of orexin neurons in mice results in narcolepsy, hypophagia, and obesity. Neuron 30(2):345–354.
13. Gerashchenko, D., Kohls, M.D., Greco, M., Waleh, N.S., Salin-Pascual, R., Kilduff, T.S., Lappi, D.A., Shiromani, P.J., 2001. Hypocretin-2–saporin lesions of the lateral hypothalamus produce narcoleptic-like sleep behavior in the rat. J. Neurosci. 21, 7273–7283.
14. Peyron C, Faraco J, Rogers W, Ripley B, Overeem S, Charnay Y, Nevsimalova S, Aldrich M, Reynolds D, Albin R, Li R, Hungs M,Pedrazzoli M, Padigaru M, Kucherlapati M, Fan J, Maki R, Lammers GJ,Bouras C, Kucherlapati R, Nishino S, Mignot E. (2000) A mutation in a case of early onset narcolepsy and a generalized absence of hypocretin peptides in human narcoleptic brains. Nat Med. 6: 991–997.

15. Thannickal T, Moore, RY, Nienhuis R, Ramanathan L, Gulyani S, Aldrich M, Cornford, M, Siegel, JM. (2000) Reduced number of hypocretin neurons in human narcolepsy. Neuron 27: 460–474.

16. Nishino S, Ripley B, Overeem S, Lammers GJ, Mignot E (2000) Hypocretin (orexin) deficiency in human narcolepsy. Lancet 355:39–40.

17. Greco MA, Lu J, Wagner D, Shiromani PJ (2000) C-Fos expression in the cholinergic basal forebrain after enforced wakefulness and recovery sleep. Neuroreport 11(3):437–440.

18. Scammell TE, Estabrooke IV, McCarthy MT, Chemelli RM, Yanagisawa M, Miller MS, Saper CB (2000) Hypothalamic arousal regions are activated during modafinil-induced wakefulness. J Neurosci. 20(22):8620–8628.

19. Estabrooke, IV, McCarthy, MT, Ko, K., Chou, TC., Chemelli, RM., Yanagisawa, M., Saper, CB., Scammell, TE., Fos expression in orexin neurons varies with behavioral state. (2001) J Neurosci 21:1656–1662.

20. Basheer, R., Sherin, J., Morgan, J, Saper, C, McCarley, RW, Shiromani, PJ. Decline in c-Fos associated with sleep. J Neurosci, 17:9746–9750, 1997

21. Shiromani PJ, Basheer R, Thakkar J, Wagner D, Greco MA, Charness ME. Sleep and wakefulness in *c-fos* and *fos B* gene knockout mice. Mol Brain Res, 80: 75–87, 2000.

22. Greco, MA, McCarley, RW and Shiromani, PJ. Choline acetyltransferase mRNA is increased during sleep in the basal forebrain of rats. Neuroscience, 93: 1369–1374, 1999.

23. Fujiki N, Yoshida Y, Ripley B, Honda K, Mignot E, Nishino S. Changes in CSF hypocretin-1 (orexin A) levels in rats across 24 hours and in response to food deprivation. Neuroreport, 2001; 12: 993–997.

24. Yoshida Y, Fujiki N, Nakajima T, Ripley B, Matsumura H, Yoneda H, Mignot E, Nishino S. Fluctuation of extracellular hypocretin-1 (orexin A) levels in the rat in relation to the light-dark cycle and sleep-wake activities. Eur.J.Neurosci., 2001; 14: 1075–1081.

25. Parmentier, R., Ohtsu, H., Djebbara-Hannas, Z., Valatx, JL., Watanabe, T., Lin, JS., Anatomical, physiology and pharmacological characteristics of histidine decarboxylase knock-out mice: evidence for the role of histamine in behavioral and sleep-wake control. (2002) J Neurosci 22: 7695–7711.

26. Scammell T, Gerashchenko D, Urade Y, Onoe H, Saper C, Hayaishi O. Activation of ventrolateral preoptic neurons by the somnogen prostaglandin D2 (1998). PNAS (U S A) 95:7754–7759.

27. Cirelli, C, Tononi, G. Differences in gene expression between sleep and waking as revealed by mRNA differential display.(1998) *Mol.Brain Res.* 56:293–305.

28. Cirelli, C, Tononi, G. Differences in gene expression during sleep and wakefulness. Ann Med 31 (2):117–124, 1999.

29. Nauta JH (1946) Hypothalamic regulation of sleep in rats. An experimental study. J Neurophysiol 9:285–316.

30. Lucas EA, Sterman MB (1975) Effect of a forebrain lesion on the polycyclic sleep-wake cycle and sleep-wake patterns in the cat. Exp Neurol 46: 368–388.

31. Szymusiak R, McGinty D (1986) Sleep suppression following kainic acid–induced lesions of the basal forebrain. Exp Neurol 94: 598–614.

31. Sallanon M, Denoyer M, Kitahama K, Aubert C, Gay N, Jouvet M (1989) Long-lasting insomnia induced by preoptic neuron lesions and its transient reversal by muscimol injection into the posterior hypothalamus in the cat. Neuroscience 32: 669–683.

32. Shoham S, Blatteis CM, Krueger JM (1989) Effects of preoptic area lesions on muramyl dipeptide-induced sleep and fever. Brain Res. 476(2):396–399.

33. Asala SA, Okano Y, Honda K, Inoue S (1990) Effects of medial preoptic area lesions on sleep and wakefulness in unrestrained rats. Neurosci Lett 114: 300–304.

34. John J, Kumar VM, Gopinath G, Ramesh V, Mallick H (1994) Changes in sleep-wakefulness after kainic acid lesion of the preoptic area in rats. Jpn J Physiol 44: 231–242.

35. Alam MN, Mallick BN (1990) Differential acute influence of medial and lateral preoptic areas on sleep-wakefulness in freely moving rats. Brain Res Brain Res 525: 242–248.

36. Sterman MB, Clemente C (1962) Forebrain inhibitory mechanisms: sleep patterns induced by basal forebrain stimulation in the behaving cat. Exp Neurol 6: 103–117.

37. Sterman MB, Clemente C (1962) Forebrain inhibitory mechanisms: cortical synchronization induced by basal forebrain stimulation. Exp Neurol 6: 9–102.

38. Eguchi K, Satoh T (1980) Characterization of the neurons in the region of solitary tract nucleus during sleep. Physiol Behav 24: 99–102.

39. Szymusiak R, McGinty D (1986) Sleep-related neuronal discharge in the basal forebrain of cats. Brain Res 370: 82–92.

40. Kaitin K (1984) Preoptic area unit activity during sleep and wakefulness in the cat. Exp Neurol 83: 347–351.

41. Findlay ALR, Hayward JN (1969) Spontaneous activity of single neurones in the hypothalamus of rabbits during sleep and waking. J Physiol 201: 237–258.

42. Koyama Y, Hayaishi O (1994) Modulation by prostaglandins of activity of sleep-related neurons in the preoptic/anterior hypothalamic areas in rats. Brain Res Bull 33: 367–372.

43. Sherin JE, Shiromani PJ, McCarley RW, Saper CB (1996) Activation of ventrolateral preoptic neurons during sleep. Science 271: 216–219.

44. Gong, H., Szymusiak, R., King, J., Steininger, T., D. McGinty. Sleep-related c-Fos protein expression in the preoptic hypothalamus: effects of ambient warming. Am J Physiol Regul Integr Comp Physiol 279 (6):R2079–R2088, 2000.

45. Sherin, JE., Elmquist, JK., Torrealba, F., Saper, CB. Innervation of histaminergic tuberomammillary neurons by GABAergic and galaninergic neurons in the ventrolateral preoptic neurons of the rats. J Neurosci 18:4705–4721, 1998.

46. Szymusiak R, Alam MN, Steininger TL, McGinty D (1998) Sleep-waking discharge patterns of ventrolateral preoptic/anterior hypothalamic neurons in rats. Brain Res 803: 178–188.

47. Lu, J, Greco, MA, Shiromani, PJ, Saper, CB. Ibotenic acid lesions of the VLPO produce insomnia, J Neurosci 20: 3830–3842, 2000.

48. Gallopin T, Fort P, Eggermann E, Cauli B, Luppi P-H, Rossier J, Audino MG, Muhlethaler M, Serafin M (2000) Identification of sleep-promoting neurons in vitro. Nature 404: 992–995.

49. Steriade M, McCarley RW (1990). Brain Stem Control of Wakefulness and Sleep. New York: Plenum Press.

50. Nitz D. and Siegel J.. GABA release in the dorsal raphe nucleus: role in the control of REM sleep. Am J Physiol 273 (1 Pt 2):R451–R455, 1997.

51. Shiromani P, Gillin JC, Henriksen SH. Acetylcholine and the regulation of REM sleep: basic mechanisms and clinical implication for affective illness and narcolepsy. Annu Rev Pharmacol Toxicol 27: 137–156, 1987.

52. Merchant-Nancy, H., Vázquez, J. Aguilar-Roblero, R. R. Drucker-Colín. C-*fos* proto-oncogene changes in relation to REM sleep duration. *Brain Res.* 579:342–346, 1992.

53. Maloney, KJ., Mainville, L., Jones, BE. Differential c-Fos expression in cholinergic, monoaminergic, and GABAergic cell groups of the pontomesencephalic tegmentum after paradoxical sleep deprivation and recovery (1999) J. Neurosci. 1999 19: 3057–3072.

54. Shiromani, PJ, Kilduff, TC, Bloom, FE, McCarley, RW. Cholinergically-induced REM sleep triggers Fos-like immunoreactivity in dorsolateral pontine regions associated with REM sleep. Brain Res, 580:351–357, 1992.

55. Shiromani, PJ, Malik, M, Winston, S, McCarley, RW. Time course of Fos-like immunoreactivity associated with cholinergically-induced REM sleep. J Neurosci, 15:3500–3508, 1995.

56. Yamuy, J., Mancillas, JR., Morales, FR, Chase, MH. C-fos expression in the pons and medulla of the cat during carbachol-induced active sleep. J Neurosci 13:2703–2718, 1993.

57. Maloney, KJ., Mainville, L., Jones, BE. C-Fos expression in GABAergic, serotonergic, and other neurons of the pontomedullary reticular formation and raphe after paradoxical sleep deprivation and recovery J. Neurosci. 2000 20: 4669–4679.

58. Shiromani, PJ, Winston, S, and McCarley, RW. Pontine cholinergic neurons show Fos-like immunoreactivity associated with cholinergically-induced REM sleep. Mol Brain Res 38:77–84, 1996.

59. Boutrel, B., Franc B., Hen R., Hamon M., and Adrien J. Key Role of 5–HT1B receptors in the regulation of paradoxical sleep as evidenced in 5–HT1B knock-out mice. J Neurosci 19: 3204–3212; 1999

60. Greenspan RJ, Tononi G, Cirelli C, Shaw PJ (2001) Sleep and the fruit fly. Trends Neurosci 24: 142–145.

61. Hendricks JC, Finn SM, Panckeri KA, Chavkin J, Williams JA, Sehgal A, Pack AI (1999) Rest in *Drosophila* is a sleep-like state. Neuron 25: 129–138.

62. Shaw, PJ., Cirelli, C., Greenspan, RJ., and Tononi, G. Correlates of sleep and waking in *Drosophila melanogaster*. Science 287: 1834–1837, 2000.

63. Hendricks JC, Williams JA, Panckeri K, Kirk D, Tello M, Yin JC, Sehgal A (2001) A noncircadian role for cAMP signaling and CREB activity in *Drosophila* rest homeostasis. Nat Neurosci 4: 1108–1115.

64. Cirelli C, Pompeiano M, Tononi G (1996) Neuronal gene expression in the waking state—a role for the locus coeruleus. Science 274: 1211–1215.

65. Shaw PJ, Tononi G, Greenspan RJ, Robinson DF (2002) Stress response genes protect against lethal effects of sleep deprivation in *Drosophila*. Nature 417: 287–291.

66. Porkka-Heiskanen T, Strecker RE, Thakkar M, Bjorkum AA, Greene RW, McCarley RW (1997) Adenosine: a mediator of the sleep-inducing effects of prolonged wakefulness. Science 276: 1265–1266.

67. Hayaishi O (2002) Invited Review: Molecular genetic studies on sleep-wake regulation, with special emphasis on the prostaglandin D(2) system. J Appl Physiol 92: 863–868.

68. Basheer R, Rainnie DG, Porkka-Heiskanen T, Ramesh V, McCarley RW (2001) Adenosine, prolonged wakefulness, and A1–activated NF-kappaB DNA binding in the basal forebrain of the rat. Neuroscience 104: 731–739.

69. Storch KF, Lipan O, Leykin I, Viswanathan N, Davis FC, Wong WH, Weitz CJ (2002) Extensive and divergent circadian gene expression in liver and heart. Nature; 417(6884):78–83

20

Mood Changes

CAMELLIA P. CLARK

University of California–San Diego, San Diego, California, U.S.A.

This chapter will focus primarily on effects of sleep deprivation (SD) on mood in healthy control subjects, since the antidepressant effects of SD (Chap. 21) and the effects of SD in other psychiatric conditions (Chap. 22) are covered elsewhere in this volume.

I. Continuous Sleep Deprivation

In contrast to antidepressant effects seen in up to 60% of depressed patients following partial SD or total SD (TSD) for one night, mood effects in healthy persons are generally of an uncomfortable or dysphoric nature when the individuals experience TSD for long periods of time.

Prolonged SD may precipitate perceptual distortions and illusions (usually visual) and, occasionally, paranoia. Following 112 hr of TSD, 7 of 350 subjects reportedly "experienced temporary states resembling acute paranoid schizophrenia" (1), although the older literature often contains vague diagnostic and syndromal impressions (if any) and does not always clearly differentiate between perceptual disturbances and full-blown waking hallucinations. Mood changes commonly include increased sleepiness, fatigue, irritability, difficulty concentrating, disorientation (2), and "dysphoria" (3). One night of TSD produced increased tension, confusion, and fatigue subscores on the Profile of Mood States (POMS) and worsening on the hostility and anxiety scales of the Multiple Affect Adjective Check List (4). However, the experimenters observed euphoria, talkativeness, increased activity, and greater socialization at approximately 4:30 A.M. to 6:00 A.M., prompting speculation of a circadian effect (5). In another study of one night's TSD, subjects were observed to decrease activity, "try to keep at rest," and "shut themselves off from all problems", including more primitive responses and less cognitive flexibility on a test of decision making and problem solving (6).

In interpreting such results, a number of factors related to the particular study paradigm and the individual subject must be considered. In a TSD study of healthy 80-year-olds and 20-year-olds, mood and performance on a vigilance task showed less deterioration in the old than in the young. Interestingly, the young group was more sleepy (as measured by the Multiple Sleep Latency Test) than the elders, raising the question of a preexisting chronic sleep deficit in this college-aged group. Alternatively, the octogenarians may have possessed an as-yet-unidentified biological resilience factor (7). In a 72-hr SD study, mood changes included "waking dreams", confusion, and decreased motivation for experimental and leisure activities, with a prominent circadian component of the mood effects as well (8).

Other factors that may influence the measures of SD in normal controls include the investigator's and subject's preconceived hypotheses or expectations. If the investigators or subjects anticipate that SD will either induce or ameliorate psychiatric signs and symptoms, the study may be biased by self-fulfilling prophecies. In addition, the subjects' response may be influenced by support or attitudes from fellow subjects or staff.

II. Effects of Sleep Disruption and Deficiency

The previous section is only a sample of the importance of human SD studies based on varying durations of TSD. While similar situations arise particularly in some occupations (e.g., military maneuvers), the problems of sleep disruption and fragmentation (by noise and other factors) and of chronically obtaining insufficient sleep in our increasingly busy culture are far more common and more likely to have major public health impacts.

One experiment involved awakening healthy subjects with noise after *every minute* of electroencephalographic sleep for two consecutive nights. Levels of sleepiness, unhappiness, and unclear thinking as measured by the Clyde mood scale showed significant worsening; mood and performance changes were described as similar to changes associated with 40–64 hr of TSD. While recognizing that this method of sleep fragmentation is not identical to apneic episodes, the authors suggested that this was a reasonable approximation of sleep and functional loss in severe sleep apnea (9).

Another paradigm featured restricting healthy young adults to 4–5 hr of sleep per night for a week, which was comparable to 50% of preferred sleep duration or 67% of habitual sleep time. Significant worsening in fatigue/vigor, confusion, and tension (POMS) subscales developed. Recovery from these deficits appeared to require two whole nights of sleep (10).

III. Personality Factors Affecting Response to Sleep Deprivation

Normal subjects with an internal locus of control, e.g., those with a strong belief that they can influence their situation, experienced less total mood disturbance than with subjects with an external locus of control, e.g. those whose thoughts and feelings are more influenced by external circumstances (11,12). Neuroticism and extroversion also correlated with mood disturbances (12), consistent with data that subjects whose mood changed most were "in general…the more conflict ridden, loosely defended neurotics" (13) and that extroverts are more susceptible than introverts to environmental motivating factors (14).

IV. Sleep Deprivation in Children and Adolescents

Disturbed and/or deficient sleep is becoming a public health problem at progressively earlier ages. An epidemiological study of students 9–14 years old found that sleep quality showed strong negative correlations with neurotic and neurosomatic complaints. Not surprisingly, better sleep was linked with more openness to teachers' influences, better self-image, and greater achievement, motivation, and self-control (15). Another study randomized children 8–15 years old to 4 or 10 hr of sleep for a night. Although sleep restriction did not increase hyperactivity or impulsivity, it definitely decreased attentiveness and increased sleepiness (16).

V. Interaction Between Emotional Response to Sleep Deprivation and Performance

This complex topic has far-reaching implications for a variety of work, education, and safety issues.

Based on projective testing using a modified Thematic Apperception Test, subjects appeared to deal with SD-induced sleepiness by denial in the absence of increased repression of themes not related to sleep (17). This is consistent with college students' lack of awareness of SD on their cognitive performance (18) as well as effects of 29–50 hr of TSD on suggestibility, accuracy, and confidence. In the latter study, subjects were aware of their deteriorating performance on "pure" cognitive paradigms, e.g., logical reasoning and Raven's matrices, which might lead sleep-deprived subjects to proceed with extra caution in "real world" situations. However, they became measurably more suggestible, "maintained confidence in their suggestible responses, and were inaccurate when responding with the highest rating of confidence." Since the suggestibility test involved a simulated topic of court testimony (e.g., a boy in a bicycle accident), the authors expressed great concern for the effects of SD on eyewitness accuracy, particularly given that jurors are influenced greatly by individual witnesses' degrees of confidence (19). Finally, a pilot study of a new scale, Evaluation of Risks, designed to measure psychological and behavioral variables in naturalistic and military settings, revealed that pilots showed increased impulsivity near the end of a long night flight (approximately 26 hr continuously awake); they noted that this could be dangerous in combat and other hazardous situations (20).

VI. Mechanisms of Mood Response to Sleep Deprivation: Potential Clues from Animal and Pharmacology Studies

A. REM Sleep Deprivation in Animals

REM SD increases movement, grooming, appetite, sexual activity, aggression, self-stimulation, and diminishes fear and anxiety in various paradigms (21). Following 96 hr of REM SD, norepinephrine concentrations in the lateral hypothalamus of rats correlated positively with food intake and performance on the Porsolt test, which measures "ability to cope with stress" and is often regarded as an animal model of antidepressant effects (22).

B. Human Pharmacology

After 48 hr of TSD in healthy men, doses up to 20 mg of *d*-amphetamine *briefly* reversed SD-induced changes in the vigor/fatigue subscale of the POMS; together with physiological measures, the authors concluded that this time course was consistent with initial catecholamine release by *d*-amphetamine (23).

In another study of healthy subjects combining 40.5 hr of TSD with catecholamine depletion by α-methylparatyrosine (AMPT), both SD and AMPT increased sleepiness and decreased alertness ratings, with a synergistic effect. Mood ratings did not change significantly with TSD or AMPT alone, but the combination produced increases in tension, depression, and anger as measured by the POMS (24).

Tryptophan depletion in patients with primary insomnia produced negative impacts on polysomnographic variables, e.g., increased % stage 1, decreased % stage 2, and increased REM density without concomitant mood changes (25).

In a study of healthy controls, patients with current major depression, and subjects with primary insomnia, norepinephrine levels were increased throughout the night only in the insomnia group. Impairments of sleep efficiency correlated with elevated norepinephrine in the insomniacs only (26).

VII. Areas for Future Study

Just as it is unlikely that one neurotransmitter is responsible for the antidepressant effects of SD, it is unlikely that changes in one neurotransmitter account for the many mood changes in normal subjects in response to SD. Studies of various forms of SD in animals have demonstrated functional changes in most of the major neurotransmitters as well as circadian variation in function of some neurotransmitters (27). However, the above information is consistent with important roles for norepinephrine. Given dopaminergic mediation of basic "drives" and the reward system, involvement of dopamine is also likely. Both chemicals are consistent with increased alertness associated with catecholaminergic agents such as amphetamines.

Further understanding of the neurobiological underpinnings of mood, behavioral, and sleepiness changes following SD may eventually lead to better treatments for insomnia, ways to make sleep loss safer where it cannot be avoided (e.g., physicians on call), and ways to compensate for SD-induced changes in function. Meanwhile, finding ways for more of the population to obtain more sleep regularly is a formidable but vital challenge.

Dedication

To Chris Gillin, M.D.—Mentor, Collaborator, Hero, Friend.

References

1. Tyler DB. Psychological changes during experimental sleep deprivation. Dis Ner System 1955; 16:293–299.
2. Johnson LC. physiological and psychological changes following total sleep deprivation. In: Kales A, editor. Sleep Physiology and Pathology. Philadelphia: JB Lippincott, 1969: 206–220.
3. Gerner TH, Post RM, Gillin JC, Bunney WE Jr. Biological and behavioral effects of one night sleep deprivation in depressed patients and normals. J Psychiatr Res 1979; 15:21–40.
4. Zuckerman M, Lubin B, Robins S. Validation of the multiple affect adjective check list in clinical situations. J Consult Psychol 1965; 29(6):594.
5. Cutler NR, Cohen HB. The effect of one night's sleep loss on mood and memory in normal subjects. Compr Psychiatry 1979; 20(1):61–66.
6. Vein AM, Dallakyan IG, Levin YI, Skakun KE. Physiological and psychological consequences of single sleep deprivation. Hum Physiol Vol 8(6) 1983; 392–396.
7. Brendel DH, Reynolds CF, III, Jennings JR, Hoch CC, Monk TH, Berman SR et al. Sleep stage physiology, mood, and vigilance responses to total sleep deprivation in healthy 80–year-olds and 20–year- olds. Psychophysiology 1990; 27:677–686.
8. Mikulincer M, Babkoff H, Caspy T, Sing H. The effects of 72 hr of sleep loss on psychological variables. Br J Psychol 1989; 80:145–162.

9. Bonnet MH. Effect of sleep disruption on sleep, performance, and mood. Sleep 1985; 8(1):11–19.

10. Dinges DF, Pack F, Williams K, Gillen KA, Powell JW, Ott GE et al. Cumulative sleepiness, mood disturbance, and psychomotor vigilance performance decrements during a week of sleep restricted to 4–5 hours per night. Sleep 1997; 20(4):267.

11. Hill DW, Welch JE, Godfrey JA3. Influence of locus of control on mood state disturbance after short-term sleep deprivation. Sleep 1996; 19:41–46.

12. Blagrove M, Akehurst L. Personality and the modulation of effects of sleep loss on mood and cognition. Indiv Diff 30(5) 2001; 819–828.

13. Loveland NT, Singer MT. Projective test assessment of the effects of sleep deprivation. J Proj Tech 23 1959; 323–334.

14. Furnham A, Forde L, Ferrari K. Personality and work motivation. Pers Indiv Diff Vol 26(6) 1999; 1035–1043.

15. Meijer AM, Habekothe HT, Van Den Wittenboer GL. Time in bed, quality of sleep and school functioning of children. J Sleep Res 2000; 9(2):145–153.

16. Fallone G, Acebo C, Arnedt JT, Seifer R, Carskadon MA. Effects of acute sleep restriction on behavior, sustained attention, and response inhibition in children. Percept Mot Skills 2001; 93(1):213–229.

17. Murray EJ. Conflict and repression during sleep deprivation. Journal of Abnormal & Social Psychology 59 1959; 95–101.

18. Pilcher JJ, Walters AS. How sleep deprivation affects psychological variables related to college students' cognitive performance. J Am Coll Health 1997; 46(3):121–126.

19. Blagrove M, Akehurst L. Effects of sleep loss on confidence-accuracy relationships for reasoning and eyewitness memory. J Exp Psychol: App 6(1) 2000; 59–73.

20. Sicard B, Jouve E, Blin O. Risk propensity assessment in military special operations. Mil–Med 2001; 166(10):871–874.

21. Vogel GW. Evidence for REM sleep deprivation as the mechanism of action of anti-depressant drugs. Prog Neuropsychopharmacol Biol Psychiatry 1983; 7:343–349.

22. Brock JW, Farooqui SM, Ross KD, Payne S, Prasad C. Stress-related behavior and central norepinephrine concentrations in the REM sleep–deprived rat. Physiol Behav 1994; 55:997–1003.

23. Newhouse PA, Belenky G, Thomas M, Thorne D, Sing HC, Fertig J. The effects of *d*-amphetamine on arousal, cognition, and mood after prolonged total sleep deprivation. Neuropsychopharmacology 1989; 2:153–164.

24. McCann UD, Penetar DM, Shaham Y, Thorne DR, Sing HC, Thomas ML et al. Effects of catecholamine depletion on alertness and mood in rested and sleep deprived normal volunteers. Neuropsychopharmacology 1993; 8:345–356.

25. Riemann D, Feige B, Hornyak M, Koch S, Hohagen F, Voderholzer U. The tryptophan depletion test: impact on sleep in primary insomnia–a pilot study. Psychiatry Res 2002; 109(2):129–135.

26. Irwin M, Clark C, Kennedy B, Gillin JC, Ziegler M. Nocturnal catecholamines and immune function in insomniacs, depressed patients and control subjects. Brain Behav Immun 2002; 17:365–372.

27. Wirz-Justice A, Tobler I, Kafka MS, Naber D, Marangos PJ, Borbely AA et al. Sleep deprivation: effects on circadian rhythms of rat brain neurotransmitter receptors. Psychiatry Res 1981; 5(1):67–76.

21

Antidepressant Effects

JOSEPH C. WU

University of California–Irvine, Irvine, California, U.S.A.

MONTE BUCHSBAUM

Mount Sinai School of Medicine, New York, New York, U.S.A.

WILLIAM BUNNEY

University of California–Irvine, Irvine, California, U.S.A.

J. CHRISTIAN GILLIN

Veterans Administration Medical Center and University of
California–San Diego, San Diego, California, U.S.A.

I. Introduction

Sleep deprivation (SD) is an effective and rapid antidepressant in a subset of depressed patients (1). The antidepressant and cerebral metabolic effects of total sleep deprivation (TSD) or partial sleep deprivation (PSD) for one night have been studied with functional neuroimaging. Despite the variations in methods and techniques, the overall findings were relatively consistent. First, in most studies, before SD, responders have significantly elevated metabolism compared with nonresponders and normal controls, in the orbital medial prefrontal cortex and especially the ventral portions of the anterior cingulate cortex. Second, after SD these hyperactive areas normalize in the responders. Ebert and colleagues (2) first reported this finding in a single photon emission computed tomography (SPECT) scan study of 10 patients (Table 1). Wu and colleagues (3) first reported this finding of higher glucose metabolic rate with PET scans in depressed responders in 1992. This initial finding was subsequently extended to a larger group of depressed patients (4). We reported that depressed responders were higher at baseline in the medial prefrontal cortex, ventral anterior cingulate, and posterior subcallosal gyrus than depressed nonresponders. However, Smith et al. (5) noted that geriatric depressed patients did not show higher anterior cingulate activity than normal controls prior to SD. One functional imaging study suggested that synaptic dopamine release was associated with the antidepressant effects of TSD;

the neurochemical implications of this finding are explored and possible neuro-transmitter mechanisms are discussed.

II. Metabolic Activity in Specific Brain Regions in Depressed Sleep Deprivation Responders

The anterior cingulate has been hypothesized to play a significant role in affect and cognition (6). The anterior cingulate can be subdivided into several regions including the infralimbic or posterior subcallosal region (BA25) which is considered the cortical center of the autonomic nervous system, which may regulate visceral motor response to stressful behavioral or emotional events. Afferents to the infralimbic regions include the amygdala, the hypothalamus, and the thalamic paraventricular nucleus.

To summarize all the findings from functional imaging studies [positron emission tomography (PET) or single photon emission computed tomography (SPECT) with hexamethylproplyeneamine oxime (HMPAO), or functional megnatic resonance imaging (fMRI) (Table 1)], five different groups with a total of six published studies reported that responders had increased relative localized metabolic activity in the general location of the ventral anterior cingulate cortex (ACC) compared with nonresponders or normal controls at baseline (2–4,7–9). In the two groups that did not report this finding, Volk and colleagues (10) did not examine subcortical areas in their 1992 study, and Smith and colleagues (5), with only six patientsm, could not compare responders and nonresponders at baseline because all the patients tended to improve. Smith later expanded her study to 12 depressed patients and did not find the increased activity in the anterior cingulate of geriatric depressed patients compared to controls. Also, all six studies in which five groups compared patients both pre- and post-sleep deprivation reported that clinical improvement was associated with normalization of increased activity in anterior cingulate/medial prefrontal regions (2–4,7–9). Consistent with this, in Smith's studies (5,11) the whole group improved and metabolic rate in the anterior cingulate decreased significantly after SD compared with baseline.

In four SD studies, clinical improvement correlated significantly with metabolic activity in specific areas. In 1992, Volk and colleagues (10) reported that the higher the baseline HMPAO perfusion in the orbitofrontal region and left temporal cortex prior to PSD, the greater the clinical improvement after PSD. Limbic structures were not studied. In 1997, using multiple regression, Volk and colleagues (7) reported a somewhat similar finding: the greater the HMPAO activity in the right orbitofrontal cingulate before PSD and in the left inferior temporal cortex after PSD, the greater the clinical improvement after PSD. In 1999, Wu and colleagues (4) reported that the greater the reduction in local cerebral glucose metabolic rate (LCGMR) in left medial prefrontal cortex and the greater the increase in the left temporal cortex, the greater the clinical improvement in clinical ratings post-TSD compared to pre-TSD ratings. Smith and colleagues (11) noted that a decrease in the right anterior cingulate was correlated with a decrease in the Hamilton depression scale score for TSD as well as for medication treatment with paroxetine.

Some but not all functional imaging studies with antidepressant medications have reported similar findings to those with TSD or PSD. Mayberg and colleagues (12) reported that metabolic activity in the ventral anterior cingulate was elevated before treatment and reduced after clinical improvement in responders to antidepressant medications. Drevets (13) also noted that there was increased activity in the medial orbital cortex and an increase in subgenual prefrontal cortex when corrected for volume. Buchsbaum and colleagues (14) also noted that the antidepressant benefit of sertraline was a decrease in cingulate metabolism in depressed patients.

III. Role of Neurotransmitter Systems in the Antidepressant Effects of Sleep Deprivation

Reduced neurotransmission of dopamine and serotonin may be responsible for an elevated metabolic rate in anterior cingulate in responders compared with nonresponders at baseline. Mobilization of the dopamine and serotonin system could hypothetically be associated with decreased metabolism in the anterior cingulate seen in responders following SD. Both neuroanatomical and neurochemical evidence suggest that the anterior cingulate is innervated by both the dopamine and serotonin system.

A. Dopamine

Evidence from both animal and human studies suggests that SD activates the dopaminergic system (15,16). Human psychophysiological studies have been conducted using blink rate in depressed patients, retinal pigment epithelial light adaptation in Parkinson's disease patients, and light-adapted corneofundal potential in depressed responders, results of which are suggestive of increased dopaminergic function. In a study of TSD in depressed and normal control subjects, concentrations of homovallic acid (HVA), a metabolite of dopamine, in spinal fluid increased from pre- to post-SD in responders but not in nonresponders or controls (17). TSD also improved symptoms of rigidity, bradykinesia, and gait in patients with Parkinson's disease for 2 weeks; these intriguing findings suggest that the dopamine system is activated by sleep deprivation (18).

Other studies challenge the role of the dopamine system in the antidepressant effects of SD. Amineptine, a dopamine agonist, when administered 6 days prior to sleep deprivation blocked rather than enhanced the antidepressant effect of sleep (19). The possibility that amineptine blocked upregulation of D2 postsynaptic receptors in the responders has been suggested. A later study by Benedetti and colleagues (20) noted that amineptine administered contemporaneously with SD resulted in an enhancement of the beneficial aspects of sleep deprivation.

Table 1 Antidepressant and Cerebral Metabolic Effects of Total Sleep Deprivation

Author	Year (Ref)	No. of depressed patients	Depressed responder	Controls	Imaging	TSD or PSD	Findings
Ebert	1991 (2)	10	5	8	SPECT	TSD	All depressed hypoperfused in lt anterolateral prefrontal cortex before and after SD
							Resp show hyperperfusion in limbic system at baseline
							Resp show reduction in limbic region after SD
Volk	1992 (10)	20	11		SPECT	TSD	Resp show significant lt temporal and rt parietal increase after SD
Wu	1992 (3)	15	4	15	PET	TSD	Resp > nonresp or normal controls in cingulate metabolism
							Resp showed decrease in cingulate to normal levels after SD
Ebert	1994 (31)	20	11		SPECT	TSD	Resp > Nonresp in rt ant cing and rt and lt ofc perfusion at baseline
							Resp also hyperperfused in hippocampus at baseline
Ebert	1994 (21)	10	5		SPECT	TSD	Resp show significant decrease of D2 rec occupancy compared to nonresp after SD
Volk	1997 (7)	15	9		SPECT	PSD	Resp > Nonresp in rt ofc/basal ganglia perfusion at baseline
							Rt ofc/cing perfusion before PSD and left inf temporal perfusion after PSD were accurate predictors of change in Hamilton
Holthoff	1999 (8)	14	8		SPECT	TSD	Resp > nonresp in ant cing perfusion at baseline
							Resp show decrease in ant cing perfusion to normal levels after SD baseline, all pts show hypoperfusion in left prefrontal cortex vs. rt; responders show normalization upon remission

Author	Year (ref)	n	Method	n	Method	Type	Findings
Smith	1999 (5)	6	PET	6	PET	TSD	Depressed pts show reduction in ant cingulate (BA24) after SD Reduction persists after recovery sleep and after anti-depressant therapy
Wu	1999 (4)	36	PET	12	PET	TSD	Resp > nonresp in ant cingulate (BA24), medial prefrontal cortex (BA32), and posterior subcallosal gyrus (BA25) at baseline Resp decreases in medial prefrontal cortex (BA32) after SD
Clark	2001 (9)	2	fMRI	1	fMRI	PSD	Resp > nonresp larger perfusion covering ventral ant cing PSD decreased perfusion in responder's hyperperfused area but did not change nonresponder's scan
Smith	2002 (11)	12?	PET	9	PET	TSD	Rt. cing decrease with Hamilton decrease with TSD and with medication No ant cing increase at baseline between depressed patients and controls Depressed patients show increase at baseline in bilateral superior frontal gyrus Depressed patients show decrease in bilateral superior frontal gyrus with TSD and decreased Hamilton

SPECT, single-photon emission computed tomography; PET, positron emission tomography; fMRI, functional magnetic resonance imaging; TSD, total sleep deprivation; PSD, partial sleep deprivation; resp, responder; nonresp, nonresponder; ant cing, anterior cingulate; ofc, orbitofrontal cortex

Evidence for dopaminergic input into the cingulate cortex comes from retrograde tracing studies, dopamine synthetic enzymes, and electron microscopic studies of dopamine axon varicosities in the cingulate. PET evidence of a functional dopaminergic response, a dopamine two-receptor presence, and a dopamine transporter presence has also been found in the anterior cingulate.

Dopaminergic activity may inhibit absolute metabolic activity in the anterior cingulate. Both cocaine and amphetamine administration reduced the rate of cerebral glucose metabolism. If dopaminergic activity is inhibitory, then decreased dopaminergic firing in responders at baseline could disinhibit metabolic rate in the anterior cingulate. In another method, using SPECT with a D2 receptor ligand (IBZM), Ebert and colleagues (21) reported that responders had significantly greater displacement of the D2 ligand after SD compared to nonresponders, suggesting that SD mobilizes the dopaminergic system in responders.

B. Serotonin

Most metabolite studies, neuronal firing studies, and human pharmacological studies suggest that SD enhances the serotonergic system (22). 5-Hydroxyindoleacetic acid (5-HIAA) levels were increased after SD. Serotonergic dorsal raphe neuron activity was increased in cats after SD (23). Benedetti and colleagues (24) noted that the long variant of 5-hydroxytryptamine transporter (5-HTT) linked polymorphisms was associated with better mood amelioration with SD. The long variant is associated with increased density of the serotonin (5-hydroxytryptamine, 5-HT) transporter. Pindolol (a 5-HT_{1A} autoreceptor blocker) enhanced antidepressant response to TSD in bipolars and blocked short term relapse (25). TSD was facilitated by paroxetine in elderly depressed patients (26). Selective serotonin reuptake inhibitors (SSRIs) reduced anterior cingulate metabolism, and this reduction was correlated with improvement in obsessive-compulsive symptoms. Lithium, which has serotonergic properties, enhances the SD effect in in depressed individuals (27).

Other studies, including metabolite, neuroendocrine, and human clinical studies, provide conflicting evidence for how the serotonergic system is affected by sleep deprivation. Rapid tryptophan depletion, which decreases brain serotonin concentration, had no acute effect on the antidepressant benefits of SD (28). Tryptophan depletion actually prevented depressive relapse, suggesting that the serotonin system might contribute to depression. Rapid-eye-movement (REM) sleep deprivation in rats resulted in reduced serotonin and 5-HIAA in the frontal cortex (29). Citalopram-stimulated prolactin release was blunted after SD in healthy male subjects, suggesting downregulation of the serotonergic system with SD.

Serotonin transporters, serotonin receptors, serotonin synthetic enzymes, serotonin release, dorsal raphe afferents, and functional markers of response to serotonin (e.g., immediate early genes, metabolic PET response to serotonin) are present in the anterior cingulate. Fenfluramine increased metabolism in the anterior cingulate in normal controls, suggesting that the serotonin system activates anterior cingulate. If this relationship were true in depressed patients, then a decrease in anterior cingulate metabolism with SD would be associated with a decrease in the serotonin system.

C. Acetylcholine

The role of the cholinergic system in the antidepressant effects of sleep deprivation is basically unknown. Cholinergic projections from the brainstem initiate and help to maintain cortical arousal during wakefulness and REM sleep. Prolonged wakefulness would presumably enhance the duration of cholinergic neurotransmission. In addition to the cerebral cortex, the cingulate gyrus receives cholinergic input from the basal forebrain, but we are not aware of data implicating cholinergic mechanisms in SD in depressed patients. Nevertheless, the cholinergic-aminergic imbalance hypothesis suggests that depression results from an increased ratio of cholinergic-to-aminergic neurotransmission in critical areas of the brain.

IV. Conclusions

This chapter has focused on the role of dopamine and serotonin in the antidepressant effects of SD, largely because these are the neurotransmitters that have been implicated in the mechanism of action of current antidepressant medications and by aminergic hypotheses for the pathophysiology of depression. The studies reviewed herein provide some weak evidence suggesting an underactivation of serotonergic and dopaminergic activity at baseline in the anterior cingulate cortex of depressed responders. SD could increase serotonergic and dopaminergic neurotransmission in the anterior cingulate of depressed responders and might be responsible for the antidepressant benefits. Nevertheless, this hypothesis is far from proven. Even if the evidence were compelling, it might be very surprising since the antidepressant effects of SD occur much more rapidly than those of antidepressant drugs, electroconvulsive therapy, bright light therapy, psychotherapy, or other established antidepressant treatments. It is not uncommon to see as much antidepressant improvement in 6–12 hr of SD as that typically seen after 4–6 weeks of conventional antidepressant treatment. None of the established treatments, which presumably work through the aminergic systems, achieve significant antidepressant effects within hours or even days. There is no a priori reason to believe the antidepressant effects of sleep deprivation depend primarily on aminergic or cholinergic mechanisms. The rapid, dramatic, and in well-established evidence-based antidepressant effect of SD might lead the way the development of new paradigms for the mechanism of action of new treatments, such as drugs, that act quickly.

Functional imaging studies of sleep deprivation first suggested in 1991–1992 that elevated cerebral metabolism in the anterior cingulate gyrus was a predictor of antidepressant response; furthermore, clinical improvement was associated with decreased metabolic activity there. As reviewed here and elsewhere (30), all the functional brain imaging studies of sleep deprivation have shown these relatively consistent findings. As mentioned briefly, some but not all antidepressant medication studies with functional brain imaging have had results that are consistent with the SD findings. Whether or not all antidepressant treatments should fit this model remains to be seen, but it should not necessarily do so because different therapies may have quite different mechanisms of action. Nevertheless, these functional imaging studies of antidepressant therapies have identified localized areas within the medial orbital prefrontal cortex and anterior cingulate that are of great interest regarding the pathophysiology and management of depression. Subtyping of depressed patients using functional brain imaging is just beginning. Further research could eventually lead to more rapid categorization of depressed patients with potentially beneficial enhancement of the appropriate selection of treatment. The augmentation of sleep deprivation with agents that enhance serotonergic activity (e.g., lithium) or dopaminergic activity could potentially make sleep deprivation more clinically useful for the management of depression.

References

1. Wu JC, Bunney WE. The biological basis of an antidepressant response to sleep deprivation and relapse: review and hypothesis. Am J Psychiatry 1990; 147:14–21.
2. Ebert D, Feistel H, Barocka A. Effects of sleep deprivation on the limbic system and the frontal lobes in affective disorders: a study with Tc-99m-HMPAO SPECT. Psychiatry Res Neuroimaging 1991; 40:247–251.
3. Wu JC, Gillin JC, Buchsbaum MS, Hershey T, Johnson JC, Bunney WE Jr. Effect of sleep deprivation on brain metabolism of depressed patients. Am J Psychiatry 1992; 149, 538–543.
4. Wu J, Buchsbaum MS, Gillin JC, Tang C, Cadwell S, Wiegand M, Najafi A, Klein E, Hazen K, Bunney WE Jr. Prediction of antidepressant effects of sleep deprivation by metabolic rates in the ventral anterior cingulate and medial prefrontal cortex. Am J Psychiatry 1999; 156:1149–1158.
5. Smith GS, Reynolds CF III, Pollock B, Derbyshire S, Nofzinger E, Dew MA, Houck PR, Milko D, Meltzer CC, Kupfer DJ. Cerebral glucose metabolic response to combined total sleep deprivation and antidepressant treatment in geriatric depression. Am J Psychiatry 1999; 156:683–689.
6. Devinsky O, Morrell MJ, Vogt BA. Contributions of anterior cingulate cortex to behaviour. Brain 1995; 118:279–306.
7. Volk SA, Kaendler SH, Hertel A, Maul FD, Manoocheri R, Weber R, Georgi K, Pflug B, Hor G. Can response to partial sleep deprivation in depressed patients be predicted by regional changes of cerebral blood flow? Psychiatry Res 1997; 75:67–74.
8. Holthoff VA, Beuthien-Baumann B, Pietrzyk U, Pinkert J, Oehme L, Franke WG, Bach O. [Changes in regional cerebral perfusion in depression.SPECT monitoring of response to treatment]. Nervenarzt 1999; 70:620–626.
9. Clark CP, Frank LR, Brown GG. Sleep deprivation, EEG, and functional MRI in depression: preliminary results. Neuropsychopharmacology 2001; 25(2):S79–84.

10. Volk S, Kaendler SH, Weber R, Georgi K, Maul F, Hertel A, Pflug B, Hor G. Evaluation of the effects of total sleep deprivation on cerebral blood flow using single photon emission computerized tomography. Acta Psychiatr Scand 1992; 86:478–483

11. Smith GS, Reynolds CF, Houck PR, Dew MA, Ma Y, Mulsant BH Pollock BG. Glucose metabolic response to total sleep deprivation, recovery sleep, and acute antidepressant treatment as functional neuroanatomic correlates of treatment outcome in geriatric depression. Am J. Geriatr Psychiatry 2002; 10:561–568.

12. Mayberg HS, Brannan SK, Tekell JT, Silva A, Mahurin RK, McGinnis S, Jerabek PA. Regional metabolic effects of fluoxetine in major depression: serial changes and relationship to clinical response. Biol Psychiatry 2000; 48:830–843.

13. Drevets WC. Neuroimaging studies of mood disorders. Biol Psychiatry 2001; 48: 813–829.

14. Buchsbaum MS, Wu J, Siegel BV, Hackett E, Trenary M, Abel L, Reynolds C. Effect of sertraline on regional metabolic rate in patients with affective disorder. Biol Psychiatry 1997; 41:15–22.

15. Ebert D, Albert R, Hammon G, Strasser B, May A, Merz A. Eye-blink rates and depression. Is the antidepressant effect of sleep deprivation mediated by the dopamine system? Neuropsychopharmacology 1996; 15:332–339.

16. Ebert D. Sleep deprivation and dopamine: The psychostimulant theory of antidepressant sleep deprivation. Adv Biol Psychiatry New Models Depression 1998; 153–169.

17. Cohen LJ. Rational drug use in the treatment of depression. Am Fam Physician 1997; 17:45–61.

18. Parry BL, Curran ML, Stuenkel CA, Yokimozo M, Tam L, Powell KA, Gillin JC. Can critically timed sleep deprivation be useful in pregnancy and postpartum depressions? J Affective Disord 2000; 60:201–212.

19. Benedetti F, Barbini B, Campori E, Colombo C, Smeraldi E. Dopamine agonist amineptine prevents the antidepressant effect of sleep deprivation. Psychiatry Res 1996; 65:179–184.

20. Benedetti F, Campori E, Barbini B, Fulgosi MC, Colombo C. Dopaminergic augmentation of sleep deprivation effects in bipolar depression. Psychiatry Res 2001; 104:239–246.

21. Ebert D, Feistel H, Kaschka W, Barocka A, Pirner A. Single photon emission computerized tomography assessment of cerebral dopamine D2 receptor blockade in depression before and after sleep deprivation—preliminary results. Biol Psychiatry 1994; 35:880–885.

22. Asikainen M, Toppila J, Alanko L, Ward DJ, Stenberg D, Porkka-Heiskanen T. Sleep deprivation increases brain serotonin turnover in the rat. Neuroreport 1997; 8:1577–1582.

23. Gardner JP, Fornal CA, and Jacobs BL. Effects of sleep deprivation on serotonergic neuronal activity in the dorsal raphe nucleus of the freely moving cat. Neuropsychopharmacology 1997; 17:72–81.

24. Benedetti F, Serretti A, Colombo C, Campori E, Barbini B, di Bella D, Smeraldi E. Influence of a functional polymorphism within the promoter of the serotonin transporter gene on the effects of total sleep deprivation in bipolar depression. Am J Psychiatry 1999; 156:1450–1452.

25. Smeraldi E, Benedetti F, Barbini B, Campori E, Colombo C. Sustained antidepressant effect of sleep deprivation combined with pindolol in bipolar depression: a placebo-controlled trial. Neuropsychopharmacology 1999; 20:380–385.

26. Bump GM, Reynolds CF, Smith G, Pollock BG, Dew MA, Mazumdar S, Geary M, Houck PR, Kupfer DJ. Accelerating response in geriatric depression: a pilot study combining sleep deprivation and paroxetine. Depress Anxiety 1997; 6:113–118.

27. Benedetti F, Colombo C, Barbini B, Campori E, Smeraldi E. Ongoing lithium treatment prevents relapse after total sleep deprivation. J. Clin Psychopharmacol 1999; 19:240–245.

28. Neumeister A, Praschak-Rieder N, Hesselmann B, Vitouch O, Rauh M, Barocka A, Tauscher J, Kasper S. Effects of tryptophan depletion in drug-free depressed patients who responded to total sleep deprivation. Arch Gen Psychiatry 1998; 55:167–172.

29. Borbely AA, Steigrad P, Tobler I. Effect of sleep deprivation on brain serotonin in the rat. Behav Brain Res 1980; 1:205–210.

30. Gillin JC, Buchsbaum M, Wu J, Clark C, Bunney WE. Sleep deprivation as a model experimental antidepressant treatment: findings from functional brain imaging. Depress Anxiety 2001; 14:37–49.

31. Ebert D, Feistel H, Barocka A, Kaschka W. Increased limbic blood flow and total sleep deprivation in major depression with melancholia. Psychiatr Res 1994; 55:101–109.

22

Personality/Psychopathologic Changes

CAMELLIA P. CLARK

University of California–San Diego, San Diego, California, U.S.A.

J. CHRISTIAN GILLIN

Veterans Administration Medical Center and University of California–San Diego, San Diego, California, U.S.A.

BARBARA L. PARRY

University of California–San Diego, San Diego, California, U.S.A.

I.   Personality

While some investigators have studied the influence of personality variables on behavioral responses to sleep deprivation (SD) (reviewed in Chap. 20), few studies have addressed the potential effects of SD on personality itself. This phenomenon is hardly surprising; personality has long been considered to be relatively stable over time, particularly beginning in adulthood. Indeed, while short-term SD paradigms do produce behavioral changes, such effects tend to be relatively brief in duration.

However, it has long been recognized by psychiatric clinicians that patients with current DSM-IV (1) Axis I disorders (e.g., significant disorders that bring patients to clinicians' attention) often behave in maladaptive ways similar to those with personality disorders. In the many patients who meet comorbidity criteria on Axis II (where personality disorders or problematic personality traits are coded), resolution of the Axis I disorder is often associated with improvement or even resolution of the "Axis II" symptoms. Other patients are relatively free of psychiatric symptoms at baseline but under conditions of extreme stress develop behaviors otherwise associated with enduring personality disorders. This observation has led to the proposal of a new syndrome, stress-induced personality disorder (2), which is similar to "personality change" previously described across five domains: affect, impulse regulation, attitudes toward self, attitudes toward others, and social/interpersonal interactions (3).

Given the increasing evidence of psychological and physiological changes associated with chronic SD, it seems reasonable to ask whether long-term SD may affect aspects of personality as well. It would also be important to explore whether shorter periods of more intense SD (e.g., firefighters working for several days at a time to extinguish wildfires) could trigger a stress-induced personality disorder. Unfortunately, a careful review of the literature failed to reveal any studies addressing possible long-term effects of SD on personality.

II. Psychopathologic Changes

In this section we briefly summarize what is known about the effects (therapeutic or otherwise) of SD on persons with psychiatric disorders and examine what is known about possible relationships between disturbed sleep and daytime symptoms.

A. Affective Disorders

Unipolar Disorders

The effects of SD on major depression are discussed elsewhere (see Chap. 21); however, the antidepressant effects of SD in special circumstances merit brief discussion here. For example, serial partial SD has been reported to be effective in management of residual insomnia after other symptoms of a major depressive episode have remitted—a common situation in clinical practice (4).

Premenstrual Dysphoric Disorder

Preliminary results look promising for the antidepressant effects of SD in premenstrual dysphoric disorder (PMDD; formerly also known as late luteal phase dysphoric disorder in DSM-III-R). However, intriguing differences exist in patterns of response compared with those seen in major depression. In contrast to SD responders with major depression, who generally relapse to baseline intensity of depression after even a few minutes of sleep (5), responders with PMDD often do not improve until after a night of "recovery" sleep ("day 2" responders). Clinical response in PMDD may last much longer as well. In contrast to the situation in major depression, in which late-night partial SD (e.g., keeping subjects awake in the latter half of the night) has generally been reported as more efficacious than early-night partial SD, differences in late- and early-night partial SD are far less pronounced in PMDD. Interestingly, polysomnographic differences in response to late- versus early-night partial SD did not correlate with clinical response (6).

Major Depression During Pregnancy and the Postpartum Period

Practitioners are becoming increasingly aware of the prevalence of major depressive episodes during these important times in a woman's life. Even pregnancy, once thought to be a time of decreased risk of depression, is now known to pose some risk of affective episodes, particularly in women with a history of psychiatric illness. Although emerging safety data for a number of antidepressant medications are encouraging, many women and their clinicians prefer not to expose infants to psychotropics in utero or through breast-feeding, and the long-term behavioral effects of these medications are not known.

Pilot data support the antidepressant efficacy of partial SD in pregnant and postpartum depressed patients. Like patients with PMDD, they were more likely to respond after a night's recovery sleep. Interestingly, pregnant subjects were the only responders to early-night partial SD and nonresponders to late-night partial SD (7). Perhaps endocrine studies in these populations will help to explain the similarities with and differences from the response patterns in PMDD and in major depression not associated with reproduction.

Psychotic Depression

Although many patients (a large portion of which were medication-free) with psychotic depression in numerous studies have been reported to improve in response to total SD (TSD) or partial SD, worsening of delusions and agitation in response to TSD was reported in five unmedicated patients (three bipolars and two unipolars) with psychotic major depression. In this small case series, there was no mention of hallucinations before or after TSD (8). Since a review of the literature failed to reveal any obvious differences between psychotic depression patients who improved and those who worsened, SD cannot be recommended as a treatment for these patients at this time.

Other Forms of Unipolar Depression

Eleven of 15 inpatients with dysthymia and 12 of 15 patients with minor depression showed good response to two applications of TSD in one week (9). The authors later obtained similar response rates with repeated partial SD, and their diagnostic criteria were rigorously applied and very similar to those in use today for dysthymia and minor depression (Z. Rihmer, personal communication, 2002).

Bipolar Disorders

Inadequate sleep for any reason has long been recognized as a common precipitant of mania and hypomania, with reports that symptomatic severity correlates with severity of sleep disturbance during manic episodes (10). In fact, prolonged SD in normal rats provides a useful model of mania, with numerous behavioral and pharmacological similarities to human mania (11). On the other hand, bipolar depression is a serious illness with relatively few optimal treatments. Some experts in bipolar disorder are already treating bipolar II patients carefully with SD for major depressive episodes (T.A. Ketter, personal communication, 1996).

While there is little doubt in the literature that SD is effective at alleviating depression in bipolar patients, the actual risk of triggering mania or hypomania is far less clear. In a study of 12 nonmedicated patients undergoing one night of TSD, 9 subjects promptly switched into mania or hypomania. Of these 9 patients, 3 reverted to depression after 1 night of "recovery" sleep; the other 6 remained manic for "days or weeks" (12). The switch rate was worse in rapid-cycling patients, in which 7 of 9 developed mania in response to TSD (13).

Another group of investigators, using three cycles of TSD in depressed bipolar inpatients, noted a 5% switch rate into mania and a 6% switch to hypomania. All patients switching into mania or hypomania were treated immediately. For example, the authors omitted the DSM-IV duration criteria in order to provide the best clinical care. Of concern, switch rates for mania or hypomania did not significantly differ for patients on mood stabilizers versus those without them, although subject numbers were relatively small (14).

Remarkably, a group of 40 medication-free depressed bipolar inpatients receiving TSD plus double-blind pindolol versus placebo exhibited no switches into mania or hypomania in either the active or placebo groups. This study excluded potential subjects for lithium use during the preceding 6 months, perhaps excluding some of the most severely unstable bipolar patients (15).

In a double-blind study of bupropion, sertraline, and venlafaxine in bipolar patients with stable adequate doses of mood stabilizers and current major depression, 13 of 95 acute trials resulted in switches (7 hypomanias, 6 full manias). In the continuation phase, 16 of 48 trials were associated with switches (10 hypomanias, 6 manias) (16). It would thus be important to obtain an accurate switch rate for SD in bipolar patients on therapeutic doses of mood stabilizers to see if SD may actually be less risky than antidepressant medications in this population. Together with colleagues at the University of California at Irvine, two of the authors (JCG and CPC) are developing such a study.

B. Anxiety Disorders

Panic Disorder

In a study of 12 patients with panic disorder (without comorbid major depression) who received one night of TSD, 7 showed heightened anxiety ratings; 4 patients showed worsened depression ratings as well. Of the 7 subjects with worse anxiety after TSD, 4 had a panic attack during the sleep-deprived day (after at least 1 week since the most recent panic attack). No mention was made of presence or severity of agoraphobia before or after SD (17).

Obsessive-Compulsive Disorder

A group of 16 patients with obsessive-compulsive disorder did not change as a group in terms of mood or obsessive-compulsive symptoms after one night of TSD, although individual results varied considerably. Four patients had concurrent major depression, with 9 others having at least one previous major depressive episode. Eight patients experienced no significant change in mood or obsessive-compulsive symptoms; 5 had improved obsessive-compulsive symptoms, while 3 experienced worsening of symptoms. Of the 5 "responders," only 1 had a concomitant antidepressant response to TSD; the other "responders" were not appreciably depressed at baseline (18).

Generalized Anxiety Disorder

Seven unmedicated patients with generalized anxiety disorder who underwent 1 night of TSD improved significantly on the Hamilton Anxiety Rating Scale as compared with normal controls; however, as measured by the Spielberger State-Trait Anxiety Inventory, the groups' responses to TSD did not differ (19).

Social Phobia

Eight medication-free social phobia patients did not differ from controls in their response to TSD as measured by the Hamilton and Spielberger scales (19).

C. Psychotic Disorders

The older literature (ca. 1970) contained considerable literature about SD, especially rapid-eye-movement (REM) SD, in schizophrenia. This research was driven by observed similarities between dream cognition and perception and waking hallucinations, delusions, and cognitive processes in schizophrenia. Although various aspects of REM "deficiency" or "daytime intrusions" causing psychosis were ingenious and quite reasonable given the state of knowledge at the time, these hypotheses were eventually abandoned based on the results of experimentation.

Unfortunately, much of the literature from that time is difficult to utilize clinically for a variety of reasons. First, the earliest papers did not use Rechtschaffen and Kales standard polysomnographic scoring criteria. Second, several other manuscripts focused almost exclusively on electroencephalographic changes but gave little information on psychotic symptoms before as opposed to after SD; where addressed, they were described very briefly, with no reports of scores on standardized rating scales, etc. Third, some laboratories used oral dexamphetamine to achieve REM SD; while effective at decreasing REM, it may well have had confounding effects on patients' behavior. Finally, like other research on psychosis at that time, studies suffered from lack of standardization of diagnoses and diagnostic criteria.

Nevertheless, a small body of literature suggests that SD may be helpful in depressive symptoms associated with psychotic disorders. In one study, TSD alleviated depressive symptoms in schizophrenic patients consisting mostly of paranoid schizophrenics, although little was said about psychotic symptoms (20). Another study, utilizing late-night partial SD in 5 paranoid schizophrenics, 6 schizoaffective patients, and 1 patient with psychotic major depression, reported no worsening of psychotic symptoms as measured by the "schizophrenic" subscale of the Association for Methodology and Documentation in Psychiatry (AMDP) Rating Scale (21). The seven subjects with antidepressant response were reported to experience "significant improvement of the . . . schizophrenic symptoms after partial SD"; nonresponders reportedly did not experience significant changes in mood or psychotic symptoms (22,23). Unfortunately, the authors did not describe in further detail specific symptoms such as hallucinations or delusions. Confounding effects of medications may also have been present. Naturally, it would be very difficult to study SD effects in such an ill patient population off medications; however, carefully designed studies of such patients on neuroleptics might yield information useful for treatment in this cohort with many refractory patients.

D. Dementia

Comorbid Depression and "Pseudodementia"

It is common for geriatric patients to present with concomitant depressive and cognitive symptoms. Although not always straightforward, it is important to distinguish between patients with endogenous depression, dementia, or both for appropriate treatment and planning. After 2 nights of REM SD, none of these three groups or normal controls experienced significant change in mood ratings. However, polysomnographic changes themselves provided important information. "Primary degenerative" dementia patients showed REM rebound during recovery sleep, although less than their healthy counterparts. Depressed subjects had very little REM rebound, suggesting impaired REM regulation in both groups (24). Patients with mixed symptoms appeared similar to dementia patients on baseline polysomnography, but their large change in phasic REM activity after REM SD suggested pathophysiological similarities to major depression. Mixed-symptom patients whose impaired cognition remained stable over time had higher REM rebound than those who went on to develop further cognitive deterioration (25).

Alzheimer's Disease

Given the well-known cholinergic degeneration and dysfunction in Alzheimer's disease (AD), it is not surprising that sleep disturbance is a common feature that frequently causes problems for patients and loved ones alike. Actigraphy data have demonstrated severe sleep-wake disruption correlating with agitation in AD patients (26,27). Chronotherapeutic agents partially restoring normal circadian rhythms, such as evening bright light (28) and melatonin (29) were associated with improvements in both sleep consolidation and behavior.

Interestingly, the prevalence of sleep-disordered breathing is elevated in dementia (30); pilot data suggest that CPAP ameliorates some cognitive deficits in patients with mild dementia. Other studies are assessing the tolerability of CPAP in early AD and its effects on cognition and sleep/wake variables (31).

Parkinson's Disease

Concomitant improvement of motor function and depression has been reported following 1 night of TSD in Parkinson's disease (32). Although Parkinson's disease is relatively common and dementia is frequently seen in PD, we are unaware of any reports of SD in Parkinson's disease that address the effects (if any) on cognitive symptoms.

E. Substance Use Disorders

Alcohol and most other "recreational drugs" are associated with sleep disturbance, whether during acute intoxication, dependence, or withdrawal. Alcohol dependence in particular is associated with disrupted, unrefreshing sleep deficient in slow-wave activity persisting for several years into sobriety. Insomnia is a common precipitant of relapse in many recovering patients, who frequently try to use alcohol or other substances to help them sleep.

Literature on the clinical effects of SD in substance use disorders is extremely limited, perhaps in part because SD could increase the risk of seizures during the withdrawal period. Alcoholic patients showed impaired slow-wave sleep rebound (compared with controls) following 1 night of early partial SD (33); however, no changes in mood or behavior were observed with the clinical scales used (M. Irwin, personal communication, 2002). These alcoholics had low baseline scores on the Hamilton Rating Scale for Depression, e.g., none had a concurrent depressive syndrome. In other words, their moods before and after partial SD were more similar to those of normal controls than to those of patients with major depression.

F. Miscellaneous Disorders

Developmental Disorders

A report of a small series (34) confirmed clinical impressions that SD tends to worsen behavioral problems in this population.

Attention-Deficit Hyperactivity Disorder (ADHD)

Naturalistic SD in children can present as hyperactivity, inattentiveness, and/or irritability (35,36). Increasing evidence has linked attention-deficit hyperactivity disorder to sleep problems (37), including one report of increased frequency of sleep-disordered breathing in children with attention-deficit hyperactivity disorder (38). In a broader context, an epidemiological study of randomly selected elementary school students demonstrated that severe sleep problems were associated with hyperactivity, poor attendance, conduct disorder symptoms (e.g., aggression, property destruction), and emotional (anxious or depressive) symptoms (39).

Given our children's increasing activities and decreasing sleep in the population as a whole, it behooves parents and educators alike to work with schools and children to encourage more healthful priorities and practices.

References

1. APA Diagnostic and Statistical Manual of Mental Disorders. IV ed. Washington, D.C.: American Psychiatric Association, 1994.

2. Reich J. Clinical correlates of stress-induced personality disorder. Psychiatr Ann 2002; 32(10):581–588.

3. Bronisch T, Klerman G. Personality functioning: change and stability in relationship to symptoms and psychopathology. J Personal Disord 1991; 5:307–317.

4. Hemmeter U, Seifritz E, Hatzinger M, Muller MJ, Holsboer-Trachsler E. Serial partial sleep deprivation as adjuvant treatment of depressive insomnia. Prog Neuropsychopharmacol Biol Psychiatry 1995; 19:593–602.

5. Roy-Byrne PG, Uhde TW, Post RM. Antidepressant effects of one night's sleep deprivation: clinical and theoretical implications. In: Post RM, Ballenger J, editors. Neurobiology of Mood Disorders. Baltimore: William & Wilkins, 1984: 817–835.

6. Parry BL, Mostofi N, LeVeau B, Nahum HC, Golshan S, Laughlin GA et al. Sleep EEG studies during early and late partial sleep deprivation in premenstrual dysphoric disorder and normal control subjects. Psychiatry Res 1999; 85(2):127–143.

7. Parry BL, Curran ML, Stuenkel CA, Yokimozo M, Tam L, Powell KA et al. Can critically timed sleep deprivation be useful in pregnancy and postpartum depressions? J Affect Disord 2000; 60(3):201–212.

8. Benedetti F, Zanardi R, Colombo C, Smeraldi E. Worsening of delusional depression after sleep deprivation: case reports. J Psychiatr Res 1999; 33:69–72.

9. Rihmer Z, Szucs R. [Differential diagnosis of mild depressions with sleep deprivation (author's translation)]. Ideggyogyaszati Szemle 1979; 32:282–284.

10. Barbini B, Bertelli S, Colombo C, Smeraldi E. Sleep loss, a possible factor in augmenting manic episode. Psychiatry Res 1996; 65(2):121–125.

11. Gessa GL, Pani L, Fadda P, Fratta W. Sleep deprivation in the rat: an animal model of mania. Eur Neuropsychopharmacol 1995; 5 Suppl:89–93.

12. Wehr TA, Sack DA, Rosenthal NE. Sleep reduction as a final common pathway in the genesis of mania. Am J Psychiatry 1987; 144(2):201–204.

13. Wehr TA, Goodwin FK, Wirz-Justice A, Breitmaier J, Craig C. 48–hour sleep-wake cycles in manic-depressive illness: naturalistic observations and sleep deprivation experiments. Arch Gen Psychiatry 1982; 39(5):559–565.

14. Colombo C, Benedetti F, Barbini B, Campori E, Smeraldi E. Rate of switch from depression into mania after therapeutic sleep deprivation in bipolar depression. Psychiatry Res 1999; 86(3):267–270.

15. Smeraldi E, Benedetti F, Barbini B, Campori E, Colombo C. Sustained antidepressant effect of sleep deprivation combined with pindolol in bipolar depression. A placebo-controlled trial. Neuropsychopharmacology 1999; 20(4):380–385.

16. Post RM, Altshuler LL, Frye MA, Suppes T, Rush AJ, Keck PE Jr. et al. Rate of switch in bipolar patients prospectively treated with second-generation antidepressants as augmentation to mood stabilizers. Bipolar Disord 2001; 3(5):259–265.

17. Roy-Byrne PP, Uhde TW, Post RM. Effects of one night's sleep deprivation on mood and behavior in panic disorder. Arch Gen Psychiatry 1986; 43:895–899.

18. Joffe RT, Swinson RP. Total sleep deprivation in patients with obsessive-compulsive disorder. Acta Psychiatr Scand 1988; 77(4):483–487.

19. Labbate LA, Johnson MR, Lydiard RB, Brawman-Mintzer O, Emmanuel N, Crawford M et al. Sleep deprivation in social phobia and generalized anxiety disorder. Biol Psychiatry 1998; 43(11):840–842.

20. Fahndrich E. [Sleep deprivation therapy of depressive syndromes in schizophrenic disorders (author's transl)]. Nervenarzt 1982; 53(5):279–293.

21. Dick P. [AMDP system and clinical psychopharmacology (author's transl)]. Acta Psychiatr Belg 1978; 78(4):583–590.
22. Hochli D, Trachsler E, von Luckner N, Woggon B. Partial sleep deprivation therapy of depressive syndromes in schizophrenic disorders. Pharmacopsychiatry 1985; 18:134–135.
23. Trachsler E, Hochli D, von Luckner N, Woggon B. Dexamethasone suppression test before and after partial sleep deprivation in depressed schizophrenic and schizoaffective patients. Pharmacopsychiatry 1985; 18:110–111.
24. Reynolds CF, III, Buysse DJ, Kupfer DJ, Hoch CC, Houck PR, Matzzie J et al. Rapid eye movement sleep deprivation as a probe in elderly subjects. Arch Gen Psychiatry 1990; 47(12):1128–1136.
25. Buysse DJ, Reynolds CF, III, Hoch CC, Houck PR, Berman SR, Matzzie J et al. Rapid eye movement sleep deprivation in elderly patients with concurrent symptoms of depression and dementia. J Neuropsychiatry Clin Neurosci 1992; 4(3):249–256.
26. Martin J, Marler M, Shochat T, Ancoli-Israel S. Circadian rhythms of agitation in institutionalized patients with Alzheimer's disease. Chronobiol Int 2000; 17(3):405–418.
27. Pat-Horenczyk R, Klauber MR, Shochat T, Ancoli-Israel S. Hourly profiles of sleep and wakefulness in severely versus mild-moderately demented nursing home patients. Aging (Milano) 1998; 10(4):308–315.
28. Ancoli-Israel S, Martin JL, Kripke DF, Marler M, Klauber MR. Effect of light treatment on sleep and circadian rhythms in demented nursing home patients. J Am Geriatr Soc 2002; 50(2):282–289.
29. Ancoli-Israel S, manuscript in preparation.
30. Ancoli-Israel S, Klauber MR, Butters N, Parker L, Kripke DF. Dementia in institutionalized eldery: relation to sleep apnea. Am Geriatr Soc 1991; 39:258–263.
31. Ancoli-Israel S, grant submitted.
32. Bertolucci PH, Andrade LA, Lima JG, Carlini EA. Total sleep deprivation and Parkinson's disease. Arq Neuro-Psiquiatria (Sao Paulo) 1987; 45:224–230.
33. Irwin M, Gillin JC, Dang J, Weissman J, Phillips E, Ehlers CL. Sleep deprivation as a probe of homeostatic sleep regulation in primary alcoholics. Biol Psychiatry 2002; 51(8):632–641.
34. Kennedy CH, Meyer KA. Sleep deprivation, allergy symptoms, and negatively reinforced problem behavior. J Appl Behav Anal 1996; 29(1):133–135.
35. Dahl RE. The development and disorders of sleep. Adv Pediatr 1998; 45:73–89.
36. Dahl RE. The impact of inadequate sleep on children's daytime cognitive function. Semin Pediatr Neurol 1996; 3(1):44–50.
37. Dagan Y, Zeevi-Luria S, Sever Y, Hallis D, Yovel I, Sadeh A et al. Sleep quality in children with attention deficit hyperactivity disorder: an actigraphic study. Psychiatry Clin Neurosci 1997; 51(6):383–386.
38. Chervin RD, Dillon JE, Bassetti C, Ganoczy DA, Pituch KJ. Symptoms of sleep disorders, inattention, and hyperactivity in children. Sleep 1997; 20(12):1185–1192.
39. Paavonen EJ, Almqvist F, Tamminen T, Moilanen I, Piha J, Rasanen E et al. Poor sleep and psychiatric symptoms at school: an epidemiological study. Eur Child Adolesc Psychiatry 2002; 11(1):10–17.

23

Age and Individual Determinants of Sleep Loss Effects

HÉLÈNE GAUDREAU

McGill University and Hôpital Sacré-Coeur, Montréal, Québec, Canada

JULIE CARRIER AND BWANGA-MUKISHI TCHITEYA

Hôpital Sacré-Coeur and University of Montreal, Montréal, Québec, Canada

I. Introduction

Sleep is a ubiquitous phenomenon that is essential for well-being. However, the exact function of sleep remains obscure. The sleep-wake cycle is under the control of a homeostatic, sleep-dependent process and a circadian, sleep-independent process. The constant interaction between these two processes allows consolidated sleep and wakefulness episodes and determines sleep propensity across the 24-hr day. Sleep undergoes marked modifications over the life span. Aging may influence homeostatic and circadian processes individually and in their interaction. In addition to aging, sleep is influenced by a variety of factors such as stress, workload, and health status. Individual differences in coping with stress throughout life will greatly influence the aging process, the sleep-wake cycle, and the vulnerability to disease later in life. Clearly, stressor exposure impairs sleep, but chronic sleep loss may also induce stress that may have an important impact on the hypothalamic-pituitary axis and consequently on stress reactivity. Therefore, it may be hypothesized that chronic sleep loss or curtailment can contribute to the acceleration of the aging process and have long-term adverse effects on health.

II. Ontogeny of Sleep Modifications

A. Age-Related Changes in Sleep Architecture

In humans, babies sleep around 16–20 hours per day, including night sleep and daytime naps. Young children's sleep pattern is characterized by important amounts of slow-wave sleep (SWS; stages 3 and 4 sleep), mostly in the first part of the night (1–3). During puberty, an important decrease in SWS occurs (1–5). Indeed, a reduction of SWS by almost 40% during the second decade of life has been reported (4). Coble and collaborators (1) showed that in 6- to 15-year-old children non-REM (NREM) sleep is marked by a progressive decrease in the percentage of SWS. Another study reported a gradual decline in SWS across the Tanner puberty stages, with approximately a 35% decline from Tanner stages 1 to 5 (6). From childhood to adolescence, sleep architecture reveals an increased proportion of stage 2 sleep, a reduction of total sleep time, and a phase delay of the sleep-wake cycle (1,3–5,7,8). Some authors have observed that the transition between childhood and adolescence is characterized by the appearance of sleep complaints and an increase in daytime sleepiness (3,7). It was thus suggested that most changes occurring between childhood and adolescence may be a consequence of pubertal or hormonal changes rather than age (4,5,9).

Slow-wave sleep undergoes another sharp decline during adulthood, mostly across the twenties (3,10,11). Young adults' sleep also presents an increase in the percentage of rapid-eye-movement (REM) sleep, a shorter latency to the first REM period, and an additional decrease in sleep duration compared with adolescents (3). As aging proceeds, sleep patterns become more disturbed, with more frequent awakenings across the night, an increase in stages 1 and 2 sleep, and a significant and gradual decline in SWS (2,3,12–14). The effect of aging on REM sleep is more controversial. Some studies have reported a reduction in REM sleep latency, less REM sleep during the night, and more REM in the first part of the sleep episode, whereas other studies have found no effects of aging on these parameters (2,15). Nocturnal sleep efficiency may decrease to 70–80% in elderly subjects. One study looked at sleep modifications in subjects from 16 to 83 years old, and reported a reduction of sleep length by 27 minutes per decade starting during middle age until the eighties (16). In this study, the sleep period time did not change across ages. Sleep timing of older people was advanced compared to that of younger individuals. Often, elderly subjects report feeling sleepy earlier during the evening and waking up earlier in the morning. Subjective sleep quality also changes in the elderly; epidemiological studies show that more than half of elderly people complain about sleep (17). Sleep of "old old" (75–87 years old) and "young old" (61–74 years old) subjects has been studied longitudinally over a 3-year period using polysomnographic recordings and sleep diaries (18,19). In the course of the study, old-old subjects showed increased sleep latency and wakefulness after sleep onset and decreased sleep efficiency and percentage of slow-wave sleep. Increased daytime napping in the old-old accompanied sleep alterations. However, habitual time in bed, daily social rhythms, or sleep apnea did not differ between groups. It is important to mention that results of polysomnographic studies in old individuals represent optimal aging and may not be representative of the general population. It was reported that in very old nursing-home patients, sleep-wake patterns are poorly consolidated and sleep episodes may spread over the entire day due to multiple daytime napping (20,21). Sleep disorders of older people may also be secondary to health problems such as depression, arthritis, cardiovascular problems, bronchitis, diabetes, sleep disordered-breathing, and restless legs syndrome (12,20).

B. Alterations of Quantitative Sleep Electroencephalograms with Aging

Quantitative analysis of the sleep electroencephalograms across the night is a powerful and sensitive tool for evaluating changes in sleep regulatory processes with advancing age. For example, slow-wave activity (SWA, spectral power between 0.75 and 4.5 Hz during NREM) increases proportionally with the number of hours of wakefulness preceding sleep; it is also an indicator of sleep intensity (22). Studies in both depressed and insomniac populations also suggest that elevated fast frequency activity during NREM sleep might be an indicator of hyperarousal and that it could be related to lower sleep quality (23,24).

We investigated the modifications in NREM sleep electroencephalographic (EEG) power in 54 subjects, from children to middle-aged adults (25). A marked decrease of absolute SWA power was observed as early as adolescence. The precocious changes in EEG SWA power between the children and adolescent groups suggest a peak associated with the maturational process, followed by the already reported decline with advancing age (Fig. 1). The early reduction of absolute SWA suggests that it may play a role in the intense physiological transformations occurring during maturation. As such, it has been proposed that the EEG changes during sleep could reflect the kinetics of the underlying metabolic processes (11,26,27). The early modifications in sleep structure across childhood and adolescence have been related to ontogenetic alterations in cortical synaptic density, which peaks in the first decade of life and then undergoes a substantial reorganization during the second decade (11,27). The higher EEG power of young subjects could also reflect a higher level of synchronization of cortical neurons compared to that of older individuals (28).

During adulthood, experimental results on quantitative sleep electroencephalograms reveal important modifications between 20 and 60 years of age. The most consistent of these age-dependent changes is a decrease in SWA, which shows that sleep of middle-aged subjects is less intense than that of younger subjects (29,30). One study assessed the effects of age on sleep EEG power spectral density in a group of 100 subjects aged 20–60 years. The effect of age varied according to frequency. The decrease in power with age was not restricted to SWA but also included theta and sigma activity. Increasing age was associated with higher power in the beta range. Dijk and collaborators showed, using forced

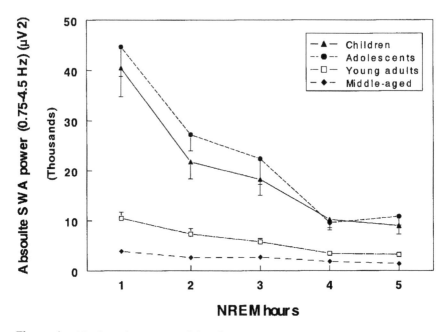

Figure 1   Absolute slow-wave activity (SWA) power across 5 NREM hr for children (black triangle), adolescents (black circles), young adults (white squares), and middle-aged adults (black diamond). (From Ref. 25.)

desynchrony experiments (in which sleep episodes were initiated at all circadian phases while homeostatic drive remained constant), that elderly people present less SWS at all circadian phases compared to young subjects (31). SWA declines throughout the sleep episode in older subjects, but the decline is less steep than the one of the young. Using the same protocol, the authors showed that sleep spindles also undergo important age-related modifications (32). Elderly subjects present decreased amplitude, duration, and incidence of spindles compared to young subjects. Moreover, the amplitude of the circadian modulation of spindles frequency (11–15 Hz) was reduced in older subjects. These sleep electroencephalogram changes may underlie the aging sleep-wake cycle system's greater difficulty adapting to challenges that ordinarily disrupt sleep.

III.   Age-Dependent Changes in Sleep Regulatory Mechanisms

According to contemporary models of sleep-wake cycle regulation, the interaction of homeostatic (process S) and circadian (process C) processes regulates the sleep-wake cycle (33–36). The two-process model predicts the timing and intensity of sleep for a variety of schedules in young subjects (total and partial sleep deprivation, shift work, constant bed rest, etc.) (37). The two independent processes are responsible for sleep regulation and the distribution of sleep and wakefulness episodes throughout the 24-hr day. The homeostatic process represents the sleep debt accumulated during wakefulness. As a result, the homeostatic process increases during waking hours and decreases exponentially during sleep. The intensity and dynamic of SWS and SWA provide a physiological estimate of the time course of the homeostatic process. Researchers have evaluated the buildup function of homeostatic sleep drive in young subjects by assessing the effects of prior wakefulness and sleep on the sleep electroencephalogram. Results of these studies have shown an enhancement of both SWS and SWA after an extension of prior wakefulness (35). SWA increases with the number of hours of wakefulness according to a saturating exponential function (buildup function), which has an estimated time constant of 18.2 hr in young subjects. The decline in SWA during NREM sleep reflects the dissipation of homeostatic sleep drive. The dissipation of process S during the night can be approximated by an exponential decay with an estimated time constant of 4.2 hr in young men (34).

The circadian process is controlled by an endogenous circadian pacemaker, located in the suprachiasmatic nucleus of the hypothalamus (38). The circadian pacemaker is responsible for the rhythmic variations of sleep propensity throughout the 24-hr days. Since it is not possible in humans to measure directly the activity of the circadian pacemaker, robust circadian rhythms such as melatonin secretion or rectal temperature are used as markers of its activity. In healthy young adults, the temperature minimum occurs in the early morning hours (around 06:00 hr) and the temperature maximum in the early evening hours (around 20:00 hr). Young subjects typically go to bed 6 hr before and awaken 2 hr after their temperature minimum. Subjects can easily initiate and maintain sleep while the biological clock promotes sleep. Subjects have difficulty falling and staying asleep when the biological clock promotes wakefulness. In a normally entrained individual, circadian sleep propensity increases during the evening (when temperature decreases) and reaches its maximum in the early morning hours, at the time of the temperature minimum. Inversely, circadian wake propensity increases during daytime (when temperature increases) and peaks at the time of the temperature maximum (which is a few hours before habitual bedtime) (39–42). The combined action of the homeostatic and circadian processes is thought to be necessary to maintain consolidated episodes of about 8 hr of sleep during the night and about 16 hr of wakefulness during the day (39). Throughout the night, increasing circadian sleep propensity counterbalances decreasing homeostatic sleep pressure. Conversely, throughout the day, increasing circadian wake propensity counterbalances increasing homeostatic sleep pressure. A nonlinear interaction of the circadian and the sleep-dependent components of sleep propensity has also been reported in forced desynchrony studies (39). These studies have shown that the last portion of a sleep episode (when homeostatic sleep pressure is low) is more vulnerable to a circadian phase of high wake propensity than is the beginning of a sleep episode (when homeostatic sleep pressure is high). A precise interaction between the homeostatic and circadian processes ensures optimal quality of both sleep and vigilance.

A. Sleep Deprivation: Effect on Sleep and Electroencephalogram Across Ages

To our knowledge, almost no information is available concerning sleep regulatory mechanisms following sleep deprivation in children and adolescents. Carskadon and collaborators (8,43,44) proposed that sleep pressure during the day starts to build up more slowly during puberty, enabling individuals to stay awake longer as adolescence progresses. They demonstrated, following sleep deprivation, a reduced amount of SWS in more mature adolescents than in less mature ones, suggesting developmental changes of homeostatic sleep-wake regulation by yet unknown mechanisms (8). However, sleep need appears not to decrease across adolescence (4,45). Time in bed is often curtailed during school days in older adolescents, reflecting progressively later bedtime but fixed wake time; weekend sleep would be more representative of their sleep need. It was reported that adolescents with higher pubertal status show longer time in bed on weekends (46), suggesting that they may actually need more sleep than prepubertal children (47). Indeed, changes in homeostatic regulation during adolescence would not reflect modifications in sleep need but would be related to biological factors.

Studies in young and old rats show that aged animals exhibit reduced responses on SWS and on EEG delta power following sleep deprivation (48,49). One study found that *c-fos* induction in the hypothalamus and cingulate cortex display a reduced response to a 6-hr and a 12-hr increase of wakefulness in aged rats compared to young ones (50). These results suggest that the mechanism of *c-fos* induction in response to wakefulness is attenuated in old rats, but the exact nature of this mechanism and the homeostatic process is still unknown. In humans, elderly subjects have been subjected to one or two nights of sleep deprivation or to sleep fragmentation. These studies showed that elderly adults respond to sleep deprivation with an increase in SWS (51–54). Some studies reported that the rebound of SWS following sleep deprivation tends to be less intense in elderly subjects than in younger ones (54,55), whereas others found no difference in the rebound of SWS/SWA between young and elderly subjects (31,53). Dijk and collaborators (31) reported that older people respond to sleep deprivation with a relative increase almost identical to that of young adults. However, absolute levels of SWA are lower for the old group, even after sleep deprivation.

We investigated the different effects of one night on complete sleep deprivation (25 hr of constant wakefulness) in young (20–39 years) and middle-aged subjects (40–60 years) (56). As measured with SWS and SWA, sleep was more intense in both groups of subjects following sleep deprivation. However, the increase of sleep intensity following sleep deprivation was less pronounced in the middle aged than in the young (Fig. 2). Therefore, it appears that even though middle-aged subjects have the ability to respond to acute sleep deprivation with an increase of deep sleep, their overall capacity to respond diminishes. These results suggest that the built-up function of the homeostatic sleep process may change during the course of life. For example, the sleep (SWA) of older people may be less sensitive to the accumulation of wakefulness than the sleep of younger subjects. In the same vein, sleep (SWA) of adolescents may be less sensitive to the accumulation of wakefulness than the sleep of children. In other words, similar increases in the number of waking hours that precede sleep will

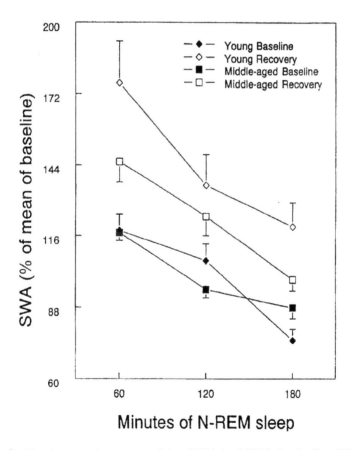

Figure 2 Hourly mean slow-wave activity (SWA) (and SEM) for the first 180 min of NREM sleep for young and middle-aged subjects. Values are expressed as a percentage of mean SWA during the first 180 min of NREM sleep for the baseline sleep episode. (From Ref. 56.)

produce different increases of SWA depending on age or hormonal status. To test this hypothesis, we should evaluate the effects of varying wake intervals on sleep in different age groups.

B.   Effects of the Accumulation of Wakefulness on Vigilance

The interaction between a homeostatic process and a circadian process also regulates vigilance levels (57–61). As reported previously, it has been suggested that the sleep (SWA) of different age groups may present a different sensitivity to the accumulation of wakefulness. If the sleep of a specific age group were less sensitive to the accumulation of wakefulness because of a reduced need for sleep, then we would not expect negative effects on vigilance (i.e., less sleep would be required to maintain optimal levels of vigilance). On the other hand, if the sleep of a specific age group is less sensitive to the accumulation of wakefulness but the need for sleep does not change, then we would expect a negative impact of sleep loss on vigilance. This would mean that sleep intensity after longer durations of wakefulness would not be sufficient to maintain optimal levels of wakefulness.

Increased daytime sleepiness and napping are frequently reported by adolescents but not by prepubertal children (4,62,63). Daytime somnolence has been evaluated in children and adolescents mostly using the Multiple Sleep Latency Test (MSLT) in the sleep laboratory. Children who had not started puberty showed a very low tendency to fall asleep during a daytime MSLT (4,64,65). Interestingly, an increased propensity to fall asleep during MSLT was observed in children from Tanner stages 3, 4, and 5 (4). Puberty appears to induce an increase in daytime sleepiness. It was proposed that maturational modifications altering the alignment of circadian and sleep-wake processes could be responsible for the increased daytime sleepiness in adolescents (44).

The majority of the few studies that have compared the effects of an acute sleep deprivation on the vigilance of young and healthy elderly subjects tended to show similar or smaller deteriorations of vigilance in the elderly during an acute sleep deprivation (53–55,66–68). To our knowledge, only one study reported that older subjects (40–49 years) exhibited more effects of an acute sleep deprivation on performance than did younger subjects (69). Together these results may indicate that the vigilance of healthy elderly subjects is less sensitive to the accumulation of wakefulness than is the vigilance of young ones. It is therefore possible that healthy elderly subjects would need less sleep than young subjects for recovery of vigilance from a similar duration of sleep deprivation, as a few studies that show similar or faster recovery rates of vigilance in healthy elderly subjects than in young subjects after recovery sleep following an acute sleep deprivation (53–55) have indicated. However, further corroboration is needed to reconcile these preliminary experimental results with the increase in sleepiness complaints accompanying increasing age seen in epidemiologic studies.

C. Age-Related Changes in Circadian Rhythms: The Phase Delay and Phase Advance Hypotheses

It has been suggested that age-dependent changes in the timing and the consolidation of sleep may be linked to age-dependent modifications in the phase of the endogenous circadian pacemaker (ECP) [reviewed in (70)]. Carskadon and collaborators (7,43) indicated that sleep phase delay, which is one of the most consistent modifications in sleep patterns between childhood and adolescence, may reflect developmental alterations in circadian timing mechanisms. In older persons, an advance in the timing of the sleep-wake cycle has been reported, and this advance was explained in terms of the ECP output signal's earlier clock time phase position. This phase advance would produce an earlier timing of the sleep episode in the evening and an earlier circadian wake signal in the morning.

Chronotype questionnaires are used to assess the tendency of an individual to be more of a morning type or an evening type by measuring the times of day that people feel their best in addition to when they prefer to wake up, to go to bed, to engage in intellectual and physical activity, and so forth (71). A change in phase preference toward eveningness is observed in older adolescents, compared to children and preadolescents, who appear to be more morning types (72). Later in life, the reverse is noted, with more older people reporting that they are morning types than young adults. This difference starts during the middle years of life (13). Research using sleep diaries on the change of habitual sleep-wake patterns in aging corroborates this age-dependent tendency toward morningness.

The delay of sleep schedule in more mature adolescents has been reported by laboratory studies (72) and longitudinal surveys (46,73). It was reported that in the sleep lab, sleep onset in adolescents was delayed by 1.5 hr, sleep offset by almost 2 hr and the onset of melatonin secretion by 1.25 hr compared with sleep recorded in the same individuals the previous school year (74). Moreover, using an elaborate experimental protocol including a constant routine, Carskadon et al. (7) proposed that the pubertal development, reflected by Tanner stages, is correlated with the phase of melatonin offset, supporting the proposition of delayed circadian timing during adolescence. These last results strengthen the proposition that the phase delay would be related to biological factors. Moreover, during laboratory experiments, adolescents are isolated from social factors (going to school) that could have influenced observations.

Researchers controlling for masking effects in adults corroborated that, in comparison with young individuals, elderly subjects show a phase advance of their temperature circadian rhythm. The phase advance of temperature circadian rhythm is associated with an earlier wake time and bedtime in elderly subjects compared with the young (75,76). In the elderly, habitual bedtime, habitual wake time, and the minimum of the circadian temperature rhythm occur 1–2 hr earlier compared with young subjects. We compared sleep patterns and unmasked circadian temperature parameters between a group of young subjects and a group of middle-aged subjects. Habitual bedtime and wake time were earlier in the middle-aged than in the young. In addition, middle-aged subjects reported a greater orientation toward morningness and showed an earlier phase of temperature rhythm (77). Circadian age-related differences were of the same magnitude as those reported in healthy elderly subjects (75,76).

Age-dependent increase in the number and duration of awakenings during sleep may also be caused by a phase angle disturbance. According to this hypothesis, the minimum of the circadian temperature rhythm (and the rising limb of the circadian temperature rhythm associated with higher wake propensity) would occur too early during the sleep episode, leading to higher amounts of wakefulness in the elderly compared to young subjects (78,79). This interpretation has led to the suggestion that changing the phase position of the circadian rhythms (through such techniques as bright light exposure) might alleviate sleep complaints among elderly subjects who have sleep difficulties (see below) (80). Studies of the healthy elderly and middle-aged population who do not complain about their sleep do not corroborate this hypothesis. In fact, some authors have reported that young and older subjects sleep at the same circadian phase, whereas others have found that elderly subjects wake up closer to the minimum of their temperature circadian rhythm (75–77). Some have interpreted the observation that elderly subjects awaken closer to the minimum of their temperature circadian rhythm as a reflection of their reduced ability to maintain sleep on the ascending limb of the temperature circadian rhythm when circadian wake propensity increases in the morning (see higher vulnerability to a phase angle misalignment below).

The mechanisms that underlie age-related phase differences of the biological clock have yet to be determined. Some authors have proposed that it is associated with a change of the endogenous period of the circadian pacemaker. However, human studies of forced desynchrony and of blind people did not report an age-dependent modification of the endogenous period (reviewed in Ref. 31). Others have suggested that age-related phase differences may be associated with the phase shifting capacity of the circadian pacemaker in response to the light-dark cycle (81). One study compared the phase shifting effects of 3 consecutive days of bright light (5 hr) exposure before (phase delay) or after (phase advance) the circadian temperature minimum in young and elderly subjects. The phase delays did not differ between the two age groups but the phase advances were attenuated in the elderly. These latest results do not explain the phase advance of the circadian pacemaker in older people (81). A complete phase-response curve and dose-response curve in different age groups is necessary to completely evaluate age-dependent changes in the phase shifting capacity of the circadian pacemaker in response to the light-dark cycle.

IV. Individual Differences in Sleep and Wakefulness

A. Gender Differences in Sleep During Aging

It is not clear when gender differences on polysomnographic sleep emerge over the aging process in healthy subjects. Gender differences in sleep architecture have been reported across the maturational process, in children and adolescents (3,64,82) and also later during adulthood and in old age (3,83,84). Some studies observed that gender differences were present in children 7–9 years, with the percentage of SWS higher in boys than girls (64). whereas others reported no gender difference in sleep patterns of prepubertal children (85). Later, boys 10 years and older presented a higher percentage of stage 3 sleep compared to girls with no change in stage 4 (3,82). Gender differences in adolescents have been associated with differences in pubertal development between boys and girls, since girls start puberty earlier than boys (47,86–89). It may be hypothesized that the higher level of SWS in boys is related to delayed or different influences of the maturational process on sleep regulatory mechanisms.

It is well recognized that there are gender differences in sleep in the elderly population. Compared to older men of the same age, older women usually show more SWS despite the fact that they complain more often of insomnia (3,83,90). These results led to the hypothesis that age might have differential effects in men and women. Gender differences in quantitative sleep EEG measures have been reported in subjects in their twenties (91,92). In our study of 110 subjects between the ages of 20 and 60 yr, we found significant gender effects for a few variables (13). Women spent significantly more time in bed than did men, as sleep diaries indicated. In the laboratory, women showed more SWS and fewer awakenings. There was no significant interaction between age and gender on any of the sleep parameters, which showed that age did not influence the sleep of men and women differently. We studied the effects of age and gender on sleep EEG power spectral density in a group of subjects aged 20–60 yr (30). Figure 3 illustrates mean power spectral densities of the women relative to the men (men = 0) for each frequency bin for the first four NREM periods. The effect of gender varied according to frequency, but no interactions emerged between age and gender, suggesting again that the aging process influences men and women in a similar fashion in a middle-aged population. Women had higher power spectral density not only in the delta and theta range (0.25–9.00 Hz), but also in the high sigma frequency range (14.25–16.00 Hz). These differences were constant across the night.

Sleep differences between men and women, especially in SWA, may be associated with gender differences in homeostatic sleep regulation. According to this hypothesis, men would be less sensitive to the accumulation of wakefulness than women. To date, there have been no cross-gender comparisons of estimates of the buildup and dissipation of homeostatic sleep pressure. One study reported that compared to young men, young women showed a higher rebound of SWA following 40-hr sleep deprivation (93). However, we showed no gender difference (or interaction with age) in the rebound of SWA/SWS following 25-hr sleep deprivation (94). These divergences stress the necessity of comparing the dynamic of homeostatic sleep-wake cycle regulation between men and women in future studies.

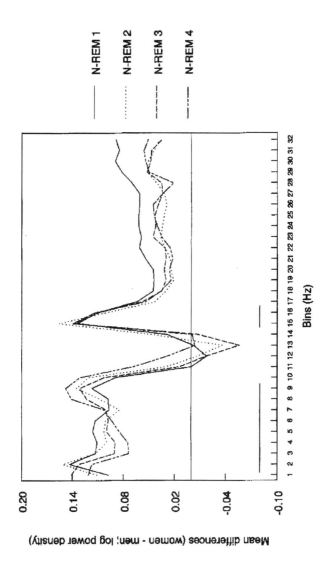

Figure 3 Mean power spectral densities of the women relative to the men (men = 0) for each frequency bin. The line represents areas where the effect of gender was significant with the regression analyses. (From Ref. 30.)

B. Effects of Aging on Sleep: Challenges to the Sleep-Wake Cycle

As noted before, one of the most important age-dependent changes in sleep architecture is the decrease in SWS and SWA. Importantly, aging is also associated with a reduction in spindle frequency and amplitudes, and with concomitant reduction in spectral power in sigma frequencies during NREM sleep. The hyperpolarization of thalamocortical and cortical neurons is a critical factor for the generation of both delta and sleep spindle oscillations, which is associated with significant changes in neurons' responsiveness to environmental stimuli (95). Although the functional role of 12- to14-Hz sleep spindles and delta waves is still obscure, some authors have suggested that they maintain NREM sleep and protect against disturbing stimuli (96). If one accepts this assumption, it is possible that with advancing age NREM sleep of older subjects will become more vulnerable to external and internal disturbing stimuli (31). Interestingly, results have demonstrated that spontaneous awakenings in older subjects are mainly related to a reduction in the consolidation of NREM sleep (97,98). The results of new studies strongly suggest that the sleep-wake cycle of healthy older subjects may be particularly vulnerable to situations that involve challenges to their sleep-wake system, such as a circadian phase misalignment and stress. However, the strength of the association between this augmented vulnerability and an inability to consolidate NREM sleep requires further elucidation.

Lower Tolerance to a Phase Angle Misalignment Between Sleep and the Circadian Timing System

To explain the increase of wakefulness during sleep associated with aging, some authors (e.g., 78) have suggested that the sleep of older subjects might be particularly vulnerable to circadian phases of high wake propensity. This hypothesis proposes that it would be more difficult for older people to sleep at the "wrong circadian phase" and might explain in part why subjective sleep problems related to jet lag and shift work increase with age. Forced desynchrony studies have corroborated this hypothesis (99). Compared to baseline sleep, both younger and elderly subjects awoke more often during their sleep episode when they were required to sleep at a circadian phase of high wake propensity. In addition, elderly subjects woke up more often during their sleep than did young subjects at all circadian phases. However, the difference between elderly and young subjects was more prominent when sleep occurred at a time of higher circadian wake propensity, such as during the day (99). These data support the hypothesis of lower tolerance to a phase angle misalignment in elderly subjects.

In our study of the effects of 25-hr sleep deprivation in young and middle-aged subjects, recovery sleep was initiated 1 hr after habitual wake time, which is a time of increasing circadian wake propensity (56). This experimental situation was similar to what night workers experience when they sleep during the day following their first night shift. Not only did the middle-aged subjects show a smaller rebound of SWS and SWA during daytime recovery sleep, but they also displayed a steeper decrease of sleep efficiency (steeper increase of wakefulness during sleep) than the young subjects. The more important reduction of sleep efficiency in the middle-aged group during daytime recovery sleep indicates that the lower tolerance to an abnormal phase angle occurs as early as the middle years of life. This age-dependent reduced tolerance to a phase angle misalignment cannot be explained solely by a circadian timing system malfunction. If that were the case, the fact that the sleep of middle-aged subjects is more sensitive to "unfavorable" circadian phases would suggest that the ECP sends a stronger signal as we get older. Results from human and animal studies do not support this idea. Studies have shown no change or even reductions in the circadian modulation of many circadian markers with increasing age (31,100–102). In our studies with the middle-aged population, we found no modification in the amplitude of the circadian temperature rhythm (77).

Knowing the nonadditive interaction between the homeostatic and the circadian processes, it is quite possible that the observed reduction in homeostatic recuperative drive following sleep deprivation in the middle-aged subjects may account for their reduced ability to maintain sleep when they have to recuperate at an abnormal circadian phase. In the middle-aged subjects, the shallower homeostatic sleep response (SWA) following sleep deprivation may not have been able to "override" the high circadian propensity for wakefulness at this time of day. This interpretation is supported by data from the forced desynchrony protocol that indicates a strong relation in older people between greater vulnerability to a phase angle misalignment and a reduction of NREM sleep consolidation (97).

C. Sleep Modifications in Aging: Neuroendocrine Factors (See Also Chap. 14)

The NREM-REM sleep cycle and the secretory pattern of the somatotropic and hypothalamic-pituitary-adrenal (HPA) axes appear to be in close temporal relationship in young healthy subjects (103–106) (see also Chapter 16). Sleep has been proposed as a regulator of neuroendocrine functions (105,107), and it is believed that the interaction between sleep and the HPA axis is bidirectional (108). Indeed, many hormones participate in the neuroendocrine and neurophysiological regulation of sleep. A temporal association has been observed between sleep alterations occurring in the course of aging and neuroendocrine changes (107,109–111) (Fig. 4).

Growth hormone (GH) secretion is under the dual control of growth hormone-releasing hormone (GHRH) and somatostatin (112,113). GH secretion is stimulated by GHRH release from the hypothalamus and is inhibited by somatostatin. GHRH is released by two groups of GHRH-containing neurons in the hypothalamus and GHRH promotes sleep and growth hormone secretion via those two different pathways. It has been proposed that the SWS-inducing effect of GHRH is mediated via projections of GHRH-containing neurons of the ventromedial hypo-

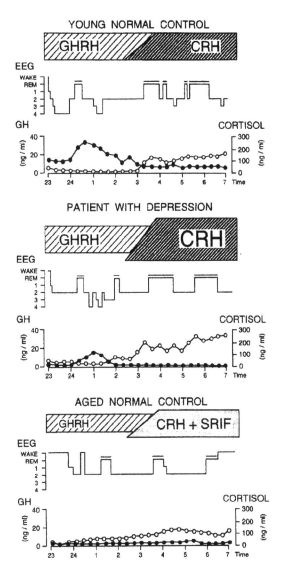

Figure 4 Hypothesized reciprocal interaction of growth hormone–releasing hormone (GHRH) and corticotropin-releasing hormone (CRH) in normal sleep regulation (young healthy control subjects), during hypothalamic-pituitary-adrenal (HPA) system hyperactivity (patients with depression), and during decreased HPA efficacy (elderly control subjects). In the elderly, somatostatin (SRIF) is believed to contribute, along with CRH, to the impairment of sleep. (From Ref. 107.)

thalamic nucleus to the preoptic area, a forebrain region implicated in sleep regulation (104,106). GHRH neurons in the arcuate nucleus of the hypothalamus project and release GHRH to the median eminence. GHRH is then transported in the bloodstream to the anterior pituitary where it induces GH production and release.

Physiological or psychological responses to stress first involve central release of corticotropin-releasing hormone (CRH), the main regulator of the HPA axis. CRH and a cosecretagogue, arginine vasopressin (AVP), originate from the parvocellular neurons of the paraventricular nucleus of the hypothalamus (114–117). CRH is released from the median eminence into the hypophyseal portal blood supply of the anterior pituitary where it stimulates adrenocorticotropic hormone (ACTH) release from proopiomelanocortin (POMC) cells. Then, ACTH travels in the systemic circulation to reach the adrenal gland, leading to glucocorticoid secretion. Another pathway involved in the stress response involved CRH neurons in the amygdala and bed nucleus of the stria terminalis. These neurons project to the locus coeruleus where they stimulate the release of noradrenaline (118–121). Those two CRH pathways are the main actors in behavioral and endocrine response to stress. Glucocorticoids, the end product of the HPA axis, stimulate an increased availability of energy substrates to the body and brain during periods of stress. Circulating glucocorticoids also feed back on the brain and pituitary to inhibit further CRH and ACTH secretion (Fig. 5) (122). This negative feedback regulation is important to avoid or limit the deleterious effects of prolonged glucocorticoid exposure.

It is now accepted that the HPA axis is involved in the regulation of vigilance states (Fig. 6). CRH, stimulating the HPA axis, is involved in a behavioral response to stress that is characterized by cortical arousal and EEG activation. CRH is also part of a general arousal mechanism; it seems to contribute to wakefulness in the absence of stressor (159,160). Cortisol and ACTH are secreted in response to hypothalamic release of CRH. Cortisol secretion appears to be mostly influenced by the circadian phase and much less by the sleep-wake cycle itself. In humans, cortisol secretion reaches its nadir in the evening, in association with sleep onset, and reaches its peak in the early morning, with the end of the nocturnal sleep episode.

Sleep and the Somatotropic Axis

The majority of the 24-hr GH release occurs usually during early nocturnal sleep, when SWS is the most abundant (123–125). The largest GH surge is seen shortly after sleep onset in young men. In women, however, GH pulses are usually smaller and more frequent (125–127). The idea of a possible mutual functional relationship between SWS and GH has been strengthened following the observation of blunted GH secretion after sleep deprivation (128,129). Moreover, the disruption of SWS by spontaneous awakenings disturbed GH secretion and is accompanied by a pulse of cortisol secretion (129,130). SWS episodes and GH release can also be dissociated since GH release is seen outside SWS episodes; about one-third of

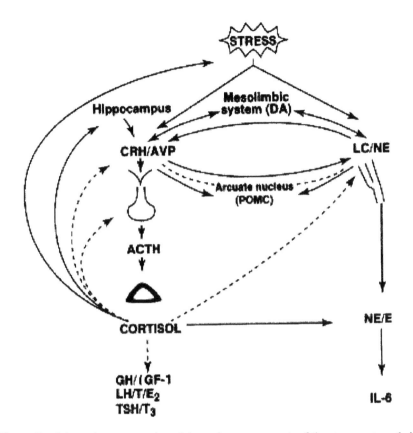

Figure 5 Schematic representation of the various components of the stress system, their functional interrelations, and their relations to other central systems involved in the stress response. The corticotropin-releasing hormone/arginine vasopressin (CRH/AVP) neurons and central catecholaminergic neurons of the locus coeruleus/norepinephrine (LC/NE) system reciprocally innervate and activate each other. The hypothalamic-pituitary-adrenal (HPA) axis is controlled by several feedback loops that tend to normalize the time-integrated secretion of cortisol, yet glucocorticoids stimulate the fear centers in the amygdala. Activation of the HPA axis leads to suppression of the growth hormone/insulin-like growth factor-1 (GH/IGF-1), luteinizing hormone (LH)/testosterone/prostaglandin E2, and thyroid stimulating hormone (TSH)/T_3 axes; activation of the sympathetic system increases interleukin-6 (IL-6) secretion. Solid lines indicate stimulation; dashed lines indicate inhibition. (From Ref. 122.)

SWS epochs occur without GH secretion, and GH increase has been seen before sleep onset (131,132). Moreover, one study using partial sleep deprivation did not show suppression or delay in the onset of GH release (133). Since the secretion of GH is stimulated by GHRH and inhibited by somatostatin, the dissociation between GH and SWS may be related to variations of the somatostatinergic control on GH secretion (112). It is also worth noting that GHRH and CRH present a

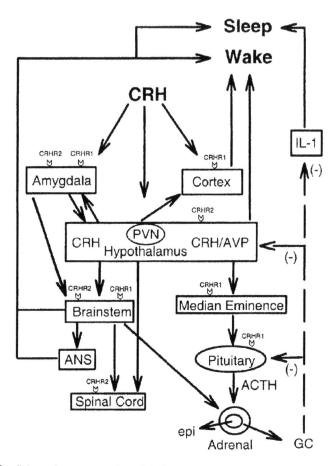

Figure 6 Schematic representation of the localization, projections, and receptor distributions of the corticotropin-releasing hormone (CRH) system as it pertains to the regulation of waking and sleep. The neuroendocrine actions of CRH involve the hypothalamic-pituitary-adrenal (HPA) axis. CRH effects on the autonomic nervous system are mediated by projections to the brainstem, specifically the locus coeruleus, A1 catecholamine cell groups, and dorsal vagal complex. Current evidence suggests interactions between CRH and the immunomodulator interleukin-1 (IL-1) as they pertain to sleep are mediated by glucocorticoid feedback mechanisms. ACTH, adrenocorticotropic hormone; AVP, arginine vasopressin; ANS, autonomic nervous system; CRHR1 and CRHR2, CRH receptor subtypes; epi, epinepinephrine; GC, glucocorticoids; PVN, paraventricular nucleus. (From Ref. 160.)

reciprocal relationship in sleep regulation; GHRH has sleep-promoting effects and CRH disrupts sleep (134). As a result, the ratio between GHRH and CRH will be an important actor in sleep-wake cycle regulation (Fig. 4).

Spontaneous GH secretion is maximal during the maturational process accompanying puberty and then starts to decrease gradually (135,136). GH is released in a series of large pulses during the day and the night in pubertal children (136). During puberty, GH is also secreted during early SWS, but not as a major GH peak as observed in adults; GH secretion occurs throughout the 24-hr day. Across puberty, an increase in the GH secretory rate occurs at an earlier pubertal stage and is more pronounced in girls than in boys (135). Van Cauter and colleagues suggested that the control of neuroendocrine release of GH during puberty would be different from the metabolic effects observed during adulthood (137).

During adulthood, an important decrease in GH secretion seems to parallel the marked SWS reduction. GH surge decreases by 75% from young adulthood to middle age, and during the same period SWS is reduced by about 80% (137). The lower GH surge in elderly individuals has been related to the lowered efficacy of GHRH in promoting GH release (138). The activity of the GHRH system has been shown to decline with aging. However, somatostatin release does not seem to be affected by aging (139). It may be hypothesized that the reduced efficacy of GHRH in promoting GH and SWS may be related to the reduced effectiveness of GHRH against inhibitory influences of somatostatin and CRH, thereby disturbing sleep. Exogenous administration of GHRH to old individuals elicited a reduced GH surge compared to young adults, but cortisol and ACTH secretion were not modified (138). Sleep was improved in old subjects after GHRH administration; a reduced number of nocturnal awakenings and an increased duration of the first NREM episode were observed, but the effect was significantly less compared to that in young individuals (140,141). In young healthy subjects, the effects of GHRH administration usually increases SWS, but the effect depends markedly on the way of administration, the time of day, and the dose used, with continuous infusion having no effect on sleep EEG (140–142). The pulsatile mode of release may best mimic the physiological release of GHRH and higher doses may inhibit GHRH via an increased GH negative feedback on GHRH release.

Surprisingly, SWS was decreased in young men after exogenous GH injection, and it was suggested that a feedback inhibition of GH on endogenous GHRH might be responsible for these effects (143). Another study observed no change of sleep architecture after systemic GH administration in young men, even if plasma GH was increased (142). However, other studies have shown in humans, rats, and cats that GH administration increased REM sleep duration (143–145).

The effect of GHRH on SWS would not be mediated by GH; GHRH seems to have direct central actions (105,107). GHRH clearly has sleep-promoting effects; however, GH would be implicated in REM sleep rebound, but not in SWS rebound. Obal and collaborators (146) showed an increase in SWS after GHRH administration in hypophysectomized rats but no change in REM sleep. In control animals, GHRH induced both SWS and REM sleep increase, suggesting that the REM sleep-promoting effect of GHRH are mediated by GH release, but GH does not affect SWS. These results point to a major role of GHRH as a sleep regulatory substance, with possible involvement of GH for REM sleep control.

D. Sleep and Stress

HPA Axis and the Stress Response. Age-Related Changes
in HPA Axis Regulation: Impaired HPA Axis "Resiliency"

The environment has a profound impact on brain development in early life, and long-term exposure to threatening environment increases vulnerability to brain damage later in life. Indeed, prolonged stress exposure has been associated with an acceleration of the aging process and with impaired stress responsivity (147,148). Excess of glucocorticoids induces hippocampal damage and synaptic loss, eventually leading to memory problems and cognitive impairments (147,149,150). Hippocampal injury appears be involved in the impaired glucocorticoid feedback regulation observed with increasing age (151). In a 4-year follow-up study, Lupien et al. (150) showed that aged humans with increasing levels of cortisol displayed a reduced hippocampal volume. The degree of hippocampal atrophy correlated strongly with both the degree of cortisol elevation over time and current basal cortisol levels.

The impaired glucocorticoid feedback results in hyperactivity of the HPA axis and reduced ability to recover from an endogenous or exogenous challenge. Such alteration of the HPA axis is observed in normal and pathological aging and in disorders such as depression and Cushing's syndrome (152). However, glucocorticoid feedback alterations during aging and increased levels of glucocorticoids are not seen in all seniors. Individual differences in coping with stress throughout life will influence greatly the aging process and the vulnerability to disease later in life (153,154). As mentioned earlier, individual differences in glucocorticoid secretion in old age are markedly influenced by life experiences (155). Accordingly, elderly individuals may present different sensitivity to negative feedback and different level of HPA axis activation following stress exposure (154). In general, elderly people show a longer stress response characterized by an increased duration of glucocorticoid secretion following stress exposure (147,156). The prolonged glucocorticoid secretion seems to be related to the inability to return to baseline values after a stressful experience, probably due to glucocorticoid receptor insensitivity (147,157). This insensitivity has been associated with the loss of glucocorticoid receptors (147,154). It has been proposed that life events increasing the activity of physiological systems induce "wear and tear" or allostatic load, resulting from overactivity of the stress responsive system (158). Accordingly, McEwens proposed that the allostatic load reflects stressful experiences but also lifestyle, including diet, exercise, and substance abuse (158).

HPA Axis, Stress, and Sleep

All of us have experienced the effect of stress on a night's sleep. The few studies available on the relationship between insomnia or "poor" sleep and stress report inconsistent results (161,162). However, it has been shown that HPA axis activity is related with the degree of sleep disturbances in chronic insomniacs (162–164). One study investigated the relationship between clinical correlates of insomnia and quantitative sleep electroencephalogram in insomniacs (165). Results showed that symptoms of stress and depression are significantly correlated with decreased delta power and increased alpha power in NREM sleep, reflecting hyperarousal during sleep. Moreover, a high level of subjective stress and intrusive thought tendencies were related to decreased delta power and tendency to increased beta power. Finally, decreased subjective sleep quality was linked to higher intrusion tendencies and symptoms of subclinical depression. The influence of stress on sleep architecture has also been studied in relation to depression. Endogenous depression is characterized by major HPA axis disturbances and sleep-wake alterations. Depressed patient's sleep is more fragmented, REM latency is shortened, SWS is reduced, and GH secretion is blunted (134,166). They also present a flattening of the sleep-wake cycle rhythms. Moreover, depressed patients exhibit hypercortisolemia, probably resulting from a chronic stress exposure. This elevated cortisol level represents a similarity between sleep and endocrine alterations in depressed patients and during normal aging (167) (Fig. 4). Hypercortisolemia and disturbed sleep characterized mostly by diminished levels of SWS are also found in Cushing's disease patients (168,169).

Exposure to chronic mild stress in rats is followed by major sleep disturbances, such as a decrease in active waking, deep sleep, and REM sleep, and the blunting of the sleep-wake cycle (170,171). On the other hand, it was observed that acute stress induced by 1 or 2 hr of immobilization at the beginning of the active period is followed by an increase in sleep duration, mostly an increase in REM sleep (172,173). These sleep changes after stress exposure have been associated with activation of a complex regulatory loop involving serotonin and POMC-derived peptides (172). Gonzales and collaborators (173) showed that lesioning the noradrenergic system of the locus coeruleus (LC) abolished sleep response to immobilization stress. Since the LC has an important role in stress response and that LC activation following stress exposure involves central action of CRH, Gonzales and Valatx looked at the possible involvement of CRH in the sleep-wake response after acute stress. They concluded that the REM sleep increase after acute stress exposure is mediated by the CRH/nonadrenaline (NA)-LC interaction (174). However, an acute stressor such as "social defeat" induced a strong rebound of SWA during SWS in rats; no effect on REM was observed (175). All of these studies suggest that the impact of stress on the sleep-wake cycle depends markedly on the type and duration of the stressor. One study looked at the effects of stress duration on sleep rebound (176). It has been shown that after 4 hr, the sleep-promoting effects of stress disappeared and sleep disturbances started. Sleep rebound after immobilization of short duration is viewed as a reactive homeostatic response to stress (176). It was also suggested that chronic stress impairs the sleep recovery process probably due to the prolonged corticosterone secretion associated with prolonged stress exposure. The deleterious effects of prolonged stress on the sleep-wake cycle may be part of other chronic stress-related health problems.

Stress in animals (and humans) influences the sleep-wake cycle with important individual differences (172,177,178). It has been shown that rats with high (high responder, HR) or low (low responder, LR) locomotor reactivity to novelty stress display different sleep-wakefulness patterns (178). Moreover, following stress exposure, animals showing hyperreactivity to novelty (HRs) had a prolonged corticosterone secretion compared to LRs. During baseline sleep recordings, LRs spent less time awake and had more SWS compared to HRs. After exposure to immobilization stress, HRs slept more than LRs, with no difference in REM sleep between groups (both showed increased REM). Previous results showed that HRs and LRs also present different dopaminergic and serotonergic activities in the nucleus accumbens, striatum and frontal cortex. The same animals exhibit different age-related decreases in cognitive abilities and sensitivities toward drug addiction (179,180). The authors concluded that the response of the sleep-wake cycle to stress is related to behavioral reactivity to stress, which is under the control of the HPA axis.

Reduced CRH synthesis has been related to a decrease in wakefulness. Central or systemic CRH administration increases EEG activation in rats, rabbits, and humans. In rats and rabbits, intracerebroventricular CRH administration decreased SWS (181,182). CRH also reduced SWS, increased REM sleep duration and prolonged sleep latency even after 72 hr sleep deprivation in rats (183). Gonzales and Valatx (174) reported no effect of α-hCRH (a CRH receptor antagonist) on spontaneous waking. However, α-hCRH blocked sleep alterations in rats after exposure to restrain stress. According to the authors (184), CRH would be mainly involved in REM sleep rebound after sleep deprivation. This study is in contrast with results of Chang and Opp showing that in rats CRH receptor antagonists (α-hCRH and astressin) injection during the dark phase decreased spontaneous waking and increased SWS, but with a different time course (185). The authors concluded that CRH is involved in normal waking mechanisms, in addition to its role in the stress response. Interestingly, genetically related rat strains presenting different synthesis and secretion of CRH present different amounts of wakefulness (186). Decreased CRH release was related to reduction of wakefulness. These last results support the view of CRH being involved in the normal regulation of wakefulness.

In humans, multiple doses of CRH (4×50 μg) to young subjects between 22 hr and 1 hr reduced SWS during the second part of the night and decreased REM sleep across all nocturnal sleep (187). Moreover, during the first part of a nocturnal sleep episode, cortisol level was increased and GH secretion was blunted. Another study using intravenous CRH injection found reduced SWS and sleep efficiency and an increase in stages 1 and 2 in normal subjects (188). A single intravenous CRH injection also affected the sleep electroencephalogram in young men. During the first three sleep cycles, an increase in sigma frequency was observed if CRH was administered either during the first episode of SWS or during wakefulness (189). It is important to note that the effects of CRH depend markedly on its dosage, timing, and route of administration.

SWS and SWA seem to exert an inhibitory influence on cortisol secretion. Indeed, a high level of SWA during sleep has been reported to be temporally related to low cortisol levels (189–191). It has still been proposed that the offset of SWS episodes may trigger the first important rise in cortisol (190). In the study by Gronfier and colleagues, REM sleep occurrence was also preceded by a decrease in cortisol secretion. They suggested that low neuroendocrine activity is a prerequisite for the increase in SWA. SWA and cortisol interaction has further been analyzed by recording sleep in two groups of young subjects sleeping at different circadian phases; one group slept during the night and sleep was delayed by 8 hr in the second group, so they slept during the day (192). The results revealed an increased SWA at the beginning of the night, when cortisol level was minimal. But when SWA and cortisol secretion were present at the same time (e.g., at the end-of-night sleep and also during daytime sleep), they were negatively correlated, and cortisol changes preceded modifications in SWA by approximately 10 min. The authors suggested that cortisol secretion and SWA have independent generators and are in-phase opposition.

In human babies, cortisol levels decrease significantly during the first weeks of life and then increase significantly reaching adult levels between 1 and 3 yrs of age (193,194). Reports on basal cortisol levels during aging have been inconclusive, some suggesting an increase, a decrease, or no change (109,111,152,195–201). More recent studies revealed that nighttime levels of glucocorticoids are somewhat increased in healthy seniors. However, the amplitude of cortisol rhythm is decreased, suggesting a flattening of circadian rhythms in old age (201,202). The morning rise in cortisol secretion is also phase advanced with advancing age (111,203). A study conducted in 149 subjects aged between 18 and 83 years reported a progressive age-related increase in the 24-hr mean level of cortisol in men and an elevation of the evening nadir (16). The increase in cortisol nadir was significant only after the age of 50 and was associated with a reduction in REM sleep and an increase in time spent awake. Van Cauter and collaborators (16) proposed that sleep alterations occurring at specific moments during aging are coupled to specific neuroendocrine changes. For example, SWS and GH decreases take place from young adulthood to middle age, whereas REM sleep and cortisol changes are not significant before the fifth decade.

Intravenous cortisol administration in young subjects, either pulsatile or continuous, induces an increase of SWS and a reduction of REM sleep (204,205). Healthy seniors who received pulsatile intravenous cortisol injection showed higher levels of SWS and SWA during NREM sleep and reduced REM sleep. Moreover, GH was increased after cortisol administration (206). The effects of exogenous cortisol on sleep (mostly SWS) are opposite to those of CRH and disagree with the idea that CRH act by stimulating cortisol release. In humans, the differential effects of cortisol on SWS and REM sleep seem to be mediated by different mechanisms. Cortisol would decrease REM sleep duration via its action on glucocorticoid receptors (GR) and increase SWS duration via mineralocorticoid receptors (204). Cortisol effects on sleep may also be mediated by its negative feedback on CRH, allowing GHRH release (206).

Sleep Loss, HPA Axis, and Stress

Chronic sleep loss or sleep restriction is a common phenomenon of our modern society promoting around-the-clock work and the reduction of time spent sleeping. Stress exposure has negative effects on sleep, and chronic sleep loss will generate a state of stress and anxiety having a deleterious impact on the HPA axis. However, different studies reported either no effect (207,208) or decreased cortisol levels (209) after total sleep deprivation. Saletu and collaborators (210) showed increased troughs and an earlier rise in cortisol levels after partial sleep deprivation. But these results were at variance with some consecutive studies. No changes in cortisol levels the day and the night following either partial (103,211) or total sleep deprivation (212–215) as well as reduced cortisol concentrations in corresponding partial (133) or total sleep deprivation (216) period have been reported. Based on their findings, Vgontzas et al. (216) suggested that sleep deprivation results in a significant reduction of cortisol secretion the next day and this reduction appears to be, to a large extent, driven by the increase of slow-wave activity during the recovery night (22,217).

On the other hand, a series of investigations support the concept of sleep deprivation being a contributor of HPA axis activation and the consequent elevation of cortisol levels (218–220). Weibel et al. (221) showed that the amount of cortisol secreted during night sleep was lower than during the corresponding period of 8 hr of sleep deprivation. In the study by von Treuer and colleagues (222), cortisol was significantly higher on the sleep deprivation night (36 hr), presumably reflecting the arousal state accompanying being awake. It was reported that sleep deprivation in young healthy men induced a modification in cortisol secretion that "mimicked" changes observed in elderly individuals, inducing a delay in the onset of the quiescent period of cortisol secretion the following evening (219). Total sleep deprivation was associated with a 2.4-fold increase in cortisol levels in the following evening. These results have been corroborated by a more chronic sleep restriction (4 hr/night for 6 days) (223). Sleep debt produced alterations in the 24-hr profile of plasma cortisol, including a shorter and delayed quiescent period and higher concentrations of cortisol in the afternoon and early evening. These findings suggest that the mechanism of HPA recovery from stimulation may be affected by sleep. The authors proposed that the prolonged sleep loss throughout life may be involved in the increase in cortisol observed in old people and that HPA axis perturbations may represent sleep and circadian alterations (105). Van Cauter and collaborators (16) also proposed that decreased sleep quality with increasing age contributes to the allostatic load. These results suggest that sleep habits throughout life may have an important impact on vulnerability to sleep disturbances and on health later in life.

It has been proposed that prolonged sleep deprivation or sleep curtailment might alter HPA axis regulation (218). They observed that rats subjected to 48 hr of sleep deprivation presented a mild increase in ACTH and a higher increase of corticosterone. During chronic sleep restriction of 20 hr each day, rats exhibited a similar increase in both ACTH and corticosterone. Moreover, sleep restriction also had an impact on response of the HPA axis to subsequent stressor presentation; following restrain stress, ACTH release was significantly decreased but corticosterone response was unchanged. The authors concluded that the effect of sleep loss on the stress system may have profound consequences since the HPA axis and glucocorticoids are responsible for a variety of processes such as metabolism, immune function, neuronal viability, and learning and memory.

HPA Axis, Sleep, and Aging

Increasing age is marked by important interindividual differences in sleep pattern. Sleep problems usually appear during the middle years of life, a period of high workload and familial occupancy. The impact of stress during middle age may be more apparent because advancing age is associated with more fragmented sleep, less SWS, and more light sleep and wakefulness. Indeed, as early as middle age, people become more vulnerable to stress-disturbing effects on sleep and report more insomnia associated with emotional stress (224). The high prevalence of insomnia with increasing age has been attributed to the high level of stress and the social situation at work (225).

The fragmentation of sleep that typically occurs in aging may play a role in the elevation of evening cortisol secretion (226). Alternatively, nocturnal exposure to increased HPA activity may produce sleep fragmentation and impair sleep quality in older people (227). To date, very few studies have tested these hypotheses. Up to now, only one study investigated the effect of age on endocrine parameters following sleep deprivation (228). Baseline GH level was lower and prolactin was higher in aged subjects than in young ones. However, GH, prolactin, and cortisol were not affected differentially by sleep deprivation in both groups of subjects. GH and cortisol secretion were unchanged after sleep deprivation and prolactin was increased in both groups. The authors concluded that the plasticity of the sleep endocrine system is preserved during aging and that modifications of the HPA and somatotropic axes with aging do not affect the response to sleep deprivation. Prinz et al. (227) showed that both aged women and men presenting higher levels of free cortisol had more beta activity and shorter stages 2, 3, and 4 during NREM sleep. Moreover, one study showed that sleep of middle-aged subjects is more sensitive to the arousing effects of CRH than that of young ones (229). One bolus of CRH (1 μg/kg IV) during the first sleep cycle (approximately 10 min after sleep onset) induced a greater increase in wakefulness and more suppression of SWS in the middle-aged than in the young subjects, despite similar elevations of ACTH and cortisol. The authors concluded that older subjects might be at higher risk of developing insomnia when faced with equivalent stressors.

V. Conclusions

Major changes of sleep and endocrine functions occur during the normal course of aging. However, the exact mechanisms that underlie many of these changes remain to be fully elucidated. For example, the phase advance hypothesis of the circadian signal has been able to predict age-dependent changes in the timing of the sleep-wake cycle. However, the neurophysiological mechanisms responsible for decreased sleep consolidation, the marked diminution of SWS and SWA during normal sleep, the lower rebound of SWS and SWA following an acute sleep deprivation, and the lower tolerance to a phase angle misalignment between sleep and the circadian signal are still unclear.

Stimulation of NREM sleep and GH secretion would be two separate effects of GHRH (106). It has been hypothesized that the relationship between SWS and GH release could be related to synchronous activity of both groups of GHRH neurons (125). As a result, the parallel decrease of both GH and SWS with aging may be a consequence of GHRH deficiency. Since during normal sleep SWS and GH are closely associated, it has been proposed that substances stimulating SWS may help to restore better sleep and also increase GH release in older people; those drugs may be used as GH secretagogues (125). However, neither GH nor GH secretagogues seems to induce a significant increase in SWS (142,230,231). Knowing GHRH involvement in regulation of sleep and endocrine functions, and since aging is related to important GHRH deficiency, drugs stimulating GHRH release may offer a way to increase SWS and help alleviate sleep problems in the elderly population.

Individual differences in the sleep of healthy adults, and even more with increasing age, may be related to the vulnerability to the sleep-disturbing effects of various factors. There is a close functional interaction between the HPA and somatotropic axes in the regulation of the sleep-wake cycle. Indeed, CRH and GHRH present an opposite relationship in sleep regulation (134). The association of decreased GH and increased CRH secretion during aging may have a major impact on sleep in healthy adults, but even more in elderly, insomniac, and depressed individuals (232). Indeed, the GHRH/CRH ratio contributes to sleep-endocrine regulation, and an increased level of CRH may favor sleep disruptions (107,134). Moreover, since somatostatin levels do not decrease (and may even increase) with age, its inhibitory influence on GHRH will further increase sleep disruptions (107,233). In addition to sleep disorders, the decreased GHRH/CRH ratio will be involved in many body alterations reported in elderly individuals, such as loss of muscle mass, increased abdominal fat with glucose tolerance, and decreased immune function (16,156,234,235).

We need to understand the precise mechanisms regulating sleep and endocrine systems to develop effective preventative and therapeutic strategies for people with sleep disturbances and in the elderly population. The impact of age-related alterations of the sleep-wake cycle and chronic sleep loss is wide and may affect physical health, cognitive functioning, quality of life, metabolism, and hormonal regulation. Moreover, acute and even more chronic stress exposure will further impair sleep, increasing health disturbances. Efforts should be invested in the research of the functional significance of the relationship between sleep and neuroendocrine systems. Understanding the age-related alterations in these inter-related systems will lead to the development of new strategies to ameliorate sleep difficulties in normal individuals and even more in insomniac and older individuals with sleep disorders.

References

1. Coble PA, Kupfer DJ, Taska LS, Kane J. EEG sleep of normal healthy children. Part I: findings using standard measurement methods. Sleep 1984; 7:289–303.
2. Feinberg I. Changes in sleep cycle patterns with age. J Psychiatr Res. 1974; 10:283–306.
3. Williams RL, Karacan I, Hursch CJ. EEG of Human Sleep: Clinical Applications. New York: John Wiley & Sons, 1974.
4. Carskadon MA. The second decade. In: Guilleminault C, ed. Sleeping and Waking Disorders: Indications and Techniques. Menlo Park, CA: Addison-Wesley, 1982:99–125.
5. Williams RL, Karacan I, Davis CE. Sleep patterns of pubertal males. Pediatric Res 1972; 6:643–648.
6. Kahn A, Dan B, Groswasser J, Franco P, Sottiaux M. Normal sleep architecture in infants and children. Review. J Clin Neurophysiol 1996; 13:184–197.
7. Carskadon MA, Acebo C, Richardson GS, Tate BA, Seifer R. An approach to studying circadian rhythms of adolescent humans. J Biol Rhythms 1997; 12:278–289.
8. Carskadon MA, Acebo C, Seifer R. Extended nights, sleep loss, and recovery sleep in adolescents. Arch Ital Biol 2001; 139:301–312.
9. Karacan I, Anch M, Thornby JI, Okawa M, Williams RL. Longitudinal sleep patterns during pubertal growth: four-year follow-up. Pediatric Res 1975; 9:842–846.
10. Feinberg I, Floyd TC. Systematic trends across the night in human sleep cycles. Psychophysiology 1979; 16(3):283–291.
11. Feinberg I. Schizophrenia: caused by a fault in programmed synaptic elimination during adolescence? J Psychiatr Res 1982; 17 (4):319–334.
12. Bliwise D. Sleep in normal aging and dementia. Sleep 1993; 16(1):40–81.
13. Carrier J, Monk TH, Buysse DJ, Kupfer DJ. Sleep and morningness-eveningness in the "middle" years of life (20y–59y). J Sleep Res 1997; 6:230–237.
14. Miles L, Dement WC. Sleep and aging. Sleep 1980; 3:119–220.
15. Reynolds CF, Hoch CC, Buysse DJ, Monk TH, Houck PR, Kupfer DJ. REM sleep in successful, usual, and pathological aging: the Pittsburgh experience 1980–1993. J Sleep Res 1993; 2:203–210.
16. Van Cauter E, Leproult R, Plat L. Age-related changes in slow wave sleep and REM sleep and relationship with growth hormone and cortisol levels in healthy men. JAMA 2000; 284:861–868.
17. Foley DJ, Monjan AA, Brown SL, Simonsick EM, Wallace RB, Blazer DG. Sleep complaints among elderly persons: an epidemiologic study of three communities. Sleep 1995; 18:425–432.

18. Hoch CC, Dew MA, Reynolds CF, Monk TH, Houck PR, Jennings JR, et al. A longitudinal study of laboratory- and diary-based sleep measures in healthy "old old" and "young old" volunteers. Sleep 1994; 17(6):489–496.

19. Hoch CC, Dew MA, Reynolds CF, Buysse DJ, Nowell P, Monk TH, et al. Longitudinal changes in diary- and laboratory-based sleep measures in health "old old" and "young old" subjects: a three- year follow-up. Sleep 1997; 20(3):192–202.

20. Phillips B, Ancoli-Israel S. Sleep disorders in the elderly. Sleep Med 2001; 2:99–114.

21. Martin J, Shochat T, Gehrman PR, Ancoli-Israel S. Sleep in the elderly. Respir Care Clin North Am 1999; 5:461–472.

22. Borbely AA, Baumann F, Brandeis D, Strauch I, Lehmann D. Sleep deprivation: effect on sleep stages and EEG power density in man. Electroencephalogr Clin Neurophysiol 1981; 51:483–493.

23. Armitage R, Hudson A, Trivedi M, Rush AJ. Sex difference in the distribution of EEG frequencies during sleep: unipolar depressed outpatients. J Affect Disord 1995; 34:121–129.

24. Merica H, Blois R, Gaillard JM. Spectral characteristics of sleep EEG in chronic insomnia. Eur J Neurosci 1998; 10:1826–1834.

25. Gaudreau H, Carrier J, Montplaisir J. Age-related modifications of NREM sleep EEG: from childhood to middle age. J Sleep Res 2001; 10:165–172.

26. Church MW, March JD, Hibi S, Benson K, Cavness C, Feinberg I. Changes in frequency and amplitude of delta activity during sleep. Electroenceph Clin Neurophysiol 1975; 39:1–7.

27. Feinberg I, Koresko RL, Heller N. EEG sleep patterns as a function of normal and pathological aging in man. J Psychiatr Res 1967; 5:107–144.

28. Astrom C, Trojaborg W. Relationship of age to power spectrum analysis of EEG during sleep. J Clin Neurophysiol 1992; 9:424–430.

29. Landolt HP, Dijk DJ, Achermann P, Borbely AA. Effect of age on the sleep EEG: slow-wave activity and spindle frequency activity in young and middle-aged men. Brain Res 1996; 738:205–212.

30. Carrier J, Land S, Buysse DJ, Kupfer DJ, Monk TH. The effects of age and gender on sleep EEG power spectral density in the "middle" years of life (20y–60y). Psychophysiology 2001; 38: 232–242.

31. Dijk DJ, Duffy JF, Czeisler CA. Contribution of circadian physiology and sleep homeostasis to age-related changes in human sleep. Chronobiol Int 2000; 17:285–311.

32. Wei HG, Riel E, Czeisler CA, Dijk DJ. Attenuated amplitude of circadian and sleep-dependent modulation of electroencephalographic sleep spindle characteristics in elderly human subjects. Neurosci Lett 1999; 260:29–32.

33. Borbely AA. A two-process model of sleep regulation. Hum Neurobiol 1982; 1:195–204.

34. Daan S, Beersma DGM, Borbely AA. Timing of human sleep: recovery process gated by circadian pacemaker. Am J Physiol 1984; 246:R161–R178.

35. Achermann P, Dijk D-J, Brunner DP, Borbély A. A model of human sleep homeostasis based on EEG slow-wave activity: quantitative comparison of data and simulations. Brain Res Bull 1993; 31:97–113.

36. Broughton RJ. SCN controlled circadian arousal and the afternoon "nap zone." Sleep Res Online 1998; 1:166–178.

37. Borbély AA, Achermann P. Sleep homeostasis and models of sleep regulation. In: Kryger MH, Roth T, Dement WC, eds. Principles and Practice of Sleep Medicine. 3rd ed. Philadelphia: WB Saunders, 2000:377–390.
38. Wexler DB, Moore-Ede MC. Circadian sleep-wake cycle organization in squirrel monkeys. Am J Physiol 1985; 248:R353–R362
39. Dijk DJ, Czeisler CA. Paradoxical timing of the circadian rhythm of sleep propensity serves to consolidate sleep and wakefulness in humans. Neurosci Lett 1994; 166:63–68.
40. Zulley J, Wever R, Aschoff J. The dependence of onset and duration of sleep on the circadian rhythm of rectal temperature. Pflugers Arch 1981; 391:314–318.
41. Lavie P. Ultrashort sleep-waking schedule. III. Gates and "forbidden zones" for sleep. Electroencephalogr Clin Neurophysiol 1986; 63:414–425.
42. Czeisler CA, Weitzman ED, Moore-Ede MC, Zimmerman JC, Knauer RS. Human sleep: its duration and organization depend on its circadian phase. Science 1980; 210:1264–1267.
43. Carskadon MA, Wolfson AR, Acebo C, Tzischinsky O, Seifer R. Adolescent sleep patterns, circadian timing, and sleepiness at a transition to early school days. Sleep 1998; 21:871–881.
44. Carskadon MA, Acebo C. Regulation of sleepiness in adolescents: update, insights, and speculation. Sleep 2002; 25:606–614.
45. Carskadon MA, Harvey K, Duke P, Anders TF, Litt IF, Dement WC. Pubertal changes in daytime sleepiness. Sleep 1980; 2(4):453–460.
46. Laberge L, Petit D, Simard C, Vitaro F, Tremblay RE, Montplaisir J. Development of sleep patterns in early adolescence. J Sleep Res 2001; 10:59–67.
47. Carskadon MA. Patterns of sleep and sleepiness in adolescents. Pediatrician 1990; 17(1):5–12.
48. Mendelson WB, Bergmann BM. EEG delta power during sleep in young and old rats. Neurobiol Aging 1999; 20:669–673.
49. Mendelson WB, Bergmann BM. Age-dependent changes in recovery sleep after 48 hours of sleep deprivation in rats. Neurobiol Aging 2000; 21:689–693.
50. Basheer R, Shiromani PJ. Effects of prolonged wakefulness on c-fos and AP1 activity in young and old rats. Brain Res Mol Brain Res. 2001; 89:153–157.
51. Bonnet MH. Effect of 64 hours of sleep deprivation upon sleep in geriatric normals and insomniacs. Neurobiol Aging 1986; 7:89–96.
52. Bonnet M. The effect of sleep fragmentation on sleep and performance in younger and older subjects. Neurobiol Aging 1989; 10:21–25.
53. Brendel DH, Reynolds CF, Jennings JR, Hoch CC, Monk TH, Berman SR, et al. Sleep stage physiology, mood, and vigilance responses to total sleep deprivation in healthy 80–year-olds and 20–year-olds. Psychophysiology 1990; 27 (6):677–685.
54. Carskadon MA, Dement WC. Sleep loss in elderly volunteers. Sleep 1985; 8:207–221.
55. Bonnet MH, Rosa RR. Sleep and performance in young adults and older normals and insomniacs during acute sleep loss and recovery. Biol Psychol 1987; 25:153–172.
56. Gaudreau H, Morettini J, Lavoie HB, Carrier J. Effects of a 25–h sleep deprivation on daytime sleep in the middle-aged. Neurobiol Aging 2001; 22:461–468.
57. Akerstedt T, Folkard S. The three-process model of alertness and its extension to performance, sleep latency and sleep length. Chronobiol Int 1997; 14:115–123.

58. Folkard S, Akerstedt T. A three-process model of the regulation of alertness-sleepiness. In: Broughton RJ, Ogilvie RD, eds. Sleep, Arousal, and Performance: A Tribute to Bob Wilkinson. Boston: Birkhauser, 1992:11–26.

59. Jewett ME, Kronauer RE. Interactive mathematical models of subjective alertness and cognitive throughput in humans. J Biol Rhythms 1999; 14:588–597.

60. Johnson MP, Duffy JF, Dijk DJ, Ronda JM, Dyal CM, Czeisler CA. Short-term memory, alertness and performance: a reappraisal of their relationship to body temperature. J Sleep Res 1992; 1:24–29.

61. Monk TH, Moline ML, Fookson JE, Peetz SM. Circadian determinants of subjective alertness. J Biol Rhythms 1989; 4:393–404.

62. Anders TF, Carskadon MA, Dement WC, Harvey K. Sleep habits of children and the identification of pathologically sleepy children. Child Psychiatry Hum Dev 1978; 9:56–63.

63. Andrade MM, Benedito-Silva AA, Domenice S, Arnhold IJ, Menna-Barreto L. Sleep characteristics of adolescents: a longitudinal study. J Adolesc Health 1993; 14:401–406.

64. Carskadon MA, Keenan S, Dement WC. Nightime sleep and daytime sleep tendency in preadolescents. In: Guilleminaut C, ed. Sleep and Its Disorders in Children. New York: Raven Press, 1987:43–52.

65. Palm L, Persson E, Elmqvist D, Blennow G. Sleep and wakefulness in normal preadolescent children. Sleep 1989; 12:299–308.

66. Bonnet MH, Arand DL. Sleep loss in aging. Clin Geriatr Med 1989; 5:405–420.

67. Smulders FT, Kenemans JL, Jonkman LM, Kok A. The effects of sleep loss on task performance and the electroencephalogram in young and elderly subjects. Biol Psychol 1997; 45:217–239.

68. Vojtechovsky M, Brezinova V, Simane Z, Hort V. An experimental approach ot sleep and aging. Human Dev 1969; 12:64–72.

69. Webb WB, Levy CM. Age, sleep deprivation, and performance. Psychophysiology 1982; 19:272–276.

70. Myers BL, Badia P. Changes in circadian rhythms and sleep quality with aging: mechanisms and interventions. Neurosci Biobehav Rev 1995; 19:553–571.

71. Horne JA, Ostberg O. A self-assessment questionnaire to determine morningness-eveningness in human circadian rhythms. Int J Chronobiol 1976; 4:97–110.

72. Carskadon MA, Vieira C, Acebo C. Association between puberty and delayed phase preference. Sleep 1993; 16:258–262.

73. Giannotti F, Cortesi F. Sleep patterns and daytime function in adolescence: an epidemiological survey of an Italian high school student sample. In: Carskadon MA, ed. Adolescent Sleep Patterns: Biological, Social and Psychological Influences. Cambridge, UK: Cambridge University Press, 2002:132–147.

74. Tzischinsky O, Wolfson AR, Darley C., Brown C, Acebo C, Carskadon MA. Sleep habits and salivary melatonin onset in adolescents. Sleep Res 1995; 24:543.

75. Carrier J, Monk TH, Reynolds CFI, Buysse DJ, Kupfer DJ. Are age differences in sleep due to phase differences in the output of the circadian timing system? Chronobiol Int 1999; 16:79–91.

76. Duffy JF, Dijk DJ, Klerman EB, Czeisler C. Later endogenous circadian temperature nadir relative to an earlier wake time in older people. Am J Physiol 1998; 275:R1478–R1487

77. Carrier J, Paquet J, Morettini J, Touchette E. Phase advance of sleep and temperature circadian rhythms in the middle years of life in humans. Neurosci Lett 2002; 320:1–4.

78. Campbell SS, Dawson D. Aging young sleep: a test of the phase advance hypothesis of sleep disturbance in the elderly. J Sleep Res 1992; 1:205–210.

79. Weitzman ED, Moline ML, Czeisler CA, Zimmerman JC. Chronobiology of aging: temperature, sleep-wake rhythms and entrainment. Neurobiol Aging 1982; 3:299–309.

80. Campbell SS, Dawson D, Anderson MW. Alleviation of sleep maintenance insomnia with timed exposure to bright light. J Am Geriatr Soc 1993; 41:829–836.

81. Klerman EB, Duffy JF, Dijk DJ, Czeisler CA. Circadian phase resetting in older people by ocular bright light exposure. J Invest Med 2001; 49:30–40.

82. Coble PA, Reynolds CF 3rd, Kupfer DJ, Houck P. Electroencephalographic sleep of healthy children. II: Findings using automated delta and REM sleep measurement methods. Sleep 1987; 10:551–562.

83. Webb WB. The measurement and characteristics of sleep in older persons. Neurobiol Aging 1982; 3:311–319.

84. Reynolds CF, Monk TH, Hoch CC, Jennings JR, Buysse DJ, Houck PR, et al. EEG sleep in the healthy "old old": a comparison with the "young old" in visually scored and automated (period) measures. J Gerontol 1991; 46:M39–M46

85. Wolfson A.R. Sleeping patterns of children and adolescents. Child Adolesc Psychiatr Clin North Am 1996; 5:549–568.

86. Rugg-Gunn A.J., Hackett A.F., Appleton D.R., Eastoe J.E. Bedtimes of 11–14–year old children in north-east England. J Biosoc Sci 1984; 16:291–297.

87. Wolfson A.R., Carskadon M.A. Sleep schedules and daytime functioning in adolescents. Child Dev 1998; 69:875–887.

88. Petersen A.C., Crockett L., Richard M., Boxer A. A self-report measure of pubertal status: reliability, validity and initial norms. J Youth Adolesc 1988; 17:117–133.

89. Lee KA, McEnany G, Weekes D. Gender differences in sleep patterns for early adolescents. J Adolesc Health 1999; 24:16–20.

90. Mourtazaev MS, Kemp B, Zwinderman AH, Kamphuisen HA. Age and gender affect different characteristics of slow-waves in the sleep EEG. Sleep 1995; 48:557–564.

91. Armitage R. Sex difference in the distribution of EEG frequencies in REM and NREM sleep stages in healthy young adults. Sleep 1995; 18:334–341.

92. Dijk D-J, Beersma DGM, Hoofdakker RH. Sex differences in the sleep EEG of young adults: visual scoring and spectral analysis. Sleep 1989; 12:500–507.

93. Armitage R, Smith C, Thompson S, Hoffmann R. Sex differences in slow-wave activity in response to sleep deprivation. Sleep Res Online 2001; 4:33–41.

94. Carrier J, Gaudreau H, Lavoie HB, Morettini J. Do middle-aged men and women differ in their ability to recuperate during the day following an acute sleep deprivation? Sleep, in press.

95. Elton M, Winter O, Heslenfeld D, Loewy D, Campbell K, Kok A. Event-related potentials to tones in the absence and presence of sleep spindles. J Sleep Res 1997; 6:78–83.

96. Steriade M, McCormick DA, Sejnowski TJ. Thalamocortical oscillations in the sleeping and aroused brain. Science 1993; 262:679–685.

97. Dijk DJ, Duffy JF, Czeisler CA. Age-related increase in awakenings: impaired consolidation of nonREM sleep at all circadian phases. Sleep 2001; 24:565–577.

98. Salzarulo P, Fagiolo I, Lombardo P, Gori S, Gneri C, Chiaramonti R, et al. Sleep stages preceding spontaneous awakenings in the elderly. Sleep Res Online 1999; 2:73–77.

99. Dijk DJ, Duffy JF, Riel E, Shanahan TL, Czeisler C. Ageing and the circadian and homeostatic regulation of human sleep during forced-desynchrony of rest, melatonin and temperature rhythms. J Physiol 1999; 516.2:611–627.

100. Monk TH, Buysse DJ, Reynolds CF, Kupfer DJ, Houck PR. Circadian temperature rhythms of older people. Exp Gerontol 1995; 30:455–474.

101. Monk TH, Buysse DJ, Reynolds CF, Kupfer DJ, Houck PR. Subjective alertness rhythms in elderly people. J Biol Rhythms 1996; 11:268–276.

102. Zeitzer JM, Daniels JE, Duffy JF, Klerman EB, Shanahan TL, Dijk D-J, et al. Do plasma melatonin concentrations decline with age? Am J Med 1999; 107:432–436.

103. Follenius M, Bradenberger J, Bandesapt JJ, Libert JP, Ehrhart J. Noctural cortisol release in relation to sleep structure. Sleep 1992; 15:21–27.

104. Krueger JM, Fang J, Hansen MK, Zhang J, Obàl F. Humoral regulation of sleep. News Physiol Sci 1998; 13:189–194.

105. Van Cauter E, Plat L, Leproult R, Copinschi G. Alteration of circadian rhythmicity and sleep in aging: endocrine consequences. Horm Res 1998; 49:147–152.

106. Obal F, Jr., Krueger JM. The somatotropic axis and sleep. Rev Neurol (Paris) 2001; 157:S12–S15

107. Steiger A, Holsboer F. Neuropeptides and human sleep. Sleep 1997; 20:1038–1052.

108. Steiger A. Sleep and the hypothalamo-pituitary-adrenocortical system. Sleep Med Rev 2002; 6:125–138.

109. Touitou Y. Some aspects of circadian time structure in the elderly. Gerontology 1982; 28(Suppl 1):53–67.

110. Sharma M., Palacios-Bois J., Schwartz G., Iskandar H., Thakur M., Quirion R., et al. Circadian rhythms of melatonin and cortisol in aging. Biol Psychiatry 1989; 25:305–319.

111. van Coevorden A, Mockel J, Laurent E, Kerkhofs M, L'Hermite-Baleriaux M, Decoster C, et al. Neuroendocrine rhythms and sleep in aging men. Am J Physiol 1991; 260:E651–E661.

112. Jaffe C.A., Turgeon D.K., Friberg R.D., Watkins P.B., Barkan A.L. Nocturnal augmentation of growth hormone (GH) secretion is preserved during repetitive bolus administration of GH-releasing hormone: potential involvement of endogenous somatostatin—a clinical research center study. J Clin Endocrinol Metab 1995; 80:3321–3326.

113. Krueger JM, Obal F, Jr. Growth hormone-releasing hormone and interleukin-1 in sleep regulation. FASEB J 1993; 7:645–652.

114. Rivier C.L., Plotsky P.M. Mediation by corticotropin releasing factor (CRF) of adenohypophysial hormone secretion. Annu Rev Physiol 1986; 48:475–489.

115. Plotsky P.M. Pathway to the secretion of adrenocorticotropin: a view from the portal. J Neuroendocrinol 1991; 3:1–9.

116. Antoni FA. Vasopressinergic control of pituitary adrenocorticotropin secretion comes of age. Review. Front Neuroendocrinol 1993; 14:76–122.

117. Whitnall MH. Regulation of the hypothalamic corticotropin-releasing hormone neurosecretory system. Prog Neurobiol 1993; 40:573–629.

118. Moga M.M., Gray T.S. Evidence for corticotropin-releasing factor, neurotensin, and somatostatin in the neural pathway from the central nucleus of the amygdala to the parabrachial nucleus. J Comp Neurol 1985; 241:275–284.

119. Koegler-Muly S.M., Owens M.J., Ervin G.N., Kilts C.D., Nemeroff C.B. Potential corticotropin-releasing factor pathways in the rat brain as determined by bilateral electrolytic lesions of the central amygdaloid nucleus and the paraventricular nucleus of the hypothalamus. J Endocrinol 1993; 5:95–98.

120. Gray TS, Bingaman EW. The amygdala: corticotropin-releasing factor, steroids, and stress. Crit Rev Neurobiol 1996; 10:155–168.

121. Valentino RJ, Curtis AL, Page ME, Pavcovich LA, Florin-Lechner SM. Activation of the locus ceruleus brain noradrenergic system during stress: circuitry, consequences, and regulation. Adv Pharmacol. 1998; 42:781–784.

122. Tsigo C, Chrousos GP. Hypothalamic-pituitary-adrenal axis, neuroendocrine factors and stress. J Psychosom Res 2002; 53:865–871.

123. Takahashi Y, Kipnis D.M., Daughaday WH. Growth-hormone secretion during sleep. J Clin Invest 1968; 47:2079–2090.

124. Sassin J.F., Parker DC, Mace JW, Gotlin GW, Johnson LC, Rossman LG. Human growth-hormone release: relation to slow-wave sleep and sleep-waking cycles. Science 1969; 165:513–515.

125. Van Cauter E., Plat L., Copinschi G. Interrelations between sleep and the somatotropic axis. Sleep 1998; 21:553–566.

126. Ho KY, Evans WS, Blizzard RM, Veldhuis JD, Merriam GR, Samojlik E, et al. Effects of sex and age on the 24–hour profile of growth hormone secretion in man: importance of endogenous estradiol concentrations. J Clin Endocrinol Metab 1987; 64:51–58.

127. Antonijevic IA, Murck H, Frieboes RM, Steiger A. Sexually dimorphic effects of GHRH on sleep-endocrine activity in patients with depression and normal controls: Part ll. Sleep Res Online 2000; 3:15–21.

128. Beck U, Hunter WM, Oswald I., Brezinova V. Plasma growth hormone and slow wave sleep increase after interruption of sheep. J Clin Endocrinol Metab 1975; 40:812–815.

129. Van Cauter E, Kerkhofs M, Caufriez A, Van Onderbergen A, Thorner MO, Copinschi G. A quantitative estimation of growth hormone secretion in normal man: reproducibility and relation to sleep and time of day. J Clin Endocrinol Metab 1992; 74:1441–1450.

130. Van Cauter E., van Coevorden A, Blackman JD. Modulation of neuroendocrine release by sleep and circadian rhythmicity. In: Yen SS, Vale W, editors. Advances in Neuroendocrine Regulation of Reproduction. Norwell: Symposia USA, 1990:113–122.

131. Steiger A, Herth T, Holsboer F. Sleep-electroencephalography and the secretion of cortisol and growth hormone in normal controls. Acta Endocrinol 1987; 116:36–42.

132. Jarrett DB, Greenhouse JB, Miewald JM, Fedorka IB, Kupfer DJ. A reexamination of the relationship between growth hormone secretion and slow wave sleep using delta wave analysis. Biol Psychiatry 1990; 27:497–509.

133. Born JSE, Schenk E, Spath-Schwalbe E, Fehm HL. Influences of partial REM sleep deprivation and awakenings on nocturnal cortisol release. Biol Psychiatry 1988; 24:801–811.

134. Ehlers CL, Kupfer DJ. Hypothalamic peptide modulation of EEG sleep in depression: a further application of the S-process hypothesis. Biol Psychiatry 1987; 22:513–517.

135. Albertsson-Wikland K., Rosberg S., Karlberg J., Groth T. Analysis of 24–hour growth hormone profiles in healthy boys and girls of normal stature: relation to puberty. J Clin Endocrinol Metab 1994; 78:1195–1201.

136. Rose SR, Municchi G, Barnes KM, Kamp GA, Uriarte MM, Ross JL, et al. Spontaneous growth hormone secretion increases during puberty in normal girls and boys. J Clin Endocrinol Metab 1991; 73:428–435.

137. Van Cauter E., Leproult R, Plat L. Age-related changes in slow wave sleep and REM sleep and relationship with growth hormone and cortisol levels in healthy men. JAMA 2000; 284:861–868.

138. Guldner J, Schier T, Friess E, Colla M, Holsboer F, Steiger A. Reduced efficacy of growth hormone–releasing hormone in modulating sleep endocrine activity in the elderly. Neurobiol Aging 1997; 18:491–495.

139. Sonntag WE, Boyd RL, Booze RM. Somatostatin gene expression in hypothalamus and cortex of aging male rats. Neurobiol Aging 1990; 11:409–416.

140. Steiger A, Guldner J, Hemmeter U, Rothe B, Wiedemann K, Holsboer F. Effects of growth hormone–releasing hormone and somatostatin on sleep EEG and nocturnal hormone secretion in male controls. Neuroendocrinology 1992; 56:566–573.

141. Marshall L, Molle M, Boschen G, Steiger A, Fehm HL, Born J. Greater efficacy of episodic than continuous growth hormone–releasing hormone (GHRH) administration in promoting slow-wave sleep (SWS). J Clin Endocrinol Metab. 1996; 81:1009–1013.

142. Kern W, Halder R, al-Reda S, Spath-Schwalbe E, Fehm HL, Born J. Systemic growth hormone does not affect human sleep. J Clin Endocrinol Metab. 1993; 76:1428–1432.

143. Mendelson WB, Slater S, Gold P, Gillin JC. The effect of growth hormone administration on human sleep: a dose-response study. Biol Psychiatry 1980; 15:613–618.

144. Drucker-Colin RR, Spanis CW, Hunyadi J, Sassin JF, McGaugh JL. Growth hormone effects on sleep and wakefulness in the rat. Neuroendocrinology 1975; 18:1–8.

145. Stern WC, Jalowiec JE, Shabshelowitz H, Morgane PJ. Effects of growth hormone on sleep-waking patterns in cats. Horm Behav 1975; 6:189–196.

146. Obal F Jr, Floyd R, Kapas L, Bodosi B, Krueger JM. Effects of systemic GHRH on sleep in intact and hypophysectomized rats. Am J Physiol 1996; 270:E230–E237

147. Sapolsky RM, Krey LC, McEwen BS. The neuroendocrinology of stress and aging: the glucocorticoid cascade hypothesis. Endocr Rev 1986; 7:284–301.

148. Meaney MJ, Diorio J, Francis D, Widdowson J, LaPlante P, Caldji C, et al. Early environmental regulation of forebrain glucocorticoid receptor gene expression: implications for adrenocortical responses to stress. Dev Neurosci 1996; 18:49–72.

149. Lupien S, Lecours AR, Lussier I, Schwartz G, Nair NP, Meaney MJ. Basal cortisol levels and cognitive deficits in human aging. J Neurosci 1994; 14:2893–2903.

150. Lupien SJ, de Leon M, de Santi S, Convit A, Tarshish C, Nair NP, et al. Cortisol levels during human aging predict hippocampal atrophy and memory deficits. Nat Neurosci 1998; 1:69–73.

151. McEwen BS, Brinton RE, Sapolsky RM. Glucocorticoid receptors and behavior: implications for the stress response. Adv Exp Med Biol 1988; 245:35–45.

152. Ferrari E, Cravello L, Muzzoni B, Casarotti D, Paltro M, Solerte SB, et al. Age-related changes of the hypothalamic-pituitary-adrenal axis: pathophysiological correlates. Eur J Endocrinol 2001; 144:319–329.

153. Sapolsky RM. Glucocorticoids, stress, and their adverse neurological effects: relevance to aging. Exp Gerontol 1999; 34:721–732.

154. Nichols NR, Zieba M, Bye N. Do glucocorticoids contribute to brain aging? Brain Res Rev 2001; 37:273–286.

155. Meaney MJ, Sharma S, Viau V. Basal ACTH, corticosterone and corticosterone-binding globulin levels over the diurnal cycle, and age-related changes in hippocampal type I and type II corticosteroid receptor binding capacity in young and aged, handled and nonhandled rats. Neuroendocrinology 1992; 55:204–213.

156. Seeman TE, Robbins RJ. Aging and hypothalamic-pituitary-adrenal response to challenge in humans. Endocr Rev 1994; 15:233–260.

157. Sapolsky R.M., Altmann J. Incidence of hypercortisolism and dexamethasone resistance increases with age among wild baboons. Biol Psychiatry 1991; 30:1008–1016.

158. McEwen BS. Protective and damaging effects of stress mediators: the good and bad sides of the response to stress. Review. Metabolism 2002; 51:2–4.

159. Opp MR. Corticotropin-releasing hormone involvement in stressor-induced alterations in sleep and in the regulation of waking. Adv Neuroimmunol 1995; 5:127–143.

160. Chang F.C., Opp M.R. Corticotropin-releasing hormone (CRH) as a regulator of waking. Neurosci Biobehav Rev 2001; 25:445–453.

161. Adams J, Folkard S, Young M. Coping strategies used by nurses on night duty. Ergonomics 1986; 29:185–196.

162. Vgontzas AN, Tsigosgontzas AN C, Bixler EO, Stratakis CA, Zachman K, Kales A, et al. Chronic insomnia and activity of the stress system: a preliminary study. J Psychosom Res 1998; 45:21–31.

163. Rodenbeck A, Huether G, Ruther E, Hajak G. Nocturnal melatonin secretion and its modification by treatment in patients with sleep disorders. Adv Exp Med Biol 1999; 467:93

164. Rodenbeck A, Huether G, Ruther E, hajak g. Interactions between evening and nocturnal cortisol secretion and sleep parameters in patients with severe chronic primary insomnia. Neurosci Lett 2002; 324:159–163.

165. Hall M, Buysse DJ, Nowell PD, Nofzinger EA, Houck P, Reynolds CF III, et al. Symptoms of stress and depression as correlates of sleep in primary insomnia. Psychosom Med 2000; 62:227–230.

166. Steiger A, Herth T, Holsboer F. Sleep EEG and nocturnal secretion of cortisol and growth hormone in male patients with endogenous depression before treatment and after recovery. J Affective Disord 1989; 16:189–195.

167. Antonijevic IA, Murck H, Frieboes RM, Barthelmes J, Steiger A. Sexually dimorphic effects of GHRH on sleep-endocrine activity in patients with depression and normal controls: Part 1. Sleep Res Online 2000; 3:5–13.

168. Krieger DT, Glick SM. Sleep EEG stages and plasma growth hormone concentration in states of endogenous and exogenous hypercortisolemia or ACTH elevation. J Clin Endocrinol Metab 1974; 39:986–1000.

169. Shipley JE, Schteingart DE, Tandon R, Pande AC, Haskett RF, Starkman MN. EEG sleep in Cushing's disease and Cushing's syndrome: comparison with patients with major depressive disorder. Biol Psychiatry 1992; 32:146–155.

170. Kant GJ, Pastel RH, Bauman RA, Maughan KR, Robinson TN III, Covington PS. Effects of chronic stress on sleep in rats. Physiol Behav1995 Feb;57(2):359–65. 1995.

171. Cheeta S, Ruigt G, van Proosdij J, Willner P. Changes in sleep architecture following chronic mild stress. Biol Psychiatry 1997; 41:419–427.
172. Rampin C, Cespuglio R, Chastrette N, Jouvet M. Immobilisation stress induces a paradoxical sleep rebound in rat. Neurosci Lett 1991; 126:113–118.
173. del C Gonzalez MM, Debilly G, Valatx JL, Jouvet M. Sleep increase after immobilization stress: role of the noradrenergic locus coeruleus system in the rat. Neurosci Lett 1995; 202:5–8.
174. Gonzalez MM, Valatx JL. Effect of intracerebroventricular administration of alpha-helical CRH (9–41) on the sleep/waking cycle in rats under normal conditions or after subjection to an acute stressful stimulus. J Sleep Res 1997; 6:164–170.
175. Meerlo P, Pragt BJ, Daan S. Social stress induces high intensity sleep in rats. Neurosci Lett 1997; 225:41–44.
176. Marinesco S, Bonnet C, Cespuglio R. Influence of stress duration on the sleep rebound induced by immobilization in the rat: a possible role for corticosterone. Neuroscience 1999; 92:921–933.
177. Bouyer JJ, Deminiere JM, Mayo W, Le Moal M. Inter-individual differences in the effects of acute stress on the sleep-wakefulness cycle in the rat. Neurosci Lett 1997; 225:193–196.
178. Bouyer JJ, Vallee M, Deminiere JM, Le Moal M, Mayo W. Reaction of sleep-wakefulness cycle to stress is related to differences in hypothalamo-pituitary-adrenal axis reactivity in rat. Brain Res 1998; 804:114–124.
179. Piazza PV, Deminiere JM, Maccari S, Mormède P, Le Moal M, Simon H. Individual reactivity to novelty predicts probability of amphetamine self-administration. Biol Pharmacol 1990; 1:339–345.
180. Piazza PV, Le Moal ML. Pathophysiological basis of vulnerability to drug abuse: role of an interaction between stress, glucocorticoids, and dopaminergic neurons. Ann Rev Pharmacol Toxicol 1996; 36:359–378.
181. Ehlers CL, Reed TK, Henriksen SJ. Effects of corticotropin-releasing factor and growth hormone–releasing factor on sleep and activity in rats. Neuroendocrinology 1986; 42:467–474.
182. Opp M, Obal F Jr, Krueger JM. Corticotropin-releasing factor attenuates interleukin 1–induced sleep and fever in rabbits. Am J Physiol 1989; 257:R528–R535
183. Marrosu F, Gessa GL, Giagheddu M, Fratta W. Corticotropin-releasing factor (CRF) increases paradoxical sleep (PS) rebound in PS-deprived rats. Brain Res 1990; 515:315–318.
184. Gonzalez MM, Valatx JL. Involvement of stress in the sleep rebound mechanism induced by sleep deprivation in the rat: use of alpha-helical CRH (9–41). Behav Pharmacol 1998; 9:655–662.
185. Chang FC, Opp MR. Blockade of corticotropin-releasing hormone receptors reduces spontaneous waking in the rat. Am J Physiol 1998; 275:R793–R802
186. Opp MR. Rat strain differences suggest a role for corticotropin-releasing hormone in modulating sleep. Physiol Behav 1997; 63:67–74.
187. Holsboer F, Von Bardeleben U, teiger A. Effects of intravenous corticotropin-releasing hormone upon sleep-related growth hormone surge and sleep EEG in man. Neuroendocrinology 1988; 48:32–38.
188. Tsuchiyama Y, Uchimura N, Sakamoto T, Maeda H, Kotorii T. Effects of hCRH on sleep and body temperature rhythms. Psychiatry Clin Neurosci 1995; 49:299–304.

189. Antonijevic IA, Murck H, Frieboes R, Holsboer TT, Steiger A. Hyporesponsiveness of the pituitary to CRH during slow wave sleep is not mimicked by systemic GHRH. Neuroendocrinology 1999; 69:88–96.

190. Born J, Kern W, Bieber K, Fehm-Wolfsdorf G, Schiebe M, Fehm HL. Night-time plasma cortisol secretion is associated with specific sleep stages. Biol Psychiatry 1986; 21:1415–1424.

191. Gronfier C, Simon C, Piquard F, Ehrhart J, Brandenberger G. Neuroendocrine processes underlying ultradian sleep regulation in man. J Clin Endocrinol Metab 1999; 84:2686–2690.

192. Chapotot F, Gronfier C, Jouny C, Muzet A, Brandenberger G. Cortisol secretion is related to electroencephalographic alertness in human subjects during daytime wakefulness. J Clin Endocrinol Metab 1998; 83:4263–4268.

193. Sippell, Dorr HG, Bidlingmaier F, Knorr D. Plasma levels of aldosterone, corticosterone, 11–deoxycorticosterone, progesterone, 17–hydroxyprogesterone, cortisol, and cortisone during infancy and childhood. Pediatric Res 1980; 14:39–46.

194. Gomez MT, Malozowski S, Winterer J, Vamvakopoulos NC, Chrousos GP. Urinary free cortisol values in normal children and adolescents. J Pediatr 1991; 118:256–258.

195. Grad B, Rosenberg GM, Liberman H., 1971. Diurnal variation of serum cortisol levels of geriatric subjects. J Gerontol 1971; 26:357

196. Andras R, Tobin J. Endocrine systems. In: Finch CE, Hayflick L, editors. Handbook of the Biology of Aging. New York: Van Nostrand, 1977:370–371.

197. Blitchert-Toft M. The adrenal gland in old age. In: Greenblatt RB, editor. Geriatric Endocrinlogy. New York: Raven Press, 1978:81

198. Tourigny-Rivard MF, Raskind M, Rivard D. The dexamethasone suppression test in an elferly population. Biol Psychiatry 1981; 16:1177–1184.

199. Drafta D, Stroe E, Neascu E. Age-related changes of plasma steroids in normal adults males. J Steroids Biochem 1982; 17:-683

200. Sherman B, Wysham C, Pfohl B. Age related changes in the circadian rhythm of plasma cortisol in man. J Clin Endocrinol Metab 1985; 61:439–443.

201. Copinschi G, Van Cauter E. Effects of ageing on modulation of hormonal secretions by sleep and circadian rhythmicity. Horm Res 1995; 43:20–24.

202. Lupien S, Schwartz G, Sharma S, Hauger RL, Meaney MJ, Nair NP, et al. Longitudinal study of basal cortisol levels in healthy elderly subjects: evidence for subgroups. Neurobiol Aging 1996; 17:95–105.

203. Czeisler CA, Dumont M, Duffy JF, Steinberg JD, Richardson GS, Brown EN, et al. Association of sleep-wake habits in older people with changes in output of circadian pacemaker. Lancet 1992; 340:933–936.

204. Born J, DeKloet ER, Wenz H, Kern W, Fehm HL. Gluco- and antimineralocorticoid effects on human sleep: a role of central corticosteroid receptors. Am J Physiol 1991; 260:E183–E188

205. Friess E, Von Bardeleben U, Wiedemann K. Effecst of pulsatile cortisol infusion on sleep-EEG and nocturnal growth-hormone release in healty men. J Sleep Res 1994; 3:73–79.

206. Bohlhalter S, Murck H, Holsboer F, Steiger A. Cortisol enhances non-REM sleep and growth hormone secretion in elderly subjects. Neurobiol Aging 1997; 18:423–429.

207. Poland R.E., Rubin R.T., Clark B.R., Gouin P.R. Circadian patterns of urine 17–OHC and VMA excretion during sleep deprivation. Dis Nerv Syst 1972; 33:456–458.

208. Kant GJ, Genser SG, Thhorne DR, Pfalser JL, Mougey EH. Effects of 72–h sleep deprivation on urinary cortisol and indices of metabolism. Sleep 1984; 7:142–146.

209. Akerstedt T, Palmblad J, DeLaTorre B, Marana R, Giuberg M. Adrenocortical and gonadal steroids during sleep deprivation. Sleep 1980; 3(1):23–30.

210. Saletu B, Dietzel M, Lesch OM, Musalek M, Walter H, Grunberger J. Effect of biologically active light and partial sleep deprivation on sleep, awakening and circadian rhythms in normals. Eur Neurol 1986; 25 Suppl 2:82–92.

211. Salin-Pascual RJ, Ortega-Soto H, Huerto-Delgadillo L, Camacho-Arroyo I, Roldan-Roldan G, Tamarkin L. The effect of total sleep deprivation on plasma melatonin and cortisol in healthy human volunteers. Sleep 1988; 11:362–369.

212. Moldofsky H, Lue FA, Davidson JR, Gorczynski R. Effects of sleep deprivation on human immune functions. FASEB J 1989; 3:1972–1977.

213. Davidson JR, Moldosfsky FA, Lue FA. Growth hormone and cortisol secretion in relation to sleep and wakefulness. J Psychiatr Neurosci 1991; 16:96–102.

214. Brun J, Chamba G, Khalfallah Y, Girard P, Boissy I, Bastuji H, et al. Effect of modafinil on plasma melatonin, cortisol and growth hormone rhythms, rectal temperature and performance in healthy subejects during a 36–h sleep deprivation. J Sleep Res 1998; 7:105–114.

215. Heiser P, Dickhaus B, Schreiber W, Clement HW, Henning J, Remschmidt H, et al. White blood cells and cortisol after sleep deprivation and recovery sleep in humans. Eur Arch Psychiatr Neurosci 2000; 250:16–23.

216. Vgontzas AN, Mastorakos G, Bixler EO, Kales A, Gold PW, Chrousos GP. Sleep deprivation effects on the activity of the hypothalamic-pituitary-adrenal and growth axes: potential clinical implications. Clin Endocrinol 1999; 51:205–215.

217. Bierwolf C, Struve K, Marshall L, Born J, Fehm H. Slow wave sleep drives inhibition of pituitary-adrenal secretion in humans. J Neuroendocrinol 1997; 9:479–484.

218. Meerlo P, Koehl M, van der Borght K, Turek FW. Sleep restriction alters the hypothalamic-pituitary-adrenal response to stress. J Neuroendocrinol 2002; 14:397–402.

219. Leproult R, Copinschi G, Buxton O, Van Cauter E. Sleep loss results in an elevation of cortisol levels the next evening. Sleep 1997; 20:865–870.

220. Tobler I, Borbély AA, Groos G. The effect of sleep deprivation on sleep in rats with suprachiasmatic lesions. Neurosci Lett 1983; 42:49–54.

221. Weibel L, Follenius M, Spiegel K, Ehrhart J, Brandenberger G. Comparative effect of night and daytime sleep on the 24–hour cortisol secretory profile. Sleep 1995; 18:549–556.

222. von Treurer K, Norman TR, Amstrong SM. Overnight human plasma melatonin, cortisol, prolactin, TSH, under conditions of normal sleep, sleep deprivation, and sleep recovery. J Pineal Res 1996; 20:7–14.

223. Spiegel K, Leproult R, Van Cauter E. Impact of sleep debt on metabolic and endocrine function. Lancet 1999; 354:1435–1439.

224. Kales A, Kales J. Evaluation of insomnia. In: Anonymous Evaluation and treatment of insomnia. New York: Oxford University Press, 1984:

225. Akerstedt T, Knutsson A, Westerholm P, Theorell T, Alfredsson L, Kecklund G. Sleep disturbances, work stress and work hours. A cross-sectional study. J Psychosom Res 2002; 53:741

226. Van Cauter E, Spiegel K. Circadian and sleep control of hormonal secretions. In: Turek F, Zee P, editors. Regulation of Sleep and Circadian Rhythms. New York: Marcel Dekker, 1999:397–425.

227. Prinz PN, Bailey SL, Woods DL. Sleep impairments in healthy seniors: roles of stress, cortisol, and interleukin-1 beta. Chronobiol Int 2000; 17:391–404.

228. Murck H, Antonijevic IA, Schier T, Frieboes RM, Barthelmes J, Steiger A. Aging does not affect the sleep endocrine response to total sleep deprivation in humans. Neurobiol Aging 1999; 20:665–668.

229. Vgontzas AN, Bixler E, Wittman AM, Zachman K, Lin HM, Vela-Bueno A, et al. Middle-aged men show higher sensitivity of sleep to the arousing effects of corticotropin-releasing hormone than young men: clinical implications. J Clin Endocrinol Metab 2001; 86:1489–1495.

230. Frieboes RM, Murck H, Maier P, Schier T, Holsboer F, Steiger A. Growth hormone-releasing peptide-6 stimulates sleep, growth hormone, ACTH and cortisol release in normal man. Neuroendocrinology 1995; 61:584–589.

231. Copinschi G, Leproult R, Van Onderbergen A, Caufriez A, Cole KY, Schilling LM, et al. Prolonged oral treatment with MK-677, a novel growth hormone secretagogue, improves sleep quality in man. Neuroendocrinology 1997; 66:278–286.

232. Blackman MR. Age-related alterations in sleep quality and neuroendocrine function: interrelationships and implications. JAMA 2000; 284:879–881.

233. Muller EE, Cella SG, Parenti M, Deghenghi R, Locatelli V, Torsello A, et al. Somatotropic dysregulation in old mammals. Horm Res 1995; 43:39–45.

234. O'Connor KO, Stevens TE, Blackman MR. GH and aging. In: Juul A, Jorgensen JO, editors. Growth Hormone in Adults. Cambridge, UK: Cambridge University Press, 1996:323–366.

235. Bengtsson BA, Brummer RJ, Bosaeus I. Growth hormone and body composition. Horm Res 1990; 33 Suppl 4:19–24.

24

Homeostatic and Circadian Influences

JOEL H. BENINGTON

St. Bonaventure University, St. Bonaventure, New York, U.S.A.

I. Introduction

The effects of sleep deprivation are commonly interpreted in terms of the homeostatic regulation of some physiological variable that is as yet unknown. Walter Cannon introduced the term *homeostasis* in 1929 to describe physiological mechanisms found in many organisms that maintain a constant internal environment. Physiological variables that are homeostatically regulated by one or more types of organism include temperature, osmolarity, pH, body mass, density, blood pressure, respiratory rate, heart rate, and tissue concentrations of numerous nutrients, waste products, and other chemicals.

The essence of homeostatic regulation is negative feedback, by means of which any significant change in the value of the physiological variable being regulated is counteracted, thus maintaining that value at a certain level. A physiological mechanism for maintaining homeostasis thus requires: (a) a *sensor* to register the value of the variable, (b) *a control center* that compares the measured value with a *set point* and triggers a response when there is a significant deviation, and (c) an *effector* mechanism that is capable of changing the value of the variable as directed by the control center. In most documented cases of homeostasis, the physiological variable being regulated is known. In some cases, information is also available concerning the cellular mechanism by which the value of this variable is sensed, the location of the control center or centers, and the nature of the effector mechanism.

Homeostatic analysis has been applied to sleep regulation since at least 1980 (1). In the case of sleep, there is considerable evidence for homeostatic regulation, but we currently have no idea what physiological variable is being regulated. By definition, we therefore also have no idea how the sensor or effector mechanisms work. And while there is some evidence that the region of the preoptic area and basal forebrain may function as a control center (2,3), this cannot be said to have been established with any certainty. Not knowing what variable is being regulated homeostatically by means of sleep/wake behavior, we of necessity speak of sleep homeostasis abstractly, in terms of the accumulation and discharge of a propensity to sleep.

The full characterization of the sleep homeostatic process is of course impossible until the physiological variable being regulated is at last identified. Until then, abstract descriptions in terms of the accumulation and discharge of sleep propensity are the best we can do. Nevertheless, modeling the effects of sleep deprivation homeostatically is of considerable value to sleep researchers. Identifying changes in the time course of sleep homeostasis in genetically altered organisms should prove a valuable tool in the search for genes involved in the regulation of sleep (4–6). Such measurements are also relevant in pharmacological studies designed to analyze neurochemical mechanisms involved in the regulation of sleep.

In this chapter, I will review: (a) the evidence for the conclusion that sleep is homeostatically regulated and (b) the models that have been developed to simulate the time course of accumulation and discharge of sleep propensity, using electroencephalographic (EEG) slow-wave activity (SWA) in non-REM (NREM) sleep as a primary measure. The remainder of the chapter will address two issues that complicate the homeostatic interpretation of sleep deprivation studies. First, sleep deprivation has been shown to alter both NREM sleep and rapid-eye-movement (REM) sleep variables to varying degrees depending on the species and duration of sleep deprivation used. There has been some controversy as to the homeostatic implications of these findings, which I will discuss. Second, the occurrence of sleep in the recovery period following sleep deprivation is influenced by the output of the circadian pacemaker. The relative contribution of homeostatic and circadian factors in sleep expression has been elegantly analyzed in an ingenious series of experiments using a "forced desynchrony" paradigm in humans to cause sleep/wake alternation to occur at all phases of the circadian cycle. I will review the findings of these studies and discuss their implications for the design and interpretation of sleep deprivation experiments.

II. Evidence for Sleep Homeostasis

The main evidence that sleep is homeostatically regulated is that sleep deprivation produces: (a) an increase in the tendency to go to sleep (sleepiness, or sleep drive) that becomes more pronounced as sleep deprivation is extended, and (b) an increase in the duration of sleep during the recovery period following sleep deprivation. Anecdotally, these observations are of course familiar to all and have been known for literally thousands of years. The increase in the tendency to go to sleep is commonly interpreted as an output of the effector mechanism, increasing the likelihood of the occurrence of sleep in proportion to the amount of accumulated sleep propensity. The increased duration of sleep during the recovery period is also consistent with homeostatic regulation, as a greater amount of sleep should be needed to fully discharge sleep propensity when it has accumulated to higher levels.

It has also been long accepted that sleep during recovery from sleep deprivation is "deeper" in that one has more difficulty waking up, and this belief has been confirmed by studies showing that there is an increase in the arousal threshold for auditory stimuli during recovery sleep (7–10). Recovery sleep has further been shown to differ from baseline sleep in being characterized by increases in both the amplitude and prevalence of slow waves in the NREM sleep electroencephalogram, corresponding to increased expression of stage 3 and 4 NREM sleep in humans (see Chap. 12). Increased EEG SWA in recovery sleep may in fact be largely responsible for the associated increase in arousal threshold, as arousal threshold has been shown to be higher during stage 3 and stage 4 NREM sleep in humans, when EEG SWA is maximal (11–13).

Some of the sleep "lost" during sleep deprivation is "recovered" through increased sleep duration following the deprivation period, but there is by no means a one-for-one recovery of sleep lost. In humans, one entire night of sleep deprivation may result in an aggregate increase of just 2–4 hr of sleep duration on the subsequent nights, at the end of which time subjects report normal low levels of subjective sleepiness. This observation is most commonly interpreted as suggesting that recovery sleep following sleep deprivation is more "intense" and therefore discharges accumulated sleep propensity more rapidly than baseline sleep does. This conclusion is consistent with the observation that recovery sleep is also "deeper" than baseline sleep, in terms of both increased arousal threshold and increased EEG SWA. However, an alternative explanation has been proposed—that only a portion of sleep ("obligatory sleep") is actually required for accomplishing the function of sleep and that the remainder ("facultative sleep") can be lost without consequences (14).

In animal studies, the magnitude of the increase in EEG SWA produced by sleep deprivation is to some extent influenced by the intervention used to deprive animals of sleep (15), but not to so great a degree that one would conclude that it is merely an artifact of the experimental interventions. Rather, one could instead argue that sleep deprivation protocols that produce smaller increases in EEG SWA may be associated with lower rates of accumulation of sleep propensity, owing to the discharge of some sleep propensity during NREM sleep and drowsy waking during the sleep deprivation period. Consistent with this hypothesis, studies reporting the smallest increase in EEG SWA in recovery NREM sleep have used sleep deprivation protocols (such as the disk-over-water method) that allow the most NREM sleep and drowsy waking during the deprivation period (15).

It has been argued that the larger increases in EEG SWA observed following more aggressive sleep deprivation protocols result in part from stress associated with the sleep deprivation intervention (15). While sleep deprivation in rodents does in some cases presumably cause some stress, just as practically any other experimental manipulation, this is unlikely to be the only or even the major cause of increases in EEG SWA during recovery sleep. Increased EEG SWA has been observed even following short sleep deprivations using gentle interventions to interrupt sleep (16). Moreover, the tight correlation between sleep loss and EEG SWA in most studies strongly suggests that the increase in EEG SWA is sleep related, and equivalent increases in EEG SWA occur following natural versus enforced waking (17), implying that whatever stress may be produced by enforced waking has at most a small effect on EEG SWA.

Following extremely long sleep deprivations in rats (lasting 18–19 days), there is a striking absence of increase in EEG SWA (15), even though one would certainly expect that accumulated sleep propensity should be considerable. It is difficult to say for certain what to make of this finding. REM sleep drive appears to be intense in the early phases of recovery and may therefore interfere with expression of deep NREM sleep. But in any event, given how radically the conditions in these experiments differ from the circumstances of normal mammalian sleep/wake behavior, one would not want to reject the well-established link between EEG SWA and the level of accumulated sleep propensity based on this one divergent finding.

If the more "intense" sleep following sleep deprivation does indeed discharge accumulated sleep propensity more rapidly, then the neurophysiological characteristics of recovery sleep may provide clues as to the physical substrate of the sleep recovery process. Increased EEG SWA in NREM sleep is associated with increased synchronized rhythmic activity in neurons throughout the brain (18,19), which is in turn thought to be caused by tonic hyperpolarization of neuronal membranes (20–22). The cellular mechanism of rhythmic neuronal activity further involves increased Ca^{2+} influx through T-type Ca^{2+} channels, followed by K^+ influx through SK Ca^{2+}-dependent K^+ channels (19). Any of these cellular events or the consequences thereof could be linked to the sleep recovery process.

III. Modeling Sleep Homeostasis

The goal of homeostatic models of sleep deprivation and recovery is to identify measurable variables that accurately reflect the accumulation and discharge of sleep propensity. Any of the known consequences of sleep deprivation could in theory be used as an indicator variable for sleep propensity as long as: (a) it can be readily and consistently quantified and (b) there is reason to believe that it reflects the level of accumulated sleep propensity at any given time. For example, the fact that sleepiness increases progressively as sleep deprivation becomes more extended suggests that the degree of sleepiness may reflect the level of accumulated sleep propensity. Using techniques such as the Multiple Sleep Latency Test to quantify the degree of sleepiness, one might therefore model the accumulation and discharge of sleep propensity based on increases and decreases in a subject's degree of sleepiness. However, sleepiness is also markedly influenced by the phase of a person's circadian rhythm, and may further be elevated in the minutes immediately after a sleep episode, as a result of "sleep inertia" (23). Moreover, the Multiple Sleep Latency Test can be rather cumbersome to perform and has only been validated in humans. For all of these reasons, degree of sleepiness is not widely used as a variable in homeostatic models of sleep deprivation and recovery.

The most commonly used variable for modeling sleep homeostasis is EEG SWA during NREM sleep (24). This variable is most often quantified using Fourier analysis to calculate spectral power in the "delta" frequency range, extending from a lower limit of 0.5–1 Hz to an upper limit of 4–5 Hz. Power in Fourier analysis is a measure of both the prevalence and amplitude of waveforms in the specified frequency range. EEG delta power in NREM sleep has been shown to increase monotonically as a function of duration of prior waking, as sleep propensity accumulates, and to decrease over the course of a sleep episode, as sleep propensity is discharged. This finding has been established in a number of different species of mammals, including humans, cats, rats and mice, dolphins, rabbits, and others (5,25–32). The increase in EEG delta power results from increases in both the prevalence and amplitude of slow waves.

The relationship between NREM-sleep EEG delta power at the beginning of a recovery period and the duration of prior waking describes an exponentially saturating function, and the decrease in NREM sleep EEG delta power over the course of the recovery period describes an exponentially decaying function (24). These mathematical relationships are in some cases obvious in recordings from a single animal, but their exponential nature often only becomes clear in group means. Over 20 years ago, these mathematical relationships were modeled in terms of a sleep homeostatic process (process S) that accumulates during waking and is discharged during sleep (33). The guiding assumption of this model is of course that NREM sleep EEG delta power is a measure of process S and thus of the level of accumulated sleep propensity.

Because the accumulation and discharge functions for process S both describe exponential curves, they can be mathematically described in terms of exponential time constants—one for accumulation and one for discharge. The accumulation time constant (τ_i) expresses the number of hours needed to achieve an increase in sleep propensity from zero to a level that is 63% of the asymptotic maximum. The discharge time constant (τ_d) expresses the number of hours needed to achieve a decrease in sleep propensity to 37% of the value at sleep onset. The values for these time constants can be established by determining a best fit between experimental observations and an exponential curve. To determine the time constant for the exponentially saturating accumulation function, this entails plotting EEG delta power at the beginning of recovery sleep as a function of the duration of the preceding sleep deprivation. To determine the time constant for the exponentially decaying discharge function, the exponential curve is fit to mean EEG delta power values for a series of time periods during recovery sleep. In recordings from a given animal, the value of these time constants is rather stable. For example, the time constant for the discharge function has been shown to be approximately the same for recovery sleep following short versus long sleep deprivations (26,34).

The accumulation and discharge of process S can be simulated for extended recordings from individual animal and human subjects (Fig. 1), and the

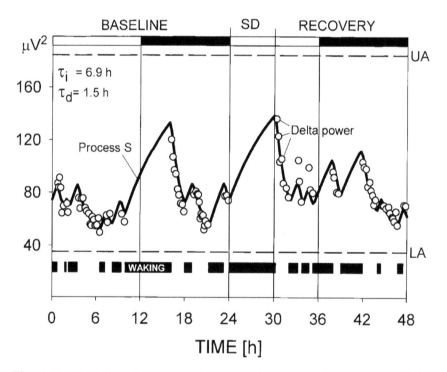

Figure 1 Simulation of process S using mouse electroencephalographic data. Circles represent median electroencephalographic delta power in NREM sleep episodes of more than 5 min in a 48-hr recording of one BALB/cByJ mouse, including 24-hr baseline, 6-hr sleep deprivation, and recovery. The solid line represents simulated level of process S, using optimized parameters shown at top left. See text for details of simulation process. (Modified from Ref. 6.)

predicted values of process S for any given time can be compared with observed levels of EEG delta power in NREM sleep (17,35,36). To do so, one merely needs to define: (a) the conditions under which process S accumulates and is discharged, (b) the initial value of process S at the beginning of the recording period (S_0), (c) the upper and lower asymptotes for the exponentially saturating and exponentially decaying curves, and (d) the time constants for accumulation and discharge (τ_i and τ_d). In some simulations, process S has been assumed to accumulate during waking and to be discharged during both NREM sleep and REM sleep, whereas in others process S has been assumed to accumulate during both waking and REM sleep and to be discharged only during NREM sleep (17,35). The upper and lower asymptotes can be arbitrarily assigned values of 1 and 0 following a linear transformation of the EEG delta power values to fit within this range, or they can be empirically determined as free parameters from the data (36). The initial value of process S can be approximated by assuming that, in the absence of experimental sleep deprivation, there is no long-term accumulation or discharge of sleep propensity from day to day, and therefore the simulated value of process S after 24 hr of recording is a retrospective measure of the initial value. Alternatively, the initial value of process S can be a free parameter in addition to τ_i and τ_d.

The optimal values of all free parameters (τ_i, τ_d, and in some simulations S_0 and/or the upper and lower asymptotes) are determined by: (a) generating a range of simulated time series for process S given various different values for each of the free parameters; (b) correlating each of those time series to the observed values for EEG delta power in NREM sleep during a recording period; and (c) establishing which set of parameters produces a simulation that best fits the observations (producing the highest correlation coefficient). The maximal correlation coefficients achieved by means of such optimization procedures with rodent data are impressively high, typically in the 0.8–0.9 range (Table 1). This implies $r^2 = 0.64$–0.81, suggesting that the simulation accounts for 64–81% of the variation in NREM sleep EEG delta power values. Similarly high r^2 values have been obtained when parameters determined from one study are applied to data in another study. This demonstrates that these values are not markedly inflated through the use of an optimization procedure that by definition permits one to choose values for each parameter that maximizes r^2 (37,38).

Simulations of process S have also been used to test hypotheses about the nature of sleep homeostasis in a variety of experimental protocols. In rats, such a simulation has provided evidence that the increase in NREM sleep EEG delta power following cold exposure can be explained based only on the amount of sleep lost during the exposure period (38). Similarly, the time constants for accumulation and discharge of process S have been shown to be unaffected when rats are maintained in 16:8 light-dark cycles versus 8:16 light-dark cycles, even though the distribution of sleep-wake states is markedly altered (37). In the latter stages of recovery sleep following sleep deprivation in rats, NREM sleep EEG delta power can actually drop *below* baseline levels, producing a "negative rebound." In both

Table 1 Sleep Homeostatic Parameters in Different Mammalian Species[a]

Species	Ref.	τ_i (hr)	τ_d (hr)
Human	35	18.2	4.2
Human	103	25.6, 26.3	
Rat	17	8.6	3.2
Rat	5	13.5 (3.8)	4.1 (1.1)
Mouse (AKR/J)	6	5.3 (0.3)	1.9 (0.1)
Mouse (BALB/cByJ)	6	7.6 (1.1)	1.6 (0.2)
Mouse (C57BL/6J)	6	8.0 (0.5)	1.8 (0.2)
Mouse (C57BR/cdJ)	6	7.7 (0.8)	1.5 (0.1)
Mouse (DBA/2J)	6	12.6 (1.6)	1.8 (0.3)
Mouse (129/Ola)	6	8.8 (1.4)	1.6 (0.2)
Mouse (129/Ola)	5	25.9 (5.6)	11.2 (3.9)
Mouse (129/SvJ)	5	3.6 (1.1)	4.1 (1.0)
Mouse (C57CL/6J)	5	4.9 (1.2)	3.3 (2.1)

[a]All values obtained using simulations of the time course of process S as described in the text. Where applicable, numbers in parentheses represent standard error of the mean. Values for τ_i and τ_d are not strictly comparable among all studies, as the details of the simulation procedures used may differ. See cited articles for details.

intact rats (17,39) and rats whose suprachiasmatic nuclei had been lesioned, eliminating the circadian pacemaker (40), simulations have demonstrated that this negative rebound is consistent with normal homeostatic processes, as recovery sleep was merely extended to the point where process S likewise fell below baseline levels. In humans, simulation of process S in recordings from long sleepers versus short sleepers has suggested that the time constants for accumulation and discharge of process S do not differ in the two groups, but instead that short sleepers habitually endure higher levels of process S (41). In an analysis of the sleep of six different inbred strains of mice, simulations of process S have suggested that the accumulation time constant varies by as much as 2:1 between strains, whereas the discharge time constant is relatively invariant (6).

While the above-described applications are noteworthy, simulations of process S have considerable untapped potential. As noted earlier, published simulations differ as to the conditions under which process S is assumed to accumulate and be discharged. Process S has been assumed either to accumulate or be discharged in REM sleep (17,35), but this question has not yet been systematically tested in one data set by determining which assumption consistently produces higher correlations between simulated and observed data. In one paper simulating process S in humans, process S has been assumed to accumulate exponentially *at all times* (in waking, REM sleep, and NREM sleep) and to be discharged in NREM sleep at a rate proportional to the level of EEG delta power (42). The nontraditional assumption that process S accumulates even during

NREM sleep was made because in the data sets on which the simulation was tested the fit between simulation and observations was improved. Similarly, an improvement in fit between simulation and observations has been achieved in rodent data by assuming different time constants for discharge of process S during the light period versus the dark period (17), based on the observation that light suppresses EEG delta power in rats (43–45). While these observations are suggestive, the conclusions that process S accumulates in NREM sleep or that there are different rates of discharge in light versus dark would be more clearly substantiated by systematic studies demonstrating significant improvements in fit between simulations and observations using these assumptions rather than others, and by replications of such findings in different species and under various experimental conditions. Ultimately, simulations may in some cases be incapable of distinguishing between alternative hypotheses, but generally they should be more widely employed as a valuable adjunct to experimental tests.

Simulations of process S have been conducted in humans, rats, and mice. The time constants for the accumulation and discharge functions in these studies are summarized in Table 1. Theoretically, findings such as these have the potential to establish how the time course of sleep homeostasis differs in different species. However, the results of these various studies cannot be directly compared with one another because the assumptions used for the simulations are not in every case the same. To facilitate such comparisons, there should be one series of analyses all of which use the same simulation.

IV. Implications of Sleep Homeostatic Models

In the above-described simulations, sleep propensity (process S) is measured in terms of EEG delta power in NREM sleep and is assumed to increase as an exponentially saturating function and to decrease as an exponentially decaying function. The success of such simulations in modeling sleep homeostasis is often taken to imply that: (a) discharge of sleep propensity is physiologically linked to the occurrence of slow waves in the NREM-sleep EEG, and (b) sleep propensity itself (the physiological basis of which is still unknown) likewise describes an exponentially saturating increase and an exponentially decaying decrease. In this section, I will consider the evidence for and against these two propositions.

The idea that discharge of sleep propensity is physiologically linked to the occurrence of slow waves in the NREM sleep EEG is intuitively appealing because the stages of NREM sleep when EEG slow waves are most prevalent are also the "deepest" and differ from waking to the greatest degree. As noted earlier, arousal threshold is highest when EEG slow waves are more pronounced (11–13), and this state is achieved only by first passing through "lighter" and less slow-wave-intensive stages of NREM sleep. Neurophysiologically, high-amplitude slow waves appear to occur only when neurons are tonically hyperpolarized, in contrast to the tonic depolarization that is characteristic of waking (20–22). It would therefore be reasonable to suppose that the function of NREM sleep is most effectively accomplished, and therefore that sleep propensity is discharged most rapidly, when slow waves are most obvious in the electroencephalogram and thus a state most unlike waking is achieved.

However, the exact relationship between EEG delta power and the discharge of sleep propensity is by no means clear. It is sometimes assumed that there is a simple linear relationship between NREM sleep EEG delta power and the rate of discharge of sleep propensity, but there is little direct evidence for this assumption. Even if there is such a correlation under normal circumstances, there may be notable exceptions. For example, discharge of sleep propensity appears to occur at normal or even above-normal levels following administration of benzodiazepine hypnotics, even though EEG slow waves in NREM sleep are markedly suppressed (46,47). This finding appears to argue against a tight relationship between the neurophysiological processes associated with the production of EEG slow waves and discharge of sleep propensity. Benzodiazepines suppress EEG slow waves presumably because benzodiazepine-induced increases in neuronal chloride conductance attenuate the membrane hyperpolarization required for rhythmic neuronal activity in the delta frequency range (reviewed in section 2.2 of Ref. 48). This effect on EEG slow waves is distinct from sleep homeostatic modulation (49), and in fact the exponential decay process in sleep persists following benzodiazepine administration (50). The persistence of discharge of sleep propensity following benzodiazepine administration, even though EEG delta power is markedly reduced, would thus suggest that the discharge function is not linked to hyperpolarization per se, though it may be linked to the cellular processes that produce hyperpolarization during deep NREM sleep in the absence of benzodiazepines. Evidence that has been cited for a causal connection between expression of EEG delta power and discharge of sleep propensity is the finding that selective deprivation of slow-wave sleep without decreasing total NREM sleep time produces a compensatory increase in EEG delta power (51). However, this effect would be expected as long as sleep that more efficiently discharges sleep propensity is *ordinarily* correlated with high EEG delta power, regardless of whether the occurrence of EEG slow waves per se is directly related to the discharge process.

The hypothesis that sleep propensity itself increases in an exponentially saturating manner and decreases in an exponentially decaying manner is implicitly based on the assumption that there is indeed a simple linear relationship between NREM sleep EEG delta power and the rate of discharge of sleep propensity. However, alternative hypotheses are easy to imagine. Conceivably, sleep propensity itself (the underlying process as opposed to process S as it is measured) may accumulate in a linear manner with no upper asymptote, and yet there may be physiological limits on the maximal prevalence and amplitude of EEG slow waves. In this case, successive linear increases in the level of sleep propensity would result in progressively smaller incremental increases in NREM sleep EEG delta power.

There is in fact evidence for linear accumulation of sleep propensity in the finding that theta power in the waking electroencephalogram increases as a linear function (when a sinusoidal circadian component is subtracted), relative to the duration of waking since the last sleep period (52,53). This is of interest because increase in waking theta power correlates with level of EEG delta power at the beginning of the subsequent sleep period, suggesting that waking theta power may be a proxy measure for sleep propensity (53). There is also evidence for linear *discharge* of sleep propensity in the finding that improvements in both performance and subjective measures of sleepiness increase as a linear function relative to duration of immediately prior sleep (54).

A heuristic argument against the idea that sleep propensity actually increases and decreases as a linear function could be based on the fact that, while NREM sleep EEG delta power describes an exponentially *saturating* increase, its decrease is exponentially *decaying*. If sleep propensity accumulates in a linear manner and an upper limit on the expression of slow waves in the electroencephalogram is responsible for the upper asymptote of the process S accumulation function, then a corresponding linear discharge of sleep propensity should produce a process S discharge function that mirrors the exponentially saturating increase. That is, initial linear decreases in sleep propensity should only result in small decreases in electroencephalographically based measurements of process S, until levels of sleep propensity become low enough that the hypothesized physiological limit on expression of EEG slow waves is no longer a factor. The fact that the process S discharge function instead describes an *exponentially decaying* decrease would, in the context of this alternative hypothesis, imply that while sleep propensity increases linearly, it decreases as a very steep exponential function, with an even greater initial rate of discharge than appears to be indicated by the rate of change in EEG delta power. While it is indeed possible that sleep propensity accumulates in a linear manner and yet is discharged in such an exponentially decaying manner, the most parsimonious hypothesis at the moment is that the accumulation and discharge of sleep propensity do in fact track the exponentially saturating and exponentially decaying increase and decrease of process S.

The hypothesis that sleep propensity describes an exponentially saturating increase and exponentially decaying decrease is consistent with the properties of other homeostatic control systems. When physiological variables such as body temperature and levels of energy reserves in tissues depart markedly from their set points, countermeasures are activated to attenuate further incremental departures. For example, marked decreases in body temperature cause peripheral vasoconstriction, thus producing an insulating layer between the body core and the external environment. Depletion of energy reserves is countered by decreases in cellular metabolic activity until the energy supply is once again sufficient to meet demand. The imposition of such countermeasures produces what would in effect be exponentially saturating increase functions for "heat propensity" or "nutrient propensity." Likewise, the behaviors that reverse such departures from the set point, such as shivering or feeding, are commonly more vigorous when the deficit to be made up is greater. As a result, the decrease functions for the applicable "propensities" should describe exponentially decaying curves.

In the case of sleep propensity, an exponentially saturating increase function could be produced by countermeasures that slow the rate of accumulation of sleep propensity in waking as sleep deprivation becomes more extended. It has been suggested that more frequent occurrence of brief NREM sleep episodes in the later stages of sleep deprivation could accomplish this (36). Increased expression of slow waves in the waking electroencephalogram has also been observed in the later stages of sleep deprivation (39,55,56) and could further contribute to a progressive reduction in the rate of accumulation of sleep propensity. An exponentially decaying decrease function would naturally occur if recovery sleep following sleep deprivation is indeed more "intense" than baseline sleep. The properties of recovery sleep certainly support this idea, even if we do not suppose that the discharge function is directly linked to the expression of EEG slow waves.

V. Effects of Sleep Deprivation on Sleep Structure

In the above sections I have focused largely on changes in NREM sleep produced by sleep deprivation. Sleep deprivation also produces rebound increases in REM sleep expression, but the effects are considerably more variable. In humans, one night of sleep deprivation often produces a *decrease* in REM sleep expression in the first recovery night, followed sometimes by an increase in the second recovery night, resulting in no net change in REM sleep expression during recovery (26,57–59). Four nights of sleep deprivation in humans, by contrast, produces robust increases in REM sleep expression during recovery (56). In rats, there is little or no increase in REM sleep expression during recovery from 3, 6, or 12 hr of sleep deprivation (60) but significant increases in REM sleep expression during recovery from 24 hr of sleep deprivation (25,39,60,61). Longer sleep deprivation periods in rats produce progressively more pronounced increases in REM sleep rebounds during recovery (15).

Following 18–19 days of sleep deprivation in rats, increased REM sleep expression is the most obvious feature of recovery sleep, so much so that there is not even a significant increase in EEG delta power in recovery NREM sleep (15). This latter effect has led some to argue that increased EEG delta power in recovery NREM sleep is not a consistent or especially relevant element of the homeostatic recovery process. Alternatively, EEG delta power may be partially suppressed in recovery NREM sleep merely because intense REM sleep drive following long sleep deprivations interferes with normal expression of EEG slow waves in NREM sleep (62–64).

Rechtschaffen and colleagues have tested for this by looking for delayed rebounds in NREM sleep EEG delta power and found none (15). But as discussed above, the normal association between sleep propensity and EEG delta power can be dissociated in particular circumstances (as following benzodiazepine administration) without apparently impairing the recovery process itself. While this is indeed evidence against a necessary connection between recovery and EEG delta power per se, these findings are consistent with the idea that the sleep recovery process is tied to some other cellular function which, under normal circumstances, promotes expression of high-amplitude EEG slow waves. It is worth emphasizing that 10 days of sleep deprivation in the rat is an extremely severe treatment, which should theoretically be equivalent to twice that much sleep loss in the human, given the ratio in process S accumulation time constants (see Table 1). There is thus every reason to believe that sleep regulatory mechanisms are seriously disturbed in the latter stages of these sleep deprivations. This need not imply that the results of these experiments are of no value, but it is cause for interpreting these findings with some caution.

A. Accumulation of REM Sleep Propensity in NREM Sleep (Benington-Heller Hypothesis)

The question remains why the magnitude of REM sleep rebound differs in humans versus rats and is so sensitive to the duration of sleep deprivation. According to one hypothesis advocated by Benington and Heller, REM sleep propensity accumulates not in waking but in NREM sleep (65). As a result, relatively short sleep deprivations (especially in humans) produce no REM sleep rebound because no REM sleep propensity has accumulated during the sleep deprivation period. But as sleep deprivation is extended, sleep drive becomes increasingly intense, increasing the number of brief periods of NREM sleep, microsleeps, and sleeplike neuronal activity in drowsy waking (6,39,56). These tendencies have all been observed in sleep deprivation experiments. In fact, following extended sleep deprivation, the waking electroencephalogram can become dominated by slow waves normally characteristic only of NREM sleep (39,56). The occurrence of brief periods of NREM sleep during sleep deprivation should, according to this hypothesis, cause an accumulation of REM sleep propensity during nominal waking, even though REM sleep propensity does not normally accumulate in that state. Since REM sleep cannot occur during the brief sleep episodes and microsleeps that occur in extended sleep deprivation, the REM sleep propensity that does accumulate cannot be discharged.

Because the rate of accumulation of REM sleep propensity during the sleep deprivation period is a function of the intensity of sleep drive at a given time, one would expect little or no accumulation during short sleep deprivations, when sleep drive is still at a relatively low level, and a progressively increasing rate of accumulation as sleep deprivation is extended and the level of sleep drive increases. This prediction is consistent with the observed levels of REM sleep rebounds following sleep deprivations of various lengths in one species. *But why is one night of sleep deprivation in humans (typically 36–40 hr) followed by no*

REM sleep rebound whereas 24 hr of sleep deprivation in rats is followed by a REM sleep rebound?

One explanation is that sleep propensity (process S) appears to accumulate about twice as quickly in rats as in humans (see Table 1). Thus, 24 hr of sleep loss in rats may result in higher levels of accumulated sleep propensity than 36–40 hr of sleep loss in humans, producing more sleep drive toward the end of the sleep deprivation period and thus a greater tendency toward brief NREM sleep episodes, microsleeps, and NREM sleep-like neuronal activity in waking. Moreover, human subjects in sleep deprivation experiments are mindful of the purpose of the experiment and so can be expected to make reasonable attempts to remain awake, whereas rats are of course unaware of the purpose of the experiment and will make every effort to sleep and be drowsy as much as they can. This too should produce a greater tendency for NREM sleep and NREM sleep-like activity to occur during sleep deprivation in rats, causing a greater accumulation of REM sleep propensity. This tendency will be especially pronounced when more "gentle" sleep deprivation protocols are used, which permit more transient expression of NREM sleep during the deprivation period. Indeed, sleep deprivation experiments using such protocols appear to result in more pronounced REM sleep rebound during recovery sleep (as they result in a lesser increase in EEG delta power, as noted earlier) (15).

This hypothesis has been debated in two recent series of papers, with Rechtschaffen et al. and Franken offering arguments against it (15,66–69). Rechtschaffen et al. have argued that the amount of NREM sleep equivalent that would have to occur during sleep deprivation to account for the increased REM sleep expression during recovery considerably exceeds the amount observed or even amounts that could reasonably be expected, particularly following 10-day sleep deprivations (66). This argument is of course predicated on the idea that sleep state scoring during deprivation adequately accounts for the amount of NREM sleep experienced in the frequent, brief episodes that occur during sleep deprivations in rodents. Moreover, one's conclusions are critically dependent on how many minutes of NREM sleep equivalent during the deprivation period are assumed to produce an amount of REM sleep propensity that would be discharged in 1 min of REM sleep, and that number is not yet known with any precision.

Franken has argued that, while slow waves do indeed appear in the waking electroencephalogram during sleep deprivation, they are of considerably lower amplitude than those observed during NREM sleep, and therefore should not cause the accumulation of more than a small amount of REM sleep propensity, even if one accepts Benington and Heller's hypothesis (67,68). This argument assumes that, were REM sleep propensity to accumulate in response to NREM sleep-like neuronal activity, the rate of accumulation would have to be a function of intensity (perhaps even a simple function of the rate of discharge of process S) and that EEG delta power and similar measures of the occurrence of EEG slow waves are reasonably adequate indices of the rate of accumulation of REM sleep propensity under all circumstances. I noted earlier that while benzodiazepines suppress EEG delta power, they do not appear to interfere with discharge of NREM-sleep propensity, suggesting that there is no direct link between expression of EEG slow waves and the sleep recovery process. Likewise, even if accumulation of REM sleep propensity is to some degree linked to the occurrence of EEG slow waves, it need not be a tight, quantifiable association. In the abnormal drowsy waking that occurs during experimental sleep deprivation, acetylcholine and other excitatory neuromodulators are released at higher levels than in NREM sleep. These neurochemicals may interfere with expression of EEG slow waves, even though the state produced bears significant similarities to NREM sleep with regard to the accumulation of REM sleep propensity. Accepting this possibility, Franken has argued in response that Benington and Heller's hypothesis that REM sleep rebounds following extended sleep deprivation are at least in part driven by the occurrence of NREM sleep-like activity in drowsy waking is thus not quantifiably testable at the moment (70). This point is well taken, but while the current impossibility of quantifying this matter is unfortunate, that is not a refutation of the hypothesis itself.

B. Accumulation of REM Sleep Propensity in Wakefulness

The alternative to Benington and Heller's hypothesis is that REM sleep rebounds following total sleep deprivation result from accumulation of REM sleep propensity in waking. According to this hypothesis, sleep deprivation causes parallel accumulation of NREM sleep propensity (resulting in increases in total sleep time and NREM sleep EEG delta power) and REM sleep propensity (resulting in increases in REM sleep time). This hypothesis requires that there be some, as yet unknown, mechanism for alternating the discharge of NREM sleep propensity and REM sleep propensity during recovery sleep. It must also account for the absence of a REM sleep rebound following 36–40 hr of sleep deprivation in humans, as well as the tendency for REM sleep rebounds to increasingly overwhelm NREM sleep recovery processes in more extended sleep deprivations. On the latter issue, one could argue that occurrence of brief NREM sleep episodes and microsleeps during more extended sleep deprivations permits some discharge of NREM sleep propensity without any discharge of REM sleep propensity. This, in turn, causes REM-sleep propensity to increase relative to NREM sleep propensity with increasing duration of sleep deprivation.

VI. Circadian Rhythms and Sleep Deprivation

In our discussions so far, we have considered sleep homeostasis independently of the body's circadian rhythms, which ordinarily consolidate sleep and waking in distinct phases of the 24-hr cycle. In mammals, circadian rhythmicity is produced by the output of neurons in the suprachiasmatic nucleus (SCN), located in the base of the hypothalamus, just dorsal to the optic chiasm (71). The mechanisms by which the output of these neurons influences sleep-wake behavior are still unknown. According to one hypothesis, the output consists of an endogenous stimulant, which is released during the active phase of the 24-hr cycle and promotes waking (72). Sleep is, according to this hypothesis, consolidated in the rest phase by default, as a result of the sleep deprivation that occurs during the active phase. Alternatively, the output of the circadian pacemaker may consist of both a stimulant, promoting waking during the active phase, and a somnolent, promoting sleep during the rest phase (73,74).

The circadian consolidation of waking during the active phase produces a natural daily sleep deprivation, which in turn drives a homeostatic response. The simulations of sleep homeostasis described earlier demonstrate that the sleep deprivation and recovery processes caused by the circadian pacemaker involve the same increases and decreases in EEG delta power as occur during experimental sleep deprivation. Therefore, the homeostatic mechanisms are presumably the same. Experimental sleep deprivations differ from these naturally occurring sleep deprivations only in that the consolidation of waking during the deprivation period is somewhat more complete and the duration of sleep deprivation can be systematically altered under experimental conditions.

The promotion of waking and/or sleep by the circadian pacemaker is a factor in the design and interpretation of sleep deprivation experiments for a number of reasons. First, baseline levels of sleep and waking systematically vary between rest and active periods, as a result of circadian consolidation of waking and sleep. Thus, sleep deprivations performed during the active period may not reduce sleep expression much, relative to control, as control levels of sleep during this period are low in the first place. This consideration is more obvious in experiments with human subjects, since waking is more completely consolidated in humans than in rodents and other experimental animals. For this reason, sleep deprivation experiments in humans generally last at least 36–40 hr, eliminating sleep for one entire night as well as the day before and after.

The output of the circadian pacemaker also influences how readily subjects can be deprived of sleep at different times of day. Assuming that the pacemaker does indeed promote release of an endogenous stimulant during the active period, it facilitates sleep deprivation by reducing the natural tendency to sleep at that time. However, this effect is lost when sleep deprivations continue into the natural rest period, when keeping subjects awake is much more difficult. As noted above, it is unclear whether this is merely because release of an endogenous stimulant ceases, exposing the underlying homeostatic sleep drive, or whether the circadian pacemaker actively promotes sleep through the release of an endogenous somnolent.

Finally, the output of the circadian pacemaker is a factor in the expression of the sleep recovery process. When sleep deprivations are timed to end at the beginning of the rest period (as is most often the case), then recovery sleep is relatively well consolidated. If, however, sleep deprivation ends at the beginning of the active period, the circadian promotion of wake at that time tends to fragment recovery sleep, even in the face of high levels of sleep propensity (75–77). For the most part, levels of EEG delta power in recovery sleep track the predicted process S function in spite of this interference, but some of the discharge of process S is deferred to the following rest period, when sleep can be more effectively consolidated.

A. The Two-Process Model

One of the earliest applications of homeostatic models of sleep expression was to explain the timing of onset and offset of sleep periods when sleep deprivation is terminated at various phases of the circadian rhythm (33,78). This was accomplished by making sleep onset and offset dependent on two processes: the process S of sleep homeostasis and a process C reflecting the output of the circadian pacemaker. In the original model, sleep onset was assumed to occur whenever process S exceeded an upper limit and sleep offset whenever process S fell below a lower limit. Process C was assumed to describe a sinusoidal function, increasing the thresholds for sleep onset and offset during the active period, and decreasing them during the rest period.

This "two-process" model has been found to be rather powerful in predicting sleep expression under a variety of naturally occurring and experimental conditions (24,79). It has also been successfully applied to predicting sleep expression in rodents, by simply narrowing the range between the upper and lower thresholds (35,78). Its power in predicting human sleep expression was increased when the shape of the process C function was changed from a pure sinusoidal one to one in which the slope of the increase in the transition from rest period to active period is greater than the slope of the decrease in the transition from active period to rest period (35). The two-process model is predicated on the assumption that changes in sleep propensity regulate both sleep onset and sleep offset. While this is certainly true in large part, as the success of this model attests, there are exceptions. For example, sleep deprivation in rodents has been shown to extend sleep time beyond what would be predicted based on sleep propensity alone, so that NREM sleep EEG delta power and process S decrease in the latter stages of recovery sleep to *below* baseline levels, producing a "negative rebound" in EEG delta power (17,39,40). Selective deprivation of slow-wave sleep in humans has been shown to increase subsequent EEG delta power without resulting in an extension of spontaneous sleep duration, as would be predicted by the two-process model (80).

B. Measures of Sleep Propensity

In our initial discussion about identifying a measurable variable to indicate the ongoing level of sleep propensity, I argued that sleepiness is not an optimal candidate for use as such a variable because it is markedly influenced by the output of the circadian pacemaker, and advocated the use of NREM sleep EEG delta power instead. The success of simulations of process S based on EEG delta power measures alone, without factoring in circadian phase, is itself an argument in favor of the idea that the output of the circadian pacemaker has little or no influence on EEG delta power. The only sleep-independent influence on EEG delta power that has been noted is a tendency in rodents for EEG delta power to be inhibited by light (45,81).

However, NREM sleep EEG delta power is not the only sleep-related variable that could conceivably be influenced by the output of the circadian pacemaker. I have already noted the obvious effect of circadian phase on sleep tendency. In addition, the increase in REM sleep expression in the late rest period is a function of circadian as well as sleep homeostatic factors (82–84). There is also a well-known association between circadian phase and core body temperature, yet this variable is also influenced by the sleep-wake state (85,86).

For these and other variables, one would like to know the relative influence exerted by sleep homeostatic versus circadian factors. An ideal protocol for eliminating circadian influences is to characterize sleep-wake behavior in the absence of the circadian pacemaker in the SCN. Such studies have been performed in SCN-lesioned rats (40,61,87), but of course the equivalent studies are impossible in humans. An alternative approach is to cause sleep to be initiated at all phases of the circadian cycle. Such a protocol provided some of the first solid evidence for circadian modulation of REM sleep expression (82,83).

C. Forced Desynchrony Protocol

More recently, the experimental design of allowing sleep to be initiated at all phases of the circadian cycle has been employed systematically in an elegant series of experiments using a "forced desynchrony" protocol (74,88). In this protocol, humans are exposed to a 28-hr light-dark cycle, to which their circadian pacemaker cannot entrain. As a result, their biological clock "free runs" at its endogenous period. Because the experimental subjects are only permitted to sleep during the dark phase of the 28-hr light-dark cycle, this protocol amounts to a series of sleep deprivations, each lasting approximately 19 hr, which begin and end at all possible phases of the circadian cycle. The protocol does not cause long-term accumulation of sleep propensity because subjects are permitted sufficient sleep time to recover each "night." Human subjects have been maintained under conditions of forced desynchrony for several weeks at a time, with recordings of EEG variables and body temperature during each rest period. Since any given point in an individual subject's record can be analyzed both in terms of the phase of the light-dark cycle and in terms of time since sleep onset, this protocol in effect enables circadian influences to be characterized independently of sleep homeostatic influences, and vice versa.

Data from these studies (Fig. 2) have demonstrated circadian promotion of wakefulness during rest periods at circadian phases normally associated with activity, and a corresponding deficit in total sleep time as well as sleep continuity at those same circadian phases (74). REM sleep (as a percentage of total sleep time) is increased at phases normally associated with the end of a rest period.

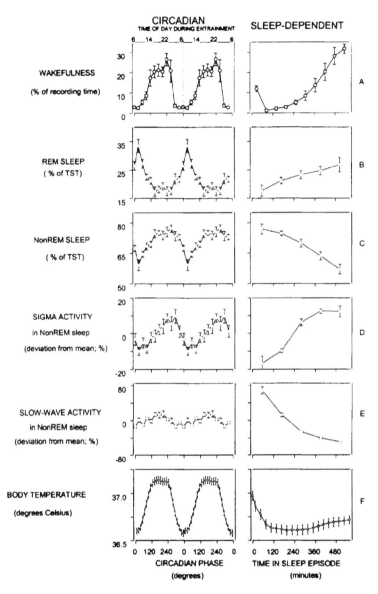

Figure 2 Separation of circadian and sleep-dependent influences on sleep/wake variables, using a forced desynchrony paradigm (see text for details). Panels on left analyze recordings relative to circadian phase, as determined by core body temperature. Data in these panels are double plotted to illustrate rhythmicity. Panels on right analyze recordings relative to time since onset of sleep episode, revealing the influence of level of accumulated sleep propensity. Wakefulness is expressed as percentage of recording time, whereas NREM sleep and REM sleep are expressed as a percentage of total sleep time (TST). Sigma (12.75–15.0 Hz) activity and delta (0.75–4.5 Hz) activity are expressed as percent deviation from mean. Core body temperature is expressed in degrees Celsius. (From Ref. 74.)

Sleep homeostatic modulation of these variables is as would be expected, with progressive decreases in NREM sleep and increases in both waking and REM sleep from the beginning to the end of a sleep episode. EEG slow-wave activity has been shown to be little affected by circadian phase, whereas activity in the sigma band (12.75-15 Hz) corresponding to the occurrence of sleep spindles is increased at phases normally associated with the active period (74). Not surprisingly, EEG delta power decreases and EEG sigma power increases from the beginning to end of a sleep episode. A corresponding increase in delta power in the waking electroencephalogram as a function of time awake has also been noted (89). Age-related changes in circadian versus homeostatic influences have been studied by comparing data from forced desynchrony experiments in elderly versus young adults (88). In comparison to young adults (20–30 years old), the elderly (65–75 years old) exhibit reduced circadian modulation of body temperature and REM sleep expression, while sleep-dependent effects on the expression of REM sleep and stage 4 NREM sleep are reduced.

VII. Conclusions

In this chapter, we have seen how noninvasive measurements of electrographic variables can provide insights into the homeostatic and circadian factors involved in the regulation of sleep. Throughout this discussion, I have described the homeostatic process in terms of increases and decreases in sleep "propensity," reflecting our current ignorance regarding the biochemical substrates of that propensity and hence the function of sleep. Considering that our ultimate goal should be to discover the biochemical substrate of the function of sleep, the analyses described in this chapter inevitably represent halfway measures. Once we know the function of sleep, abstract analyses in terms of propensity will in retrospect appear inadequate.

Yet in our present state of ignorance, these analyses are critically important. In one sense, they enable us to describe prospectively key characteristics of this function. For example, there is reason to believe that the biochemical substrate in question accumulates and is discharged exponentially. We can also predict with some confidence the time course of accumulation and discharge in different species, and the relative rates of accumulation and discharge between species may provide clues as to the nature of that substrate. These and the other insights made possible by means of homeostatic and circadian modeling of sleep regulation should not be neglected in our ongoing search for the function of sleep.

The analyses described in this chapter should play an important role also in the analysis of data in experiments focused on the search for the biochemical substrate of sleep function. Molecular genetic studies of sleep in rodents are currently underway in a number of laboratories (5,6,29,90–101). Following recent evidence that rest in *Drosophila* may be homologous to mammalian sleep (8,102), molecular genetic studies of this process have likewise been undertaken (4). The goal of such studies is the identification of specific genes involved in the regulation of sleep, either through genetic linkage analysis or through the identification of mutant alleles that markedly alter sleep regulation. Identification of such genes will hopefully lead us to proteins that contribute to the biochemical processes underlying sleep regulation, and the further investigation of interactions between these proteins and other proteins should eventually enable us to describe these processes in some detail.

In these investigations, sleep homeostatic models should play a central role. Variables such as time spent awake, time spent in sleep, or time spent in specific sleep states would of course be altered by mutations of proteins involved in sleep regulation, but they could also be altered by mutations of proteins that are only tangentially related to the sleep regulatory process. For example, any mutations that increase an animal's excitability or stress response should decrease sleep time under the somewhat artificial conditions in which sleep is recorded in rodents, and REM sleep expression is likely to be particularly sensitive to such an effect. However, such mutations are unlikely to alter homeostatic variables such as the time course of accumulation and discharge of process S. These latter variables should be much more selectively affected only by mutations in proteins more closely involved in the regulation of sleep per se. This is especially so in the case of the discharge function, which represents processes taking place *in* sleep. For this reason, simulations of process S such as I have described in this chapter should be routinely performed in experiments designed to identify and characterize sleep-related mutations, just as Franken and colleagues have done in the characterization of sleep in genetically distinct mouse strains (93).

Acknowledgments

Paul Franken provided considerable guidance and insight at every stage in the production of this chapter, and it practically could not have been written without his assistance. Alex Borbely read and commented on an earlier draft of the chapter. I thank them both.

References

1. Borbely AA. Sleep: circadian rhythm versus recovery process. In: Koukkou M, Lehmann D, Angst J, eds. Functional States of the Brain: Their Determinants. Amsterdam: Elsevier, 1980:151–161.
2. Suntsova N, Szymusiak R, Alam MN, Guzman-Marin R, McGinty D. Sleep-waking discharge patterns of median preoptic nucleus neurons in rats. J Physiol 2002; 543:665–677.
3. Szymusiak R, Steininger T, Alam N, McGinty D. Preoptic area sleep-regulating mechanisms. Arch Ital Biol 2001; 139:77–92.
4. Shaw PJ, Tononi G, Greenspan RJ, Robinson DF. Stress response genes protect against lethal effects of sleep deprivation in *Drosophila*. Nature 2002; 417:287–291.

5. Huber R, Deboer T, Tobler I. Effects of sleep deprivation on sleep and sleep EEG in three mouse strains: empirical data and simulations. Brain Res 2000; 857:8–19.

6. Franken P, Chollet D, Tafti M. The homeostatic regulation of sleep need is under genetic control. J Neurosci 2001; 21:2610–2621.

7. Rosa RR, Bonnet MH. Sleep stages, auditory arousal threshold, and body temperature as predictors of behavior upon awakening. Int J Neurosci 1985; 27:73–83.

8. Shaw PJ, Cirelli C, Greenspan RJ, Tononi G. Correlates of sleep and waking in *Drosophila melanogaster*. Science 2000; 287:1834–1837.

9. Bonnet MH. Effect of sleep disruption on sleep, performance, and mood. Sleep 1985; 8:11–19.

10. Frederickson CJ, Rechtschaffen A. Effects of sleep deprivation on awakening thresholds and sensory evoked potentials in the rat. Sleep 1978; 1:69–82.

11. Williams HL. The problem of defining depth of sleep. Res Publ Assoc Res Nerv Ment Dis 1967; 45:277–287.

12. Williams HL, Tepas DI, Morlock HCJ. Evoked responses to clicks and electroencephalographic stages of sleep in man. Science 1962; 138:685–686.

13. Williams HL, Hammack JT, Daly RL, Dement WC, Lubin A. Responses to auditory stimulation, sleep loss and the EEG stages of sleep. Electroenceph Clin Neurophysiol 1964; 16:269–279.

14. Horne JA. Sleep function, with particular reference to sleep deprivation. Ann Clin Res 1985; 17:199–208.

15. Rechtschaffen A, Bergmann BM, Gilliland MA, Bauer K. Effects of method, duration, and sleep stage on rebounds from sleep deprivation in the rat. Sleep 1999; 22:11–31.

16. Tobler I, Borbely AA. The effect of 3-h and 6-h sleep deprivation on sleep and EEG spectra of the rat. Behav Brain Res 1990; 36:73–78.

17. Franken P, Tobler I, Borbely AA. Sleep homeostasis in the rat: simulation of the time course of EEG slow-wave activity. Neurosci Lett 1991; 130:141–144.

18. Calvet J, Fourment A, Thieffry M. Electrical activity in neocortical projection and association areas during slow wave sleep. Brain Res 1973; 52:173–187.

19. Steriade M, McCormick DA, Sejnowski TJ. Thalamocortical oscillations in the sleeping and aroused brain. Science 1993; 262:679–685.

20. Hirsch JC, Fourment A, Marc ME. Sleep-related variations of membrane potential in the lateral geniculate body relay neurons of the cat. Brain Res 1983; 259:308–312.

21. Steriade M, Curro Dossi R, Nunez A. Network modulation of a slow intrinsic oscillation of cat thalamocortical neurons implicated in sleep delta waves: cortically induced synchronization and brainstem cholinergic suppression. J Neurosci 1991; 11:3200–3217.

22. Dossi RC, Nunez A, Steriade M. Electrophysiology of a slow (0.5–4 Hz) intrinsic oscillation of cat thalamocortical neurones in vivo. J Physiol 1992; 447:215–234.

23. Dinges DF. Are you awake? Cognitive performance and reverie during the hypnopompic state. In: Bootzin RR, Kihlstrom JF, Schacter D, eds. Sleep and Cognition. Washington, DC: American Psychological Association, 1990:159–175.

24. Borbely AA, Achermann P. Sleep homeostasis and models of sleep regulation. In: Kryger MH, Roth T, Dement WC, eds. Principles and Practice of Sleep Medicine. Philadelphia: WB Saunders, 2000:377–390.

25. Borbely AA, Neuhaus HU. Sleep-deprivation: effects on sleep and EEG in the rat. J Comp Physiol 1979; 133:71–87.

26. Borbely AA, Baumann F, Brandeis D, Strauch I, Lehmann D. Sleep deprivation: effect on sleep stages and EEG power density in man. Electroenceph Clin Neurophysiol 1981; 51:483–493.

27. Tobler I, Scherschlicht R. Sleep and EEG slow-wave activity in the domestic cat: effect of sleep deprivation. Behav Brain Res 1990; 37:109–118.

28. Tobler I, Franken P, Scherschlicht R. Sleep and EEG spectra in the rabbit under baseline conditions and following sleep deprivation. Physiol Behav 1990; 48:121–129.

29. Franken P, Malafosse A, Tafti M. Genetic variation in EEG activity during sleep in inbred mice. Am J Physiol 1998; 275:R1127–1137.

30. Strijkstra AM, Daan S. Dissimilarity of slow-wave activity enhancement by torpor and sleep deprivation in a hibernator. Am J Physiol 1998; 275:R1110–1117.

31. Deboer T, Tobler I. Slow waves in the sleep electroencephalogram after daily torpor are homeostatically regulated. Neuroreport 2000; 11:881–885.

32. Oleksenko AI, Mukhametov LM, Polyakova IG, Supin AY, Kovalzon VM. Unihemispheric sleep deprivation in bottlenose dolphins. J Sleep Res 1992; 1:40–44.

33. Borbely AA. A two-process model of sleep regulation. Human Neurobiol 1982; 1:195–204.

34. Dijk D-J, Brunner DP, Borbely AA. Time course of EEG power density during long sleep in humans. Am J Physiol 1990; 27:R650–R661.

35. Daan S, Beersma DGM, Borbely AA. Timing of human sleep: recovery process gated by a circadian pacemaker. Am J Physiol 1984; 246:R161–R178.

36. Franken P, Chollet D, Tafti M. The homeostatic regulation of sleep need is under genetic control. J Neurosci 2001; 21:2610–2621.

37. Franken P, Tobler I, Borbely AA. Varying photoperiod in the laboratory rat: profound effect on 24–h sleep pattern but no effect on sleep homeostasis. Am J Physiol 1995; 269:R691–701.

38. Franken P, Tobler I, Borbely AA. Effects of 12–h sleep deprivation and of 12–h cold exposure on sleep regulation and cortical temperature in the rat. Physiol Behav 1993; 54:885–894.

39. Franken P, Dijk D-J, Tobler I, Borbely AA. Sleep deprivation in rats: effects on EEG power spectra, vigilance states, and cortical temperature. Am J Physiol 1991; 261:R198–R208.

40. Trachsel L, Edgar DM, Seidel WF, Heller HC, Dement WC. Sleep homeostasis in suprachiasmatic nuclei–lesioned rats: effects of sleep deprivation and triazolam administration. Brain Res 1992; 589:253–261.

41. Aeschbach D, Cajochen C, Landolt H, Borbely AA. Homeostatic sleep regulation in habitual short sleepers and long sleepers. Am J Physiol 1996; 270:R41–53.

42. Achermann P, Dijk DJ, Brunner DP, Borbely AA. A model of human sleep homeostasis based on EEG slow-wave activity: quantitative comparison of data and simulations. Brain Res Bull 1993; 31:97–113.

43. Tobler I, Franken P, Alfoldi P, Borbely AA. Room light impairs sleep in the albino rat. Behav Brain Res 1994; 63:205–211.

44. Trachsel L, Tobler I, Borbely AA. Sleep regulation in rats: effects of sleep deprivation, light, and circadian phase. Am J Physiol 1986; 251:R1037–R1044.

45. Alfoldi P, Tobler I, Borbely AA. The effect of light on sleep and the EEG of young rats. Pflügers Arch 1990; 417:398–403.

46. Borbely AA, Mattmann P, Loepfe M, Strauch I, Lehmann D. Effect of benzodiazepine hypnotics on all-night sleep EEG spectra. Human Neurobiol 1985; 4:189–194.

47. Achermann P, Borbely AA. Dynamics of EEG slow wave activity during physiological sleep and after administration of benzodiazepine hypnotics. Human Neurobiol 1987; 6:203–210.

48. Benington JH, Heller HC. Restoration of brain energy metabolism as the function of sleep. Prog Neurobiol 1995; 45:347–360.

49. Landolt HP, Finelli LA, Roth C, Buck A, Achermann P, Borbely AA. Zolpidem and sleep deprivation: different effect on EEG power spectra. J Sleep Res 2000; 9:175–183.

50. Borbely AA, Achermann P. Ultradian dynamics of sleep after a single dose of benzodiazepine hypnotics. Eur J Pharmacol 1991; 195:11–18.

51. Dijk DJ, Beersma DG, Daan S, Bloem GM, Van den Hoofdakker RH. Quantitative analysis of the effects of slow wave sleep deprivation during the first 3 h of sleep on subsequent EEG power density. Eur Arch Psychiatr Neurol Sci 1987; 236:323–328.

52. Dumont M, Macchi MM, Carrier J, Lafrance C, Hebert M. Time course of narrow frequency bands in the waking EEG during sleep deprivation. Neuroreport 1999; 10:403–407.

53. Finelli LA, Baumann H, Borbely AA, Achermann P. Dual electroencephalogram markers of human sleep homeostasis: correlation between theta activity in waking and slow-wave activity in sleep. Neurosci 2000; 101:523–529.

54. Jewett ME, Dijk DJ, Kronauer RE, Dinges DF. Dose-response relationship between sleep duration and human psychomotor vigilance and subjective alertness. Sleep 1999; 22:171–179.

55. Borbely AA, Tobler I, Hanagasioglu M. Effect of sleep deprivation on sleep and EEG power spectra in the rat. Behav Brain Res 1984; 14:171–182.

56. Berger RJ, Oswald J. Effects of sleep deprivation on behavior, subsequent sleep, and dreaming. J Ment Sci 1962; 108:457–465.

57. Carskadon MA, Dement WC. Effects of total sleep loss on sleep tendency. Percept Mot Skills 1979; 48:495–506.

58. Carskadon MA, Harvey K, Dement WC. Sleep loss in young adolescents. Sleep 1981; 4:299–312.

59. Brendel DH, Reynolds CF, Jennings JR, Hoch CC, Monk TH, Berman SR, Hall FT, Buysse DJ, Kupfer DJ. Sleep stage physiology, mood, and vigilance responses to total sleep deprivation in healthy 80–year-olds and 20–year-olds. Psychophysiology 1990; 27:677–685.

60. Tobler I, Borbely AA. Sleep EEG in the rat as a function of prior waking. Electroenceph Clin Neurophysiol 1986; 64:74–76.

61. Mistlberger RE, Bergmann BM, Waldenar W, Rechtschaffen A. Recovery sleep following sleep deprivation in intact and suprachiasmatic nuclei–lesioned rats. Sleep 1983; 6:217–233.

62. Beersma DGM, Dijk DJ, Blok CGH, Everhardus I. REM sleep deprivation during 5 hours leads to an immediate REM sleep rebound and to suppression of non-REM sleep intensity. Electroenceph Clin Neurophysiol 1990; 76:114–122.

63. Brunner DP, Dijk D-J, Tobler I, Borbely AA. Effect of partial sleep deprivation on sleep stages and EEG power spectra: evidence for non-REM and REM sleep homeostasis. Electroenceph Clin Neurophysiol 1990; 75:492–499.

64. Brunner DP, Dijk D-J, Borbely AA. Repeated partial sleep deprivation progressively changes the EEG during sleep and wakefulness. Sleep 1993; 16:100–113.

65. Benington JH, Heller HC. Does the function of REM sleep concern non-REM sleep or waking? Prog Neurobiol 1994; 44:433–449.

66. Rechtschaffen A, Bergmann BM. Sleep rebounds and their implications for sleep stage substrates: a response to Benington and Heller. Sleep 1999; 22:1038–1043.

67. Franken P. Long-term vs. short-term processes regulating REM sleep. J Sleep Res 2002; 11:17–28.

68. Benington JH. Debating how REM sleep is regulated (and by what). J Sleep Res 2002; 11:29–31; discussion 31–23.

69. Benington JH, Heller HC. Implications of sleep deprivation experiments for our understanding of sleep homeostasis. Sleep 1999; 22:1033–1037.

70. Franken P. Response to "Debating how REM sleep is regulated (and by what)." J Sleep Res 2002; 11:31–33.

71. Reppert SM, Weaver DR. Coordination of circadian timing in mammals. Nature 2002; 418:935–941.

72. Edgar DM, Dement WC, Fuller CA. Effect of SCN lesions on sleep in squirrel monkeys: evidence for opponent processes in sleep-wake regulation. J Neurosci 1993; 13:1065–1079.

73. Dijk DJ, Czeisler CA. Paradoxical timing of the circadian rhythm of sleep propensity serves to consolidate sleep and wakefulness in humans. Neurosci Lett 1994; 166:63–68.

74. Dijk DJ, Czeisler CA. Contribution of the circadian pacemaker and the sleep homeostat to sleep propensity, sleep structure, electroencephalographic slow waves, and sleep spindle activity in humans. J Neurosci 1995; 15:3526–3538.

75. Akerstedt T, Gillberg M. The circadian variation of experimentally displaced sleep. Sleep 1981; 4:159–169.

76. Dijk DJ, Brunner DP, Beersma DG, Borbely AA. Electroencephalogram power density and slow wave sleep as a function of prior waking and circadian phase. Sleep 1990; 13:430–440.

77. Dijk DJ, Brunner DP, Borbely AA. EEG power density during recovery sleep in the morning. Electroencephalogr Clin Neurophysiol 1991; 78:203–214.

78. Borbely AA. The sleep process: circadian and homeostatic aspects. In: Obal F, Benedek G, eds. Advances in Physiological Sciences, vol 18 Environmental Physiology. Oxford, UK: Pergamon Press, 1981:8591.

79. Borbely AA, Achermann P. Sleep homeostasis and models of sleep regulation. J Biol Rhythms 1999; 14:557–568.

80. Dijk DJ, Beersma DG. Effects of SWS deprivation on subsequent EEG power density and spontaneous sleep duration. Electroencephalogr Clin Neurophysiol 1989; 72:312–320.

81. Trachsel L, Tobler I, Borbely AA. Sleep regulation in rats: effects of sleep deprivation, light, and circadian phase. Am J Physiol 1986; 251:R1037–1044.

82. Weitzman ED, Czeisler CA, Zimmerman JC, Ronda JM. Timing of REM and stages 3 + 4 sleep during temporal isolation in man. Sleep 1980; 2:391–407.

83. Czeisler CA, Zimmerman JC, Ronda JM, Moore-Ede MC, Weitzman ED. Timing of REM sleep is coupled to the circadian rhythm of body temperature in man. Sleep 1980; 2:329–346.

84. Czeisler CA, Weitzman ED, Moore-Ede MC, Zimmerman JC, Knauer RS. Human sleep: its duration and organization depend on its circadian phase. Science 1980; 210:1264–1267.

85. Franken P, Tobler I, Borbely AA. Sleep and waking have a major effect on the 24–hr rhythm of cortical temperature in the rat. J Biol Rhythms 1992; 7:341–352.

86. Folkard S. The pragmatic approach to masking. Chronobiol Int 1989; 6:55–64.

87. Tobler I, Borbely AA, Groos G. The effect of sleep deprivation on sleep in rats with suprachiasmatic lesions. Neurosci Lett 1983; 42:49–54.

88. Dijk DJ, Duffy JF, Czeisler CA. Contribution of circadian physiology and sleep homeostasis to age-related changes in human sleep. Chronobiol Int 2000; 17:285–311.

89. Cajochen C, Wyatt J, Czeisler C, Dijk D. Separation of circadian and wake duration–dependent modulation of EEG activation during wakefulness. Neurosci 2002; 114:1047.

90. Dugovic C, Turek FW. Similar genetic mechanisms may underlie sleep-wake states in neonatal and adult rats. Neuroreport 2001; 12:3085–3089.

91. Naylor E, Bergmann BM, Krauski K, Zee PC, Takahashi JS, Vitaterna MH, Turek FW. The circadian clock mutation alters sleep homeostasis in the mouse. J Neurosci 2000; 20:8138–8143.

92. Kolker DE, Turek FW. The search for circadian clock and sleep genes. J Psychopharmacol 1999; 13:S5–9.

93. Franken P, Malafosse A, Tafti M. Genetic determinants of sleep regulation in inbred mice. Sleep 1999; 22:155–169.

94. Kapfhamer D, Valladares O, Sun Y, Nolan PM, Rux JJ, Arnold SE, Veasey SC, Bucan M. Mutations in Rab3a alter circadian period and homeostatic response to sleep loss in the mouse. Nature Genet 2002; 32:290–295.

95. Veasey SC, Valladares O, Fenik P, Kapfhamer D, Sanford L, Benington J, Bucan M. An automated system for recording and analysis of sleep in mice. Sleep 2000; 23:1025–1040.

96. Tafti M, Franken P, Kitahama K, Malafosse A, Jouvet M, Valatx JL. Localization of candidate genomic regions influencing paradoxical sleep in mice. Neuroreport 1997; 8:3755–3758.

97. Tafti M, Chollet D, Valatx JL, Franken P. Quantitative trait loci approach to the genetics of sleep in recombinant inbred mice. J Sleep Res 1999; 8 (Suppl) 1:37–43.

98. Tafti M, Franken P. Invited review: genetic dissection of sleep. J Appl Physiol 2002; 92:1339–1347.

99. Toth LA. Identifying genetic influences on sleep: an approach to discovering the mechanisms of sleep regulation. Behav Genet 2001; 31:39–46.

100. Toth LA, Williams RW. A quantitative genetic analysis of slow-wave sleep in influenza-infected CXB recombinant inbred mice. Behav Genet 1999; 29:339–348.

101. Toth LA, Williams RW. A quantitative genetic analysis of slow-wave sleep and rapid-eye movement sleep in CXB recombinant inbred mice. Behav Genet 1999; 29:329–337.

102. Hendricks JC, Finn SM, Panckeri KA, Chavkin J, Williams JA, Sehgal A, Pack AI. Rest in *Drosophila* is a sleep-like state. Neuron 2000; 25:129–138.

103. Brunet D, Nish D, MacLean AW, Coulter M, Knowles JB. The time course of "process S": comparison of visually scored slow wave sleep and power spectral analysis. Electroencephalogr Clin Neurophysiol 1988; 70:278–280.

Index

α-agonists, cardiovascular drugs, effect
    on sleep, 178
Acetylcholine
    antidepressant effects, sleep
        deprivation and, 427
    wakefulness and, 403
Acute alcohol intoxication,
    effect on sleep, 168, 170
Acute stress, sleep deprivation and, 71
Acute total sleep deprivation, effects of,
    299–302
Adam, Kristin, function(s) of sleep, 40
ADHD (attention deficit hyperactivity
        disorder)
    central nervous system stimulants,
        175
    psychopathology, changes from sleep
        deprivation, 437
Affective disorders, and sleep
        deprivation, 432–434
Affymetrix GeneChip technology, 389
Age, sleep deprivation, 441–467

Age-dependent changes in sleep
    chronotype questionnaires, 449
    circadian process, 445
    elderly subjects, 449
    homeostatic process, 445
    HPA axis "resiliency," 460
    HPA axis regulation 460
    middle-aged subjects, 449
    phase preference, 449
    Process C, 444
    Process S, 444
    sleep architecture, 442–443
    sleep regulatory mechanisms, 444–450
    sleep schedule, adolescents, 449
Aging, sleep deprivation and,
    circadian timing system, 453–454
    HPA axis, sleep, 465
    NREM sleep, 443
    REM sleep, 442
        short wave sleep (SWS) in, 451–453
        sleep EEGs, 443–444
        sleep modifications in,

NREM (*contd.*)
    circadian timing system, 453–454
    corticotropin-releasing hormone
        (CRH), 455–456
    growth hormone (GH), 454
    neuroendocrine factors, 454–459
    somatotropic axis, 456–457
    slow-wave activity (SWA), 443
    SWA, 451–453
Agostini, Ceasare, sleep deprivation,
    early studies, 32
Aircraft noise, effect of, on sleep,
    134–135
AIR$_G$, sleep deprivation and, 310
Albert, Ira, theories on function(s) of
    sleep, 42
Alcohol
    γ-hydroxybutyrate and, 171
    as antidepressant, 170
    and barbiturates, 170
    as CNS depressants, 168–170
    REM sleep deprivation and, 168
    sedative effects of, 168
    sleep and, 167–181
Alcohol-dependent subjects, sleep loss
    and immune dysregulation,
    378–379
Alertness, as component of sustained
    attention, 204–205
Alpha rhythm, wakefulness and EEG
    activity, 226
Altitude, sleep at, 137–138
Alzheimer's disease, psychopathology
    changes with sleep deprivation,
    436
Ambient temperature
    body temperature, 322
    environmental factors, 130–131
Amineptine, antidepressant effects, 423
Aminergic receptor sensitivity, 345
Aminergic system, sleep deprivation and,
    344–345
Aminoketones, as antidepressants, 172
Amphetamines, as central nervous system
    stimulants, 175
Animal models, sleep deprivation in,
    47–58
Anterior attention network, 205

Anterior cingulated, antidepressant
    effects, sleep deprivation, 422
Antiarrhythmic drugs, effect on sleep,
    179
Antidepressant drugs, and sleep
    deprivation, 421–428
    acetylcholine, 427
    amineptine, 423
    aminoketones, 172
    anterior cingulated, 422
    antidepressant medications, 423
    bupropion, 172
    cerebral metabolic, 424–425
    dopamine, 423–427
    effect on sleep, 171–173
    fluoxetine, 172
    metabolic activity, 422–423
    mirtazapine, 173
    monamine oxidase inhibitors (MAOIs),
        173
    nefazondone, 173
    neurotransmitter systems, 423–427
    paroxetine, 172
    phenethylamines, 173
    phenethylamines, 173
    selective serotonin reuptake inhibitors
        (SSRIs), 171–172
    serotonin, 426–427
    sleep-conserving, 173
    SSSD studies, 89
    studies in, 422–423
    trytophan, 426
    venlafaxine, 173
Antihypertensives, cardiovascular drugs,
    effects on sleep, 178
Antiparkinsonian medications
    effect on sleep, 177
    medications, selegiline,177
Antipsychotics, effect on sleep, 173–174
Antisense technology, sleep research, 275
Anxiolytics, effects on sleep, 174
Appetite, sleep deprivation and, 13, 306,
    308
Appetite suppressants
    insomnia, 177
    sleep, 177
Arctic, sleep
    in, 135–137

Arithmetic, sleep deprivation, effect on learning, 249–250

Arousal technique, animal studies of REM sleep deprivation, 280

Arousal types, sleep fragmentation, 112–114

Arylsulfotransferase (AST), sleep deprivation and, 393

Aserinsky, Eugene, sleep deprivation, early studies, 37

Attention, sleep deprivation effects, on alertness, 204
changes in, 199–213
cognitive function and, 204

Attention deficit hyperactivity disorder (ADHD)
central nervous system stimulants, 175
psychopathology, changes from sleep deprivation, 437

Auditory arousal threshold, sleep fragmentation, 110

Auditory processing, during sleep, 123–125

Auditory stimulation, sleep deprivation and brainstem neurons, 340

Autoimmune disorders, sleep loss, 380
rheumatoid arthritis, 380

Autonomic thermoregulation, 322–323

β-Blockers, cardiovascular drugs, effects on sleep, 178

BDNF, synaptic plasticity genes and, 22

Behavioral responsiveness
long-term memory, 124
during sleep, 122–127
tones, during sleep, 123

Behavioral thermoregulation, 323–324

Benca, Ruth, theory of sleep function(s), 41

Benington, Joel, theory of sleep function(s), 42

Benington-Heller hypothesis, 493–495

Benzodiazepines, effect on sleep, 174

Bergmann, Bernard, theory of sleep function(s), 41

Beta oscillations, wakefulness and EEG activity, 228

Biochemical changes, sleep deprivation, 339–350

Biomoleculary marker, sleep loss, 349–350

Biomolecules, changes in,
blood, 341–343
brain, sleep deprivation, 343–347
sleep deprivation, 346–349

Bipolar disorders, psychopathology changes, sleep deprivation, 433

Blood, sleep deprivation and, 342

Blood oxygenation level dependent (BOLD) response, 232, 250–251

Body restitution hypothesis
Oswald, Ian, 40
sleep, function(s) of, 40

Body temperature, 325
and ambient temperature, 322
and circadian rhythms, 325
and EEG activity, 234–235
regulation, and sleep deprivation, 320–325
and wakefulness, 231–232

BOLD (blood oxygenation level dependent) response
EEG activity during wakefulness, 251
sleep deprivation and, 250–251

Borbely's Two-Process Model, 9–10

Brain
body fluid changes, and sleep deprivation, 340
electrical stimulation of, total sleep deprivation methods, 68
sleep and, 223–224

Brain cell death, sleep deprivation and, 393–394

Brain injury, REM sleep, 19–20

Brain lesions, REM sleep-depression, 19–20

Brain maturation, theory of sleep and, 17

Brain metabolic function
during continuous performance, 246
during sleep, 247
during wakefulness, 246

Brain tissue, 342

Brainstem, wake-active regions, gene expression, 403

Bronchodilators, effect on sleep, 180
Bupropion, as antidepressant, 172

Caenorhabditis elegans, sleep
 deprivation, animal models of, 55
Calcium channel blockers, effect on
 sleep, 178
Capillary hemorrhages, 341
Carbohydrate tolerance, 310
Cardian sympathovagal balance, index of,
 311
Cardiovascular drugs, effect on sleep,
 178
 α-agonists, 178
 β-blockers, 178
 antiarrhythmic, drugs, 179
 antihypertensives, 178
 bronchodilators, 180
 calcium channel blockers, 178
 cimetidine, 179
 histamine$_2$ antagonists, 179
 hormones, 180
 hyperthyroidism, 180
 hypolipidemic drugs, 179
 lovastatin, 179
 pravastatin, 179
 rantidine, 179
 salbutamol, 180
 sleep deprivation and, 266–267
 steroids, 180
 theophylline, 180
Cardiovascular effects, sleep
 fragmentation and, 109
Carrington, Patricia, theory of sleep,
 function(s), 42
Carskadon, Mary, sleep deprivation, early
 studies, 39
Catecholamine levels, sleep deprivation
 and, 266–267, 311
Cellular immunity, and partial sleep
 deprivation, 375
Central nervous system depressants
 acute alcohol intoxication, 168, 170
 alcohol, 168–170
 effect on sleep, 168–171
Central nervous system stimulants
 amphetamines, 175

attention deficit hyperactivity disorder
 (ADHD), 175
 codeine, 177
 heroin, 177
 methadone, 177
 methylphenidate, 175
 modafinil, 175
 morphine, 177
 narcolepsy, 175
 nicotine, 176
 phenylpropanolamine (PPA), 175
 pseudoephedrine, 175
 and sleep, 174–175
Cerebral metabolism, total sleep
 deprivation and, 424–425
Cerebral restitution hypothesis, 40
c-fos, in sleep, 346, 404, 405
 REM sleep, gene expression in, 406
 sleep-wake circuitry, gene expression,
  401–403
 wakefulness and, 404
Chemical stimulation, total sleep
 deprivation methods of, 68
Choline acetyltransferase, effects of
 sleep, 404
Cholinergic neurons, 344
Cholinergic system, sleep deprivation
 and, 345
Chronic stress, sleep deprivation and,
 71–73
Cimetidine, effect on sleep, 179
Circadian influences
 desynchronization, 230–231
 sleep deprivation, 481–500
 wakefulness and, 230–232
Circadian modulation, EEG activity,
 233–234
Circadian pacemaker
 effect on sleep/waking, 496
 output, 496
 Process C, 497
Circadian rhythm, 294
 age-related changes, 445, 449–450
 definition of, 230
 endocrine functions, 294–298
 metabolic functions, 294–298
 sleep deprivation and, 495–500
  two-process model, 495–497

sleep, function(s) of, 43
suprachiasmatic nucleus (SCN), 495
Circadian timing system, and aging, 453–454
City traffic, sleep, effect of, 134–135
Classic single platform, SSSD animal studies, 86–88
Classifying genes, criteria, 403
Clock genes, role of, in sleep, 401
Clonidine, effect on sleep, 178
Clyde mood scale, sleep disruption, 416
CNS development, sleep, function(s) of, 43
Cocaine, effect of, 176
Cockroach, in sleep deprivation studies, 55
Codeine, effects of, 177
Cognition, fast oscillations, wakefulness and EEG activity, 228
Cognitive function
    attention, 204
    memory, 203–204
    and sleep, 202–213
        protocols for studying, 205–213
Cognitive load, increased, effects on, 206–207
Cognitive operations, definition of, 202–205
Comorbid depression, sleep deprivation and, 436
Conduction coefficients, 320
Consecutive interbeat intervals (rRR), index of, 311
Core temperature fall, waking to NREM sleep, 324
Cortical changes, during sleep, 223–255
Corticotropic axis, sleep deprivation, 304–306
Corticotropin-releasing hormone (CRH) system, 458
    aging and neuroendocrine factors, 455–456
Cortisol, 342
    levels, in human babies, 463
    REM sleep, 463
    sleep deprivation and, 297–298
    sleep onset and, 304
    SWS, 463
    total sleep deprivation and, 464

Cosleeping, 133
CRH synthesis, wakefulness and, 462
Cytochrome *c* oxidase, wakefulness and, 390
Cytokines, 342
    anti-inflammatory, 366
    behavioral effects of, 361–362
    immunity and, 361
    partial sleep deprivation studies, 377–378
    in physiological regulation of sleep, 364
    production, total sleep deprivation and, 370
    proinflammatory, 366
    sleep and, 13–16, 364–367

Daddi, Lamberto, early studies of sleep deprivation, 32
Danio rerio. See Zebrafish.
Daytime alertness
    sleep fragmentation effects, 105–106
    sleep loss and sleep deprivation, early studies, 39
De Manaceine, Marie, early studies of sleep deprivation, 32
Declarative memory, 203
Delta power, 9–10, 294
Dement, William C., early studies of sleep deprivation, 37
Dementia, psychopathology and sleep deprivation, 436
Depression
    during pregnancy and postpartum, sleep deprivation and, 432–433
    sleep loss, immune dysregulation and, 379
Deprivation method, function(s) of sleep, 339
Desynchronization, of biorhythms, 230
Developmental disorders, psychopathology changes, and sleep deprivation, 437
Developmental plasticity, theory of sleep, 17
Dewan, E.M., theory on function(s) of sleep, 42

Direction of shift rotation, 163
Disk-over-water method. *See* DOW
    method.
Disordered sleep, prevalence, 359
Distal extremities, temperature of, 324
Divided attention
    component of alertness, 205
    and sleep deprivation, 249–250
Dopamine, antidepressant effects, sleep
    deprivation, 423–427
Dorsal raphe cells, neurmodulatory
    systems, gene expression, 393
DOW method, 65–66
    energy metabolism in, 277
    in gene expression studies, 389
    REM sleep deprivation studies, 91
        biomolecules in blood, 348
        neurophysiological effects, on
            animals, 280
    sleep deprivation studies, 5, 276–277,
        328, 484
    SSSD, 90–91
    stress, and sleep deprivation, 71
    SWS deprivation with, 91
    syndrome, 73–74
    thermoregulation, 277
    in total sleep deprivation studies,
        65–66
        animal studies, 328
Drosophila, sleep deprivation studies,
    54–55, 406–407
Drugs of abuse, and sleep, 167–181

EEG, changes during sleep, 223–255
    arousals, definition of, 103
    body temperature and, 233, 234–235
    changes during sleep, 224
    frontal predominance, 243
    homeostatic process in waking, 235
    sensitivities of, 233
    sleep and performance, 122
    sleep deprivation, total, 270
    sleep fragmentation and, 110
    sleep spindles, 200
    sleep studies, 3, 22
    theta powers, local increase of, 243–245

EEG markers
    of sleep, 239–245
    of sleep homeostasis, 239–242, 243
        SWA and, 485
        two-process model, 240
    of wakefulness, 239–245
EEG theta activity
    with attention and effort, 245
    with prolonged wakefulness, 242–243
Elderly subjects
    age-related changes, 449
    sleep deprivation, vigilance, 448
    wakefulness, vigilance, 448
Electrical stimulation technique, SSSD
        studies, 89
Endocrine changes
    circadian rhythmicity, 294–298
    sleep deprivation, 293–312
    sleep-wake cycle, 294–298
Endogenous circadian pacemaker (ECP),
        449
Endogenous sleep-promoting substances,
        342
Endogenous somnogens, 16–17
Endotoxin, sleep and infectious agents,
        362
Energy expenditure (EE), in animal sleep
        studies, 328
Energy metabolism
    DOW method, 277
    sleep deprivation and, 13
Enforced locomotion, sleep deprivation
        study methods, 4
Environmental factors
    bed partners, 133
    bed surfaces, 131–133
    performance, 141–142
    sleep/sleep deprivation, 121–145
Ephron, H.D., theory of sleep function(s),
        42
Epilepsy, sleep deprivation and, 271
Epinephrine, 342
    sleep deprivation, animal studies of,
        329
Excessive sleepiness, psychomotor
        stimulants, 175
Exogenous somnogens, 16–17

Expressed sequence tags (ESTs), and
   wakefulness
   gene expression, 391

Facultative sleep, 483
Fast oscillations, wakefulness and EEG
   activity, 228
Fenfluramine, antidepressant effects,
   sleep deprivation, 426
Flower pot technique, sleep deprivation,
   REM 278, 280
fMRI (functional magnetic resonance
   imaging), 224
Forced desynchrony
   paradigm, sleep/wake variables, 499
   protocol, 498–499
Forced locomotion techniques, TSD
   methods, 64–67
Forebrain, wake-active regions, gene
   expression, 403
Fruit fly
   sleep and genetics in, 406
   sleep deprivation, animal models of,
   54
Function(s) of sleep, deprivation method,
   339
Functional analysis
   sleep, effect on gene expression, 391
   wakefulness, effect on gene expression,
   391
Functional magnetic resonance imaging
   (fMRI), 224

GABAergic system, sleep deprivation,
   345–346
Gamma oscillations, wakefulness and
   EEG activity, 228
Gardner, Randy, sleep deprivation studies,
   36–37
Gastrointestinal effects, of sleep
   deprivation, 268
Gender differences and aging, sleep,
   450–452
Gene expression studies
   disk-over-water (DOW) method in, 389

GeneChip technology in, 389
   mRNA differential display (mRNA
   DD) in, 389
   nylon membrane arrays in, 389
Gene expression
   changes in, 387
   immediate early genes (IEGs), 388
   neuromodulatory systems, 392–393
   REM sleep and, 406
   sleep deprivation, effect on, 393
   sleep and, 388–392
   sleep-active regions and, 405
   sleep-wake circuiting and, 401–406
   wake-active regions and, 403–405
   wakefulness and, 388–392
      long periods of, 391–392
      short periods, 390–391
   whole-genome analysis of, 389
GeneChip technology, gene expression
   studies, 389
Generalized anxiety disorder,
      psychopathology changes, sleep
      deprivation, 435
Genes, classification, sleep vs. wake,
   399–409
Genetics, function of sleep, 22
Gentle handling technique, TSD methods,
   63–64
GH (growth hormone), 342
   neuroendocrine factors, sleep
      modification, and aging, 454
   sleep deprivation and, 303–304
GH (growth hormone) secretion
   in adulthood, 459
   in puberty, 458
   in women, 456
   in young men, 456
Ghrelin levels, sleep deprivation, 306
Gilbert, J. Allen, early studies of sleep
      deprivation, 35
Glucocorticoid feedback, elderly,
   460
Glucose metabolism
   brain, 308
   sleep deprivation, 297–298, 308
Goodnow, Jacqueline, early studies of
      sleep deprivation, 35

Granulocytes, 342
    immune system, 361
Growth hormone. *See* GH.

Hallucinogens
    lysergic acid diethylamide (LSD), 176
    marijuana, 176
    sleep and, 176
HCRT/ORX, wakefulness, 403
Heart rate variability, sleep deprivation,
    311
Heat dissipation, 323
Heat gain/retention, 323
Heat retention mechanisms, sleep
    deprivation, 326
Heat transfer, 320–321
Hebb theory, 21
Heroin, 177
Hippocampal volume, elderly, 460
Histamine, wakefulness, 403
Histamine$_2$ antagonists, cardiovascular
    drugs, effect on sleep, 179
HIV, sleep loss, immunodeficiency, 380
Homeostasis, definition, 230, 481–482
Homeostatic drives, sleep deprivation, 57
Homeostatic influences
    desynchronization, 230–231
    on sleep deprivation, 481–500
    wakefulness and, 230–232
Homeostatic model, sleep, function(s) of,
    42
Homeostatic process
    age-dependent changes, 445
    in waking, EEG, 235
Homeostatic rate markers
    for sleep, SWA, 241
    for waking, theta activity, 241
Honeybees, sleep deprivation, animal
    models, 55
Hormonal effects, sleep fragmentation
    and, 109–111
Hormones, and cardiovascular drugs,
    180
Horne, Jim, theory of sleep function(s),
    40
HPA axis

activity, insomnia and, 460
    regulation of, age-related, 460
    "resiliency," age-related, 460
    sleep, and aging, 465
    stress response, 460
    stress, sleep loss and, 460–465
Human babies, cortisol levels, 463
Human studies, sleep deprivation,
    325–327
Humoral factor(s), sleep deprivation, 341
Hypercatabolic state, 369
    lymph nodes, 363
    symptoms, 363
Hyperphagia, sleep deprivation, 306
Hypertension and sleep fragmentation,
    115
Hypertensive patients, sleep deprivation,
    266–267
Hyperthyroidism, cardiovascular drugs in,
    effect on sleep, 180
Hypnagogic state, 227
Hypnotics, effect on sleep, 174
Hypnotoxin blood, sleep deprivation, 341
Hypnotoxin theory, sleep deprivation, 35
Hypocretin (HCRT)
    narcolepsy and, 403
    "wake gene," 404
    wakefulness and, 403–404
Hypolipidemic drugs, cardiovascular,
    effect on sleep, 179
Hypomania, psychopathology changes in
    sleep deprivation, 433
Hypothalamo-pituitary hormones, sleep
    deprivation, 301–306
Hypothalamus, 293
Hypothermia, 341
Hypothesis, sequential, of sleep function,
    213

IEGs/transcription factors, wakefulness,
    390
IL-2, and partial sleep deprivation, 376
IL-6, and partial sleep deprivation, 377
Illness, sleep, 16–17
Immediate early genes (IEGs), gene
    expression of, 388

Immobilization, theory of sleep, function(s), 40
Immune function, sleep and, 13–16
Immune system
    cellular components of, 360–361
    fluctations in normal sleep, 367–369
    granulocytes, 361
    innate immunity, 360
    leukocytes, 360
    lymphocytes, 360
    macrophages, 360
    monocytes, 360
    specific immunity, 360
Immunity
    cytokines in, 361
    sleep, effects on, 362–367
    sleep deprivation, 369–378
        total, 369–375
    sleep loss, clinical samples, 378–381
Immunodeficiency and sleep loss, 380
Immunologic changes, sleep deprivation, 359–381
Individual determinants, sleep deprivation, 441–467
Individual differences
    sleep, 450–465
    wakefulness, 450–465
Individual neurons, behavior, sleep deprivation, 340
Infection
    sleep deprivation and, 362–364
    sleep processes, 362–364
Infectious agents, sleep, 362
Innate immunity, 360
Insomnia, 212
    appetite suppressants and, 177
    HPA axis activity, 460
    stress and, 460
    tryptophan depletion, 418
Insulin, sleep deprivation, 297–298
Integumentary effects, sleep deprivation, 269
Intracellular cascades, sleep-wake regulation, 400
Intralaminar nuclei, wakefulness and, 225
Intravenous glucose tolerance test (IVGTT), after sleep restriction, 309

Invertebrates, sleep deprivation, animal models, 55
Ishimori, Kuniomi, sleep deprivation, early studies of, 35

K complexes, sleep fragmentation, arousal types, 114
Kleitman, Nathaniel, sleep deprivation, early studies, 32, 37
Korean War, studies of sleep deprivation, 35
Krueger, James, theory of sleep, function(s), 41

Learning, sleep deprivation effects, 42–43
Legendre, Rene, sleep deprivation, early studies of, 35
Leptin levels, sleep deprivation and, 306
Leukocytes, immune system and, 360
Light, exposure, effects on sleep, 129
Light, nocturnal, effects on performance, 141–142
Long-term memory, 203
Lovastatin, effect on sleep, 179
Lubin, Artie, sleep deprivation, early studies of, 35
Lymph nodes, hypercatobolic state, 363
Lymphoctyes, 342, 360
Lysergic acid diethylamide (LSD), 176

Macrophages, in immune system, 360
Maintenance of Wakefulness Test (MWT), 107
Mammalian models, sleep deprivation studies, 52–54
Mania, sleep deprivation effects, 433
MAO (monoamine oxidase), 344
Marijuana, 176
Meddis, R., theory of sleep function(s), 40
Medical intensive care units, sleep in, 135
Medications, sleep and, 167–181
Melatonin, in adolescents, 449
Memory, and sleep loss,
    changes, 199–213
    cognitive functions, 203–204

Memory (*contd.*)
  consolidation, 18
  declarative, 203
  long-term, 203
  nondeclarative, 203
  priming, 203
  procedural, 203
  reinforcement, theory of sleep, 17–20
  short-term, 203
  sleep, function(s) of, 42–43
  systems, organization and substrates of, 204
  traces during sleep, strengthening of, 210–211
  working circuit, 203
  working, 203
Men, gender differences in sleep, 451
Mesencephalic reticular formation (MRF), wakefulness and, 225
Metabolic activity, antidepressant effects, 422–423
Metabolic changes, sleep deprivation and, 293–312
Metabolic effects, and sleep fragmentation, 110
Metabolic functions
  circadian rhythmicity, 294–298
  sleep-wake cycle, 294–298
Methadone, CNS stimulants, 177
Methyldopa, cardiovascular drugs, effect on sleep, 178
Methylphenidate, central nervous system stimulants, 175
Microsleep, 2, 233
  total sleep deprivation and, 65
Middle-aged subjects, age-related changes, 449
Mirtazapine, as antidepressant, 173
Mitochondrial genes, wakefulness and, 390
Modafinil, central nervous system stimulants, 175
Monoamine oxidase (MAO), 344
Monamine oxidase inhibitors (MAOIs)
  antidepressants, 173
  memory and, 19
Monocytes, immune system, 360
Mood changes, sleep deprivation and, 415–419

Morphine, as central nervous system stimulants, 177
Moruzzi, Giuseppe, theory of sleep function(s), 42
mRNA differential display (mRNA DD), gene expression studies, 389
MSLT (Multiple Sleep Latency Test), 39, 202
  in children and adolescents, 448
  sleep fragmentation and, 105
Mu rhythm, wakefulness and EEG activity, 226–227
Multiple platform technique, SSSD studies in animals, 88
Multiple Sleep Latency Test. *See* MSLT.
Muscle tone, during sleep, 308
Muscle, level, sympathetic nerve activity (MSNA), 311
MWT (Maintenance of Wakefulness Test), 107
  sleep fragmentation and, 107

Narcolepsy, 212
  and central nervous system stimulants, 175
  hypocretin in, 403
Nefazondone, antidepressants, 173
Neonatal animals, SSSD studies in, 89
Neural correlates, wakefulness and, 224–226
Neuroendocrine factors, corticotropin-releasing hormone (CRH), 455–456
  sleep modifications, aging, 454–459
  somatotropic axis, and aging, 456–457
Neuroimaging studies, sleep deprivation, total, 273
Neuromodulatory systems
  gene expression, 392–393
    dorsal raphe cells, 393
    norepinephrine, 392
Neuronal activity during sleep, POA, 405
Neuronal circuitry diagram
  non-REM sleep, 402
  REM sleep, 402
  wakefulness, 402
Neuronal plasticity, 20–22

Neuronendocrine factors, aging and
    growth hormone (GH), 454
Neurophysiological effects
  REM sleep deprivation, 279
  sleep deprivation, 269
Neurotransmitter, sleep and, 343
Neurotransmitter systems, antidepressant
    effects, 423–427
Nicotine, as central nervous system
    stimulants, 176
NK cells
  partial sleep deprivation, 376
  total sleep deprivation,and, 370
Noise, effects on performance, 141
Nondeclarative memory, 203
Non-REM. *See* NREM.
Noradrenergic neurons, 343
  sleep deprivation and, 73–74
Norepinephrine, 342
  neuromodulatory systems, gene
    expression, 392
  sleep deprivation, animal studies, 329
  wakefulness, 403
Normal day shifts, shift work and sleep,
    159
Normal sleep, fluctuations in the immune
    system, 367–369
NREM rebound, 74–75
NREM sleep
  aging, 443
  deprivation, effects of, 281–282
  heart rate variability, 310
  neuronal circuitry diagram, 402
  REM sleep propensity in, 493–495
  sleep rebound, humans, 274
  stress and, 461–462
Nursing homes, sleep in, 135
Nylon membrane arrays, gene expression
    studies, 389

Obligatory sleep, 483
Obsessive-compulsive disorder, sleep
    deprivation and, 434
Obstructive sleep apnea (OSA), 10
Obstructive sleep apnea syndrome
    (OSAS), 212
Olfactory processing, during sleep, 125

Opioids, effect on sleep, 176
Orexin, wakefulness, 403
OSA (obstructive sleep apnea), 10
OSAS (obstructive sleep apnea
    syndrome), 212
Osler test, sleep fragmentation, arousal
    types, 113
Oswald, Ian, body restitution hypothesis,
    40
Oxidative cell damage, sleep deprivation
    and, 394
Oxidative stress, sleep deprivation and,
    393–394

Panic disorder, sleep deprivation and, 434
Paradoxical sleep, 1
Parametric mapping, during waking, 239
Parkinson's disease, sleep deprivation,
    177, 436
Partial SD (partial sleep deprivation),
    81–95
  causes of, 82
  cellular immunity and, 375
  cytokines, 377–378
  definitions of, 81–82
  IL-2, 376
  IL-6, 377
  memory and attention, 208–209
  NK cells, 376
  studies in humans, 82–83
Patrick, George Thomas White, early
    studies of, 35
Pearson correlation, 105
Peptides, 342
Performance
  alcohol, effects on, 170
  awakenings, from various sleep stages,
    211–212
  brain metabolic function during, 246
  sleep, assessment of, 122
Periodic limb movement (PLM), sleep
    fragmentation and, 115–116
Permanent shifts, shift work and sleep,
    159
Personality
  changes, sleep deprivation and,
    431–437

Personality (*contd.*)
  DSM-IV Axis I and II disorders, 431
  sleep deprivation, 431–432
PET (positron emission tomography)
    studies, 224
  fMRI studies, neural correlates of
      alertness and performance,
      245–248
Phase preference, age-related, 449
Phenethylamines, as antidepressant, 173
Phenylpropanolamine (PPA), central
    nervous system stimulants, 175
Physiological functions of sleep, 41–42,
    201
  changes in, with sleep deprivation,
      347–349
Pieron, Henri, early studies of, 35
Pindolol, and bipolar disorders, 434
Pink noise
  definition of, 127
  REM sleep, 127–128
  vs. white noise, 141
Pituitary hormone release, sleep-wake
    states, 295
Plasma cortisol
  in sleep debt, 305
  sleep deprivation and, 304–306
Plasma glucose levels, 308
Plasma melatonin, drowsiness and, 228
POA (preoptic area), sleep cener, 405
Pons, wakefulness, 403
Positron emission tomography. *See* PET.
Posterior attention network, 205
Postpartum depression, sleep deprivation
    and, 432–433
Pravastatin, effect on sleep, 179
Pregnancy, sleep deprivation and,
    432–433
Premenstrual dysphoric disorder, sleep
    deprivation and, 432
Preoptic area (POA), sleep center, 405
Priming memory, 203
Priming task, performance, 211
Procedural memory, 203
Process C
  age-dependent changes, 444
  circadian pacemaker, 497
  and Process S, 497

Process S, 9, 10, 294
  age-dependent changes, 444
  EEG delta power, 490
  fluctuations, 490
  and Process C, 497
  simulation of, sleep homeostasis,
      486–487, 489
  SWS and, 489
Prolonged wakefulness, systemic
    infection, 343
"Pseudodementia," sleep deprivation and,
    436
Pseudoephedrine, 175
Psychological effects, sleep deprivation,
    269
Psychomotor stimulants, excessive
    sleepiness, 175
Psychopathology changes, sleep
    deprivation, 432–437
  affective disorders, 432–434
  Alzheimer's disease, 436
  attention-deficit hyperactivity disorder
      (ADHD), 437
  bipolar disorders, 433
    pindolol and, 434
  comorbid depression, 436
  dementia, 436
  depresson, pregnancy and postpartum,
      432–433
  developmental disorders, 437
  generalized anxiety disorder, 435
  hypomania, 433
  mania, 433
  obsessive-compulsive disorder, 434
  panic disorder, 434
  Parkinson's disease, 436
  premenstrual dysphoric disorder, 432
  "pseudodementia," 436
  pregnancy and postpartum depression,
      432–433
  psychotic depression 433
  psychotic disorders, 435–436
  schizophrenia, 435
  social disorders, 435
  substance use disorders, 437
  unipolar disorders, 432
Psychotic depression, sleep deprivation,
    433, 435–436

Pulmonary effects, of sleep fragmentation, 109
Punitive methods, TSD methods, 67
Putative sleep-promoting substances, 365

Rantidine, cardiovascular drugs, effect on sleep, 179
Rapid-eye-movement. *See* REM.
Rat Genome Project, 22
Rebound insomnia, 174
Recall
explicit vs. implicit, 203
Rechtschaffen, Allan, thory of sleep function(s), 41
Recovery sleep
duration, 483
intensity, 483–484
need for, 244–245
sleep homeostasis, evidence for, 483
Red blood cell count, 341
REM sleep, 82
in adults, 442
aging and, 442
cortisol, 463
gene expression in, 406
c-fos expression, 406
heart rate variability, 310
memory, 18–19
neuronal circuitry diagram, 402
propensity
NREM sleep, 493–495
wakefulness and, 495
stress and, 461–462
studies of, 3–4
REM sleep rebound, 10–11, 74–75, 274, 279
animal studies, 418
arousal technique, 280
disk-over-water (DOW) technique, 91, 280
neurophysiological effects, 279, 280–281
SSD studies86–88
DOW method, 91, 280
human studies, 83–84
REM sleep deprivation, 278–282
Renal effects, of sleep deprivation, 268

Respiratory effects, of sleep deprivation, 267–268
Respiratory response, to tones during sleep, 124
Reticular activating system, wakefulness and, 225
Rheumatoid arthritis, autoimmune disorders, sleep loss, 380
Richardson, Gary et al., early studies, 39
Rotating shifts
direction of shift rotation, 163
shift work and sleep, 161
speed of shift rotation, 162
time of shift, 161

Salbutamol, effect on sleep, 180
SCN (suprachiasmatic nucleus), 293, 294
SD studies, in animals, 85–86
Selective attention
component of alertness, 205
sleep deprivation, 248–249
Selective NREM, sleep deprivation and, 281–282
Selective serotonin reuptake inhibitors. *See* SSRIs.
Selective sleep deprivation, effects on memory and attention, 209–210
Selegiline, as antiparkinsonian medication, 177
Semantic priming task, performance, 211
Sensory neurophysiology, during sleep, 122–127
Sequential hypothesis of sleep function, 213
Serotonin, 345
antidepressant effects, 426–427
wakefulness and, 403
Shift length, shift work and sleep, 163
Shift work
sleep, permanent shifts, 159
on-duty alertness, 157
sleep, effect on, 157–164
direction of shift rotation, 163
normal day shifts, 159
permanent evening shifts, 159
permanent shift, 158
rotating shift, 158, 161

Shift work (*contd.*)
    shift length, 163
    speed of shift rotation, 162
    time of shift, 161
Short-term memory, 203
SIDS (sudden infant death syndrome),
    267
Simulated aircraft noise, effect on sleep,
    128–129
Simulated traffic noise, effect on sleep,
    128–129
Sleep
    and alcohol, 167–181
    in altered environments, 133–141
    altitude, 137–138
    ambient temperature, environmental
        factors, 130–131
    in the Artic, 135–137
    auditory processing during, 123–125
    bed partners, as environmental factor,
        133
    bed surfaces, as environmental factor,
        131–133
    behavioral responsiveness during,
        122–127
    brain metabolic function, 223–224, 247
    c-fos gene expression, 388–389, 404
    choline acetyltransferase, 404
    cognitive functions and, 202–213
    cytokines, 364–367
    definition of, 1, 21
    drugs of abuse, 167–181
    EEG markers of, 239–245
    environmental factors, 127–133
        light exposure on, 129
        noise making stimuli, 127
        simulated aircraft noise, 128–129
        simulated traffic noise, 128–129
    function of, 2–3, 39–43
    function, theories of
        Adam, Kristin, 40
        Albert, Ira, 42
        Benca, Ruth, 41
        Bergmann, Bernard, 41
        body restitution hypothesis, 40
        Carrington, Patricia, 42
        cerebral restitution hypothesis, 40
        circadian rhythm, 43

Sleep (*contd.*)
        CNS development, 43
        Dewan, E.M. 42
        Ephron, H.D., 42
        homeostatic model, 42
        Horne, Jim, 40
        immobilization theory, 40
        Krueger, James, 41
        Learning theory , 42–43
        Meddis, R., 40
        Meddis, Ray, 40
        memory, 42–43
        Moruzzi, Giuseppe, 42
        physiological function, 41–42
        Rechtschaffen, Allan, 41
        Vogel, Gerald, 42
    gender differences during aging,
        450–452
    gene expression in, 388–392
    genetics, in *Drosophila*, 406–407
    HPA axis, stress, 460–464
    illness, 16–17
    immunity, 362–367
    individual differences in, 450–465
    infectious agents, 362
    long periods of, effect on gene
        expression, 391–392
    medical intensive care units, 135
    medications, 167–181
    nursing homes, 135
    olfactory processing during, 125
    performance, assessment of, 122
    physiological functions of, 201
    protein content changes, 387–388
    respiratory response to tones during,
        124
    RNA changes, 387–388
    sea level vs. altitude, 137
    sensory neurophysiology during,
        122–127
    shift work, 157–164
    somatosensory processing during,
        126–127
    space, 138–141
    stress, 460–465
    theories of, 17–20
    thermoregulation, 12–13
    visual processing during, 127

whole-genome analysis, gene
    expression, 389–390
Sleep apnea
    sleep fragmentation, 109
        clinical effects of 115–116
Sleep architecture
    age-related changes in, 442–443
    stress and, 461–462
Sleep attacks, Parkinson's, 177
Sleep center, preoptic area (POA) as, 405
Sleep continuity theory, 213
Sleep cycles, 201
Sleep data vs. waking data, 224
Sleep debt, plasma cortisol, 305
Sleep deficiency, effects of, 416–417
Sleep deprivation
    acetylcholine, 427
    acute, sleep following, 298–301
    acute stress, 71
    adaptation, 250
    affective disorders, 432–434
    age, 441–467
    AIR$_G$, 310
    Alzheimer's disease, 436
    amineptine, 423
    aminergic system, 344–345
    animal models of, 47–58, 327–333
        Caenorhabditis elegans, 55
        cockroach, 55
        cost-benefit analysis, 50–52
        disk-over-water method, 328
        drosophila, 54–55
        energy expenditure (EE), 328
        epinephrine, 329
        fruit fly, 54
        higher vertebrates, 49–50
        historical overview, 48–49
        honeybees, 55
        invertebrates, 55
        mammalian models, 52–54
        nonmammalian species, 50
        norephinephrine, 329
        simple models, 54–56
        TSD rats, 328
        zebrafish, 55
    antidepressant effects, 421–428
    appetite, 13
        increase, 308

regulation, 306
arithmetic, effect on learning, 249–250
attention-deficit hyperactivity disorder,
    437
biochemical changes, 339–350
biomolecules, changes in, 347–349
    blood, 341–343
    body fluids, brain, 340
    brain, 343–347
bipolar disorders, 433
body temperature regulation, 320–325
BOLD response, 250–251
brain metabolic function, 247
brain slice studies, 56
carbohydrates, 309
cardiovascular effects, 266–267
catecholamine levels, 266–267
cerebral metabolic effects, 424–425
in children and adolescents, 417
cholinergic system, 345
chronic stress, 71–73
circadian influences, 481–500
circadian rhythms, 495–500
comorbid depression, 436
compensation for, 250
computer models, 56
continuous
    age-related, 416
    circadian effect, 416
    mood changes, 415–416
    Multiple Affect Adjective Check
        List, 416
    paranoia, 415
    perceptual distortions, 415
    Profile of Mood States (POMS), 415
corticotropic axis, 304–306
cortisol, 297–298
definition of, 1–2
dementia, 436
developmental disorders, 437
disk-over-water (DOW) method, 5
divided attention, 249–250
dopamine, 423–427
early studies of, 32–37
early studies
    Agostini, Ceasare, 32
    Aserinsky, Eugene, 37
    Carskadon, Mary, 39

Sleep deprivation (*contd.*)
  Daddi, Lamberto, 32
  De Manaceine, Marie, 32
  Dement, William C. 37
  Gilbert, J. Allen, 35
  Goodnow, Jacqueline, 35
  Ishimori, Knuiomi, 35
  Kleitman, Nathaniel, 32
  Kleitman, Nathaniel, 37
  Korean War, 35
  Legendre, Rene, 35
  Lubin, Artie, 35
  Patrick, George Thomas White, 35
  Pieron, Henri, 35
  Richardson, Gary et al., 39
  Tarozzi, Giulio, 32
  Tripp, Paul, 35
  Williams, Hal, 35
  effects
    on brainstem neurons, auditory
      stimulation, 340
    on metabolic functions, 310–312
    on memory and attention,
      207–210
  endocrine changes, 293–312
  energy metabolism, 13
  fenfluramine, 427
  frontal brain, 244
  GAGAergic system, 345–346
  gastrointestinal effects, 268
  gender differences, 451
  generalized anxiety disorder, 435
  ghrelin levels, 306
  glucose, 297–298
  glucose metabolism, 308
  growth hormone (GH), 297–298,
    303–304
  heat retention mechanisms, 326
  history of, 31–43
  homeostasis, 481
  homeostatic drives, 57
  homeostatic influences, 481–500
  human pharmacology, 418
  human studies, 270–273, 325–327
  humoral factor(s), 341
  hypertensive patients, 266–267
  hypnotoxin theory of, 35
  hypomania, 433

Sleep deprivation (*contd.*)
  hypothalamo-pituitary hormones,
    301–306
  immunologic changes in, 359–381
  individual determinants, 441–467
  insulin, 297–298
  integumentary effects, 269
  leptin levels, 306
  long periods of
    arylsulfotransferase (AST), 393
    brain cell death, 393–394
    effect on gene expression, 393
    oxidative cell damage, 39
    oxidative stress, 393–394
  mania, 433
  metabolic changes, 293–312
  methods for study, 3–8
  microsleeps, 2
  in middle-aged adults, 446–447
  mood changes, 415–419
    animal and pharmacology studies, 418
  neural correlates of alertness and
    performance
    PET studies, 245–248
    fMRI studies, 245–248
  neurophysiological effects, 269
  noradrenergic system, 73–74
  NREM vs. REM rebound, 74–75
    and obsessive-compulsive disorder,
      434
  in older adults, 447
  panic disorders, 434
  Parkinson's disease, 436
  performance, emotional response, 417
  personality, effect on, 417, 431–432
  personality/psychopathologic changes,
    431–437
  physiological effects of, 266–269,
    347–349
  pindolol, 434
  plasma cortisol, 304–306
  premenstrual dysphoric disorder, 432
  "pseudodementia," 436
  psychiatric consequences, 37–39
  psychological effects, 269
  psychopathology changes, 432–437
  psychotic disorders, 433
  REM rebound, 279

Sleep deprivation (*contd.*)
REM, 278–282
REM, flower pot technique, 278, 280
renal effects, 268
research design and procedures, 91–92
respiratory effects, 267–268
schizophrenia, 435
selective attention, 248–249
selective NREM, 281–282
serotonin, 426–427
sleep recovery, acute total, 299
sleep structure, 492–495
REM sleep expression, 492
sleep-state selective. *See* SSSD.
social disorder, 435
somatotropic axis, 303–304
stress, 57–58, 71
substance use disorder, 437
sudden infant death syndrome (SIDS),
267
symptoms of, 15
temporal issues, recovery from, 56–57
thermoregulation, 272–273
thermoregulatory changes, 319–334
thyrotropic axis, 304
thyrotropin (TSH), 297–298
total, 63–75, 270–278
EEG effects, in animals, 270, 274–275
epilepsy, 271
neuroimaging studies, 273
neuronal activity studies, 277–278
thermoregulation in animals, 275–277
tryptophan 426
TSH, 304
unipolar disorder, 432
verbal learning, effects on, 249–250
vigilance, effects on, 448
in young adults, 446–447
Sleep deprivation vs. fragmentation,
111–112
Sleep deprivation studies
in animals
effectiveness and specificity of, 93
interpretation of findings, 92–95
stress reactivity and responses, 94
subject selection bias, 93–94
Gardner, Randy, 36–37
in humans

procedures, 85
research design, 85
interpretive and methodological issues,
56–58
Sleep deprivation syndrome, 69
Sleep disruption
Clyde mood scale, 416
effects of, 416–417
Parkinson's disease, 177
Sleep EEGs, aging, 443–444
Sleep fluctuations
cytokines, 367
IL-2, 367
NK cells, 367
Sleep fragmentation, 103–07
animals, 104
arousal types, 112–114
cardiovascular measures, , 112
Epworth Sleepiness Scale (ESS),
112–113
Osler test, 113
scoring paradigms, , 112
visual vigilance, 113
clinical effects of, 115–116
periodic limb movements, 115–116
sleep apnea, 115–116
daytime alertness, 105–106
definition of, 103
memory and attention, effects on, 209
experimental controls for, 107–109
hypertension, 115
Maintenance of Wakefulness Test
(MWT), 107
mood, 106
multiple sleep latency test (MSLT),
105
physiological and behavioral measures,
109–111
auditory arousal threshold, 110
cardiovascular effects, 109
EEG effects, 110
hormonal effects, 109–111
metabolic effects, 110
pulmonary effects, 109
vs. sleep deprivation, 111–112
studies, history of, 104–15
Sleep function(s) of, Benington,
Joel, 42

Sleep genes
  classification of, 399–409
  criteria for classifying, 407–409
Sleep homeostasis
  definition of, 230
  EEG markers, 239–242
    two-process model, 240
  EEG SWA during NREM sleep, 485
  evidence for, 482–484
    recovery sleep, 483
    slow-wave activity (SWA), 483–484
  goal of, 484–485
  implication of models, 489–492
  mammalian species, 488
  modeling, 484–489
  Process S, 485–487 489
    simulation of, 486, 487
Sleep loss
  African-American ethnicity, alcohol
    dependence, 379
  autoimmune disorders, 380
  biomolecular marker, 349–350
  early studies, daytime sleepiness, 39
  HPA axis, stress, 464–465
  hypercatabolic state, 362–363
  immune dysregulation
    alcohol-dependent subjects,
      378–379
    depressed subjects, 379
  immunodeficiency, 380
  psychiatric conditions, 378
  psychological stress, 378
  systemic infection, 13–16
Sleep modification, and aging
  growth hormone (GH),
      neuronendocrine factors, 454
  HPA axis, 465
  neuroendocrine factors, 454–459
    corticotropin-releasing hormone
      (CRH), 455–456
  "old old," 442
  sleep-wake cycle, 453–454
  somatotropic axis, 456–457
  "young old," 442
Sleep modifications, ontogeny of,
    442–444
Sleep organization, 200–201
Sleep processes, infection, 362–364

Sleep propensity. *See* Process S.
Sleep recovery, acute total sleep
    deprivation, 299
Sleep regulatory mechanisms, age-
    dependent changes, 444–450
Sleep restriction
  NREM sleep, 301
  partial, sleep following chronic,
    298–301
Sleep schedule, adolescents, age-related
    changes, 449
Sleep signs, waking EEG, 242
Sleep spindles, EEG, 200
Sleep stages, 298–299
  and EEG sleep stage scoring activity,
    200–201
Sleep state-selective deprivation. *See*
    SSSD.
Sleep structure, sleep deprivation,
    492–495
Sleep vs wakefulness, theta activity, EEG,
    200
Sleep vs. wake genes, classification of,
    403
Sleep-wake circuiting, gene expression,
    401–406
Sleep/sleep deprivation, environmental
    influences on, 121–145
Sleep/wake variables, forced desynchrony
    paradigm, 499
Sleep-active regions, gene expression in,
    405
Sleep-conserving antidepressants,
    antidepressants, 173
Sleep-deprived subjects, exercise, cold
    and hot environments, 326
Sleepiness, puberty and, 448
Sleep-promoting factor, 342
Sleep-wake circuiting, gene expression,
    c-fos, 401–403
Sleep-wake cycle
  aging, 453
  endocrine functions, 294–298
  metabolic functions, 294–298
  stress, 461–462
Sleep-wake homeostasis, 294
Sleep-wake regulation, intracellular
    cascades, 400

Sleep-wake-dependent influences, 233
Slow-wave activity (SWA), 9–10, 240, 294
  aging, 443
  sleep homeostasis, evidence for, 483–484
Slow-wave sleep (SWS), 9–10, 82
  in adulthood, 442
  in children and young adults, 442
  infectious agents and, 362
Social phobia, psychopathology changes, sleep deprivation, 435
Somatosensory processing, during sleep, 126–127
Somatostatin, 342
Somatotropic axis
  sleep deprivation, 303–304
  aging and 456–457
Somnogens
  endogenous, 16–17
  exogenous, 16–17
Space environment, sleep, 140
Space, sleep in, 138–141
Specific immunity, immune system, 360
Speed of shift rotation, 162
Spindle activity, IQ, 206
SSRI
  discontinuation syndrome, 172
  antidepressants, 171
  withdrawal from, 172
SSSD
  definitions of, 81–82
  DOW method, 90–91
SSSD studies
  in animals, 86–91
    classic single platform, 86–88
    methods in, 88
    multiple platform techniques, 88
    neonatal animals, methods in, 89
    REM sleep deprivation, platform techniques, 86–88
  antidepressant drugs in, 89
  cold ambient environment, 89
  electrical stimulation technique, 89
  in humans, 83–84
  pendulum or swing technique, 89
Steroids, cardiovascular drugs, effect on sleep, 180

Stress reactivity and responses, sleep deprivation studies, in animals, 94
Stress response, HPA axis, 460
Stress system, neuroendocrine response, 457
Stress
  insomnia, 460
  NREM sleep, 461–462
  REM sleep, 461–462
  sleep and, 460–465
  sleep architecture, 461–462
  sleep deprivation, 57–58, 71
    DOW studies method, 71
  sleep loss, HPA axis, 464–465
  sleep-wake cycle, 461–462
Subject selection bias, studies in animals, 93–94
Substance use disorders, sleep deprivation, 437
Sudden infant death syndrome (SIDS), sleep deprivation, 267
Suprachiasmatic nucleus (SCN), 293, 294
  circadian rhythms, 495
  role of, in sleep, 401
Sustained attention, component of alertness, 205
SWA (slow wave activity), 240
  aging, 451–453
  cortisol, 463
  homeostatic rate markers, 241
SWS (slow wave sleep)
  and aging, 451–453
  cortisol and, 463
  deprivation studies, DOW method, 91
  infectious agents, 362
  studies in humans, 84
  young men, 459
Synaptic consolidation, 20–22
Synaptic plasticity genes, BDNF, 22
Systemic infection, sleep loss, 13–16

Tarozzi, Giulio, sleep deprivation, early studies, 32
Temperature, distal extremities, 324
Temporal issues, recovery from, sleep deprivation, 56–57

Test performance, factors affecting,
  191–197
  behavioral observations, 195
  clinical interview, 195
  cooperation, 191
  motivation and alertness, 196
  subject characteristics, 192–193
  subject factors, 191–194
  subject rapport, 194–195
  test administration, 196
  test session structure, 195
  testing environment, 194–197
TH (tyrosine hydroxylase) activity, 344
Theophylline, cardiovascular drugs, effect
  on sleep, 180
Thermoregulation, autonomic, 322–323
  DOW method, 277
  resting body, 272
  during sleep, 324
  sleep deprivation, 272–273
  sleep, 12–13
  sweating, 272
Thermoregulatory changes, sleep
  deprivation and, 319–334
Theta activity
  during wakefulness, 236–237
  EEG, sleep vs wakefulness, 200
Theta power
  topographic distribution, 238
  wakefulness, 237–239
Theta rhythm
  monotonous tasks, 227
  NREM sleep stage 1, 227
  operant conditioning, 227
  wakefulness and EEG activity, 227
Thyroid hormone concentration, 342
Thyrotropic axis, sleep deprivation, 304
Thyrotropin (TSH), sleep deprivation,
  297–298
Time awake
  changes in performance with, 228–232
  electrophysiological changes, 232–239
Time of shift, 161
Total sleep deprivation (TSD)
  cortisol, 464
  cytokines, in vivo vs. ex vivo
    production, 375
  IL-6, 373–375

memory and attention, 207
  NK responses, 370
  studies on immunity, 369–375
  thermoregulatory pathways, 319–320
Traditional sleep stage scoring, 103
Transcription factors, wakefulness, short
  periods, 390
Triazolam, effect on sleep, 174
Tricyclic antidepressants (TCA), memory,
  19
Tripp, Paul, sleep deprivation, early
  studies, 35
Tryptophan depletion, insomnia, 418
Tryptophan, antidepressant effects, sleep
  deprivation, 426
TSD (total sleep deprivation), 63–75
  effects of, 69
TSD methods
  advantages and disadvantages, 63–69
  brain electrical stimulation, 68
  chemical stimulation, 68
  disk-over-water (DOW) method,
    65–66
  forced locomotion techniques, 64–67
  gentle handling technique, 63–64
  punitive methods, 67
  yoked control, 70
TSD rats, sleep deprivation, 328
TSH, nocturnal rise, 304
TSH, sleep deprivation, 304
Two-Process Model, Borbely's, 9–10
Tyrosine hydroxylase (TH) activity, 344

Unipolar disorders, sleep deprivation and,
  432
Urine, 342

Venlafaxine, antidepressants, 173
Verbal learning, sleep deprivation effects
  on, 249–250
Vigilance, sleep deprivation
  effect on, 448
  elderly subjects, 448
Viral infections, 16
Visual processing, during sleep, 127
Vogel, Gerald, sleep, function(s) of, 42

"Wake gene"
  classification of, 399–409
  hypocretin, 404
Wake maintenance zone, 231
Wake vs. sleep genes, classification of,
  403
Wake-active regions
  gene expression in, 403–405
    brainstem, 403
    forebrain, 403
Wakefulness
  acetylcholine, 403
  alertness and circadian phase,
    231–232
  body temperature, 231–232
  brain metabolic function during, 246
  c-fos gene expression, 388–389, 404
  circadian influences, 230–232
  constant routine protocol, 232–233
  CRH synthesis, 462
  cytochrome *c* oxidase, 390
  EEG activity and, 226–228, 232
    alpha rhythm, 226
    beta oscillations, 228
    desynchronized activity, 228
    EEG spectrum 226
    fast oscillations, 228
    gamma oscillations, 228
    mu rhythm, 226–227
    theta rhythm, 227
  EEG markers of, 239–245
  EEG, BOLD response, 251
  frequency-specific circadian phase
    manner, 233–234
  gene expression in, 388–392
  HCRT/ORX, 403
  histamine, 403
  homeostatic influences, 230–232
  hypocretin (HCRT), 403, 404
  IEGs/transcription factors, 390
  individual differences in, 450–465
  intralaminar nuclei, 225
  long periods, effect on gene expression,
    391–392
    expressed sequence tags (ESTs),
      391
    functional analysis, 391
    known transcripts, 391

mesencephalic reticular formation
  (MRF), 225
mitochondrial genes, 390
neural correlates of alertness and
  performance, PET studies,
  245–248
fMRI studies, 245–248
neuronal circuitry diagram, 402
norepinephrine, 403
orexin, 403
pons, 403
REM sleep propensity in, 495
reticular activating system, 225
serotonin, 403
short periods of
  effect on gene expression, 390–391
  mitochondrial genes, 390
  transcription factors, 390
theta activity during, 236–237
theta power, 237–239
time spent awake, 235–236
vigilance, effect on, 448
whole-genome analysis, gene
  expression, 389–390
Waking (theta activity), homeostatic rate
  markers, 241
Waking data vs. sleep data, 224
Waking EEG, sleep signs in, 242
Waking state, electrophysiology of,
  224–228
White noise
  definition of, 127
  vs. pink noise, 141
  REM sleep, 127–128
Whole-genome analysis, gene expression,
  389
Williams, Hal, sleep deprivation, early
  studies of, 35
Women, and sleep, gender differences,
  451
Working memory, 203

Xanthines, effect on sleep,174

Yoked control, TSD methods, 70

Zebrafish, sleep deprivation, animal
  models of, 55